MEDICAL RADIOLOGY

Diagnostic Imaging and Radiation Oncology

Springer
Berlin
Heidelberg
New York
Barcelona
Budapest
Hong Kong
London
Milan
Paris
Santa Clara
Singapore
Tokyo

Thermoradiotherapy and Thermochemotherapy

Volume 2: Clinical Applications

Contributors

M. Abe · F. Ambesí Impiombato · M. Amichetti · M. Anza · G. Arcangeli
M.A. Astrahan · L. Baert · J.M.C. Bull · A. Callopoli · A. Capua · S. Carlini
F. Cavaliere · R. Cavaliere · T.A. Colacchio · P.M. Corry · P. Debicki
M.W. Dewhirst · F. Di Filippo · F. d'Oleire · J. Erb · H.J. Feldmann
P.T. Finger · R. Garinei · F.A. Gibbs · G. Giovinazzo
D. González González · W. Havers · M. Hiraoka · R.D. Issels · K. Kitamura
G. Klautke · R.G.F. Knol · K. Leopold · D. Machin · J. Overgaard
P. Perri · Z. Petrovich · A. Psaila · R. van Heek-Romanowski · T.P. Ryan
S.A. Sapareto · M. Schiratti · J. Schorcht · M.H. Seegenschmiedt · R. Seidel
P.K. Sneed · P.R. Stauffer · B. Stea · K. Sugimachi · R. Valdagni
J. van der Zee · C.C. Vernon · J. Whaley · M. Zimmermann

Edited by

M.H. Seegenschmiedt, P. Fessenden, and C.C. Vernon

Foreword by

L.W. Brady and H.-P. Heilmann

With 115 Figures, 2 of Them in Color and 155 Tables

Springer

Priv.-Doz. Dr. M. HEINRICH SEEGENSCHMIEDT
Strahlentherapeutische Klinik und Poliklinik
Universität Erlangen-Nürnberg
Universitätsstraße 27
91054 Erlangen, Germany

PETER FESSENDEN, PhD
Professor Emeritus, Radiation Oncology
Stanford University Medical Center
Room S-044
Stanford, CA 94305, USA

CLARE C. VERNON, MA, FRCR
Department of Clinical Oncology
Hammersmith Hospital
Du Cane Road
London W12 OHS, UK

MEDICAL RADIOLOGY. Diagnostic Imaging and Radiation Oncology

Continuation of
Handbuch der medizinischen Radiologie
Encyclopedia of Medical Radiology

ISBN-13:978-3-642-64613-3 e-ISBN-13:978-3-642-60938-1
DOI:10.1007/978-3-642-60938-1

Library of Congress Cataloging-in-Publication Data. Thermoradiotherapy and thermochemotherapy/contributors, J.C. Bolomey . . . [et al.]; edited by M.H. Seegenschmiedt, P. Fessenden, and C.C. Vernon; foreword by L.W. Brady and H.-P. Heilmann. p. cm. - (Medical radiology) Includes bibliographical references and index. Contents: v. 1. Biology, physiology, and physics. 1. Cancer - Thermotherapy. 2. Cancer - Chemotherapy. 3. Cancer - Radiotherapy. 4. Cancer - Adjuvant treatment. I. Bolomey, J.C. (Jean-Charles) II. Seegenschmiedt, M.H. (Michael Heinrich), 1955-. III. Fessenden, P. (Peter) IV. Vernon, C.C. (Clare C.) V. Series. [DNLM: 1. Neoplasms - therapy. 2. Hypothermia, Induced. 3. Radiotherapy, Adjuvant. 4. Chemotherapy, Adjuvant. QZ 266 T412 1995] RC271. T5T44 1995 616.99'406—dc20 DNLM/DLC for Library of Congress 95-11653

Softcover reprint of the hardcover 1st edition 1996

Cover design: Springer-Verlag, E. Kirchner

Typesetting: Best-set Typesetter Ltd., Hong Kong

SPIN: 10126955 21/3135/SPS - 5 4 3 2 1 0 - Printed on acid-free paper

Foreword

Hyperthermia has been found to be of great benefit in combination with radiation therapy or chemotherapy in the management of patients with difficult and complicated tumor problems. It has been demonstrated to increase the efficacy of ionizing radiation when used locally but also has been of help in combination with systemic chemotherapy where hyperthermia is carried out to the total body. Triple modality (thermo-chemo-radiotherapy) or other treatment combinations have not been fully evaluated and may demonstrate extended clinical applications in the future.

Problems remain with regard to maximizing the effects of hyperthermia as they are influenced by a variety of external and intrinsic factors including bloodflow, microenvironment etc.

While the previous volume has summarized more theoretical aspects of hyperthermia, i.e. biology, physiology and physics, the present volume compiles the current knowledge relative to the clinical applications of hyperthermia in combination with radiation therapy and/or chemotherapy, providing a comprehensive overview of its use in cancer management.

Philadelphia/Hamburg, June 1995

L.W. Brady
H.-P. Heilmann

Preface

In an attempt to overcome tumor resistance, hypoxia, or unfavorable tumor conditions, oncological research has come to focus on gene therapy, immunotherapy, new cytotoxic agents, and increasingly sophisticated radiotherapy. Radiation research has been directed towards heavy particle therapy and modification of the radiation response by either protecting or sensitizing agents. Improved dose localization using conformal strategies has also been implemented. Recently, changes in radiation fractionation schedules have shown promise of better results. *Hyperthermia in cancer therapy* can be viewed similarly as another means to increase the sensitivity of tumors to radio- and chemotherapy.

Hyperthermia (i.e., the application of heat to attain elevated tumor temperatures, usually in the range of 41°–44°C) as an *adjuvant* to chemo- and radiotherapy is primarily employed to improve local control, while its combination with systemic chemotherapy aims at the control of systemic metastases as well. It is in *local control of the primary lesion* that hyperthermia will have the greatest impact, and it is *in combination with radiotherapy* that hyperthermia appears to have its greatest potential. Therefore it should be implemented in patients in whom the rate of local failure is high, such as those with the common tumors of the brain, breast, lung, oropharynx, upper gastrointestinal tract, and pelvis including the prostate, uterus, cervix, ovary, and bladder. Even if the impact on survival from improved local control were to be as low as 5%, this increase would still represent a very significant number of patients saved from a cancer death.

In cases where no hope for better survival can be expected from improved local control, many patients could still benefit from alleviation of the extremely unpleasant effects of uncontrolled local disease (bleeding, pain, infection, etc.). This is particularly true for breast cancer patients who experience a local failure at the operated breast or chest wall, such failure often being associated with a variety of very distressing symptoms and circumstances. Thus, *palliation of uncontrolled local disease* is another important indication for hyperthermia.

A general rationale for the use of hyperthermia began to evolve from the laboratory in the early 1960s, but the actual task of inducing and monitoring the heat application clinically proved to be much more technically difficult than was anticipated. Nevertheless, even early clinical trials using crude heating equipment achieved encouraging results when hyperthermia and appropriate radiotherapy were combined.

More recently we have seen some very positive clinical results emerging from well-controlled phase III randomized trials (including malignant brain tumors, melanomas, head and neck and breast tumors) where good quality assurance has been assured. Most of these trials were of multi-institutional design to recruit sufficient numbers of patients within a reasonable period. Studies involving heat in combination with chemotherapy and even tripe-modality therapy are now underway for tumors with a high tumor growth fraction or high metastatic potential. Innovative and invasive techniques, such as interstitial and intracavitary hyperthermia, have become available to our oncological armamentarium. Presently unresolved questions point to the following areas of research:

1. *Biologists* may deepen or even complete our insight into the development of thermotolerance, and specific assays of heat shock proteins may provide us with information about the optimal treatment schedule.
2. *Physiologists and pharmacologists* may induce artifical alterations of the cellular environment by means of specific thermosensitizers, vasodilators, or the infusion of glucose to alter the pH. Using positron emission tomography or magnetic resonance spectroscopy, the induced changes might easily be monitored and used for the prediction of tumor response.
3. *Physicists and engineers* may improve present heating systems: applicators are now being designed to provide broader field sizes; improved control of power deposition, thermal homogeneity and heat delivery to areas of limited access; better protection of sensitive adjacent normal tissues; better conformity to curved body surfaces; improvement of overall treatment comfort for patients; and improved equipment and computer operation for staff.
4. There is a further need for noninvasive thermometry techniques, e.g., microwave or ultrasound radiometry, applied potential tomography, or magnetic resonance imaging.
5. *Clinical oncologists* (surgeons, radiotherapists, and medical oncologists) must cooperate to an even greater extent in multicenter trials and quality control, and design appropriate controlled clinical studies for suitable tumors and body sites.

Despite this "work-in-progress situation" there is no doubt that the addition of hyperthermia to chemo- and radiotherapy provides a significant and worthwhile improvement in cancer control for selected body sites.

In the two volumes of *Thermoradiotherapy and Thermochemotherapy* we have aimed to bring together a group of experts to present up-to-date knowledge and future perspectives in the fields of hyperthermic biology, physiology, and physics (volume 1) and clinical options for combined hyperthermia and ionizing radiation or chemotherapy (volume 2). The two volumes include 45 contributions (21 chapters in volume 1 and 24 chapters in volume 2) which demonstrate the advanced state of this multidisciplinary field. We have structured the contents of the volumes into six sections: historical review, biological principles, pathophysiological mechanisms, physical principles and engineering, clinical applications, and multicenter trials and future research.

The logical order of the chapters, the figures and tables, the concise tabulation of parameters for hyperthermia data evaluation, and the subject index provide a clear orientation in the field. The reader will find the important aspects summarized and highlighted at the end of each chapter. The two volumes are designed to allow the specialist as well as the interested newcomer to start with any desired topic or preferred area of research and then easily to proceed to any other topic of interest.

In publishing these two volumes we hope to promote further scientific exchange among the countries of Europe, America, Asia and other areas in order to stimulate the diffusion of knowledge of thermoradio- and thermochemotherapy in all specialized oncological fields. Biological research, technical improvements, and new clinical concepts and therapeutic ideas may pave the way for a broad spectrum of oncological and even nononcological applications. We hope that you will find this book interesting, informative, and stimulating: it certainly was for all three of us as we participated in the writing and editing of it.

Erlangen/Stanford/London

M. Heinrich Seegenschmiedt
Peter Fessenden
Clare C. Vernon

Contents

Clinical Applications of Hyperthermia

Multicenter Trials and Future Clinical Research

Clinical Applications of Hyperthermia

1 Clinical Rationale for Thermoradiotherapy

M.H. SEEGENSCHMIEDT and H.J. FELDMANN

CONTENTS

1.1 Introduction

Oncological research has advanced in many areas, including surgery, chemotherapy (CT), radiotherapy (RT), and immunotherapy, but only in a few cancers has long-term control of locally advanced and disseminated disease been routinely attained. For most cancers, *local tumor control* is still the primary treatment goal, and determines long-term outcome.

Cancer prevention is the best but still an unrealistic way of overcoming this oncological dilemma. Another option, tumor screening and early detection of small tumors, allows treatment of patients with organ preservation and yields excellent functional results and long-term relapse- or disease-free survival, if not cure. Unfortunately, however, only one-third of all cancers are detected in an early, still operable stage. The other tumors are advanced at the time of diagnosis and there is little possibility of cure. Even aggressive surgery or CT is unable to prevent local tumor progression or subsequent tumor relapse, and high-dose RT also may not provide sufficient control of bulky tumors. In addition, recurrent tumors are even more difficult to control by any means and are often "heralds" of distant metastases (SUIT and WESTGATE 1986).

Data of the American Cancer Society for 1991 show that two-thirds of cancer patients die with persistent local disease, while local failure contributes directly to death in almost one-third. In many tumors the ratio is much higher, such as brain and CNS tumors and cancers of the head and neck, esophagus, ovaries, prostate, cervical or endometrial uterus, and bladder, but even in colorectal or lung cancer, where local failure accounts for a small proportion of deaths (23% and 11% respectively), about 30000 (14000 and 15600 respectively) patients could benefit from improved local treatment (SUIT 1982) (Table 1.1). In particular, stigmatized patients with uncontrolled local tumor growth and tumor-related symptoms require improved oncological therapy to yield a better quality of life or improved local control (KAPP 1986; SEEGENSCHMIEDT et al. 1993).

New strategies have combined surgery and RT (e.g., neoadjuvant RT for advanced soft

M. HEINRICH SEEGENSCHMIEDT, MD, Klinik und Poliklinik für Strahlentherapie, Universität Erlangen-Nürnberg, Universitätsstraße 27, D-91054 Erlangen, FRG
HORST J. FELDMANN, MD, Klinik und Poliklinik für Strahlentherapie und Radiologische Onkologie der Technischen Universität München, Klinikum rechts der Isar, Ismaninger Straße 22, D-81675 München, FRG

Table 1.1. Impact of tumor control on overall survival (American Cancer Society: Cancer facts and figures – 1991)

Tumor type	Annual death rate (in 1990) (*n*)	Estimated local failures as major cause of death[a] [*n* (%)]
Brain and CNS tumors	11 100	10 500 (95%)
Ovarian carcinoma	12 400	10 400 (84%)
Skin carcinoma	8 800	6 100 (69%)
Prostatic carcinoma	30 000	18 300 (61%)
Cervical carcinoma	6 000	3 600 (60%)
Endometrial carcinoma	4 000	2 350 (59%)
Esophageal carcinoma	9 500	5 600 (59%)
Bladder carcinoma	9 700	5 250 (54%)
Head and neck cancer	16 700	6 850 (41%)
Colorectal cancer	60 900	14 000 (23%)
Breast carcinoma	44 300	6 200 (14%)
Malignant lymphoma	28 700	3 450 (12%)
Bronchial carcinoma	142 000	15 600 (11%)
Total	384 100	108 200 (29%)

[a] Relative numbers and percentages are based on Rubin and Carter (1976)

tissue sarcomas) or CT and RT (e.g., RT-CT for advanced esophageal, rectal, or head and neck tumors); with regard to biology and physiology, new RT schedules (e.g., hyperfractionation) and radiosensitizers (e.g., misonidazole) have been recommended. Another new treatment strategy is to use combined heat (HT) and RT (thermoradiotherapy, HT-RT) or heat and CT (thermochemotherapy, HT-CT). The principles, rationale, and potential of this new oncological modality are reviewed in this chapter based on several comprehensive journal (Kapp 1986; Overgaard 1989, 1993; Seegenschmiedt et al. 1993) and textbook articles (Gerner and Cetas 1993; Hall 1988; Gautherie 1990; Perez et al. 1992; Seegenschmiedt and Sauer 1993).

Although for almost 5000 years heat has been employed in all cultures as a remedy for many diseases, including cancer, it was not until the 1960s, after modern radiobiological knowledge had increased and better research tools had become available, that serveral laboratories independently confirmed experimentally that heat was useful in the treatment of malignant tumors. Biologists studied the biochemical, cellular, and physiological effects of HT in various tissues. Physicists and engineers developed methods to apply heat to many body sites and to refine treatment planning and thermal monitoring. Clinical researchers tested the feasibility and efficacy of HT using different combinations of heat with RT or CT for palliative and curative treatments. Recently, physiological research on tissue perfusion and metabolism (pH, pO_2, energy status) has gained momentum and had a substantial impact on HT research. Each of these research fields has contributed good arguments to support the clinical rationale for HT-RT.

1.2 Biological Effects

Biological mechanisms which support the clinical rationale for HT-RT have been extensively reviewed (Hall 1988; Overgaard 1989; Streffer and van Beuningen 1987; vol. 1, Chap. 2: Streffer; Chap. 4: Konings). In vitro and in vivo studies and clinical observations suggest that heat preferentially damages tumor cells and sensitizes them to RT and CT. The biological rationale is convincing and one of the major arguments for combining both modalities. There are two basic mechanisms involved, namely direct *hyperthermic cytotoxicity* and indirect *hyperthermic radiosensitization*. The principal mechanisms are depicted in Fig. 1.1.

1.2.1 Thermal Cytotoxicity

Heat at high temperatures (beyond 42.5°–43°C) destroys cells directly. In principle, this effect does not differ quantitatively between tumor and normal cells, as it leads directly to protein denaturation, which represents a different destructive mechanism than the cytotoxic effects of radiation, which preferentially damages the DNA. Consensus as to the molecular mechanisms of thermal killing has not yet emerged, but the postulated targets of induced damage are the plasma membrane, cytoskeleton, and nucleus (Hall 1988; vol. 1, Chap. 2: Streffer; Chap. Konings).

The damage to the *plasma membranes* is based on observations that membrane-active agents (e.g., local anesthetics) and alcohols act synergistically with heat. Some studies show a relationship between the membrane lipid composition and thermal cell death. With regard to the *cytoskeleton*, heat has been shown to alter the structure and function of cytoplasmic organelles, including mitochondria, lysosomes, and the protein synthesis apparatus. Heat also leads to

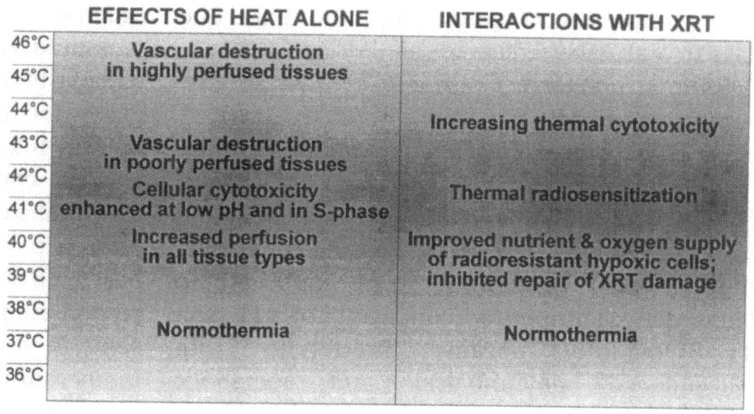

Fig. 1.1. Principal mechanisms of thermal radiosensitization and cytotoxicity

alteration and disruption of *nuclear functions*. The nucleolus appears to be a very heat-sensitive structure and undergoes marked changes at temperatures which leave other cytoplasmic organelles unaffected, and accumulation of the nuclear protein content occurs upon heat exposure. Other studies also implicate the presence of excess proteins in the nucleolus with the inhibition of DNA replication and DNA repair (HALL 1988; vol. 1, Chap. 3: BURGMAN et al.).

Generally, thermal cytotoxicity is enhanced in a nutrient-deprived tissue microenvironment which is characterized by insufficient blood supply, energy-deprived nutrition, and increased acidity due to anaerobic metabolism. Bulky tumors can present these features, which often render them radioresistant but also highly heat-sensitive. Under such conditions, even relatively low temperatures of 40.5°–41°C may lead to the destruction of tumor cells while not causing damage to cells in a "normal" cellular microenvironment (Fig. 1.1).

1.2.2 Thermal Radiosensitization

Heat exposure during or shortly before or after RT radiosensitizes cells even at lower temperatures. This phenomenon has been studied more in combination with low LET than with high LET radiation (STREFFER et al. 1983; GERNER et al. 1976), but the complex mechanisms of radiosensitization are even now not fully understood. One important factor seems to be the accumulation of proteins in the nucleus which bind to the nuclear matrix after heat exposure. Heat-exposed cells cannot repair the radiation-induced single-strand breaks and chromosome aberrations. This translates into the inability to repair sublethal (SLD) and potentially lethal damage (PLD) (OVERGAARD 1989; BEN-HUR et al. 1974).

Also, a complementary synergism across the cell cycle is observed when HT and RT are combined (WESTRA and DEWEY 1971): cells in Gl phase are less sensitive to heat than cells in S phase, while the opposite is true for cellular sensitivity to RT (WESTRA and DEWEY 1971). This almost complementary interaction of HT and RT on the cellular and molecular level is another major factor contributing to the "biological rationale" for the clinical implementation of combined HT and RT (OVERGAARD 1989; PEREZ et al. 1992).

1.2.3 Thermal Enhancement

The enhancement of cell killing by combined HT-RT as compared to RT alone is defined by the *thermal enhancement ratio* (TER), that is, the ratio of the RT dose required to yield a defined biological endpoint and the RT dose plus HT required to achieve the same endpoint. Experimentally, TER values are based on isoeffect calculations, while in most clinical studies they are related to isodose levels, that is, rates of clinical response after combined HT-RT versus RT alone. Another important parameter can be derived from the isoeffect TER values; it is defined as the ratio of TERs in tumor versus normal tissue. This *therapeutic gain factor* (TGF) is measured by generating RT dose-response curves with or without HT for tumor and normal tissues. Thus, a TGF greater than 1 generally implies that the thermal enhancement of RT is more pronounced in tumor than in normal tissue (Overgaard 1989; Perez et al. 1992).

1.2.4 *Sequencing of Heat and Irradiation*

To optimize the interaction between HT and RT and to yield a high therapeutic effect under clinical conditions, it is important to define the appropriate sequencing of HT and RT. Obviously, negative interference with heat-induced physiological and metabolic conditions is to be avoided (Streffer 1985). Experimental data suggest that the highest TER is observed for *simultaneous* application of HT and RT. In this situation the TER depends on the duration and achieved thermal level during HT. The TER in tumor and normal tissue decreases rapidly when HT is applied more than 30–60 min before or after RT.

Sequential application reduces the response to combined HT-RT treatment. This reduction is probably independent of the sequence of application. While simultaneous application of HT and RT can provide TER values beyond 2, sequential applications provide a lower TER of 1.5–2 in tumors when intervals are ≥4 h, independently of the treatment schedule. This can provide a therapeutic gain even when normal tissues and tumors are at the same temperature. If tumors are heated exclusively and normal tissue is completely spared from the heat exposure, simultaneous application gives the best TER and a high TGF (Overgaard 1989).

However, for typical schedules of fractionated HT combined with low LET radiation at 2- to 4-Gy dose fractions no detailed radiobiological data exist. It must be assumed that under these conditions only a suboptimal interaction is achieved. This calls for improvements, including optimized schedules (e.g., simultaneous HT-RT, continuous modest-temperature HT-RT), use of step-down heating, and application of heat sensitizers (e.g., pH sensitization, sulfhydryl agents, flavonoids, amino acid analogs) (Hahn 1993).

1.2.5 *"Thermal Dose" Description*

Experimental and clinical data indicate that thermal sensitization exponentially increases with both time and temperature. In contrast to the radiation dose prescription, which is defined and measured by a physical unit that directly correlates with the biological effect, no such agreed definition exists for the "thermal dose" (vol. 1, Chap. 6: Dewhirst). One proposed "thermal dose" concept converts the heat exposure at various temperatures to equivalent times at a defined reference or index temperature (usually 43°C) based on biologically derived time-temperature response curves (Sapareto and Dewey 1984). In some in vitro and in vivo experiments this time-temperature conversion has been found to be a prognostic indicator for tumor response, but nowadays many additional factors are known to modulate this biological effect, including step-down heating, thermotolerance, specific HT-RT interactions, and physiological and metabolic tissue factors (blood flow, pH, bioenergetic status, etc.) (Hall 1988; Overgaard 1989; Perez et al. 1992; Song 1984, 1993; Vaupel and Jain 1991; vol. 1, Chap. 7: Song et al.; Chap. 8: Vaupel and Kelleher; Chap. 9: Prescott).

1.3 Physiological Effects

Heat exposure can induce, alter, and maintain various metabolic conditions at the cellular and tissue level which are closely interrelated with the superordinated physiological changes at the tissue level. Physiological conditions can help to enhance thermal effects on tissues and to achieve a "therapeutic differential" between tumor and normal tissue (Molls et al. 1992; vol. 1, Chap. 7: Song et al.; Chap. 8: Vaupel and Kelleher; Chap. 9: Prescott).

1.3.1 *Changes in Blood Perfusion*

The thermal level obtained in tumor and normal tissues during HT depends on the *balance between heat (energy) efflux and heat (energy) influx*. Heat efflux is mainly represented by blood flow and to a lesser extent by thermal conduction. Whether or not tumors are *preferentially* heated compared to normal tissues depends on relative and absolute perfusion rates in these tissues (Waterman et al. 1987). Several studies in humans underscore the importance of blood flow and address its variability in tumors and normal tissues (Mäntyla 1979; Milligan et al. 1983; Nyström et al. 1969; Reinhold and Endrich 1986; Vaupel et al. 1989;

VAUPEL and JAIN 1991). Quantitative perfusion studies have been conducted using positron emission tomography, isotope clearance techniques, laser Doppler flowmetry, and thermal washout measurements (ACKER et al. 1990; BEANEY et al. 1984; ITO et al. 1982; LAGENDIJK 1982; LAGENDIJK et al. 1988; LAHTINEN et al. 1979; LAMMERTSMA et al. 1985; MÄNTYLA et al. 1988; VAUPEL et al. 1990).

Blood flow varies remarkably depending upon tumor type, volume, and site of growth, and influences the thermal response in two ways: (a) by causing heat to dissipate from the heated tumor mass, and (b) by creating a metabolic micromilieu which modulates the heat sensitivity. Clinical data show that there is a significant difference between relative blood flow rates of the tumor center and the periphery, indicating a considerable heterogeneity within the treatment volume (FELDMANN et al. 1992; SAMULSKI et al. 1987; WATERMAN et al. 1987); this can be explained by the heterogeneous vascular density in tumors (JIRTLE 1988). Generally, in human tumors an inverse correlation exists between relative tissue perfusion rates and achieved steady state temperatures; thus, favorable and limiting tissue conditions have to be accounted for in achieving the prescribed temperature.

Some experiments suggest that poorly perfused tissues are more heat-sensitive than highly perfused tissues, which are protected by heat dissipation. Heat "accumulates" in poorly perfused areas, be they well confined (tumor core) or highly scattered throughout the target volume. Low blood flow during heat exposure deprives the tissues of nutrients (e.g., oxygen, glucose), enhances the accumulation of waste products, and influences the metabolic environment (e.g., leading to hypoxia, acidosis, and energy depletion), which in itself increases the cytotoxic effects of HT (STREFFER 1985; VAUPEL et al. 1989). This *dual role of blood flow* is illustrated in Fig. 1.2.

In summary, the expected biological response to heat exposure may be quite different even in the same tumor depending upon local metabolic tissue and perfusion conditions. Tumor blood flow may increase in some areas, while in others it may steadily decrease, but the extent and direction of blood flow changes do not correlate significantly with tumor type, site, or volume.

1.3.2 Changes in Tissue pH

In vivo studies reveal that induction of *acute intracellular acidosis (low pH)* increases the cellular sensitivity to heat by reducing the stability of cellular proteins. This phenomenon is observed with a single HT exposure as well as during fractionated HT (SONG 1984, 1993). The intracellular pH falls in a "dose"-dependent manner, thereby increasing thermal cytotoxicity and inhibiting the development of thermal tolerance and repair of thermal damage. The following pathogenetic mechanisms are assumed to be responsible for this tissue acidification: (a) accumulation of lactic acids, (b) change in chemical equilibria of the intra- and extracellular buffer systems, (c) increase in adenosine triphosphate (ATP) hydrolysis, (d) increase in pCO_2 levels, and (e) inhibition of the Na^+/H^+ ion pumps (STREFFER and VAN BEUNINGEN 1987). In summary, preclinical data confirm experimental observations that low pH enhances the effect of HT (VAN DEN BERG et al. 1989).

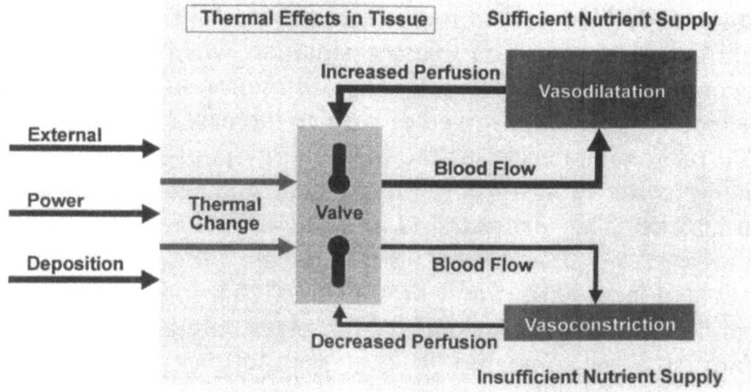

Fig. 1.2. Physiological modification of thermal effects in highly and poorly perfused tissues. (From SEEGENSCHMIEDT et al. 1994)

1.3.3 Changes in Tissue Oxygenation

Both acutely induced and prolonged hypoxia increases the thermal sensitivity of malignant tumors. Whether hypoxia plays a direct or indirect role is still under discussion, but in general tumor oxygenation is closely related to the efficiency of tumor microcirculation: changes in the perfusion rate are directly followed by changes in the tissue oxygenation. The application of high temperatures in *low-flow* tissues provokes a blood flow decline or even disruption, leading to increasing hypoxia, while oxygenation of *high-flow* tumors can even improve upon heating. Thus, the heterogeneous blood flow response during HT is expected to be the main modulator of the induction, maintenance, and even enhancement of pO_2 gradients between low- and high-flow areas within the same tumor volume as well as between normal and tumor tissues. Preliminary clinical data show that a decrease in the average pO_2 in comparison with the initial pO_2 is observed 24 h after heat exposure. It has been speculated that this is due to the developing edema and a higher interstitial pressure following the HT application.

1.3.4 Changes in Bioenergetic Status

A reduction in the bioenergetic status in conjunction with other physiological mechanisms can contribute to thermal sensitization, as tumors can develop decreased glucose levels and undergo thermal sensitization during HT. Studies in *high-flow* tumors indicate that this does not always occur, and even increased glucose concentrations may be observed, as high perfusion can increase glucose availability and lead to a better distribution of the substrate. Another aspect is important: intratumoral lactic acid levels increase, since the citric acid cycle but not the glycolysis is inhibited during HT, and an 18-fold decrease in ATP yield occurs as compared to the situation when glucose oxidation is present. This difference in the bioenergetic status together with an increased ATP turnover rate causes the high-energy phosphates to decay in a "dose"-dependent manner during the heat exposure (LILLY et al. 1985; OKUNIEFF and PARDO 1993; SIJENS et al. 1989; VAUPEL et al. 1990). It may be concluded that for high-flow tumors energy deprivation plays only a minor role as compared to that seen in fast-growing low-flow tumors.

1.3.5 Manipulation of Physiological Parameters

Efforts to improve thermal efficacy have led to various attempts to modulate physiological parameters either directly or indirectly; the modulators most often studied have been tumor pH and blood flow. Blood flow is the main target, as it influences not only tumor temperatures during HT, but also oxygen availability and nutrient delivery to and waste product removal from the tumor, which subsequently also influences the cellular pH level (DEWHIRST et al. 1990b; MOLLS et al. 1992; PRESCOTT et al. 1992; vol. 1, Chap. 7: SONG et al.; Chap. 8: VAUPEL and KELLEHER; Chap. 9: PRESCOTT).

The cellular pH can be reduced through induction of hyperglycemia (stimulation of glycolysis), intake of ion channel blockers (e.g., amiloride), or modulation of perfusion by means of peripheral vasodilators (hydralazine, sodium nitroprusside) (DEWHIRST et al. 1990b; PRESCOTT et al. 1992; vol. 1, Chap. 8: VAUPEL and KELLEHER; Chap. 9: PRESCOTT). In all instances, either thermal sensitization of tumor or thermal protection of normal tissues is expected to occur. Presently the experimental data on the implementation of physiological heat response modifiers are very promising, but testing under clinical conditions has not yet been performed.

1.3.6 Conclusions

In summary, the differential heat sensitivity of tumors as compared to normal tissues is more the consequence of differential physiological effects in tumor and normal tissues, including perfusion patterns, nutrient supply or energy deprivation, and tissue acidosis, than a result of the intrinsic state of the tumor cells themselves. Environmental conditions which enhance thermal damage are typically those which will reduce radiation damage. Tumor areas resistant to RT are likely to be sensitive to HT, while well-perfused tumors (and a normal environment) are sensitive to RT but relatively resistant to HT. This almost *complementary interaction* is the most attractive reason for combining HT and RT, and is most indicative of its potential.

1.4 Technical Instrumentation

The goal of HT treatment is to maximize the volume of tissue in which optimal "therapeutic" temperatures are induced. This maximization should be accomplished while keeping the temperature of the normal tissues at risk for thermal toxicity below a specified level (ROEMER 1991). Nevertheless, the nature of the heat-tissue interaction, tissue composition, and blood flow effects implies that technically uniform heating cannot be achieved. Thus, different physical agents and HT devices have to be utilized for the various tumor sizes, configurations, and tumor locations (GAUTHERIE 1990; PEREZ et al. 1992; SEEGENSCHMIEDT and SAUER 1993). The HT techniques which are already used in the clinic, such as microwaves (MW), radiofrequency (RF) waves, and ultrasound (US) waves, reflect the tremendous technical progress made by physicists and engineers over the past decades, but they also mirror the complexity of specific clinical situations. Presently, no single universal HT technique allows the heating of any desired target volume to 43°C in a reliable and reproducible way. Thus, in contrast to biology and physiology, the physical principles of heating do not favor the application of combined HT-RT.

1.4.1 Physical Agents

The physical agents used for HT are electromagnetic (EM) fields at high (300–2450 MHz), lower (60–120 MHz), and very low frequencies (0.1–27 MHz), or ultrasound (US) at 0.5–5.0 MHz. *Conductive* or *resistive* methods rely on RF currents driven between pairs of electrodes. Heating is produced through collisions of moving ions with cellular molecules. *Dielectric* or *capacitive heating* is achieved by polarization charges induced through capacitive electrodes with the tissue in between acting as dielectric. *Inductive heating* is induced by magnetic fields via large RF coil applicators around the target volume. US devices create *mechanical* waves at frequencies above the audible range and heat through mechanical forces, that is, compression and decompression of molecules within tissue. Heat transfer in tissue is mediated by thermal conduction or thermal convection (blood flow). In clinical practice, EM and US modalities are plagued by problems of controllable energy deposition which are related to the heterogeneous tissue composition and the differential physiological (perfusional) responses to heat.

1.4.2 Factors Affecting Power Deposition

Adequate heating depends on four parameters: (a) the anatomical site, (b) the biophysical tissue properties, (c) the physiological conditions, and (d) the employed HT technique. The first two parameters are set conditions, such that small surface lesions are more amenable and offer better conditions for homogeneous heating than bulky or deep-seated tumors. In the case of heat production via RF and MW devices, biophysical tissue properties will modify the power deposition due to differential absorption in tissues with high (e.g., muscle) or low water content (e.g., fat, bone). Tissue boundaries (e.g., fat-muscle, muscle-bone) also influence energy absorption and may cause development of "cold" and "hot spots" due to interference or reflection phenomena. The biophysical heterogeneities are even more complicated by the fact that energy deposition depends on the direction of the incident EM fields. Thus, the selection of adequate HT techniques is probably the single most important parameter that can be influenced such that it produces a differential impact on tumor and normal tissues.

1.4.3 Technical Options

The different physical agents and modalities for heating are listed in Table 1.2. Usually, energy from a generator is propagated into waveguides, electrodes, antennas, transducers, or coils, which are coupled to the patient. The basic components of a modern HT system are shown in Fig. 1.3. It consists of a power source (generator), one or several adjustable HT applicators, interposed coupling media, invasive multipoint thermometry, and an operator-controlled computer for data recording, feedback control during HT, and data evaluation.

In clinical practice, a distinction is often made between "superficial" and "deep heating": *superficial HT* is considered to reach a therapeutic level (42°–43°C) up to 3 cm in depth, while *deep HT* refers to target volumes which extend beyond the effective heating depths of simple HT devices and

Table 1.2. Physical heating methods and heating techniques

Parameters	Type of hyperthermia	Description and specification
Depth of heating penetration	Superficial hyperthermia	Penetration depth up to 3 cm (skin, subcutis, superficial muscles)
	Medium-depth hyperthermia	Penetration depth between 3 and 6 cm (deep muscles, extremities)
	Deep-body hyperthermia	Penetration depth up to body center (thorax, abdomen, pelvis)
Dimensions of body region	Local or focal hyperthermia (LH)	Small localized tumor volumes
	Regional hyperthermia (RHT)	Large and deep penetrating tumors
	Whole-body hyperthermia (WBH)	Systemic temperature elevation for diffuse and metastatic tumors
Type of technical HT application	External hyperthermia (EHT)	External coupling of HT applicators, partly with cooled bolus material
	Interstitial hyperthermia (IHT)	Direct coupling of IHT applicators, partly with cooled surface
	Intracavitary hyperthermia (ICHT)	Direct and indirect coupling of ICHT applicators with cooled surfaces
	Hyperthermic perfusion (HTP)	Extracorporeal heating of blood
Physical agent and HT principle	Electromagnetic (EM) techniques:	
	a) Lower radiofrequencies (RF) (0.5–27 MHz)	Resistive and capacitive coupling: condensators and electrical currents Inductive coupling: magnetic induction and eddy currents
	b) Microwaves (UHF-RF) (60–120, 434, 915, 2450 MHz)	Radiative coupling of antennas
	Ultrasound (US) techniques: (0.5–5.0 MHz)	Acoustic – mechanical coupling of stationary and mobile transducers
Clinical mode of HT application	Thermoradiotherapy (HT-RT)	Clinical applications in all body regions (EHT, IHT, ICHT)
	Thermochemotherapy (HT-ChT)	Clinical applications in a few tumors: sarcomas, pelvic and head and neck tumors
	Combined HT-ChT-RT ("HCR")	Clinical applications in a few tumors: breast and esophageal carcinoma
	Combined intraoperative HT-RT (IOHT-IORT)	Clinical applications in a few tumors: pancreatic and rectal carcinoma

require complex HT technologies. In addition, "invasive" and "noninvasive" HT methods are distinguished: *noninvasive* HT devices are positioned externally to the patient and power is deposited through the intact skin, similarly to external beam RT, while *invasive* HT devices produce HT directly within the target volume, similarly to brachytherapy. In the latter case, power is deposited either within natural body cavities (intracavitary HT), in intraluminal sites (endoluminal HT), or directly within the tumor by means of implanted probes (interstitial HT). The set-up of these techniques is illustrated by Fig. 1.4.

Among the HT methods, interstitial HT and intracavitary HT have several theoretical and practical advantages over external HT: (a) well-defined energy deposition in tumors and better sparing of normal tissues; (b) access to localized deep-seated tumors; (c) improved homogeneity of power deposition and heating characteristics due to feedback control of all HT applicators; (d) option of invasive thermometry for good heating reliability. Although interstitial HT techniques are difficult to operate, they provide the greatest therapeutic potential and come closest to fulfilling the demand for complete thermal coverage of a defined target volume.

Methods for regional HT are at a developmental stage. Sites most amenable to regional HT are the pelvis, extremities, abdomen, and chest wall. Capacitive 13.56- or 8-MHz applicators, which are mostly utilized in Japan, produce electrical fields which are predominantly perpendicular to the body surface and deep tissue layers (Koga et al. 1985). The excessive power deposition in

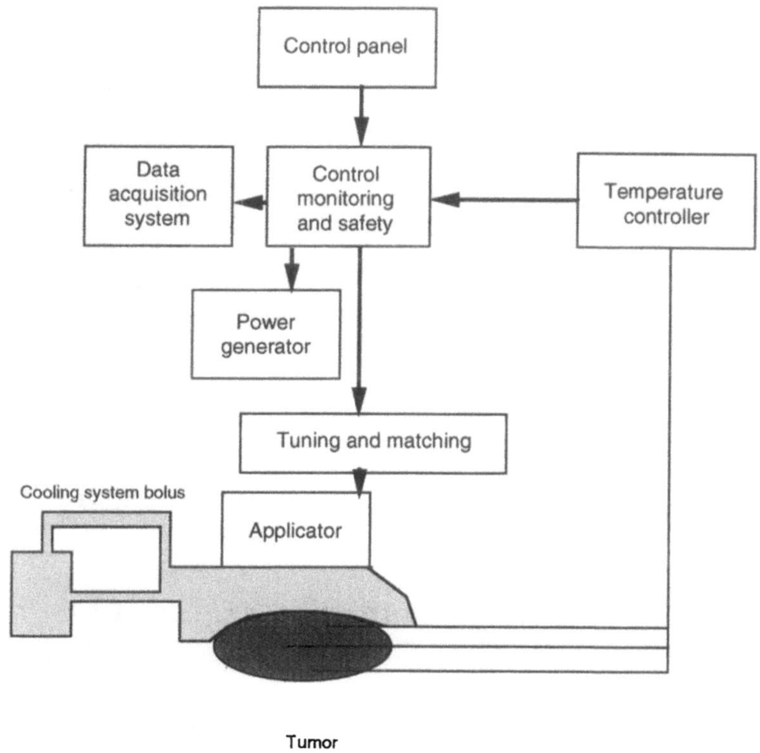

Fig. 1.3. Schematic diagram of the basic components of a clinical HT system. The operator applies the treatment manually or automatically by means of a PC which controls the power deposition through feedback thermometry control

fatty tissues can often limit the efficacy of this technique (HIRAOKA et al. 1985). As current flow and density are not controllable, undesired "hot spots" can arise anywhere in the human body (KATO et al. 1985; OLESON and CETAS 1982). In contrast, inductive concentric coil RF devices produce electric fields parallel to the skin and superficial tissues, but clinical studies have shown that this technique is ineffective for deep-seated tumors (OLESON et al. 1984, 1986).

Radiative devices such as the annular phased array systems (APAS) and the TEM applicator (DELEEUW and LAGENDIJK 1987; TURNER 1984 a,b; TURNER and SCHAEFERMEYER 1989) are techniques in which the E-field is parallel to the skin and deeper body tissues and aligns with the patient's longitudinal axis. The devices operate at frequencies of less than 100 MHz and through constructive interference attain a significant power deposition in the center of the human body. Clinical research activities in Europe and United States have concentrated on these applicators (GIBBS and STEWART 1985; MYERSON et al. 1991; OLESON et al. 1988; PETROVICH et al. 1989; SAPOZINK et al. 1984). Focused ultrasonic devices, another means of deep heating, operate at short wavelengths (≤1 cm) and can be more precisely directed than EM devices, but they are compromised by "hot spots" and reflection phenomena at tissue interfaces (bone, air).

1.4.4 Temperature Monitoring

Invasive thermal monitoring constitutes the only reliable method of treatment verification and is obligatory for quality control and evaluation of results in clinical HT (FELDMANN et al. 1992, 1993a; ISSELS et al. 1990; KAPP et al. 1988). Obviously, the requirement does not enhance the applicability of HT as a routine treatment. In clinical practice, it is important to monitor the whole thermal range in the target volume, including the minimum and maximum temperatures. Regions of tumor necrosis usually yield the highest temperatures, while well-perfused tumors, tumor periphery, and normal tissues often yield the lowest temperatures (FELDMANN et al. 1992; SAMULSKI et al. 1987). Computed tomography-guided insertion of closed-tip

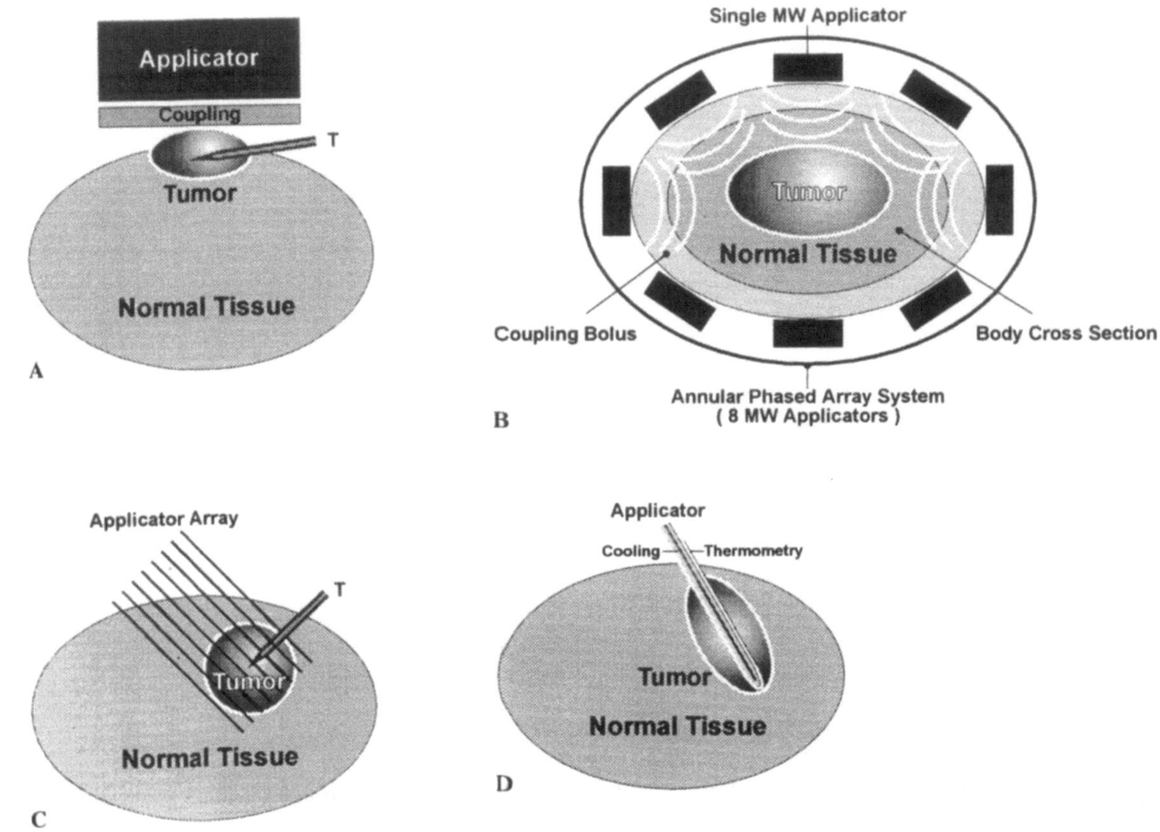

Fig. 1.4. **A** Superficial local HT setup with an external HT applicator. The invasive thermometry probes (*T*) monitor intratumoral temperatures. Additional thermometry is required in normal tissues. The coupling bolus can be cooled with perfused liquids. **B** Regional HT setup with an annular phased array system (APAS) using eight independently controlled microwave (MW) sources. Several other regional HT techniques are possible. Invasive thermometry (not included in the schematic drawing) is also implemented. **C** Interstitial HT setup with an array of implanted independently powered heating sources. Additional invasive probes are required for thermal monitoring (*T*). Power sources may be microwave antennas, radiofrequency electrodes, hot source tubes, laser sources, and even miniaturized ultrasound devices. **D** Intracavitary HT setup in a body cavity with an inserted heating source which incorporates both cooling (perfused liquids) and thermometry at the surface of the HT device. Additional invasive thermometry probes are recommended. (All figures from SEEGENSCHMIEDT et al. 1994)

catheters into deep-seated lesions is a well-tolerated method to place thermometry devices. They can be mechanically or automatically mapped through tumor and normal tissues during the HT treatment (BERGER et al. 1988; MÜLLER et al. 1988; PIROTH and BRINKMANN 1988). Few side-effects have been observed when using this invasive technique (FELDMANN et al. 1993b; VAN DER ZEE et al. 1992).

Methods of invasive thermometry include electrically conducting probes (thermistors, thermocouples), minimally conducting probes (high-impedance thermistors), and nonconducting optical probes (gallium arsenide). Noninvasive thermometry methods may become routinely available in the future, including infrared thermography, microwave radiometry, ultrasound, and magnetic resonance reconstructions (GAUTHERIE 1990), but even then HT will not be a simple "switch on and off" treatment modality.

1.4.5 Planning and Thermal Modeling

HT treatment planning and thermal modeling are means of detecting and overcoming technical insufficiencies and allow an a priori optimization of the treatment. This can be carried out as in RT, through measurements in phantoms and calculations within models of tissue heating. However, the fabrication of patient-equivalent phantoms is far more difficult to achieve in HT than in RT owing to the inability to simulate adequately the conductive and convective heat transfer under various conditions. Mapping of electrical (or acoustic) fields is performed in liquid phantoms and absorbed power density patterns are derived from the initial slopes of temperature curves at selected points in semiliquid or solid phantoms. This provides valuable data about specific types, sizes, required number, and exact placement of HT applicators and which HT applicators are best suited for a specific clinical application. However, it does not account for actual blood flow changes and heat dissipation during an ongoing HT treatment in an individual patient.

1.5 Clinical Options

A survey of different options of clinical HT applications is provided in Table 1.3. Review papers have discussed clinical results obtained with superficial, regional, and interstitial HT (Feldmann et al. 1995; Overgaard 1989, 1993; Perez et al. 1992; Seegenschmiedt et al. 1993; Seegenschmiedt and Sauer 1993). So far worldwide more than 50 000 patients have been treated with combined HT-RT or HT plus chemotherapy. An excellent survey on the present status of laboratory and clinical research related to HT was provided at the last International Congress on Hyperthermic Oncology (ICHO) in Tucson (USA), where about 30% of more than 450 presentations addressed clinical studies and HT applications (Gerner and Cetas 1993). Comparisons with the types of presentations at previous international meetings clearly demonstrate the increasing number and diversification of clinical HT studies (Fig. 1.5). Nevertheless, the hyperthermia scientific community has still not come forth with the necessary clinical studies and convincing proof of its specific importance and role in oncology.

1.5.1 Treatment Indications

The rationale for the use of combined HT-RT in clinical trials is twofold: HT has an evident role as

Table 1.3. Options for clinical hyperthermia applications

Type of application	Clinical indications for hyperthermia
Superficial hyperthermia: EM and US applicators	*Superficially located, confined tumors (0–3 cm):* Skin cancer, melanoma, Kaposi's sarcoma, Subcutaneous relapses and metastases of solid tumors; breast and other carcinomas and small metastases; superficial relapses of head and neck tumors
Medium-depth hyperthermia: EM and US applicators	*More deeply situated, confined tumors (3–6 cm):* N3 neck node metastases; chest wall recurrences of breast carcinoma and primary breast carcinomas Small pelvic and thoracic tumors
Regional deep hyperthermia: EM and US applicators	*More deeply situated bulky tumors (>6 cm):* Primary advanced and recurrent pelvic tumors: colorectal, uterus, prostate, and bladder carcinomas Pediatric and adult soft tissue and bone sarcomas
Interstitial hyperthermia: EM, US, hot source applicators	*Confined implantable tumors:* Accessible head and neck, breast, chest wall and abdominal wall, and trunk tumors Small pelvis: colorectal, uterus, prostate, and bladder carcinomas; brain tumors: astrocytoma, glioblastoma
Intracavitary hyperthermia: EM, US, hot source applicators	*Confined intraluminal cancers:* Esophagus, central bronchus, bile duct, urethral, distal rectum, and anal canal carcinoma Carcinoma of the vagina, cervix, and corpus uteri
Whole-body hyperthermia: Extracorporeal blood heating	*Diffuse and systemically spread cancers:* Metastasized solid carcinomas Advanced soft tissue and bone sarcomas Diffuse lymphomas and leukemias

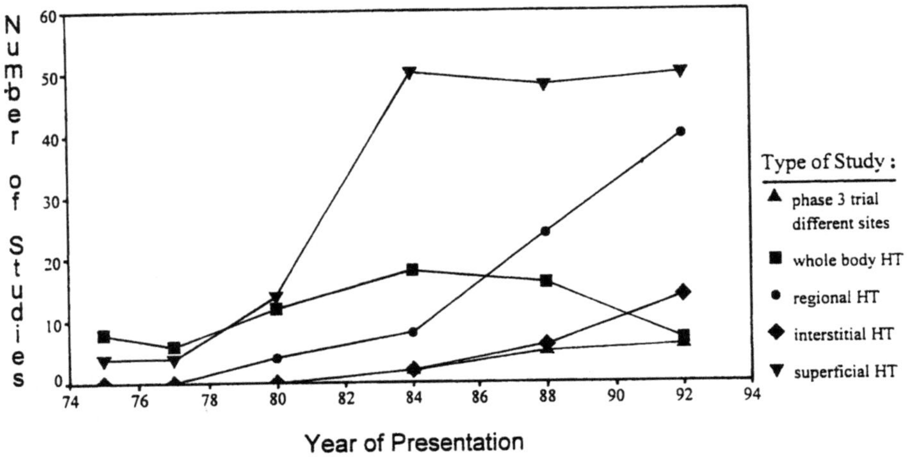

Fig. 1.5. Development of clinical HT applications demonstrated as clinical studies presented at previous international hyperthermia meetings in Washington, USA (1975), Essen, Germany (1977), Fort Collins, USA (1980), Aarhus, Denmark (1984), Kyoto, Japan (1988), and Tucson, USA (1992). The rate of clinical studies is increasing and clinical approaches become more complex, including regional and interstitial HT. Due to insufficient HT equipment the number of controlled phase III studies is still low. (Modified from OVERGAARD (1993))

palliative therapy for primary advanced and preirradiated recurrent tumors, which are difficult to control by other modalities. However, even then the clinical implementation of HT should always be preceded by adequate evaluation of other treatment alternatives. Another indication would be to use HT with *curative intent* in the treatment of primary tumors in which better local control is expected to improve curability and survival. Neither strategy has yet been fully implemented in clinical research, as despite strong biological and physiological arguments to support them, clinical application is still limited by insufficiencies of HT technology. One of the most crucial parameters which limits clinical implementation is the inability to homogeneously heat any circumscribed target volume, but this drawback applies more to diffusely spread or deep-seated tumors than to well-confined and accessible tumors.

1.5.2 Design of Clinical Studies

While the "gold standard" for drug evaluation in clinical trials is well established, including the method of randomized testing, for HT-RT applications sophisticated testing has been rather difficult to achieve. Since the major challenge has been the *technical feasibility* of using HT devices, the majority of clinical studies have been conducted as phase I trials, which simply address treatment feasibility and toxicity. Although these studies are still necessary to evaluate new HT devices, they are inappropriate for definition of a possible therapeutic gain. Unfortunately, many clinical studies provide only a poor description of the most relevant tumor and treatment variables, including RT parameters and a clear definition of the selected treatment endpoints.

Only well-designed controlled phase II and phase III studies which have utilized appropriate heating techniques, invasive thermometry, and quality assurance steps deserve to be further evaluated when addressing the question of whether combined HT-RT offers a *therapeutic advantage* over RT alone in a given treatment situation. If these stipulations are not met, such studies will fail, owing to inappropriate clinical and technical application rather them inefficacy of the method (PEREZ et al. 1991). The different types and specific goals of HT-related clinical studies are cited in Table 1.4.

1.5.3 Treatment Endpoints

The credibility of combined HT-RT depends on it having objective proven advantages as compared with the best standard RT treatment. This requires prospective definition of relevant treatment endpoints. Most radiobiological studies evaluate treatment response by comparing the damage to the most resistant tumor cell population with that

Table 1.4. Types and specific goals of HT-RT clinical trials (modified from SEEGENSCHMIEDT et al. 1993)

Type of study	Specific goals of the study (and approximate number of subjects required)
"Phase 0":	Equipment development – technical feasibility (about 20 subjects) (1) Basic equipment development: technical specifications, design and construction (2) Technical evaluation of equipment: Safety requirements, testing on phantoms (3) Clinical evaluation of equipment: Clinical testing on selected number of "signal tumors"; specification of evaluation criteria and "thermal dose" measures
Phase 1:	Clinical feasibility – treatment toxicity (about 20–100 subjects) (1) Corresponding to clinical phase 1 study: Determination of toxicity; "thermal dose" – response relationship (2) Improvement of technical equipment: Improved heating performance; reduced treatment toxicity; improved user's device handling and data analysis
Phase 2:	Specific suitability – clinical efficacy (about 100–200 subjects) (1) Corresponding to clinical phase 2 study: Evaluation of tumor suitability and effectiveness; identification of confounding and prognostic factors (2) Further optimization of technical equipment: Optimized heating performance; minimal treatment toxicity; optimized user's device handling; optimized data analysis
Phase 3:	Controlled randomized testing (about 100–400 subjects) (1) Corresponding to clinical phase 3 study: Randomization and controlled comparison between standard treatment and investigational treatment concept (2) Multicenter design with reference center (quality control): "Routine clinical handling" with optimized technical equipment

to the most sensitive ("critical") normal tissue. Most clinical studies apply WHO criteria to assess tumor response and EORTC/RTOG criteria to score normal tissue reactions. Endpoints like "complete tumor disappearance" or "sustained tumor control" have been used in most HT-RT studies, but subjective impairment and symptom-related reduced quality of life have rarely been evaluated. The most important criteria for treatment response evaluation in curative and palliative clinical HT-RT trials are summarized in Table 1.5 (NIELSEN et al. 1992).

1.5.4 Results of Clinical Trials

The majority of the published clinical HT–RT trials can be characterized as single-institutional uncontrolled phase I/II trials with retrospective data analysis. Most of these studies have been inadequately performed, using poor heating and thermometry techniques, practicing inconsistent patient accrual, not providing detailed reporting of all relevant treatment parameters, treatment toxicity, or treatment outcome, and lacking careful analysis of possible confounding factors and prognostic parameters.

The presented overview on site-specific clinical trials (Table 1.6) has been intentionally restricted to those HT-RT studies which fulfil the following "quality criteria":

1. The clinical trial has been published within the last 10 years and was designed as a controlled (randomized) study.
2. Especially for those trials including "matched pair" comparisons in the same patient, a similar distribution of all relevant tumor stratification factors (e.g., tumor volume, site, histology) and treatment variables (e.g., RT dose; HT-RT schedule) has to have been achieved.
3. The overall number of patients, the numbers in each treatment arm (HT-RT vs RT alone), and the frequencies yielding the treatment endpoint "CR" have been completely reported.
4. The employed RT and HT treatments have been well documented.
5. By modern oncological standards all patients had a reasonable chance of being adequately treated.

For this specific overview, only the "CR" was considered as relevant treatment endpoint.

Obviously, clinical HT-RT trials for *deep-seated lesions* which have been treated with regional HT do not meet these eligibility criteria due to clinical problems and inherent technical insufficiencies. In contrast, clinical studies using

Table 1.5. Criteria for treatment response in HT-RT clinical trials (modified from NIELSEN et al. 1992)

Response criteria	Specific variables
Tumor response	1. WHO criteria: complete/partial response, no change, progressive disease; locoregional recurrence 2. Local tumor control: freedom from progression, time to relapse, duration of local response 3. Radiological criteria (imaging studies): low-density areas in post-treatment CT scans
Normal tissue response	1. Organ-specific acute and late treatment toxicity 2. Radiation- versus hyperthermia-induced toxicity 3. Duration of recovery from treatment sequelae
Survival analysis	1. Overall (actuarial) survival, median survival 2. Disease-free survival and relapse-free survival 3. Symptom-free survival (especially for palliative trials)
Assessment of symptoms	1. Linear analogue self-assessment (LASA) analogue scales 2. Scoring systems for symptoms (pain, hemorrhage, neurological deficit, etc.; categorical scales) 3. Analgesic drug medication or other medical requirements
Quality of life	1. Karnofsky performance scale (KPS), WHO performance grading 2. Functional and emotional status (EORTC): functional status, psychological distress, sickness impact profile (SIP) 3. Measures for general and treatment-specific symptoms, e.g., Functional Living Index Cancer (FLIC) Scales

interstitial and intracavitary HT applications (brain, head and neck, breast, pelvic, and other tumors) have been technically refined and have yielded very encouraging results, but a comparative trial of combined HT-RT and RT alone is still lacking (SEEGENSCHMIEDT and SAUER 1992, 1993).

Thus, only *superficial tumors* treated with external HT devices have stood a reasonable chance of being adequately heated by better HT techniques and sufficiently controlled with regard to confounding factors in prospective clinical studies. Table 1.6 shows the site-specific results of tumors located in the breast and chest wall, on the skin (melanomas), in the head and neck, and in other superficial sites. The CR rates of both treatments are given, together with the TER and the odds ratio (plus mean and range) of each trial (references for the listed trials are provided in four recent publications: OVERGAARD 1989, 1993; PEREZ et al. 1992; SEEGENSCHMIEDT et al. 1993).

With only a few exceptions (PEREZ et al. 1991), studies have shown better results for combined HT-RT than for RT alone. This is substantiated when the data are subjected to meta-analysis methods, with the results from all studies being analyzed jointly (although not all the criteria of a meta-analysis are fulfilled, e.g., lack of medline search, inhomogeneous eligibility criteria, and some variability of patient or treatment data). Overall, these selected results indicate a clear biological advantage of combined HT-RT as compared to RT alone, and it is concluded that the biological rationale behind these studies seems valid and justified.

1.5.5 *Prognostic Parameters*

Several interrelated parameters can influence the tumor response when applying external or interstitial HT-RT (FELDMANN et al. 1993a; ISSELS et al. 1990; KAPP et al. 1988, 1991; LEOPOLD et al. 1992, 1993; MYERSON et al. 1990; OLESON et al. 1993; OVERGAARD 1989; PEREZ et al. 1992; SEEGENSCHMIEDT et al. 1989, 1993; VALDAGNI et al. 1988). Recognition of these parameters is important for the design of controlled HT-RT studies and the development of quality assurance criteria for patient and tumor selection and treatment control. The following types of prognostic parameters have to be distinguished: (a) parameters associated with the initial tumor characteristics; (b) patient parameters prior to the actual treatment initiation; (c) treatment parameters related to both RT and HT; and (d) factors related to tumor biology and tumor physiology. All these factors can influence treatment outcome independently of the HT quality. Clinical HT-RT studies indicating relevant prognostic factors are compiled in Table 1.7.

1.5.5.1 Tumor Parameters

Clinical data to date do not reveal any influence of tumor histology and tumor site on the response

Table 1.6. Overview of site-specific results of combined HT-RT versus RT alone[a]

Study	Type[b]	Number of cases			Complete response		TER: RT + HT / RT alone	Odds ratio	
		Total	RT	RT + HT	RT[b]	RT + HT[c]		Mean ± SD	Range
Chest wall									
BICHER et al. (1986)	R	12	5	7	3 (35)	6 (86)	1.43	4.00 ± 4.11	0.25–63.95
EGAWA et al. (1989)	R	19	10	9	4 (40)	6 (67)	1.67	3.00 ± 2.60	0.46–19.59
GONZALES GONZALES (1988)	R	18	9	9	3 (33)	7 (78)	2.33	7.00 ± 2.91	0.86–56.90
KJELLEN et al. (1989)	R	44	22	22	6 (27)	15 (68)	2.50	5.71 ± 1.94	1.56–20.93
LI et al. (1985)	C	56	22	34	8 (36)	22 (65)	1.78	3.21 ± 1.77	1.05–9.81
PEREZ et al. (1989)	R	20	9	11	3 (33)	6 (55)	1.64	2.40 ± 2.54	0.39–14.88
PEREZ et al. (1990)	R	23	10	13	4 (40)	4 (31)	0.78	0.67 ± 2.42	0.12–3.76
SCOTT et al. (1984)	R	34	17	17	8 (47)	16 (94)	2.00	18.00 ± 3.13	1.93–168.0
VAN DER ZEE et al. (1988)	C	41	10	31	2 (20)	18 (58)	2.90	5.54 ± 2.39	1.01–30.50
		267	114	153	41 (36)	100 (65)	1.81	4.41 ± 1.41	2.25–8.62
Melanoma									
ARCANGELI et al. (1987)	R	38	17	21	9 (53)	16 (76)	1.43	2.84 ± 2.03	11.35–0.71
EMAMI et al. (1988)	C	121	77	44	16 (21)	29 (66)	3.17	7.37 ± 1.53	3.21–16.93
ESHO 3-85/OVERGAARD (1993)	R	123	62	61	18 (29)	27 (44)	1.52	1.94 ± 1.46	0.92–4.09
GONZALES GONZALES (1986)	C	46	8	38	3 (38)	19 (50)	1.33	1.67 ± 2.22	0.35–7.98
KIM et al. (1984)	R	108	63	45	26 (41)	31 (69)	1.67	3.15 ± 1.51	1.41–7.06
OVERGAARD et al. (1987)	R	99	56	43	28 (50)	29 (67)	1.35	2.07 ± 1.52	0.91–4.73
		535	283	252	100 (35)	151 (60)	1.71	2.46 ± 2.10	0.57–10.56
Head and neck									
ARCANGELI et al. (1985)	R	81	43	38	18 (42)	20 (53)	12.6	1.54 ± 1.57	0.64–3.72
DATTA et al. (1990)	R	52	24	28	3 (13)	11 (39)	3.14	4.53 ± 2.07	1.09–18.89
RTOG 81-04/PEREZ et al. (1990)	R	22	14	8	7 (50)	3 (38)	0.75	0.60 ± 2.47	0.10–3.54
SCOTT et al. (1984)	R	18	9	9	2 (22)	8 (89)	4.00	28.00 ± 3.78	2.07–379.2
VALDAGNI et al. (1988)	R	36	19	17	7 (37)	14 (82)	2.24	8.00 ± 2.21	1.69–37.95
		209	109	100	37 (34)	56 (56)	1.64	6.98 ± 1.65	2.60–18.71
Miscellaneous									
ARCANGELI et al. (1984)	C	163	74	89	28 (38)	66 (74)	1.96	4.71 ± 1.41	2.42–9.19
DUNLOP et al. (1986)	C	54	32	22	16 (50)	19 (86)	1.73	6.33 ± 2.04	1.56–25.71
HOWARD et al. (1987)	R	41	21	20	7 (33)	9 (45)	1.35	1.64 ± 1.91	0.46–5.80
LI et al. (1984)	C	124	31	93	9 (29)	50 (54)	1.85	2.84 ± 1.56	1.18–6.83
MYERSON et al. (1990)	C	53	19	34	4 (21)	21 (62)	2.93	6.06 ± 1.94	1.65–22.27
RTOG 81-04/PEREZ et al. (1990)	R	10	4	6	0 (0)	4 (67)	–	–	–
SCOTT et al. (1984)	R	62	31	31	12 (39)	27 (87)	2.25	1.92 ± 10.69	2.99–38.24
		507	212	295	76 (36)	196 (66)	1.83	4.86 ± 1.99	1.26–18.77
Overall total number		1518	718	800	254 (35)	503 (63)			

[a] Detailed references are given in: OVERGAARD (1989, 1993), PEREZ et al. (1992), and SEEGENSCHMIEDT et al. (1993)
[b] R = Randomized clinical trial, C = Controlled clinical trial
[c] Percentages are given in parentheses

to combined HT-RT, although histology and site are mutually associated in trials using superficial HT. Often tumor volume has been negatively correlated with response to combined HT-RT, but the volume effect is less pronounced than with the application of RT alone. It certainly depends on the technical ability of a given HT device to encompass the whole target volume with adequate power deposition. The development of optimized HT technology should allow the influence of volume to be reduced considerably.

1.5.5.2 Treatment Parameters

Clinical studies suggest that no limitation of the radiation dose is required when RT is combined with HT to avoid increased toxicity in normal

Table 1.7. Survey of types of prognostic parameters in HT-RT clinical trials with selected references

Type of prognostic parameter	Specific variable	Reference
1. *Factors associated with initial patient and tumor conditions:*		
Genetic Precondition	Positive family history	KAPP et al. (1991)
Initial tumor extension	Tumor stage	(overview)
Initial tumor control	Time to relapse, disease-free interval	KAPP et al. (1991)
Prior treatment	Adjuvant chemotherapy (breast cancer)	KAPP et al. (1991)
2. *Factors associated with actual patient and tumor conditions:*		
Patient's age	Menopausal status (breast cancer)	KAPP et al. (1991)
Performance status (Karnofsky)	KPS < 70 vs KPS > 70	(overview)
Presence of distant metastases	M1 vs M0	SEEGENSCHMIEDT et al. (1989)
Actual tumor size	Small vs large tumors	VALDAGNI et al. (1988)
3. *Factors associated with actual HT-RT treatment parameters:*		
Applicator characteristics	Effective field size Penetration depth: 25%/50% iso-SAR coverage	KAPP et al. (1988) CORRY et al. (1988) MYERSON et al. (1990)
Concurrent RT dose (prior RT exposure)	Low concurrent RT dose (<30 Gy) compared to high RT dose (>30 Gy)	VALDAGNI et al. (1988) (overview)
4. *Thermal parameters*	Thermal dose (equivalent min) Maximum, minimum, and mean tumor temperatures T_{20}, T_{50}, T_{90} percentiles EQ MIN T_{90} 43°C	VALDAGNI et al. (1988) LEOPOLD et al. (1989) ISSELS et al. (1991) FELDMANN et al. (1993) OLESON et al. (1993)
5. *Development of low-density areas (LDA)*	Low-density-areas of 80%–100% after treatment	TAKESHITA et al. (1993)
6. *Intrinsic and external conditions (tumor biology, physiology):*		
Tumor perfusion	CT contrast medium enhancement: blood perfusion pattern	MOLLS and FELDMANN (1991) FELDMANN et al. (1992)
Modification of blood flow	Application of vasoactive drugs: nitroprusside, dihydralazine, etc.	DEWHIRST et al. (1990b) PRESCOTT et al. (1992)
Metabolic status and regulation	Cellular parameters: glycolysis, cytogenetic activity, intra-/extracellular pH	VAUPEL et al. (1989) MOLLS et al. (1992)
Tumor oxygenation	Intra-/extracellular pO_2	FELDMANN et al. (1994)

tissues, while in tumor tissue, thermal enhancement can be achieved even with lower RT doses. With the exception of melanomas, no influence is observed for RT fraction size. With regard to timing and sequence of HT-RT, several studies indicate that maximum sensitization of tumor and normal tissue is observed when HT and RT are applied simultaneously – which is difficult to achieve in practice – and that if an interval is introduced between the modalities, thermal radiosensitization decreases more rapidly in normal tissues than in the tumor. An optimum number of HT fractions has not been established, and a large number of HT sessions may not be required, although this is disputed (OLESON et al. 1993; SAPOZINK 1986). Certainly treatment success is strongly related to the achieved thermal distribution in the tumor.

1.5.5.3 Thermal Parameters

Striking correlations of thermal parameters with tumor response (for minimum temperatures) and toxicity (for maximum temperatures) have been observed in many clinical studies. In the treatment of superficial tumors, initial and long-term responses often correlate with mean or minimum intratumoral temperatures. Recently, LEOPOLD et al. (1993) have shown that, in addition to histology, tumor volume, and RT dose, the cumulative minutes that the temperature achieved by 90% of the measured tumor sites (T_{90}) was ≥40°C correlated significantly with tumor response. In deep-seated tumors the correlation between thermal parameters and tumor response is much less evident due to the poor thermometric representation of the whole tumor volume. In these sites computed tomographic imaging has proved useful: TAKESHITA et al. (1993) found that development of low-density areas representing tumor necrosis after HT-RT treatment was closely correlated with the tumor response and also the achieved tumor temperatures. Similarly, LEOPOLD et al. (1992) found that histopathological changes after combined HT-RT correlated with tumor response and average $T_{50} \geq 41.5$°C. Other clinical researchers have confirmed these observations (ISSELS et al. 1990; OLESON et al. 1993). However, the applicability of any "thermal dose" formulas to the treatment of human tumors is still controversial and needs to be further validated by prospective clinical trials.

1.5.6 Practical Considerations

Relevant considerations in respect of the selection of treatment sites are summarized in Table 1.8. However, to enhance the clinical applicability of HT as an oncological treatment, other criteria also have to be fulfilled: (a) availability of an adequate HT device; (b) reliable heating performance of the available HT system; (c) clinical practicability; (d) consistent implementation of quality assurance measures, and (e) overall cost-effectiveness including calculations regarding manpower and time expenditure. In current HT practice, at least the first two criteria are insufficiently addressed. With regard to clinical practicability, routine clinical availability in oncological centers still needs to be established and requires the availability of several HT modalities and thermometry systems, a well-trained team, and interdisciplinary cooperation. Quality assurance has recently been well addressed by task force groups, and consensus reports have been published on the subject (DEWHIRST et al. 1990a; HAND et al. 1989). Research and public funding are still essential to support the ongoing developments until reimbursement has been established, but this also holds true for many other oncological and nononcological treatments that have already been "accepted" by the medical community.

Table 1.8. Selection of treatment sites for HT-RT: relevant considerations, treatment intent, and appropriate trial designs

Primary advanced tumors:
Tumor control is poor using conventional therapies (ralapse rate >20%–25%)
→ curative intent: prospective randomized trials recommended

Persistent primary tumors:
Tumors prone to regrowth after completion of conventional therapy
→ curative intent: prospective randomized trials recommended

Local recurrent tumors:
Retreatment of relapses after full-dose RT or RT–CT regimens
→ palliative intent: controlled trial design recommended

Local metastatic tumors:
Inoperable lesions in patients with good physical condition
→ palliative intent: controlled trial design recommended

Residual microscopic disease:
→ curative intent: prospective randomized trials recommended

1.6 Future Perspectives

Biological and physiological arguments for HT-RT are strong, but clinical realization is hampered by intrinsic physical difficulties and insufficiently developed techniques for applying heat consistently and effectively. Nevertheless, HT-RT has gained some importance in clinical oncology, although it still needs to be integrated in multidisciplinary oncological treatment concepts.

Presently, HT is only indicated clinically as second-line therapy. In respect of *palliation*, HT has helped to boost treatment outcome far beyond what could have been expected with conventional therapies. On the other hand, it is still too early to draw a final conclusion as to what extent HT may be integrated into *adjuvant* treatments for malignant diseases that are poorly managed with "classical" oncological tools. The further development of HT technology is essential to improve clinical applications and results, especially for deep-seated tumors. Certainly, much more basic research and clinical work deserves to be performed on the combined effects of HT, RT, and chemotherapy. Improved heating performance may be achieved by using drugs to modulate physiological parameters, but so far this approach has not been fully developed and clinically tested. Consistently applied quality assurance of technical and clinical performance in controlled multicenter trials will help to boost the credibility of HT-RT.

1.7 Summary

- Hyperthermia is used to induce effective thermal radiosensitization in malignant tumors, which can be of special value in the treatment of advanced, persistent, and recurrent tumors, and when standard oncological treatments fail to yield satisfactory results.
- Major biological and physiological justifications for thermoradiotherapy and important technical aspects of HT and their impact on various clinical applications are outlined.
- Superficial HT techniques are relatively simple to apply and have contributed to satisfactory practice and reasonable clinical results. Interstitial, intracavitary, and endoluminal HT techniques have great potential, as they are well-advanced techniques applied to tumor volumes which are usually well confined. In the treatment of deep-seated malignancies, HT technology and clinical handling lag behind the required needs.
- Presently, clinical use of HT is established for *palliative care* of patients with a poor prognosis. Although most studies have been performed with suboptimal HT techniques and insufficient treatment control, the clinical results have been encouraging.
- An overview of well-designed controlled (randomized) trials in different body sites (breast and chest wall, superficial sites, melanomas, and head and neck tumors) reveals advantages of combined HT-RT over RT alone in the treatment of these tumors.
- Clinical use of HT depends on improved technologies to achieve homogeneous HT of any desired volume. Controlled clinical studies are needed to confirm the initial encouraging results and to define the role of HT in adjuvant treatments with a *curative intent*.

References

Acker JC, Dewhirst MW, Honore GM, Samulski TV, Tucker JA, Oleson JR (1990) Blood perfusion measurements in human tumors: evaluation of laser doppler methods. Int J Hyperthermia 6: 287–304

Beaney RP, Lammertsma AA, Jones T, McKenzie CG, Halnan KE (1984) Positron emission tomography for invivo measurement of regional blood flow, oxygen utilisation, and blood volume in patients with breast carcinoma. Lancet 1: 131–134

Ben-Hur E, Elkind MM, Bronk BV (1974) Thermally enhanced radioresponse of cultured Chinese hamster cells: inhibition of repair of sublethal damage and enhancement of lethal damage. Radiat Res 58: 38–51

Berger H, Markl G, Issels RD, Lissner J (1988) Percutaneous placement of catheters for temperature measurement during hyperthermia. Recent Results Cancer Res 107: 263–266

Corry PM, Jabboury K, Kong JS, Armour EP, McCraw FJ, LeDuc T (1988) Evaluation of equipment for hyperthermia treatment of cancer. Int J Hyperthermia 4: 53–74

De Leeuw AAC, Lagendijk JJW (1987) Design of a clinical deep-body hyperthermia system based on the coaxial TEM applicator. Int J Hyperthermia 3: 413–421

Dewhirst MW, Phillips TL, Samulski TV, et al. (1990a) RTOG quality assurance guidelines for clinical trials using hyperthermia. Int J Radiat Oncol Biol Phys 18: 1249–1259

Dewhirst MW, Prescott DM, Clegg S, et al. (1990b) The use of hydralazine to manipulate tumor temperatures during hyperthermia. Int J Hyperthermia 6: 971–983

Emami B, Myerson RJ, Cardenes H, et al. (1992) Combined hyperthermia and irradiation in the treatment of superficial tumors: results of a prospective randomized trial of hyperthermia fractionation (1/wk vs. 2/wk). Int J Radiat Oncol Biol Phys 24: 145–152

Feldmann HJ, Molls M, Höderath A, Krümpelmann S, Sack H (1992) Blood flow and steady state temperatures in deep seated tumors and normal tissues. Int J Radiat Oncol Biol Phys 23: 1003–1008

Feldmann HJ, Molls M, Heinemann HG, Romanowski R, Stuschke M, Sack H (1993a) Thermoradiotherapy in locally advanced deep seated tumors – thermal parameters and treatment results. Radiother Oncol 26: 38–44

Feldmann HJ, Höderath A, Molls M, Sack H (1993b) Problems with CT guided catheter insertions. Int J Hyperthermia 9: 219–225

Feldmann HJ, Molls M, Füller J, Stüben G, Sack H (1994) Changes in oxygenation patterns of locally advanced recurrent tumors under thermoradiotherapy. In: Vaupel P, Zander R, Bruley DF (eds) Oxygen transport to tissue, vol XV. Plenum Press, New York, pp 479–483

Feldmann HJ, Seegenschmiedt MH, Molls M (1995) Hyperthermia – its actual role in radiation oncology. III. Clinical rationale and results in deep seated tumors. Strahlenther Onkol 171: 251–264
Gautherie M (ed) (1990) Methods of external hyperthermic heating. Clinical Thermology Series, Springer, Berlin Heidelberg New York
Gerner EW, Cetas TC (eds) (1993) Hyperthermic oncology 1992, vol 2. Plenary and symposia lectures. Arizona Board of Regents, Tucson, Az
Gerner EW, Leith JT, Boone MLM (1976) Mammalian cell survival response following irradiation with 4 MV X-rays or accelerated helium ions combined with hyperthermia. Radiology 119: 715–720
Gibbs FA, Stewart JR (1985) Regional hyperthermia in the treatment of cancer: a review. Cancer Invest 3: 445–452
Hahn G (1993) Biological rationale for new clinical trials. In: Gerner EW, Cetas TC (eds) Hyperthermic oncology 1992, vol 2. Plenary and symposia lectures. Arizona Board of Regents, Tucson, Az, pp 79–81
Hall EJ (ed) (1988) Hyperthermia. In: Hall EJ (ed) Radiobiology for the Radiologist, 3rd edn. Lippincott, Philadelphia, pp 293–329
Hand JW, Lagendijk JJW, Bach Andersen J, Bolomey JC (1989) Quality assurance guidelines for ESHO protocols. Int J Hyperthermia 5: 421–428
Hiraoka M, Jo S, Takahashi M, Abe M (1985) Effectiveness of RF capacitive heating in the heating of human deep-seated tumors. In: Abe M, Takahashi M, Sugahara T (eds) Hyperthermia in cancer therapy. Mag Bros, Tokyo, pp 98–99
Issels RD, Prenninger SW, Nagele A, et al. (1990) Ifosfamide plus etoposide combined with regional hyperthermia in patients with locally advanced sarcomas: a phase II study: J Clin Oncol 8: 1818–1829
Issels RD, Mittermüller J, Gerl A, et al. (1991) Improvement of local control by regional hyperthermia combined with systemic chemotherapy (ifosfamide plus etoposide) in advanced sarcomas: updated report on 65 patients. J Cancer Res Clin Oncol 117 (Suppl. IV), pp 141–S147
Ito M, Lammertsma AA, Wise RJS, et al. (1982) Measurement of regional cerebral blood flow and oxygen utilisation in patients with cerebral tumors using ^{15}O and positron emission tomography: analytical techniques and preliminary results. Neuroradiology 23: 63–74
Jirtle RL (1988) Chemical modifications of tumor blood flow. Int J Hyperthermia 4: 355–371
Kapp DS (1986) Site and disease selection for hyperthermia clinical trials. Int J Hyperthermia 2: 139–156
Kapp DS, Fessenden P, Samulski TV, et al. (1988) Stanford University institutional report. Phase I evaluation of equipment for hyperthermia treatment of cancer. Int J Hyperthermia 4: 75–115
Kapp DS, Petersen IA, Cox RS (1990) Two or six hyperthermia treatments as an adjunct to radiation therapy yield similar tumor responses: results of a randomized trial. Int J Radiat Oncol Biol Phys 19: 1481–1495
Kapp DS, Cox RS, Barnett TA, Lee ER, Lohrbach A, Fessenden P (1991) Hyperthermia and radiation therapy of local-regional recurrent breast cancer: prognostic factors for response and local control of diffuse or nodular tumors. Int J Radiat Oncol Biol Phys 20: 1147–1164
Kato H, Hiraoka M, Nakajima T, Ishida T (1985) Deep-heating characteristics of an RF capacitive heating device. Int J Hyperthermia 1: 15–28
Koga S, Maeta M, Shimizu N, et al. (1985) Clinical effects of total-body hyperthermia combined with anticancer chemotherapy for far-advanced gastrointestinal cancer. Cancer 55: 1641–1647
Lagendijk JJW (1982) The influence of blood flow in large vessels on the temperature distribution. Phys Med Biol 27: 17–23
Lagendijk JJW, Schellekens M, Schipper J, van den Linden PM (1984) A three dimensional description of heating patterns in vascularised tissues during hyperthermic treatment. Phys Med Biol 29: 495–507
Lagendijk JJW, Hofman P, Schipper J (1988) Perfusion analyses in advanced breast carcinoma during hyperthermia. Int Hyperthermia 5: 479–495
Lahtinen T, Karjalainen P, Alhava M (1979) Measurement of bone blood flow with a ^{133}Xe washout method. Eur J Nucl Med 4: 435–439
Lammertsma AA, Wise RJS, Cox TCS, Thomas GT, Jones T (1985) Measurement of blood flow, oxygen utilisation, oxygen extraction ratio, and fractional blood volume in human brain tumors and surrounding oedematous tissue. Br J Radiol 58: 725–734
Lilly MB, Katholi CR, Ng TC (1985) Direct relationship between high-energy phosphate content and blood flow in thermally treated murine tumors. J Natl Cancer Inst 75: 885–889
Leopold KA, Harrelson J, Prosnitz L, Samulski TV, Dewhirst MW, Oleson JR (1989) Preoperative hyperthermia and radiation for soft tissue sarcomas: advantage of two vs one hyperthermia treatments per week. Int J Radiat Oncol Biol Phys 16: 107–115
Leopold KA, Dewhirst M, Samulski TV, et al. (1992) Relationships among tumor temperature, treatment time, and histopathological outcome using preoperative hyperthermia with radiation in soft tissue sarcomas. Int J Radiat Oncol Biol Phys 22: 989–998
Leopold KA, Dewhirst M, Samulski TV, et al. (1993) Cumulative minutes with T90 greater than $Temp_{index}$ is predictive of response of superficial malignancies to hyperthermia and radiation. Int J Radiat Oncol Biol Phys 25: 841–847
Mäntyla MJ (1979) Regional blood flow in human tumors. Cancer Res 39: 2304–2306
Mäntyla MJ, Heikkonen J, Licphil M, Perkkiö J (1988) Regional blood flow in human tumors measured with argon, krypton and xenon. Br J Radiol 61: 379–382
Milligan AJ, Conran PB, Ropar MA, McCulloch HA, Ahuja RK, Dobelbower RR (1983) Predictions of blood flow from thermal clearance during regional hyperthermia. Int J Radiat Oncol Biol Phys 9: 1335–1343
Molls M, Feldmann HJ (1991) Clinical investigations on blood flow in malignant tumors of the pelvis and abdomen. In: Vaupel P, Jain RK (eds) Tumor blood flow supply and metabolic microenvironment: characterization and implications for therapy. Funktionsanalyse biologischer Systeme 20. Fischer, Stuttgart, pp 143–153
Molls M, Feldmann HJ, Streffer C (1992) Physiological, glycolytic and cytogenetic parameters as predictors for heat treatment. In: Dewey WC, Edington M, Fry RJM, Hall EJ, Whitmore GF (eds) Radiation research – a twentieth-century perspective, vol II. Academic Press, San Diego, pp 946–950
Müller RD, Feldmann HJ, Molls M, John V, Stuschke M (1988) Computertomographisch gesteuerte positionierung von Kathetern zur temperaturmessung bei

der Hyperthermie maligner Tumoren. Strahlenther Onkol 164: 593–601
Myerson RJ, Perez CA, Emami BN, Straube W, Kuske RR, Leybovich L (1990) Tumor control in long-term survivors following superficial hyperthermia. Int J Radiat Oncol Biol Phys 18: 1123–1129
Myerson RJ, Leybovich L, Emami BN, Grigsby PW, Straube W, von Gerichten D (1991) Phantom studies and preliminary clinical experience with the BSD 2000. Int J Hyperthermia 7: 937–951
Myerson RJ, Emami B, Perez CA, Straube W, Leybovich L, von Gerichten D (1992) Equilibrium temperature distributions in uniform phantoms for superficial microwave applicator: implications for temperature-based standards of applicator adequacy. Int J Hyperthermia 8: 11–21
Nielsen OS, Munro AJ, Warde PR (1992) Assessment of palliative response in hyperthermia. Int J Hyperthermia 8: 11–21
Nyström C, Forssman L, Roos B (1969) Myometrial blood flow studies in carcinoma of the corpus uteri. Acta Radiol Ther 8: 193–198
Oleson JR, Cetas TC (1982) Clinical hyperthermia with RF currents. In: Nussbaum GH (ed) Physical aspects of hyperthermia. American Institute of Physics, New York, pp 280–306
Oleson JR, Sim DA, Manning MR (1984) Analysis of prognostic variables in hyperthermia treatment of 161 patients. Int J Radiat Oncol Biol Phys 10: 2231–2239
Oleson JR, Sim DA, Conrad J, Fletcher AM, Gross EJ (1986) Results of a phase I regional hyperthermia device evaluation: microwave annular array versus radiofrequency induction coil. Int J Hyperthermia 2: 327–336
Oleson JR, Calderwood SR, Coughlin CT, Dewhirst MW, Gerweck LE, Gibbs FA, Kapp DS (1988) Biological and clinical aspects of hyperthermia in cancer therapy. Am J Clin Oncol 11: 368–380
Oleson JR, Samulski TV, Leopold KA, Clegg ST, Dewhirst MW, Dodge RK, George SL (1993) Sensitivity of hyperthermia trial outcomes to temperature and time: implications for thermal goals of treatment. Int J Radiat Oncol Biol Phys 25: 289–297
Okunieff P, Pardo F (1993) ^{31}P-NMR studies of hyperthermia and comparisons with radiation and other nonsurgical therapies. In: Gerner EW, Cetas TC (eds) Hyperthermic oncology 1992, vol 2. Plenary and symposia lectures. Arizona Board of Regents, Tucson, Az, pp 153–156
Overgaard J (1989) The current and potential role for hyperthermia in radiotherapy. Int J Radiat Oncol Biol Phys 16: 535–549
Overgaard J (1993) The future of hyperthermic oncology. In: Gerner EW, Cetas TC (eds) Hyperthermic oncology 1992, vol 2. Plenary and symposia lectures. Arizona Board of Regents Tucson, Az, pp 87–92
Perez CA, Pajak T, Emami B, Hornback NB, Tupchong L, Rubin P (1991) Randomized phase III study comparing irradiation and hyperthermia with irradiation alone in superficial measurable tumors. Am J Clin Oncol 14: 133–141
Perez CA, Emami B, Myerson RJ, Roti JL (1992) Hyperthermia. In: Perez CA, Brady LW (eds) Principles and practice of radiation oncology, 2nd edn. Lippincott Philadelphia, pp 396–446
Petrovich Z, Langholz B, Gibbs FA, et al. (1989) Regional hyperthermia for advanced tumors: a clinical study of 353 patients. Int J Radiat Oncol Biol Phys 16: 601–607
Piroth HD, Brinkmann G (1988) CT-guided placement of temperature probes in pulmonary cancer. Recent Results Cancer Res 107: 267–271
Prescott DM, Samulski TV, Dewhirst MW, Page RL, Thrall DE, Dodge RK, Oleson JR (1992) Use of nitroprusside to increase tissue temperatures during local hyperthermia in normal and tumor-bearing dogs. Int J Radiat Oncol Biol Phys 23: 377–385
Reinhold HS, Endrich B (1986) Tumour microcirculation as a target for hyperthermia. Int J Hyperthermia 2: 117–137
Roemer RB (1991) Optimal power deposition in hyperthermia. I. The treatment goal: the ideal temperature distribution: the role of large blood vessels. Int J Hyperthermia 7: 317–341
Rubin P, Carter SR (1976) Combination radiation therapy and chemotherapy: a logical basis for their clinical use. CA Cancer J Clin 26: 274–292
Samulski TV, Fessenden P, Valdagni R, Kapp DS (1987) Correlations of thermal washout rate, steady state temperatures, and tissue type in deep seated recurrent or metastatic tumors. Int Radiat Oncol Biol Phys 13: 907–916
Sapareto SA, Dewey WC (1984) Thermal dose determination in cancer therapy. Int J Radiat Oncol Biol Phys 10: 787–800
Sapozink MD (1986) The application of thermal dose in clinical trials. Int J Hyperthermia 2: 157–164
Sapozink MD, Gibbs FA, Gates KS, Stewart JR (1984) Regional hyperthermia in the treatment of clinically advanced deep seated malignancy: results of a pilot study employing an annular array applicator. Int J Radiat Oncol Biol Phys 10: 775–786
Seegenschmiedt MH, Sauer R (1992) The current role of interstitial thermoradiotherapy. Strahlenther Onkol 168: 119–140
Seegenschmiedt MH, Sauer R (eds) (1993) Interstitial and intracavitary thermoradiotherapy. Medical Radiology Series, Diagnostic Imaging and Radiation Oncology. Springer, Berlin Heidelberg New York
Seegenschmiedt MH, Karlsson UL, Sauer R, et al. (1989) Superficial chestwall recurrences of breast cancer: prognostic treatment factors for combined radiation therapy and hyperthermia. Radiology 173: 551–558
Seegenschmiedt MH, Feldmann HJ, Molls M (1993) Hyperthermia – its actual role in radiation oncology. II. Clinical fundamentals and results in superficial tumors. Strahlenther Onkol 169: 635–654
Seegenschmiedt MH, Martus P, Vernon CC (1994) Can hyperthermia improve cancer therapy? I. rationale and techniques. Curr Oncol 1: 34–39
Sijens PE, Bovee WM, Koole P, Schipper J (1989) Phosphorous NMR study of the response of a murine tumor to hyperthermia as a function of treatment time and temperature. Int J Hyperthermia 5: 351–357
Song CW (1984) Effect of local hyperthermia on blood flow and microenvironment. Cancer Res (suppl) 44: 4721s–4730s
Song CW (1993) Effect of hyperthermia on the blood flow in tumors and normal tissues and vascular adapation to repeated heating. In: Gerner EW, Cetas TC

(eds) Hyperthermic oncology 1992, vol 2. Plenary and symposia lectures. Arizona Board of Regents, Tucson, Az, pp 87–92

Streffer C (1985) Review: metabolic changes during and after hyperthermia. Int J Hyperthermia 1: 305–319

Streffer C, van Beuningen D (1987) The biological basis for tumor therapy by hyperthermia and radiation. In: Streffer C (ed) Hyperthermia and the therapy of malignant tumors. Springer, Berlin Heidelberg New York, pp 24–70

Streffer C, van Beuningen D, Bertholdt G, Zamboglou N (1983) Some aspects of radiosensitization by hyperthermia: neutrons and X-rays. In: Kato E (ed) Fundamentals of cancer therapy by hyperthermia, radiation and chemicals. Mag Bros, Tokyo, pp 121–134

Suit HD (1982) Potential for improving survival rates for the cancer patient by increasing the efficacy of treatment of the primary lesion. Cancer 50: 1227–1234

Suit HD, Westgate SJ (1986) Impact of improved local tumor control on survival. Int J Radiat Oncol Biol Phys 12: 453–458

Takeshita N, Tanaka Y, Matsuda T (1993) Evaluation of CT images, tumor response and prognosis after thermoradiotherapy for deep seated tumors. Int J Hyperthermia 9: 1–17

Turner PF (1984a) Hyperthermia and inhomogeneous tissue effect using an annular phased array. IEEE Trans Microwave Theory Tech 34: 1131–1139

Turner PF (1984b) Regional hyperthermia with an annular phased array. IEEE Trans Biomed Eng 31: 106–114

Turner PF, Schaefermeyer T (1989) The BSD 2000 approach for deep local and regional hyperthermia: clinical utility. Strahlenther Onkol 165: 700–704

Valdagni R, Lui EF, Kapp DS (1988) Important prognostic factors influencing outcome of combined radiation and hyperthermia. Int J Radiat Oncol Biol Phys 15: 959–972

van den Berg AP, Wike-Hooley JL, Broekmeyer-Reurink MP, van der Zee J, Reinhold HS (1989) The relationship between the unmodified initial tissue pH of human tumours and the response to combined radiotherapy and local hyperthermia treatment. Eur J Cancer Clin Oncol 25: 73–78

van der Zee J, Veeze-Kuijpers B, Wiggers T, van der Merwe SA, Treurniet-Donker AD (1992) Risk of tumour growth along thermometry catheter track: a case report. Int J Hyperthermia 8: 625–629

Vaupel P, Jain RK (eds) (1991) Tumor blood flow supply and metabolic environment – characterization and implication for therapy. Fischer, Stuttgart, pp 123–141

Vaupel P, Kallinowski F, Okunieff P (1989) Blood flow, oxygen and nutrient supply, and metabolic microenvironment of human tumors: a review. Cancer Res 49: 6449–6465

Vaupel P, Okunieff P, Neuringer LJ (1990) In vivo ^{31}P-NMP spectroscopy of murine tumors before and after localized hyperthermia. Int J Hyperthermia 6: 15–31

Waterman FM, Nerlinger RE, Moylan III DJ, Leeper DB (1987) Response of human tumor blood flow to local hyperthermia. Int J Radiat Oncol Biol Phys 13: 75–82

Westra A, Dewey WC (1971) Heat shock during the cell cycle of Chinese hamster cells in vitro. Int J Radiat Biol 19: 467–477

World Health Organization (1979) Handbook for reporting results of cancer treatment. World Health Organization, Geneva

2 Clinical Rationale for Thermochemotherapy

R.D. Issels

CONTENTS

2.1 Introduction

In general, locally advanced malignant tumors present a dual management problem: local control and prevention of distant metastases. In most cases, no curative treatment can be offered to patients with distant metastases already present at the time of first presentation (diagnosis). For improvement of local control interdisciplinary treatment strategies have been more recently employed using preoperative radiation and/or chemotherapy followed by appropriate radical surgery. The concept of neoadjuvant (preoperative) chemotherapy targets the elimination of distant microscopic disease which is not detectable with common diagnostic procedures but is assumed to be present a priori due to several high risk factors (e.g., tumor size, tumor grade, mitotic activity).

Major approaches to enhance the therapeutic effectiveness of chemotherapy include: (a) the application of alternated cycles of multidrug combined regimens, (b) increasing the conventional dose and dose intensity by the use of growth factors (e.g., G-CSF, GM-CSF), and (c) the use of high-dose chemotherapy followed by transplantation of autologous bone marrow or by transplantation of peripheral blood progenitor cells separated from the individual patient before starting ablative chemotherapy.

The results of extensive research into the biology of malignant tumors show that intrinsic drug resistance of tumor cells dependent upon environmental conditions (e.g., hypoxia) and acquired multidrug resistance (MDR) after repeated exposure to MDR-inducing cytotoxic agents are biological limitations which might explain the low rate and short duration of clinical responses often seen with conventional chemotherapy alone in the majority of malignant solid tumors. Whether or not the above-mentioned dose-intensifying concepts will overcome such drug resistance of tumors is an open question.

Another approach to synergistically enhance the efficacy of chemotherapeutic agents is their simultaneous clinical application with hyperthermia (thermochemotherapy). Beside direct cytotoxicity (>42.5°C), hyperthermia causes thermal enhancement even at moderate temperatures (range of 40°–44°C), which leads to an increased kill of tumor cells by chemotherapeutic agents if one compares their effect at 37°C alone.

The concept of thermochemotherapy and its clinical rationale in solid tumors will be addressed using soft tissue sarcomas as an example for such a clinical strategy. In the last decade the current standard of either limb-sparing surgery plus radiation therapy or radical resection (often amputation) has largely improved local control rates. However, the anatomical location and invasiveness of sarcomas often prevent resection with adequate margins, and toxicity of radiotherapy limits the use of potentially curative doses. In addition, patients with large, high-grade sarcomas are at high-risk for recurrent local disease and

R.D. Issels, MD, PhD, GSF-Institut für Klinische Hämatologie, Marchioninistraße 25, D-81377 München, FRG, and Medizinische Klinik III, Klinikum Großhadern, Marchioninistraße 15, D-81377 München, FRG

development of distant metastases. Despite multimodality management for the disease, currently 40%–60% of patients die within 5 years. In cases of complete resection, adjuvant chemotherapy intended to eradicate occult micrometastatic disease already present at diagnosis has not been shown to benefit patients in terms of overall survival. The rationale for the simultaneous application of hyperthermia and chemotherapy in sarcomas rests on the assumption that heat exposure (40°–44°C) will increase tumor-cell kill by direct thermal cytotoxicity (>42.4°C) and/or thermal chemosensitization (40°–44°C) within different areas of the same tumor depending on blood perfusion. The consequence of use of such combined therapy should be better functional and cosmetic results at comparable or higher local control rates than are achieved by standard treatment procedures. In addition, the simultaneous systemic effect of thermochemotherapy should lead to an improvement in the overall survival by controlling distant microscopic disease.

In this chapter, based upon clinical results of chemotherapy alone in soft tissue sarcoma, the most active single agents will be defined and preclinical data on their potential for use in thermochemotherapy will be given. Then, different heating techniques used for the application of thermochemotherapy in sarcomas will be discussed, with an overview of the clinical data of several institutions.

2.2 Preclinical Aspects

2.2.1 General Considerations

Hyperthermia (temperature range 40°–44°C) shows supra-additive interactions with selected chemotherapeutic drugs or causes toxicity of compounds that are nontoxic at 37°C (thermosensitizer). Excellent reviews of the interactions of hyperthermia with a wide range of drugs (e.g., doxorubicin, bleomycin, cisplatin, nitrosoureas, cyclophosphamide) in models employing cells in tissue culture and animal tumors have been presented by Hahn (1982), Marmor (1979), Engelhardt (1987), and Dahl (1988) and the phenomenon of thermal enhancement dependent upon timing or sequencing is well documented. In most of the preclinical studies the classification of the type of interaction (e.g., additive, synergistic or supra-additive) is based upon a phenomenological analysis of the data obtained. The term "additive" for the increased effect is used but might being simply the product of the lethal effect of the separate agents. To describe effects in which the continued application (e.g., heat and drug) have been shown to be better than this product the terms such as supra-additive, synergistic, and enhanced are appropriate. However there are serious conceptual problems in demonstrating greater-than-additive effects whenever dose-response curves are nonlinear (Steel et al. 1979). Maximal effects have been found when the chemotherapeutic agents are scheduled simultaneously with hyperthermia either in vitro (end-point: clonogenic cell survival) or in vivo (endpoint: tumor growth delay). In tissue culture studies, hyperthermia has also been demonstrated to enhance drug cytotoxicity in cell lines rendered resistant to individual drugs including doxorubicin (Wallner and Li 1986; Bates and Mackillop 1986), cisplatin (Wallner et al. 1986), and mitomycin C (Wallner et al. 1987).

2.2.2 Doxorubicin

In vitro studies with CHO cells have shown thermal enhancement of the response to doxorubicin only at temperatures above 42.0°–43°C and heat exposure durations shorter than 30 min (Hahn and Strande 1976). In rat cells, at 41°C synergism with doxorubicin was present for exposure durations shorter than 1 h, but at 42°C synergism persisted even for 2-h heat treatments (Dahl 1982). More generally, such differences might reflect the heterogeneity in the intrinsic thermochemosensitivity of different cell lines. In vitro thermochemosensitivity screening of human tumors has been reported more recently by Calabro et al. (1989). Hyperthermia alone for 2 h at 42.5°C but not at 40.5°C decreased the in vitro growth of 83% (15/18) of all tumors, including the six biopsy specimens obtained from human sarcomas, at a maximum of heat exposure (120 min). Doxorubicin plus heat was synergistic in only 15% of heat-drug combinations that were randomly distributed among the tumors; i.e., no specific pattern was evident for either temperature level or exposure time. Development of heat-doxorubicin antagonism occurred with longer hyperthermic exposure. In contrast, Akiyoshi et al. (1989) reported a much higher rate (31%) of synergistic interaction in biopsies of 13 human tumors treated with 42°C hyperthermia plus doxorubicin at three different doses.

Although the aforementioned data cannot be extrapolated to clinical practice without considering the possible influence of the in vivo effects of hyperthermia, in vitro thermochemosensitivity screening of human tumors may assist in the selection of appropriate chemotherapeutic agents, including doxorubicin, prior to the clinical application of combined treatment regimens including hyperthermia.

2.2.3 Ifosfamide

The ability of hyperthermia to increase the sensitivity of human-derived tumor xenografts in nude mice to ifosfamide was extensively investigated by Wiedemann et al. (1992). Both ifosfamide and cyclophosphamide alone caused only a transient growth delay of the xenografted tumors comparable with the effect of hyperthermia (43°C, 1 h), while the combination of the same dose of the chemotherapeutic agents with heat resulted in complete remissions ($P = 0.001$). Moreover, the authors could demonstrate that tumor oxygenation was improved, not decreased, during hyperthermia, most likely due to an increase in tumor blood flow. An extension of this study using human sarcoma xenografts has recently been reported by the same authors (Wiedemann et al. 1993). The results for ifosfamide at different doses showed a strong *synergistic effect* with hyperthermia at clinically relevant temperatures (40°–43°C) using tumor-free survival of treated mice as the endpoint for the analysis. These in vitro data confirm previous results on the enhancement of ifosfamide toxicity at mild (41°C) temperature elevations (Voth et al. 1988).

2.2.4 Cisplatin

Hyperthermia has been shown to increase the cellular uptake of cisplatin (Alberts et al. 1980), the amount of DNA cross-linking (Mean et al. 1980) and the cytotoxic actions of cisplatin (Douple et al. 1982; Herman et al. 1982). More recent results on pharmacokinetics and toxicity also provide a rationale for hyperthermic enhancement of cisplatin effects in vivo (Zakris et al. 1987).

2.2.5 Etoposide

Although the drug etoposide (VP-16, epipodophyllotoxin) had been previously shown to have only minor activity against sarcomas, its combination with alkylating agents was found to result in synergistic effects (Miser et al. 1987). A positive effect has been observed in vitro for etoposide combined with heat exposure (Ikegami et al. 1988), and a preclinical in vivo study has shown the potential of etoposide to increase the effectiveness of cisplatin under hyperthermia conditions (Pfeffer et al. 1989).

In conclusion, there is substantial evidence from preclinical data that the antitumoral cytotoxicity of chemotherapeutic agents can be enhanced by combining them with appropriate heat exposure to cells or the tumor tissue (Table 2.1).

2.3 Systemic Thermochemotherapy

As most cancers refractory to conventional therapy are systemic diseases, the proposal that *whole-body hyperthermia (WBH) in combination with systemic chemotherapy* be used to treat metastatic disease is an inherently attractive approach. Several different physical techniques have been utilized for the induction of WBH. One technique involves the placement of an arteriovenous shunt and heating of the shunted blood through a countercurrent heat exchanger (Parks 1982). The most common techniques induce WBH by transfer of heat through the skin surface (Robins et al. 1985). The temperature distributions that develop during WBH are presumably more uniform than those that can be achieved with locoregional heating, although they are limited to a maximum of 41.8°–42°C. A recent detailed study on the temperature distributions in dogs undergoing WBH

Table 2.1. Rationales and different approaches for thermochemotherapy

- Systemic Chemotherapy combined with Whole Body Hyperthermia (WBH)
  - for metastatic disease
- Isolated Hyperthermic Antiblastic Perfusion (HAP)
  - for regional advanced disease of extremities (e.g. melanoma, soft tissue sarcoma)
- Systemic Chemotherapy combined with Regional Hyperthermia (RHT)
  - for local advanced tumors at different sites (e.g. pelvic, abdomen, extremities)

procedures has verified this general conclusion (THRALL et al. 1986). Importantly, and depending upon the method used, the several monitored internal temperatures (e.g., tumor, nasal, esophageal, bladder, rectal) can be less than the maximum by 1°C or more. The measured intratumoral temperatures were found to be statistically lower ($P = 0.0028$) and more variable than rectal temperature during the plateau phase of WBH (THRALL et al. 1990). From clinical experience, systems for WBH have warm-up times (time to reach the body target temperature of 41.8°C) of about 1–2h, and this period may induce the phenomenon of thermotolerance in tumors, as has been shown experimentally (MEYER et al. 1985). The physiological and metabolic stresses of WBH have been described in detail (PAGE et al. 1987) and recent improvements in anesthetic management have resulted in less severe direct complications of this therapy (CRONAU et al. 1984).

Rather limited information is currently available on the antitumor effects of WBH combined with chemotherapy. This is largely because the majority of the studies published have been phase I studies (ROBINS 1984). Only limited information has been provided on the effects of systemic thermochemotherapy for sarcomas. An objective response rate of 36% in 11 patients with soft tissue sarcomas was observed when doxorubicin (45 mg/m^2) was administered at the beginning of WBH (41.8°–43.0°C for 2h) followed by cyclophosphamide (1000 mg/m^2) after 6h and courses repeated 4-weekly (GERAD et al. 1984). Beside the two non-responding patients with mesothelioma, it is of note that three of three patients [one complete response (CR)/two partial responses (PRs)] with liposarcoma and one of two patients with leiomyosarcoma (one CR) showed objective responses. However, the observed response rate for these patients who had not received prior chemotherapy is similar to that which one might expect from chemotherapy alone. The authors also reported that the mean leukocyte nadir of patients receiving systemic thermochemotherapy was not significantly different from that of patients treated subsequently with chemotherapy alone. This is in contrast with the results reported by ENGELHARDT et al. (1986), who observed a significant increase ($P = 0.044$) of bone marrow toxicity with the addition of WBH to systemic chemotherapy (doxorubicin, cyclophosphamide, and vincristine) in a small randomized study of small cell lung cancer.

At the University of Texas, Jabboury and colleagues (1985) treated 17 patients with metastatic soft tissue sarcomas and osteosarcomas who had previously failed surgery, radiotherapy, and prior chemotherapy regimens. WBH (41.8°–42.0°C for 2h) was given for a median of three treatments at 6- to 8-week intervals plus BCNU chemotherapy. Tumor response was seen in four patients (one CR/three PRs), but duration of response was only 4 months.

More recently the potential positive interaction between interferon (IFN) and hyperthermia has been clinically tested by Robins et al. at the Wisconsin Clinical Cancer Center (ROBINS et al. 1989). The results of the phase I trial using WBH (40.5°C for 75 min) combined with escalated doses of IFN (maximum 10×10^6 units/m^2) in advanced cancer patients including five with sarcomas showed no statistically significant difference in toxicity or biological response modulation (e.g., natural killer cell cytotoxicity) between IFN alone and combined modality therapy. Two patients refractory to conventional treatments showed an objective response (two PRs) and three other patients (including two with leiomyosarcomas) showed long-lasting stable disease. Prior preclinical data demonstrating the thermal enhancement of the antiproliferative effects of IFN (GROVEMAN et al. 1984) together with the clinical safety reported in this phase I study encourage further investigations.

First experience with the combination of WBH and chemotherapy used for refractory cases of malignant tumors in 17 children (including five with sarcomas) has been reported by WILLNOW et al. (1989). WBH (41.8°–42.0°C for 2–3h) was induced by extracorporeal blood warming. Vincristine (1.5 mg/m^2) and actinomycin D (0.4 mg/m^2) was given during WBH while cyclophosphamide (600–800 mg/m^2) was applied 1h before starting the WBH procedure. Objective regression of metastatic disease was found in 6 of 12 evaluable cases (one CR/five PRs). Observed systemic toxicity was severe in two children in whom body temperature exceeded 42°C (42.3°–42.7°C). One of the two children died within 48h after the WBH procedure (irreversible cardiac arrest). The authors also noted acute cardiotoxicity in the first two children receiving doxorubicin (20 mg/m^2) plus WBH.

A multi-institutional trial in Japan for the clinical evaluation of WBH using an extracorporeal circuit combined with chemotherapy (cisplatin, doxorubicin, mitomycin C) for advanced miscellaneous cancer recruited 168 patients (Maeta et al. 1987). Of these patients, 88% had received prior chemotherapy and/or radiation therapy. Overall response rate was 29.5% (39 of 132 evaluable patients), the most favorable results being achieved in the subgroup of 14 patients with soft tissue sarcomas. Seven of these patients showed objective regression of their advanced disease. Performance status was the most critical prognostic factor for either response or the occurrence of complications. Due to the high incidence of severe complications (19.6%), with treatment-related death in 24 patients, the authors stated: "We should reconsider the bases for selection of patients for treatment with total body hyperthermia and we should pay greater attention to the possible development of fatal complications."

In reviewing these WBH trials it is difficult to draw any firm conclusions due to the variation in tumor grade, histology, drug(s) administered, drug dose and intensity, heating techniques, and patient history. More carefully designed phase I/II studies are warranted in order to give an indication of the value of systemic thermochemotherapy.

2.4 Isolated Hyperthermic Antiblastic Perfusion

Administration of cytotoxic drugs by hyperthermic perfusion is currently used predominantly for the treatment of malignant melanoma but also for soft tissue sarcoma of the limbs. Treatment techniques for hyperthermic antiblastic limb perfusion, the specific rationale, the clinical trials at several institutions and their results for different stages of melanoma, and the complications as well as side-effects of the procedure have been recently reviewed (Truchetet et al. 1990). The same rationale has guided the extension of this management to the treatment of soft tissue sarcomas.

The concept and technique of regional chemotherapy using intra-arterial infusion of a cytotoxic drug – as already proposed in 1950 by Klopp et al. – was introduced into clinical use for the first time in 1957, by Creech and colleagues (Creech et al. 1958). Stehlin (1969) proposed the association of hyperthermia with regional perfusion chemotherapy, stressing the importance of a synergistic effect of hyperthermia and chemotherapy. The particular technique of isolated hyperthermic limb perfusion using an extracorporeal circuit, as already described for WBH, allows high doses of a selected drug to be delivered to a precise region. At the same time no systemic toxicity (e.g., bone marrow) should occur because blood escape via collateral circulation towards the general circulation is prevented by placing a tourniquet above the arteriovenous access.

There are optimistic early reports of perfusion of limbs with L-PAM (L-phenylalanine mustard = melphalan) and actinomycin D for soft tissue sarcomas. Thirty-seven patients with soft tissue sarcomas of the extremities (nine liposarcomas, seven synovial sarcomas, six rhabdomyosarcomas, four fibrosarcomas, and 11 other histological subtypes) were entered in a multidisciplinary trial utilizing hyperthermic perfusion and external irradiation combined with radical local excision (Stehlin et al. 1975). Improvement of local tumor control, permitting limb-sparing procedures, has been claimed but no data on objective regressions at the time of local treatment have been presented. The overall local control rate was 80% and the amputation rate, 10%. As reference treatment for comparison with these results the authors discussed their previous results gained using the perfusion technique not altered to include heated blood. Lethi et al. (1986) reported on 64 patients with soft tissue sarcomas of the extremities using regional hyperthermic perfusion (40.0°C for 1 h) with L-PAM and actinomycin D either before (37 patients) or after (27 patients) surgical resection of the tumor. Postoperatively, about half of the patients received (50 Gy) external beam radiation. For all patients local recurrence rate was 3.4% at 2 years and 11.1% at 5 years. Overall 5-year survival rate was 67%. Unfortunately, no data on objective tumor response were presented for patients who received hyperthermic antiblastic perfusion before definitive surgery. The group at the University of Groningen (Hoekstra et al. 1987) treated 14 patients (eight with primary and six with recurrent high-grade soft tissue sarcomas) with isolated hyperthermic (39°–40°C for 1 h) or normothermic (two cases) perfusion (L-PAM and actinomycin D) followed by wide excision. None of the patients received systemic adjuvant chemotherapy or external-beam radiotherapy. During the follow-up (median, 13 years) five patients developed distant metastases and one other patient showed recurrent local disease after 48 months. The actuarial 5-year and 10-year survival was 69%.

In a small series (LEJEUNE et al. 1988) of 15 patients with limb sarcomas treated by hyperthermic perfusion (39°–40°C for 1 h) with L-PAM and actinomycin D, local recurrence was seen in four of eight patients with recurrent disease at presentation, but in none of six patients with primary sarcomas after 30 months' follow-up.

In an attempt to search for agents other than L-PAM or actinomycin D that can be safely utilized, the group of Fletcher and colleagues used cisplatin for hyperthermic limb perfusion in soft tissue sarcoma and melanoma of the extremities (POMMIER et al. 1988). Of 35 patients with primary soft tissue sarcoma, 15 had high-grade tumors and 20 tumors were greater than 5 cm in diameter. The applied doses of cisplatin ranged from 0.75 to 2 mg/kg during perfusion at 40°C for 1 h. Among the 29 patients who underwent hyperthermic perfusion before definitive resection was performed (approximately 1 month later), only 17 were evaluable for local response due to the lack of measurable disease in the other patients. Objective response was observed in eight patients [three PRs and five minimal responses (MRs)], where MR was defined as less than 50% reduction in the product of the dimensions of the measured lesion. At last follow-up (mean 16 months), none of the 35 sarcoma patients had locoregional recurrence but five patients had developed distant metastases.

A detailed description of the clinical results at the Regina Elena Cancer Institute using isolated hyperthermic limb perfusion for extremity sarcomas has been previously reported (DI FILIPPO et al. 1988). In a pilot study recruiting 22 patients, hyperthermic perfusion without chemotherapy but at a minimum temperature of 42°C for at least 2–4 h was performed with satisfactory tumor regressions (11 of 22 patients) but unacceptable mortality (four patients suffered postoperative toxic deaths). In consecutive studies, L-PAM (0.8 mg/kg) and actinomycin D (0.015 mg/kg) or cisplatin (2.5–5 mg/kg) were employed as antineoplastic drugs combined with a less aggressive regimen of hyperthermic perfusion (41°–41.5°C for 2 h). In 68 patients treated, two toxic deaths occurred (2.9%) and two other patients underwent amputations due to severe late complication. After cisplatin doses of 3.2 mg/kg during hyperthermic perfusion, the patients showed no significant local or systemic toxicity while high-dose cisplatin (5.0 mg/kg) was associated with severe complications in two patients.

In a first series of 30 patients, following hyperthermic antiblastic perfusion (HAP) definitive surgery was performed with an amputation rate of 42%. As local tumor response to HAP and duration of loco-regional control were unsatisfactory, the protocol was modified to include continuous intra-arterial (i.a.) doxorubicin infusion (10 mg/24 h for 10 days) generally initiated within 10 days after HAP followed by delayed surgery (in the 10th week) after three cycles. Alternatively, patients received only 45–60 Gy external beam radiation within 4 weeks after HAP administration prior to surgery. According to the most recent retrospective analysis on 70 evaluable patients presented by DI FILIPPO et al. (1991), the radiotherapy-including protocol resulted in an amputation rate of 0% and locoregional control of 94%; this is better than with the HAP + i.a. doxorubicin regimen, but overall 5-year survival of patients is comparable (70% vs 73%). From these results it has also become clear that HAP alone is insufficient for local control and for improvement of long-term survival in patients with stage III–IVA recurrent soft tissue sarcomas (see also Sect. 19.4.2).

In general, because there is no control group, treated with normothermic antiblastic perfusion, in either of the reported studies, we do not know to what extent the hyperthermic enhancement of drug effects or direct thermal cytotoxicity of hyperthermia has contributed to the overall therapeutic effect of the combined modalities. The role of hyperthermia in perfusion therapy for soft tissue sarcomas needs to be more clearly defined in controlled trials.

2.5 Regional Hyperthermia Combined with Systemic Chemotherapy

Regional hyperthermia (RHT), by the clinical use of an annular phased array system for deep-seated malignancy, has previously been studied (for review see MEYERS et al. 1989). The annular array (AA) consists of eight pairs of radiating horn-type resonant cavities in an octagonal geometry with apertures surrounding the patient's abdomen and pelvis (Sigma-60 AA) or limbs (Sigma-30 AA) in a similar manner to that used for computed tomographic scanning. Fairly uniform power deposition by this device has been observed in static phantoms and large animals. As a result of the clinical pilot studies, temperatures in the therapeutic range near 42°C have in general been achieved in pelvic rather than in upper abdominal tumors (SAPOZINK et al. 1986). However, nonuniformity of temperature distributions with large temperature gradients has been found as a general heating characteristic of deep-seated sites, this being most likely dependent on variation in local blood flow during heating.

In regard to site and disease selections for hyperthermia trials, soft tissue sarcomas and malignant bone tumors of the pelvis and the extremities are excellent candidates for the application of RHT combined with systemic chemotherapy (Table 2.2).

The most important aspect of this form of thermochemotherapy is the advantage of applying full-dose systemic standard chemotherapy at the same time as the tumor temperature is elevated. Several consecutive clinical trials have been performed at our institution (1986–1993) and impressive results have been obtained (see also Chap. 11).

2.6 Conclusion

In the application of thermochemotherapy one may use, for example, systemic heating (WBH), isolated perfusion of extremities, and regional heating of the tumor-bearing area of the body, as shown in solid tumors like soft tissue sarcomas. The choice of heating technique is strongly dependent upon the specific characteristics of the tumor to be treated. The selection of chemotherapy should be based upon preclinical data showing thermal enhancement of its antiproliferative activity under heating conditions. The dose and dose intensity of chemotherapy in clinical heating protocols should be comparable to standard regimens of medical oncology.

Table 2.2. Effects of Preoperative Systemic Chemotherapy combined with Regional Hyperthermia upon Solid Tumors

1. Systemic Chemotherapy:
   - early control of micro-metastases by chemotherapy alone
2. Simultaneous Local Treatment:
   - improvement of local control by direct thermotoxicity or thermal enhancement of chemotherapy at the site of tumor
   - time for preplanning optimal surgery/radiation
   - potential of conservative surgical approach
   - potential of inducing stress response (hsp) and modulation of antigen presentation within the tumor tissue

2.7 Summary

- There is substantial evidence from preclinical and clinical data that efficacy of chemotherapy can be enhanced by the simultaneous application of hyperthermia.
- Tumor characteristics (e.g., grade, size, site) as well as stage of disease are determining the special application forms of hyperthermia combined with chemotherapy within a multidisciplinary treatment approach.
- Beside improvement of local control the application of thermo-chemotherapy should be further tested in prospective clinical trials in regard to its impact on survival.

References

Akiyoshi T, Wanda T, Arinaga S, et al. (1989) Enhanced chemosensitivity of cells from malignant effusions under condition of exposure to high temperature. Jpn J Surg 16: 323–329

Alberts DS, Peng YM, Chen G, et al. (1980) Therapeutic synergism of hyperthermia and cisplatin in a mouse tumor model. J Natl Cancer Inst 65: 455–460

Bates DA, Mackillop WJ (1986) Hyperthermia, adriamycin transport and cytotoxicity in drug sensitive and -resistant Chinese hamster ovary cells. Cancer Res 46: 5477–5481

Calabro A, Singletary E, Tucker S, et al. (1989) In vitro thermo-chemosensitivity screening of spontaneous human tumors: significant potentiation for cisplatin but not adriamycin. Int J Cancer 43: 385–390

Creech O, Krementz ET, Ryan RF, et al. (1958) Chemotherapy of cancer: regional perfusion utilizing an extracorporal circuit. Ann Surg 148: 616–632

Cronau LH Jr, Bourke DL, Bull JM (1984) General anesthesia for whole body hyperthermia. Cancer Res (suppl) 44: 4873–4877

Dahl O (1982) Interaction of hyperthermia and doxorubicin on a malignant, neurogenic rat cell line (BT_4C) in culture. J Natl Cancer Inst 61: 251–253

Dahl O (1988) Interaction of hyperthermia and chemotherapy. Recent Results Cancer Res 107: 157–169

Di Filippo F, et al. (1988) Role of hyperthermic perfusion as a first step in the treatment of soft tissue sarcoma of the extremities. World J Surg 12: 332–339

Di Filippo F, Psaila G, Botti C, et al. (1991) Hyperthermic antiblastic perfusion for limb sarcoma. Abstract at the International Meeting in Aviano, Italy, pp 78–82

Douple EB, Strohbehn JW, de Sieyes DC, et al. (1982) Therapeutic potentiation of cis-dichlordiammineplatinum and radiation by interstitial microwave hyperthermia in a mouse tumor. Natl Cancer Inst Monogr 61: 259–262
Engelhardt R (1987) Hyperthermia and drugs. Recent Results Cancer Res 104: 136–203
Engelhardt R, Neumann NA, Weth-Simon R, et al. (1986) Randomized trial in small cell lung CA (SCLC) pts chemotherapy (CT) without vs with whole body hyperthermia (WBH). Abstract for the 34th annual meeting of the Radiation Research Society, 16
Gerad H, Echo D, Whitacre M, et al. (1984) Doxorubicin, cyclophosphamide, and whole body hyperthermia for treatment of advanced soft tissue sarcoma. Cancer 53: 2585–2591
Groveman DS, Borden EC, Merritt JA, et al. (1984) Augmented antiproliferative effects on interferons at elevated temperatures. Cancer Res 44: 5517–5521
Hahn GM (1982) Hyperthermia and cancer. Plenum Press, New York
Hahn GM, Strande DP (1976) Cytotoxic effects of hyperthermia and adriamycin on Chinese hamster cells. J Natl Cancer Inst 57: 1063–1067
Herman LS, Sweets CC, White DM, et al. (1982) Effect of heating on lethality due to hyperthermia and selected chemotherapeutic drugs. J Natl Cancer Inst 68: 487–491
Hoekstra HJ, Schraffordt Koops H, Molenaar WM, et al. (1987) Results of isolated regional perfusion in the treatment of malignant soft tissue tumors of the extremities.
Ikegami T, Kubota N, Watai K, et al. (1988) The enhancement of hyperthermic effect by etoposide (VP-16) on rat hepatoma 3924A cells (abstract). Proc Int Hyperthermia Oncol, Kyoto, Japan, vol 13, p 186
Jabboury K, Mansfield B, Bull JMC (1985) Whole body hyperthermia (WBH) + BCNU in advanced sarcoma. Abstract for the 34th annual meeting of the Radiation Research Society, 16
Klopp CT, Alford TC, Bateman J, et al. (1950) Fractionated intraarterial cancer chemotherapy with methylbis-amine hydrochloride: a preliminary report. Ann Surg 132:811–832
Lejeune FJ, Lienard D, Ewalenko P (1988) Hyperthermic isolation perfusion of the limbs with cytostatics after surgical excision of sarcomas. World J Surg 12: 345–348
Lethi PM, Moseley HS, Janoff K, et al. (1986) Improved survival for soft tissue sarcoma of the extremities by regional hyperthermic perfusion, local excision and radiation therapy. Surg Gynecol Obstet 162: 149–152
Maeta M, Koga S, Wada J, et al. (1987) Clinical evaluation of total-body hyperthermia combined with anticancer chemotherapy for far-advanced miscellaneous cancer in Japan. Cancer 59: 1101–1106
Marmor JB (1979) Interactions of hyperthermia and chemotherapy in animals. Cancer Res 39: 2269–2276
Mean RG, Corry PM, Fletcher SE, et al. (1980) Thermal enhancement of DNA damage in mammalian cells treated with cisdiamminedichloroplatinum (II). Cancer Res 40: 1136–1139
Meyer JL, Van Kersen I, Becker B, et al. (1985) The importance of thermotolerance after 41.0°C hyperthermia: in vitro and in vivo tumor and normal tissue investigations. Int J Radiat Oncol Biol Phys 11: 973–981
Meyers JL, Kapp DS, Fessenden P, et al. (1989) Hyperthermic oncology: current biology, physics and clinical results. Pharmacol Ther 42: 251–288
Miser JS, Kinsella TJ, Triche TJ, et al. (1987) Ifosfamide with mesna uroprotection and etoposide: an effective regimen in the treatment of recurrent sarcomas and other tumors of children and young adults. J Clin Oncol 5: 1191–1198
Page RL, Meyer RE, Thrall DE, et al. (1987) Cardiovascular and metabolic response of tumor bearing dogs to whole body hyperthermia. Int J Hyperthermia 3: 513–525
Parks LC (1982) Clinical evaluation: induction of systemic hyperthermia by extracorporal circulation as primary and adjuvant treatment of advanced solid tumor malignancies. In: Nussbaum GH (ed) Physical aspects of hyperthermia. American Institute of Physics, New York, pp 660–632
Pfeffer MR, Herman TS, Teicher BA, et al. (1989) Preclinical studies of etoposide and cis-diamminedichloroplatinum (II) in combination with radiation and hyperthermia in the FSA IIc fibrosarcoma (abstract). Int J Radiat Oncol Biol Phys 17: 180
Pommier RF, Moseley HS, Cohen J, et al. (1988) Pharmacokinetics, toxicity, and short-term results of cisplatin hyperthermic isolated limb perfusion for soft tissue sarcoma and melanoma of the extremities. Am J Surg 155: 667–671
Robins HI (1984) The role of whole body hyperthermia in the treatment of neoplastic disease, its current status and future prospects. Cancer Res (suppl) 44: 4878–4883
Robins HI, Dennis WH, Neville AJ, et al. (1985) A nontoxic system for 41.8°C whole body hyperthermia: results of a phase I study using a radiant heat device. Cancer Res 45: 3937–3944
Robins HI, Sielaff KM, Storer B, et al. (1989) Phase I trial of human lymphoblastoid interferon with whole body hyperthermia in advanced cancer. Cancer Res 49: 1609–1615
Sapozink MD, Gibbs FA, Egger MJ, et al. (1986) Regional hyperthermia for clinically advanced deep-seated pelvic malignancy. Am J Clin Oncol 9: 162–169
Steel G, Peckham MJ (1979) Exploitable mechnanisms in combined radiotherapy or chemotherapy: the concept of additivity. Int J Raddiat Oncol Biol Phys 5: 85–91
Stehlin JS (1969) Hyperthermic perfusion with chemotherapy for cancers of the extremity. Surg Gynecol Obstet 129: 305–308
Stehlin JS, De Ipolyi PD, Giovanella BC, er al. (1975) Soft tissue sarcomas of the extremity. Am J Surg 130: 643–646
Thrall DE, Page RL, Dewhirst MW, et al. (1986) Temperature measurements in normal and tumor tissue of dogs undergoing whole body hyperthermia. Cancer Res 46: 6229–6235
Thrall DE, Dewhirst MW, Page RL, et al. (1990) A comparison of temperature in canine solid tumours during local and whole-body hyperthermia administered alone and simultaneously. Int J Hyperthermia 6: 305–317
Truchetet F, Grosshans E, Kretz JC, et al. (1990) Combined hyperthermia and chemotherapy for malignant melanoma of the limbs. In: Gautherie M (ed) Intersitital, endocavitary and perfusional hyperthermia. Springer, Berlin Heidelberg New York, pp 77–87
Voth B, Sauer HJ, Wilmanns W (1988) Thermostability of cytostatic drugs in vitro and thermosensitivity of cultured human lymphoblasts against cytostatic drugs. Recent Results Cancer Res 107: 170–176

Wallner KE, Li GC (1986) Adriamycin resistance, heat resistance and radiation response in Chinese hamster fibroblasts. Int J Radiat Oncol Biol Phys 12: 829–833
Wallner KE, deGregorio MW, Li GC (1986) Hyperthermia potentiation of cis-diamminedichloroplatinum (11) cytotoxicity in Chinese hamster ovary cells resistant to the drug. Cancer Res 46: 6242–6245
Wallner KE, Banda M, Li GC (1987) Hyperthermic enhancement of cell killing by mitomycin C in mitomycin C-resistant Chinese hamster ovary cells. Cancer Res 47: 1308–1312
Wiedemann G, Roszinski S, Biersack A, et al. (1992) Local hyperthermia enhances cyclophosfamide, ifosfamide and cis-diamminedichloroplatinum cytotoxicity on human-derived breast carcinoma and sarcoma xenografts in nude mice. J Cancer Res Clin Oncol 118: 129–135
Wiedemann G, Knocks D, Mentzel M, et al. (1993) Effects of temperature on the therapeutic efficacy and pharmakokinetics of ifosfamide. Cancer Res 53: 1–5
Willnow U, Lindner H, Brock D, et al. (1989) Behandlung konventionell inkurabler Tumorerkrankungen im Kindesalter mit Ganzkörperhyperthermie und Chemotherapie. Dtsch Med Wochenschr 114: 208–213
Zakris EL, Dewhirst MW, Riviere JE, et al. (1987) Pharmacokinetics and toxicity of intraperitoneal cisplatin combined with regional hyperthermia. J Clin Oncol 5: 1613–1620

3 Thermoradiotherapy for Advanced and Recurrent Breast Tumours

J. VAN DER ZEE and C.C. VERNON

CONTENTS

3.1 Introduction

Among types of cancer, breast cancer has one of the highest incidences in the Western world. Tumour stage at initial diagnosis, especially the axillary nodal status, is the predominant indicator of the patient's prognosis with regard to both local control and survival (BONADONNA and VALAGUSSA 1987). More aggressive local treatment, such as the addition of hyperthermia to radiotherapy, at any time following diagnosis, will be beneficial mainly with regard to the situation within the treatment volume. Nevertheless, the achievement of tumour control within the specific volume can be of great importance for the quality of the patient's remaining life.

The opportunity to achieve local control with radiotherapy is positively related to the total radiotherapy dose applied and negatively to the tumour size (BEDWINEK et al. 1981a). The radiation dose that can be applied is limited by the surrounding normal tissues. The value of combining radiotherapy with chemotherapy is controversial with regard to local control.

A local failure generates costs, both at the individual level by negatively influencing the quality of life, and to the society in general by necessitating additional expensive treatments. On the basis of the strong biological rationale for the combination of radiotherapy and hyperthermia, together with the relatively high incidence of patients with (recurrent) breast cancer and the often superficial location of the tumour, this patient group forms the majority of patients treated with superficial hyperthermia since its clinical application was started.

3.2 Inoperable Tumours

3.2.1 General Remarks

For some patients the risk of local recurrence after mastectomy is unacceptably high (over 60% – HAAGENSEN 1943a,b) and survival is poor. Certain features of the primary breast carcinoma are particularly associated with the development of local recurrence, and the first five listed in Table 3.1 are regarded as absolute contraindications to mastectomy as the local relapse rate exceeds 50% and none of the patients survive disease-free for more than 5 years.

J. VAN DER ZEE, MD, PhD, Hyperthermia Oncologist, Department of Hyperthermia, Dr. Daniel den Hoed Cancer Center, Groene Hilledijk 301, 3075 EA Rotterdam, The Netherlands
C.C. VERNON, MA, FRCR, Clinical Oncologist, Department of Clinical Oncology, Hammersmith Hospital, Du Cane Road, London W12 0HS, United Kingdom

Table 3.1. Clinical features associated with a high risk of local recurrence and/or poor survival based on data from the Presbyterian Hospital, 1915–1932 (HAAGENSEN 1943)

Clinical feature	No. of patients	Local recurrence %	Disease-free for 5 years (%)
Extensive oedema of skin over breast (>one-third)	51	61	0
Satellite nodules	7	57	0
"Inflammatory carcinoma"	25	60	0
Parasternal or supraclavicular nodes	16	56	0
Oedema of arm	4	50	0
Oedema of skin over breast (≤one-third)	75	32	23
Skin ulceration	14	14	36
Fixation of tumour to chest wall	20	40	5
Axillary lymph nodes ≥2.5 cm diameter	24	13	38
Fixed axillary lymph nodes	8	13	13

Currently any patient with T3b–T4, N2 or N3–M0 is regarded as having locally advanced breast cancer and therefore as inoperable (WILLIAMS and BUCHANAN 1987).

3.2.2 Results with Irradiation Alone

High-dose irradiation has been shown to be capable of eradicating disease (FLETCHER and MONTAGUE 1966), and Bruckman's series in 1979 gave a total local control of 64% with those receiving >60 Gy having 78% local control and those receiving <60% only 39% local control, but despite local control only 22% remained disease-free at 5 years. FLETCHER and MONTAGUE, in their extensive review of the literature in 1966, confirmed that local failure increases with decreasing radiation total dose and increasing tumour size. Many of these studies have used additional interstitial radiotherapy. It has been suggested that even for breast cancer improvement of local control can lead to improved survival (SUIT 1982).

Results reported in the last decade have been collated and two useful clinical conclusions can be drawn:

1. When irradiation is used alone in inoperable breast cancer, the results are poor, with 12%–70% locoregional relapse.
2. Even when local relapse does not occur, there is a high rate of distant failure (5-year FF survival 12%–40%) and overall and disease-free long-term survival is poor.

These results suggest that (a) local control needs to be improved and (b) an effective systemic therapy is additionally needed. The addition of chemotherapy does lead to improved local control, but as yet few studies have shown improvement in survival as well, indicating that for some of these patients the tumour burden is too much even for chemotherapy to be effective (WILLIAMS and BUCHANAN 1987).

3.2.3 Results of Radiotherapy plus Hyperthermia

Locally advanced breast cancer which is deemed inoperable by the surgeons has been treated in the past with radical irradiation and more recently with combinations of radical irradiation and chemotherapy. However, the results have in general been poor (AMALRIC et al. 1982; ARRIAGADA et al. 1985; BOUCHARD 1985) and the addition of hyperthermia could be beneficial, if it is possible to heat these tumours adequately. However, adequate heating has been a problem in several studies (HOFMAN et al. 1989; SCOTT et al. 1988).

SAVCHENCKO et al. in 1987 published a large randomised trial comparing preoperative radiotherapy alone with combined radiotherapy and hyperthermia for stage II and III breast cancer. This study showed that the combined treatment produced a significantly improved local control rate and a non-significant tendency toward improved survival – 77% versus 87%, giving a thermal enhancement ratio (TER) of 1.13 (Table 3.2).

VORA et al. in 1986 reported treatment of ten patients with advanced breast cancer with external irradiation, brachytherapy, and interstitial hyperthermia, with complete response in nine, and emphasised the effectiveness of the combined treatments.

Table 3.2. Results of a randomised study of 507 patients comparing preoperative radiotherapy alone and combined radiotherapy and hyperthermia for stage II and III breast cancer (SAVCHENKO et al. 1987)

Stage and endpoint (507 patients)	Radiation alone (%)	Radiation and heat (%)	Isodose (TER)
Recurrence-free 2 year survival			
Stage II	75	94	1.25
Stage III	64	79	1.23
Recurrence-free survival			
At 3 years	77	87	1.13
At 5 years	67	73	1.09

Note: Response after treatment with same radiation dose given either alone or combined with hyperthermia
Radiation: 20 Gy/5 fx of 4 Gy

Other more recent phase III trials treating inoperable breast tumours with radical radiotherapy and hyperthermia have not shown such encouraging results. In the ESHO trial, which closed in 1994, patients did not show positive results for the hyperthermia arm; however, thermal parameters to assess the adequacy of the hyperthermia treatments are awaited (GONZÁLEZ GONZÁLEZ, personal communication, 1994).

The MRC Hyperthermia Group randomised 30 similar such patients as part of the much larger [Medical Research Council (MRC), European Society for Hyperthermic Oncology (ESHO), Dutch Hyperthermia Group (DHG), Princess Margaret Hospital (PMH)] trial of superficial hyperthermia for breast cancer which was completed in 1993, with overall positive results. However, for this subgroup the results were negative, with 67% complete response for radiation alone and 56% for the combined treatments (VERNON et al. 1994). Although the primary tumours were much deeper and bigger on average than the recurrent ones, there was no apparent significant difference in the thermal parameters between the two groups, indicating the same levels of heating for both.

Trimodality studies have also been performed using combined irradiation, hyperthermia and chemotherapy. ZAMBOGLOU et al. (1993) treated 65 patients with radiochemotherapy (using mitoxantrone) ± interstitial hyperthermia, followed by salvage surgery some 8–10 weeks after completion of the primary therapy. Of the 65 patients, 35 showed pathological complete remission and the remaining 30 had microscopic disease only (Table 3.3). These results were superior to a control group of 40 patients who had the same average tumour diameter size and were treated with the same regimen, excluding hyperthermia. However, this study was not a randomised trial.

Table 3.3. Histologically confirmed responses in the ZAMBOGLOU et al. (1993) study

	HT+RT+CT	RT+CT
Av. tumour diameter	7.3 cm	7.6 cm
Pathological CR	35/65 (54%)	6/40 (15%)

Table 3.4. Primary response to radiation combined with local hyperthermia for locally advanced breast cancer compared with irradiation alone (FUWA and MORITA 1986)

Maximal tumour size	Combined therapies		Radiotherapy alone[a]		
	CR	PR	CR	PR	NC
<7 cm	0		8	1	
7–10 cm	3	0	1	6	0
>10 cm	5	2	1	0	1

CR, complete response; PR, partial response; NC, no change

FUWA et al. (1986) treated ten patients with primary advanced (T3–4) breast cancers with trimodality therapy (using cyclophosphamide, 5-fluorouracil (5-FU), methotrexate and tamoxifen); eight achieved complete response and two, partial response (Table 3.4). Despite the small number of cases, this study is reported as being statistically significant. Although eight of the original ten patients died of distant metastases, no local recurrences were observed.

3.2.4 Discussion

The complete response rates and local control durations following radiotherapy plus hyperthermia in inoperable breast cancer are within the ranges reported for radiotherapy alone. One of the main problems that still exists is adequate heating at depth. Toxicity does not seem to have been severe and generally no worse than with irradiation alone. Definite conclusions can only result from comparative studies, such as the ESHO 1-85. Possible advantages of the combination are increase in local control rate, and thereby better quality of life. It may also be possible to achieve increased duration of disease-free and overall survival time.

3.3 Recurrent Tumours

3.3.1 Introduction

Of the patients with isolated local-regional recurrences, 81%–93% eventually develop distant metastases, of which about half appear within 18 months (BEDWINEK et al. 1981b; SOLIN 1992). The 5-year-survival rate following the occurrence of local-regional recurrent disease varies from 21% to 38% (BEDWINEK et al. 1981b), depending on the extent of disease at the time of recurrence and the disease-free interval since the primary treatment. The incidence of local-regional recurrence is about 10%–15% following radical primary surgery for node-negative patients. The incidence in patients with positive axillary lymph nodes may be as high as 26%–40% (LEVITT 1983; ROSENMAN et al. 1986; BEDWINEK 1984).

The incidence of local-regional recurrences can be decreased by both postoperative radiotherapy and postoperative chemotherapy, and possibly even more by the postoperative application of a combination of radiotherapy plus chemotherapy (BUZDAR et al. 1990), although results from other studies do not confirm this finding (BEDWINEK 1984). Local-regional recurrences may result in symptoms that considerably decrease the quality of life, such as pain, ulceration, bleeding, brachial plexus neuropathy and lymphoedema of the ipsilateral arm, as BEDWINEK et al. (1981a) found in 62% of their patients. Furthermore, growth

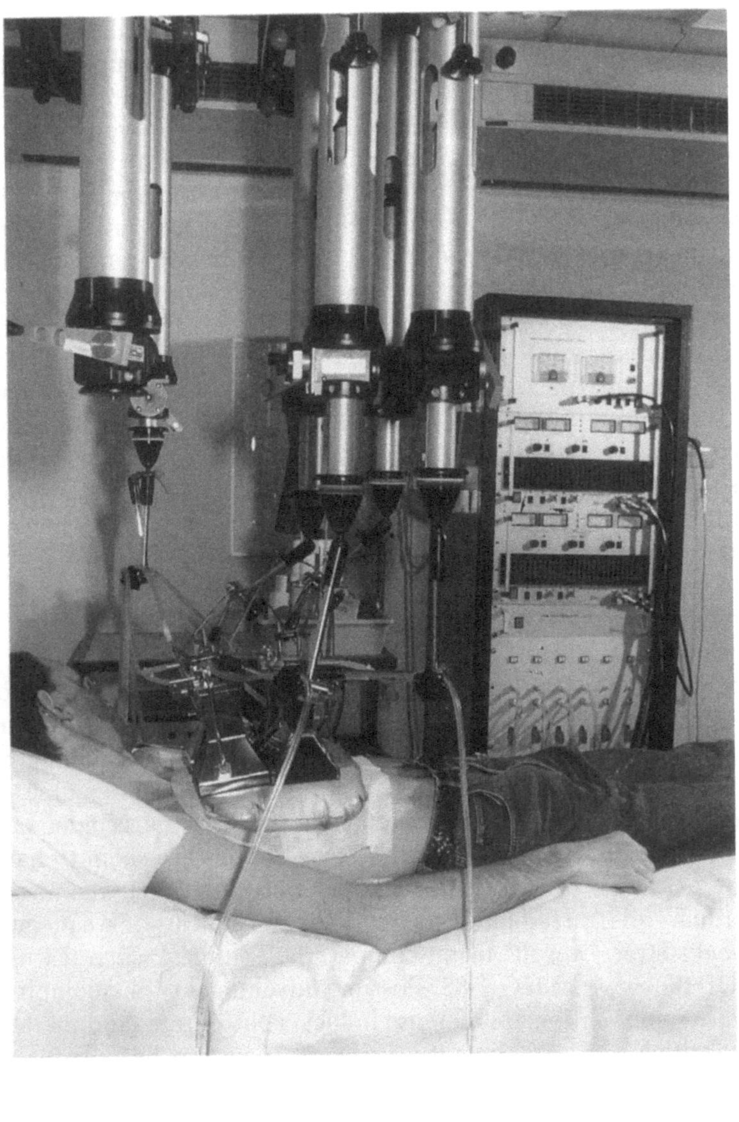

Fig. 3.1. Example of a clinical hyperthermia treatment set-up for a patient with a chest wall tumour. In this situation a 433-MHz multi-applicator multi-generator system with water-filled waveguides is used, including a perfused water bolus to control skin temperature

through the thoracic wall can be the origin of carcinomatous pleuritis in about 40% of the patients (HIRN-STADLER and EILENBERGER 1990). The treatment of an uncontrolled local-regional recurrence may cost society US$ 430 (HURLEY et al. 1992). So, both quality of life and economic arguments exist to justify optimization of local treatment for recurrent breast cancer.

About half of the patients treated with (superficial) hyperthermia suffer from chest wall tumours (International Consensus Meeting on Hyperthermia, Final Report 1990), of which the majority will be recurrent breast cancer (see Fig. 3.1 for an example of a clinical hyperthermia treatment set-up for a patient with a chest wall tumour; a schematic representation of the set-up is shown in Fig. 3.2). In most cases, hyperthermia is added to radiotherapy, which may be either a first treatment with radiation or re-irradiation. There is also ample experience with radiotherapy alone in recurrent breast cancer.

VAN DER ZEE et al. (1993) have screened the literature on radiotherapy alone, hyperthermia alone and radiotherapy plus hyperthermia in superficially located recurrent breast cancer for reports on complete response in locoregional recurrent breast cancer. Where sufficient information was available, the published data were grouped for various radiotherapy doses and for each group the average value was calculated or estimated. For radiotherapy alone, 18 datapoints were distinguishable and for radiotherapy plus hyperthermia, 31 datapoints (references listed in Table 3.5).

3.3.2 *Results of Radiation Alone*

A total of eight publications were identified reporting complete response rates following radiotherapy alone. In general, the complete response chances increased with higher radiation doses and smaller tumours.

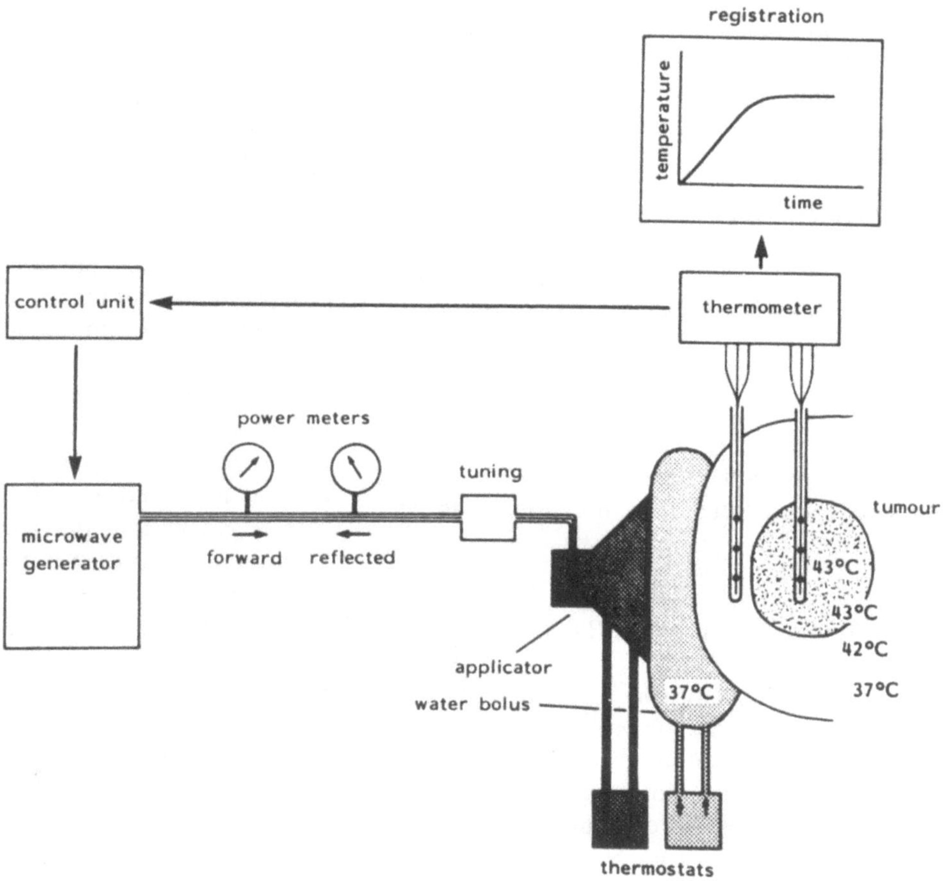

Fig. 3.2. Schematic representation of hyperthermia treatment set-up

Table 3.5. References from which data on complete response rates following radiotherapy with or without hyperthermia were collected

AMICHETTI et al. 1989[a]		
CHU et al. 1976	JO et al. 1987	RUY YING et al. 1990
DEUTSCH et al. 1986	KAPP et al. 1991	SANNAZZARI et al. 1989
DRAGOVIC et al. 1989	KJELLEN et al. 1988	SCHWAIBOLD et al. 1991
DUBOIS et al. 1990	LARAMORE et al. 1978	SCOTT et al. 1984
DUNLOP et al. 1986	MANNING et al. 1982	SCOTT et al. 1985
GABRIELE et al. 1987	MYERSON et al. 1990	SEEGENSCHMIEDT et al. 1989
GONZÁLEZ GONZÁLEZ et al. 1988	PEREZ et al. 1986	STORME and VAN DEN BERGE 1988[a]
HETZEL and MATTIELO 1988	PEREZ et al. 1989	U et al. 1980
HOFMAN et al. 1984	PHROMRATANAPONGSE et al. 1991	VAN DER ZEE et al. 1988
HORWICH 1981	PODGORSAK et al. 1981	VAN DER ZEE et al. 1993A

[a] Personal communication

The total number of treatment fields was 530 (3–98 per datapoint). Radiotherapy doses varied from 20 to 61 Gy, with a mean value of 44.4 Gy. Reported complete response rates ranged from 7% to 85%; the accumulated complete response rate was 56% (296/530).

3.3.3 *Results of Hyperthermia Alone*

For hyperthermia alone, complete response rates varying from 0% to 40% had been reported for various tumours. These data were combined, giving a complete response rate of 15% (60/412).

3.3.4 *Results of Radiation plus Hyperthermia*

In a total of 24 publications, the total number of treatment fields was 1237 (1–197 per datapoint). Radiotherapy doses given in addition to hyperthermia ranged from 10 to 65 Gy, with a mean value fo 31.5 Gy. Reported complete response rates varied from 15% to 84% (one publication mentions complete response in 1/1); the accumulated complete response rate was 59% (732/1237).

3.3.5 *Thermal Enhancement Ratio*

A logistic analysis of the published data was performed to estimate the probability of complete response versus radiotherapy dose for both radiotherapy alone and radiotherapy plus hyperthermia. Equal slopes were assumed for the two dose-effect curves. The 50% effective doses (ED_{50}) with the 95% confidence intervals were calculated from the results of these logistic analyses (Fig. 3.3). The TER was calculated by dividing the ED_{50} for radiotherapy alone by the ED_{50} for radiotherapy plus hyperthermia. For radiotherapy alone, the $ED_{50} \pm$ SE value was 42.4 ± 2.98 Gy. For radiotherapy plus hyperthermia, it was 24.7 ± 1.85 Gy. The corresponding TER value was 1.72 (95% confidence interval 1.48–1.99).

3.3.6 *Discussion*

The outcome of the retrospective analysis performed on recurrent breast carcinoma treatments should be interpreted with care. Major pitfalls are uncertainties about tumour dimensions, radiotherapy dose scheduling and previous treatments with radiotherapy. In the combined treatment groups, many, but not all, patients had previously received radiation in the field under study. In the radiotherapy-alone groups, most patients had not received radiotherapy previously. Details on radiation fractionation are not always given and hence a comparison between biologically equivalent radiation schedules cannot be performed. In various publications, a range of total radiotherapy doses was reported, from which a rough estimate of average value(s) was derived.

Tumour size has a very important influence on the result of treatment, especially for radiotherapy and, perhaps to a lesser extent, also for hyperthermia. It was not easily possible to distinguish groups of patients with smaller or larger tumour dimensions from most publications, with corresponding complete response rates. One other problem is that it is not always possible to see whether patients are reported a second time in a subsequent publication from the same group.

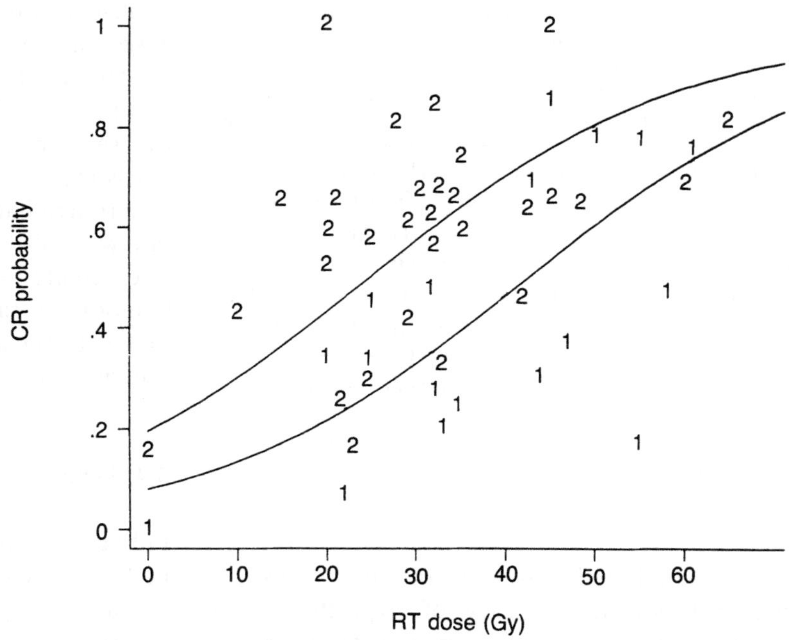

Fig. 3.3. Radiotherapy (RT) with or without hyperthermia (HT) in recurrent breast cancer (data from references in table 3.3.1). Probability of complete response in relation to radiotherapy total dose. (1) RT alone; ED50 = 42.4 Gy. (2) RT + HT; ED50 = 24.7 Gy. The thermal enhancement ratio (TER) at the ED50 level is 1.72

The number of publications reporting on results of radiotherapy alone may appear surprisingly low. The difficulty is that RT-alone publications generally report on long-term results (local control), whereas RT+HT publications mostly report on complete response rates; only a few of the latter were found to report long-term results. For this comparison of complete response rates, most of the radiation-alone publications could not be used. Nevertheless, the high complete response rate following low-dose radiotherapy plus hyperthermia, and a TER of 1.72 derived from comparison of reported results following radiation alone versus results following combined treatment, are promising. However, convincing evidence can only result from randomised trials.

3.3.6.1 Results of Randomised Studies

Five randomised trials addressing the question of whether hyperthermia in addition to radiotherapy is beneficial for breast cancer patients were started between 1988 and 1991 by the DHG (Dutch Hyperthermia Group), MRC (Medical Research Council), ESHO (European Society of Hyperthermic Oncology) and PMH (Princess Margaret Hospital/Ontario Cancer Institute). In these trials patients were eligible if they had advanced primary or recurrent breast cancer. The primary endpoint of all trials was local complete response. Slow recruitment led to the decision to collaborate and combine the trial results. There were 317 lesions randomised in 307 patients. The final analysis was conducted in June 1994 on 306 lesions in 306 patients. The tumour was primarily inoperable in 30 patients, recurrent in 66 patients and recurrent following previous radiotherapy to the same area in 210 patients.

The applied radiotherapy and hyperthermia treatment schedules were different in the various trials and depended on previous treatments and institutional standards (Table 3.6). As a consequence, the achieved complete response rates following both radiation alone and radiation plus hyperthermia showed a wide variation (Table 3.7). The overall complete response rate for radiotherapy alone was 41% and for the combined treatment arm, 59%, giving, after stratification by trial, an odds ratio of 2.3 (manuscript submitted for publication). Not all trials demonstrated an advantage of the combined treatment although the 95% confidence intervals of the different trials all contain the pooled OR. The greatest effect from additional hyperthermia was observed in patients with recurrent lesions in previously irradiated areas.

Table 3.6. Overview of randomised breast cancer trials of which the data were combined

Study	No. of patients	Tumour type	RT schedule	HT sessions
DHG	39	Recurrent	8 × 4 Gy/4 wks 25 × 2 Gy + boost	4–8 4–8
MRC BrR	150	Recurrent	8 × 3.6 Gy/2 wks 25 × 2 Gy + boost	3 6
ESHO	55	Recurrent	8 × 4 Gy/4 wks	4–8
PMH	32	Recurrent	18 × 1.8 Gy/4 wks 25 × 2 Gy + boost	2 2
MRC BrI	30	Inoperable	25 × 2 Gy + boost	6

For abbreviations, see text

The combined result of the five trials has demonstrated the efficacy of hyperthermia in addition to radiotherapy in the treatment of recurrent breast cancer. The implication of these results is that hyperthermia has an important role in the clinical management of this disease and should be used more widely.

3.3.6.2 Results of Trimodality Treatment

There is only limited experience with trimodality treatment in recurrent breast cancer. BORNSTEIN et al. (1993) reported on treatment results in 29 patients with 34 evaluable fields. Chemotherapy consisted of cisplatin, bleomycin or the combination of etanizole and cisplatin and was given intravenously once weekly, prior to hyperthermia. A radiation dose of 4 Gy was applied following combined chemotherapy and hyperthermia. The fraction size on other days was 2 Gy, 3–4 times a week in patients who had not received prior radiation therapy, and 0–1 time per week in cases of re-irradiation. The mean radiotherapy total dose ranged from 12 to 66 Gy with a mean of 50 Gy. Hyperthermia-related toxicity was observed in 54% of the fields. Persisting ulceration was seen in 50% of the fields. The incidence of persisting ulceration was higher in patients treated with re-irradiation. The overall complete response rate was 53%. This percentage is within the range of complete response rates reported for the combination of radiotherapy and hyperthermia, so that a beneficial effect of additional chemotherapy remains doubtful.

3.4 Toxicity

Publications in which (the majority) of patients had breast cancer were scanned for toxicity following combined radiotherapy and hyperthermia (DRAGOVIC et al. 1989; DUBOIS et al. 1990; EMAMI et al. 1992; GONZÁLEZ-GONZÁLEZ et al. 1988; MASANUGA et al. 1990; PHROMRATANAPONGSE et al. 1991; SEEGENSCHMIEDT et al. 1989; VAN DER ZEE et al. 1993). Two types of toxicity can be discriminated following thermoradiotherapy, i.e. *direct heat-induced damage* and *enhancement of radiation toxicity*. The percentage of second-degree burns reported varies from 7% to as high as 49%. In general, these burns heal spontaneously within 1–2 months. Third-degree burns, which may also be described as ulceration or soft tissue necrosis, are reported in 8%–19% of the patients. Such burns usually require skin grafts or long healing periods. A further direct heat-induced complication is the development of subcutaneous fat tissue necrosis; this has been observed in 3%–12% of the treated fields.

The risk of second- or third-degree burns appears to be related to the heating technique used, and specifically the use of a perfused water

Table 3.7. Summary of treatment results in combined randomised breast cancer trials

	DHG			MRC BrI			MRC BrR			ESHO			PMH			Overall		
	n	CRs	%	*n*	CRs	%	*n*	CRs	%	*n*	CRs	%	*n*	CRs	%	*n*	CRs	%
Treatment																		
RT, no HT	19	14	74	12	8	67	59	17	29	29	11	38	16	5	31	135	55	41
RT+HT	19	14	74	18	10	56	90	51	57	27	21	78	17	5	29	171	101	59
OR (95% CI)	1.00 (0.24–4.2)			0.63 (0.31–2.9)			3.23 (1.6–6.5)			5.73 (1.8–18.6)			0.92 (0.21–4.0)			2.10 (1.4–3.8)		

For abbreviations, see text

bolus to control skin temperature. LINDHOLM et al. (1987) observed a decrease in the frequency of burns from 45% to 13%, and VAN DER ZEE et al. (1993) a decrease from 69% to 30%, upon changing from air cooling to water bolus cooling (Table 3.8), and PHROMRATANAPONGSE et al. (1991) also mentioned less toxicity following the introduction of a water bolus cooling system. Several authors have suggested a relationship between the maximum temperature achieved during treatment and the risk of inducing a burn (KAPP et al. 1992; SEEGENSCHMIEDT et al. 1989).

The relatively high risk of inducing burns in patients with recurrent breast cancer is probably related to the specific local situation. The presence of bone at the bottom of the target volume may be responsible for the development of standing waves, by reflection, and thereby create high power densities. The sensitivity to pain induced by high temperatures can be decreased by previous surgery. On the other hand, decreased sensitivity is advantageous when such burns have developed: they do not cause pain. A remarkable further finding is that especially second-degree burns do heal spontaneously within, generally, a relatively short time, even in heavily pretreated areas. Altogether, thermal toxicity is considered acceptable, provided that the treatment is effective.

There is only little information on the enhancement of radiation toxicity by additional hyperthermia in breast cancer and the data are conflicting: GONZÁLEZ-GONZÁLEZ et al. (1988) observed an enhanced acute skin reaction in seven of nine patients in whom the radiotherapy field had been larger than the hyperthermia field. VAN DER ZEE et al. (1988) described 28 similar patients; in none of these patients was the score for acute skin reaction higher in the combined treated field. The absence of thermal enhancement was reported to be related to the time interval between radiotherapy and hyperthermia. Also the five combined trials on breast cancer have shown that, besides direct hyperthermia-related toxicity, the side-effects in patients receiving combined treatment were similar to those following radiotherapy alone.

Table 3.8. Complete tumour response and acute toxicity in relation to treatment technique (VAN DER ZEE et al. 1993)

	433-MHz technique perfused water bolus ($n = 86$)	2450-MHz technique air cooling ($n = 26$)
Burns: No or first degree	61	6
2nd degree	19 = 22%	15 = 58%
3rd degree	7 = 8%	3 = 12%
Subcutaneous	4	0
Complete response		
Max. tumour diameter <3 cm	91%	92%
Max. tumour diameter ≥3 cm	75%	31%

3.5 Practical Considerations for Hyperthermia

3.5.1 *Tumour-Specific Efficacy of Hyperthermia*

For breast cancer, there is some clinical evidence that hyperthermia has a tumour-specific efficacy. LYNG et al. (1991a) found in breast tumours preoperatively treated with thermoradiotherapy, that the hyperthermia dose, defined as equivalent time at 43°C, required to induce either direct tissue damage (50% necrosis) or vessel damage was lower for tumour tissue than for the surrounding normal tissue. In addition, "secondary cell kill" through vessel damage appeared less frequent in normal tissue than in tumour tissue. So, even with equal temperature distributions over the whole volume at risk, tissue damage might be induced to a greater extent in tumour tissue than in normal tissue.

3.5.2 *Treatment of Macroscopic Tumour Only, or Total Volume "at Risk"*

In the past, within the Dr. Daniel de Hoed Cancer Center, additional hyperthermia was directed at the macroscopic tumour. In several cases where the radiotherapy field had been larger than the hyperthermia field, tumour re-recurrence was observed in the radiation-alone part of the treated volume, whereas at the same time the part of the volume treated with the combined modality was free of tumour. This finding changed the treatment standards: applicator arrays are now chosen such that the whole radiation field is widely covered by the hyperthermia field (Fig. 3.4). A more recent finding is that the temperature within the normal tissue is predictive for local control duration (publication in preparation). A theoretical advantage of heating a larger volume is that the blood entering the

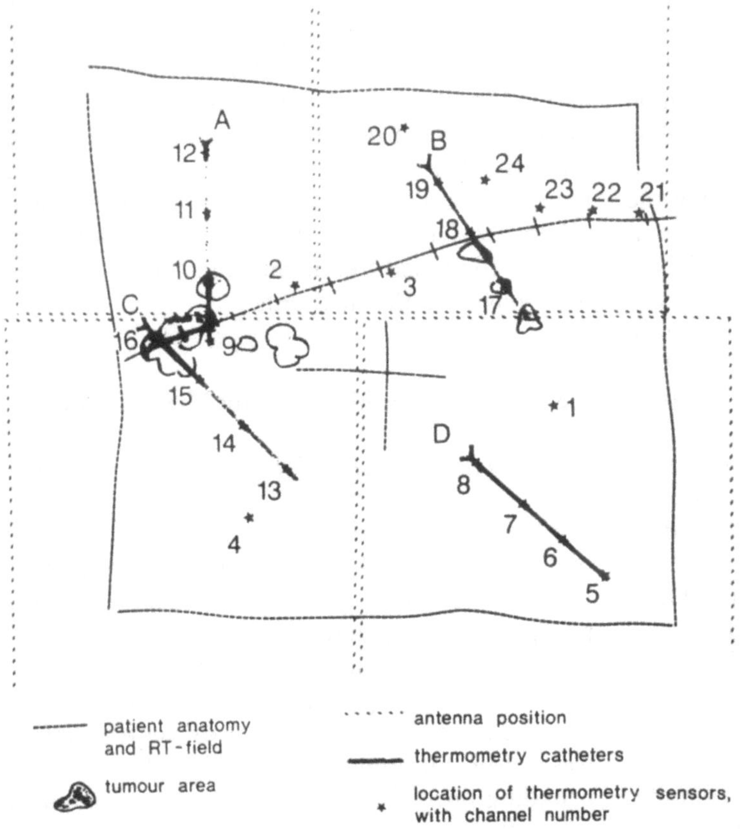

Fig. 3.4. Example of treatment area in a patient with locally recurrent breast cancer under treatment with reirradiation plus hyperthermia (Broekmeyer-Reurink et al. 1992)

treatment area is preheated, which may result in a more homogeneous temperature distribution.

3.5.3 Number of Treatments

There are several publications reporting comparative studies between a high and a low number of hyperthermia treatments (reviewed by Kapp and Meyer 1990). In most of these studies no significant differences were found, although in some a trend toward a better outcome following more treatments was indicated (Arcangeli et al. 1991; Lindholm et al. 1992). The finding by Lyng et al. (1991b) that thermal dose parameters increase with increasing fraction number supports the idea that more hyperthermic treatments may result in a better treatment outcome.

3.5.4 Prognostic Factors

The clinical outcome of hyperthermic treatment has been related to various prognostic factors (Kapp and Meyer 1990). One important factor concerns the *quality of the treatment*, which depends on the hyperthermia technique and may be represented by hyperthermia dose parameters such as temperature achieved at the coldest spot within the tumour. A further factor reported to be important is *tumour size*.

A recent study (van der Zee et al. 1993) suggests that the results achieved in larger tumours can be improved by the use of better heating techniques. In a group of 112 patients all treated with the same radiation schedule, there were 53 patients with tumours of which the maximum diameter was larger than 3 cm. In patients in whom hyperthermia had been induced with 2450 MHz ($n = 13$), the complete response rate was 31%, whereas the complete response rate in patients treated with 433 MHz was 75%. In the 59 patients with tumours smaller than 3 cm, the complete response rate was 92%, irrespective of the hyperthermia technique used. It can be hypothesized that tumour size will no longer influence the response to thermoradiotherapy when optimum treatment techniques become available for any volume of tissue.

3.5.5 *"Patchwork" Heating*

In cases where the volume to be treated is too large to be covered by one applicator set-up, the so-called patchwork heating technique has been applied. In the Rotterdam experience, two hyperthermia treatments of 1 h each, one immediately after the other and each covering half of the treatment volume, is tolerated well by patients in a relatively good general condition. When the treatment volume is too large to be covered by two applicator set-ups, there are two possible approaches. One is to divide the treatment volume into more parts and decrease the treatment time per applicator set-up; the other is to treat only part of the treatment volume per session. The latter may be preferable, as the time-consuming procedure of treatment equipment set-up and the heating time required to reach the desired temperature distribution otherwise will become larger in relation to the actual treatment time. In patients who are not fit enough to tolerate two treatment sessions of 1 h, this procedure may be the only way to treat the whole volume. That an approach in which a series of hyperthermia treatments is applied, during each session, to only part of the tumour volume, and in which each part of the tumour receives only one or a few treatments, can be very successful, has been demonstrated by ENGIN et al. (1993). In a group of 23 patients treated in combination with radiation doses of 32–58 Gy (mean 42.4 Gy) a 91% complete response rate was achieved.

3.6 The Future for Hyperthermia in Breast Cancer

It is of prime importance for the efficacy of hyperthermia to be established in randomized studies, for both primarily inoperable and recurrent tumours.

One possible situation where thermoradiotherapy may become standard is that of a recurrent tumour in a previously irradiated area. There appears to be a trend toward a decreasing incidence of such patients. This can be explained by the increased application of conservative therapy as the primary treatment. A local recurrence following conservative treatment will be treated by breast amputation. By the time a secondary recurrence has developed, the chance that the patient will have developed distant metastases too will be increased, simply due to the longer disease history. Systemic treatment will then be preferable. Nevertheless, it can be expected that there will always be a group of patients for whom thermoradiotherapy can be used with the aim of improving local palliation.

As a result of the screening programs ongoing in many countries in the Western world, the incidence of inoperable breast cancer will decrease as well. When the efficacy of hyperthermia has been proven, additional hyperthermia may be added to radiotherapy in less advanced cases, too, with the aim of increasing the possibilities for conservative therapy and/or improving cosmetic results. The latter could be the case when the radiation doses needed to achieve local control can be decreased, with a concomitant reduction in the development of late toxicity.

3.7 Conclusion

For many years it has been claimed that hyperthermia has a beneficial effect when given in conjunction with radiotherapy in patients with breast cancer. Such a beneficial effect has been indicated by (a) treatment outcomes in comparisons of response to radiotherapy alone versus combined treatment, (b) comparisons of combined treated patients with historical controls and (c) positive dose-effect relationships for hyperthermia dose parameters. However, only recently has a beneficial effect of additional hyperthermia been convincingly proven for patients with breast cancer recurring in previously irradiated areas. For patients with recurring or primarily inoperable breast cancer, treated in combination with full-dose radiotherapy, the data are less convincing. In these patient groups, more results of larger randomised studies are warranted.

3.8 Summary

- Most of the patients treated with superficial hyperthermia suffer from breast cancer. In this type of tumour, local control is important, mainly for the patient's quality of life.
- Overall, the side-effects of additional hyperthermia appear acceptable. Radiation toxicity observed following combined treatment generally is similar to that following radiation alone. Thermal burns, which mainly develop in

areas with decreased sensitivity, therefore cause only slight inconvenience to the patient and often do not require intensive treatment.

- For the combination of hyperthermia with relatively low doses of re-irradiation for recurrent breast cancer, there is convincing evidence of a worthwhile beneficial effect of hyperthermia. At present, the combined treatment has therefore become standard for this situation in various institutes.
- For hyperthermia in combination with a primary, conventionally scheduled full dose of radiotherapy, more results from randomised studies in patients with either recurrent or primarily inoperable breast cancer are necessary. One problem concerning these patient groups may be the inadequacy of the treatment techniques used to induce hyperthermia.
- So far, standard addition of chemotherapy to radiation plus hyperthermia is not indicated, since an increase in local control rate has not been demonstrated and the toxicity may be enhanced by this third modality.
- The hyperthermia treatment technique, concerning both the achieved SAR distribution within the tissues and the technique of skin temperature control, appears of considerable importance for both probability of local control and toxicity.

References

Amalric R, Santamaria F, Robert F, et al. (1982) Radiation therapy with or without primary limited surgery for operable breast cancer: a 20 year experience at the Marseilles Cancer Institute. Cancer 49: 30–34

Arcangeli G, Casale C, Colistro F, Benassi M, Lovisolo G, Begnozzi L (1991) One versus four heat treatments in combination with radiotherapy in metastatic mammary carcinoma. Int J Radiat Oncol Biol Phys 21: 1569–1574

Arriagada R, Mouriesse H, Sarrazin D, Clark RM, Deboer G (1985) Radiotherapy alone in breast cancer. I. Analysis of tumor parameters, tumor dose and local control: the experience of the Gustave-Roussy Institute and the Princess Margaret Hospital. Int J Radiat Oncol Biol Phys 11: 1751–1757

Bedwinek JM (1984) Adjuvant irradiation for early breast cancer. An ongoing controversy. Cancer 53: 729–739

Bedwinek JM, Fineberg B, Lee J, Ocwieza M (1981a) Analysis of failures following local treatment of isolated local-regional recurrence of breast cancer. Int J Radiat Oncol Biol Phys 7: 581–585

Bedwinek JM, Lee J, Fineberg B, Ocwieza M (1981b) Prognostic indicators in patients with isolated local-regional recurrence of breast cancer. Cancer 47: 2232–2235

Bonadonna G, Valagussa P (1987) Current status of adjuvant chemotherapy for breast cancer. Semin Oncol 14: 8–22

Bornstein BA, Scott Zouranjian P, Hansen JL, Teicher BA, Svensson GK, Fraser SM, Gelwan LA (1992) Combined radiation therapy, hyperthermia, and systemic therapy in patients with local-regional recurrence of breast cancer. In: Gerner EW, Cetas TC (eds) Hyperthermic oncology, vol II. Arizona Board of Regents, pp 329–331

Bouchard J (1985) Advanced cancer of the breast treated primarily with irradiation. Radiology 84: 823–842

Broekmeyer-Reurink MP, Rietveld PJM, van Rhoon GC, van der Zee J (1992) Some practical notes on documentation of superficial hyperthermia treatment. Int J Hyperthermia 8: 401–406

Bruckman JE, Harris JR, Levene MB, et al. (1979) Results of treating stage III carcinoma of the breast by primary radiation therapy. Cancer 43: 985–993

Buzdar AU, McNeese MD, Hortobagyi GN, et al. (1990) Is chemotherapy effective in reducing the local failure rate in patients with operable breast cancer? Cancer 65: 394–399

Chu FCH, Lin FJ, Kim JH, Huh SH, Garmatis CJ (1976) Locally recurrent carcinoma of the breast. Results of radiation therapy. Cancer 37: 2677–2681

Deutsch M, Parsons JA, Mittal BB (1986) Radiation therapy for local-regional recurrent breast carcinoma. Int J Radiat Oncol Biol Phys 12: 2061–2065

Dragovic J, Seydel HG, Sandhu T, Kolosvary A, Blough J (1989) Local superficial hyperthermia in combination with low-dose radiation therapy for palliation of locally recurrent breast carcinoma. J Clin Oncol 7: 30–35

DuBois JB, Hay M, Bordure G (1990) Superficial microwave-induced hyperthermia in the treatment of chest wall recurrences in breast cancer. Cancer 66: 848–852

Dunlop PRC, Hand JW, Dickinson RJ, Field SB (1986) An assessment of local hyperthermia in clinical practice. Int J Hyperthermia 2: 39–50

Emami B, Myerson RJ, Cardenes H, et al. (1992) Combined hyperthermia and irradiation in the treatment of superficial tumors: results of a prospective randomized trial of hyperthermia fractionation. Int J Radiat Oncol Biol Phys 24: 145–152

Engin K, Tupchong L, Waterman FM, Komarnicky L, Mansfield CM, Leeper DB (1993) "Patchwork" fields in thermoradiotherapy for extensive chest wall recurrences of breast carcinoma. Breast Cancer Res Treat 27: 263–270

Fletcher GH, Montague ED (1966) The primary management of breast cancer. In: Fletcher GH (ed) Textbook of radiotherapy. Lea & Febiger, Philadelphia, pp 336–362

Fuwa N, Morita K, Kimura C, Aoyama K, Muroga M, Yamamoto A (1986) Combined treatment of radiotherapy and local hyperthermia using 8 MHz R-F wave for advanced carcinoma of the breast. In: Onoyama Y (ed) Hyperthermic Oncology '86 in Japan. Proceedings of the 23rd annual meeting of the Japanese Society of Hyperthermic Oncology, pp 337–338

Gabriele P, Orecchia R, Ozzello F, Melano A, Tseron V, Perotti B (1987) Hyperthermia alone or combined with radiotherapy in the treatment of recurrences of pretreated tumours (110 sites). Int J Hyperthermia 3: 562–563

González-González D, van Dijk JDP, Blank LECM (1988) Chestwall recurrences of breast cancer: results of combined treatment with radiation and hyperthermia. Radiother Oncol 12: 95–103

Haagensen CD, Stout AP (1943a) Carcinoma of the breast. II. Criteria of operability (cont). Ann Surg 118: 859–870

Haagensen CD, Stout AP (1943b) Carcinoma of the breast. II. Criteria of operability (cont). Ann Surg 118: 1032–1051

Hetzel FW, Mattielo J (1988) Interactions of hyperthermia with other modalities. In: Paliwal BR, Hetzel FM, Dewhirst MW (eds) Medical physics monograph no. 16. Biological, physical and clinical aspects of hyperthermia. American Institute of Physics, pp 30–56

Hirn-Stadler B, Eilenberger M (1990) Pleural effusion in patients with isolated chest wall recurrences of breast cancer. Strahlenther Onkol 166: 784–786

Hofman P, Lagendijk JJW, Schipper J (1984) The combination of radiotherapy with hyperthermia in protocolized clinical studies. In: Overgaard J (ed) Hyperthermic oncology 1984, vol 1. Taylor & Francis, London Philadelphia, pp 379–382

Hofman P, Knol RGF, Lagendijk JJW, Schipper J (1989) Thermoradiotherapy of primary breast carcinoma. Int J Hyperthermia 5: 1–12

Horwich A (1981) The role of radiotherapy in locally advanced and metastatic breast cancer. In: Coombes RC, Powles TJ, Ferd HT, Gazet JC (eds) Breast cancer management: the experience of the combined breast clinic. Academic Press, London, pp 227–266

Hurley SF, Huggins RM, Snyder RD, Bishop JF (1992) The cost of breast cancer recurrences. Br J Cancer 65: 449–455

International Consensus Meeting on Hyperthermia, Final Report (1990) Int J Hyperthermia 6: 837–877

Jo S, Hiraoka M, Akuta K, Nishimura Y, Nagata Y, Takahashi M, Abe M (1987) Clinical results of thermoradiotherapy for breast cancer. In: Onoyama Y (ed) Hyperthermic oncology '86 in Japan. Mag Bros Inc., pp 339–340

Kapp DS, Mever JL (1990) Clinical hyperthermic practice: non-invasive heating. In: Field SB, Hand JB (eds) An introduction to the practical aspects of clinical hyperthermia. Taylor & Francis, London, pp 143–171

Kapp DS, Cox RS, Fessenden P, Meyer JL, Prionas SD, Lee ER, Bagshaw MA (1992) Parameters predictive for complications of treatment with combined hyperthermia and radiation therapy. Int J Radiat Oncol Biol Phys 22: 999–1008

Kapp DS, Barnett TA, Cox RS, Lee ER, Lohrbach A, Fessenden P (1991) Hyperthermia and radiation therapy of local-regional recurrent breast cancer: prognostic factors for response and local control of diffuse or nodular tumors. Int J Radiat Oncol Biol Phys 20: 1147–1164

Kjellen E, Lindholm CE, Nilsson P (1988) Radiotherapy in combination with hyperthermia in recurrent or metastatic mammary carcinomas. In: Sugahara T, Saito M (eds) Hyperthermic Oncology 1988, vol 2. Taylor & Francis, London, pp 426–429

Laramore GE, Griffin TW, Parker RG, Gerdes AJ (1978) The use of electron beams in treating local recurrence of breast cancer in previously irradiated fields. Cancer 41: 991–995

Levitt SH (1983) Patterns of failure in breast cancer. Cancer Treat Symp 2: 123–131

Lindholm CE, Kjellen E, Nilsson P, Hertzman S (1987) Microwave-induced hyperthermia and radiotherapy in human superficial tumours: clinical results with a comparative study of combined treatment versus radiotherapy alone. Int J Hyperthermia 3: 393–411

Lindholm CE, Kjellen E, Nilsson P (1992) A randomized trial on one versus two hyperthermia sessions per week combined with low dose radiotherapy in superficial malignant tumours. In: Gerner EW (ed) Hyperthermic Oncology 1992, vol I. Arizona Board of Regents, Tucson, Az, p 372

Lyng H, Monge OR, Bohler PJ, Rofstad EK (1991a) Relationships between thermal dose and heat-induced tissue and vascular damage after thermoradiotherapy of locally advanced breast carcinoma. Int J Hyperthermia 7: 403–415

Lyng H, Monge OR, Bohler RJ, Rofstad EK (1991b) Changes in temperatures and thermal doses with fraction number during hyperthermic treatment of locally advanced breast carcinoma. Int J Hyperthermia 7: 815–825

Manning MR, Cetas TC, Miller RC, Oleson JR, Connor WG, Gerner EW (1982) Clinical hyperthermia: results of a phase 1 trial employing hyperthermia alone or in combination with external beam or interstitial radiotherapy. Cancer 49: 205–216

Masanuga S, Hiraoka M, Takahashi M, et al. (1990) Clinical results of thermoradiotherapy for locally advanced and/or recurrent breast cancer – comparison of results with radiotherapy alone. Int J Hyperthermia 6: 487–497

Myerson RJ, Perez CA, Emami B, Straube W, Kuske RR, Leybovich L, Von Gerichten D (1990) Tumor control in long-term survivors following superficial hyperthermia. Int J Radiat Oncol Biol Phys 18: 1123–1129

Overgaard J (1989) The current and potential role of hyperthermia in radiotherapy. Int J Radiat Oncol Biol Phys 16: 535–549

Perez CA, Kuske RR, Emami B, Fineberg B (1986) Irradiation alone or combined with hyperthermia in the treatment of recurrent carcinoma of the breast in the chest wall. A non-randomized comparison. Int J Hyperthermia 2: 179–187

Perez CA, Gillespie B, Pajak T, Hornback NB, Emami B, Rubin P (1989) Quality assurance problems in clinical hyperthermia and their impact on therapeutic outcome: a report by the radiation therapy oncology group. Int J Radiat Oncol Biol Phys 16: 551–558

Phromratanapongse P, Steeves RA, Severson SB, Paliwal BR (1991) Hyperthermia and irradiation for locally recurrent previously irradiated breast cancer. Strahlenther Onkol 167: 93–97

Podgorsak EB, Pla M, Kim TH, Freeman CR (1981) Center-blocked field technique for treatment of extensive chest wall disease. Int J Radiat Oncol Biol Phys 7: 1465–1471

Rosenman J, Bernard S, Kober C, Leland W, Varia M, Newsome J (1986) Local recurrences in patients with breast cancer at the North Carolina Memorial Hospital (1970–1982). Cancer 57: 1421–1425

Ruy Ying L, Shi-yin L, Tian-ze Z (1990) Assessment of combined thermoradiotherapy in recurrent or advanced carcinoma of the breast. In: Bicher HI (ed) Consensus on hyperthermia for the 1990's. Plenum Press, New York, pp 521–523

Sannazzari GL, Gabriele P, Orecchia R, Tseroni V (1989) Results of hyperthermia, alone or combined with irradiation, in chest wall recurrences of breast cancer. Tumori 75: 284–288

Savchenko NE, Zhakov IG, Fradkin SZ, Zhavrid EA (1987) The use of hyperthermia in oncology (in Russian). Med Radiol (Mook) 32: 19–23

Schwaibold F, Fowble BL, Solin LJ, Schultz DJ, Goodman RL (1991) The results of radiation therapy for isolated local regional recurrences afrer mastectomy. Int J Radiat Oncol Biol Phys 21: 299–310

Scott RS, Johnson RJR, Story KV, Clay L (1984) Local hyperthermia in combination with definitive radiotherapy: increased tumor clearance, reduced recurrence rate in extended follow-up. Int J Radiat Oncol Biol Phys 10: 2119–2123

Scott RS, Perez CA, Johnson RJR, Hornback, NB, Luk KH (1985) Hyperthermia and radiotherapy in the treatment of recurrent adenocarcinoma of the breast. Int J Radiat Oncol Biol Phys 11

Scott R, Gillespie B, Perez CA, et al. (1988) Hyperthermia in combination with definitive radiation therapy: results of a phase I/II RTOG study. Int J Radiat Oncol Biol Phys 15: 711–716

Seegenschmiedt MH, Karisson UL, Sauer R, et al. (1989) Superficial chest wall recurrences of breast cancer: prognostic treatment factors for combined radiation therapy and hyperthermia. Radiology 173: 551–558

Solin LJ (1992) The treatment of local-regional recurrence of carcinoma of the breast after mastectomy. Int J Radiat Oncol Biol Phys 23: 473–475

Suit HD (1982) Potential for improving survival rates for the cancer patient by increasing the efficacy of treatment of the primary lesion. Cancer 50: 1227–1234

UR, Noell T, Woodward KT, Worde BT, Fishburn RI, Miller LS (1980) Microwave-induced local hyperthermia in combination with radiotherapy of human malignant tumors. Cancer 45: 638–646

van der Zee J, Treurniet-Donker AD, The SK, et al. (1988) Low dose reirradiation in combination with hyperthermia: a palliative treatment for patients with breast cancer recurring in previously irradiated areas. Int J Radiat Oncol Biol Phys 15: 1407–1413

van der Zee J, van Rhoon GC, Verloop-van 't Hof EM, van der Ploeg SK, Rietveld PJM, van den Berg AP (1992) The importance of adequate heating techniques for therapeutic outcome. In: Gerner EW, Cetas TC (eds) Hyperthermic oncology 1992, II, pp 349–352

van der Zee J, Koper PCM, van den Berg AP (1993) Results of hyperthermia and radiotherapy in recurrent breast cancer. In: Gerner EW, Cetas TC (eds) Hyperthermic oncology 1992, vol II. pp 317–319

Vernon CC, van der Zee J (1993) Update on the combined MRC/ESHO randomized phase III trial. In: Gerner EW, Cetas TC (eds) Hyperthermic oncology 1992, vol II: Arizona Board of Regents, pp 335–338

Vernon CC, van der Zee J, Liu FF (1994) Hyperthermia as an addition to radiation vs radiation alone in the treatment of breast carcinoma – results of a collaborative phase III trial. Abstract, 14th ESHO

Vora N, Shaw S, Forell B, et al. (1986) Primary radiation combined with hyperthermia for advanced stage III–IV and inflammatery carcinoma of the breast. Endocuritherap Hyperthermia Oncol 2: 101–106

Williams CJ, Buchanan RB (eds) (1987) The medical management of breast cancer. Castle House Publications, England

Zamboglou N, Kolotas C, Audretsch M, Rezal K, Muskalla K, Schnabel G, Schmidt G (1993) Hyperthermia and simultaneous radio-chemotherapy with mitoxantrone followed by salvage surgery in locally advanced breast cancer. Abstracts of the Hyperthermia in Clinical Oncology Meeting, Munich, Germany

4 Thermoradiotherapy for Head and Neck Tumors

R. VALDAGNI and M. AMICHETTI

CONTENTS

4.1 Introduction

Local or regional failure in patients with head and neck tumors strongly conditions survival and adversely influences quality of life. Several therapeutic modalities used alone or, as is more usual, in combination, including hyperthermia, have been explored as means of improving clinical results and avoiding local-regional failures, particularly in patients with advanced lesions.

The early experience with modern hyperthermia for head and neck tumors dates back to the mid-1970s with the Australian report by HOLT (1975). Although criticisms were raised concerning "the disparate treatment regimens" utilized and "uncertainties about the precise temperature elevations achieved" (CALDWELL 1979), Holt and co-workers' reports showed superior local control and crude survival in patients treated with the combination of external hyperthermia and irradiation as compared with patients receiving irradiation alone (HOLT and NELSON 1985; HOLT and STANFORD 1986). However, Arcangeli's clinical work on head and neck lymph nodes in the late 1970s (ARCANGELI et al. 1980a) is considered by the oncology community to be the first real evidence of the effectiveness of external hyperthermia in combination with radiation therapy.

The interest generated by the attempt to improve local control rates in bulky and locally advanced lesions using the cytotoxic and radiosensitizing properties of hyperthermia has led in the past decade to a flourishing of clinical studies. Most have focused on the treatment of lymph nodes: in fact it was at once recognized that state of the art external technology could not homogeneously heat a target positioned at a depth greater than 3–4 cm. To overcome the limited penetration depth of the external approach, the utilization of interstitial heating, possibly combined with external hyperthermia, has also been proposed (TUPCHONG et al. 1988; PEREZ and EMAMI 1989; MITTAL et al. 1990). These techniques are described in Chap. 15.

Heating of head and neck primaries is still hampered by both technological and thermometry limitations. The invasiveness of thermal measurement procedures continues to represent a significant clinical problem with respect to treatment complexity and reproducibility and patient tolerance. Nonetheless, the routine application of rigorous quality assurance procedures (DEWHIRST et al. 1990; HAND 1990), the optimization of hyperthermia treatments with respect to catheter placement (ENGIN et al. 1992b), treatment planning (CRISTOFORETTI et al. 1989), and the development of site-specific applicators (GROSS et al. 1990; LEYBOVICH et al. 1990; NISHIMURA et al.

R. VALDAGNI, MD, Divisione di Radioterapia Oncologica, Clinica S. Pio X, Via F Nava 31, I-20159 Milano, Italy, and Istituto per la Ricerca Scientifica e Tecnologica, Trento, Italy
M. AMICHETTI, MD, Centro Oncologico, Ospedale S. Chiara, I-38100 Trento, Italy

1990) should optimize hyperthermic treatments of head and neck tumors.

As mentioned above, because of their superficial or semideep location, the greatest experience of hyperthermia in the head and neck region is in the treatment of locally advanced inoperable neck lymph nodes, where hyperthermia is used as an adjuvant to conventional or hypofractionated palliative radiation and to conventional radical radiation (VALDAGNI and KAMATA 1989; VALDAGNI 1990). The utilization of heat alone (SANNAZZARI et al. 1989) or in combination with non-conventional fractionated irradiation (ARCANGELI et al. 1980b) has rarely been explored. Similarly, clinical studies of hyperthermia combined with chemotherapy utilized with cytotoxic intent (ARCANGELI et al. 1980c) or as a radiosensitizer (ARCANGELI et al. 1980b) are scanty.

In the 1990s there has been renewed interest in non-conventional irradiation fractionation schemes (COX et al. 1990; FOWLER 1992; HORIOT et al. 1992; PETERS and ANG 1992) and in the combination of cytotoxic chemotherapy with surgery and/or irradiation (VOKES 1992; JASSEM et al. 1992; DIMERY and HONG 1993), and the utilization of hyperthermia in patients with head and neck primaries and metastatic regional disease will have to be confronted and possibly integrated with these emerging therapeutic modalities.

4.2 Clinical Experience with Hyperthermia Alone

The first evidence of the efficacy of heat alone in the treatment of head and neck tumors was provided by the 1866 report by Busch, who observed the clinical regression of a facial sarcoma as a consequence of hyperpyrexia caused by erysipelas.

The cytotoxic activity of hyperthermia alone has been sporadically studied in the clinic. Table 4.1 summarizes clinical experience reported in the literature, revealing that the average complete response rate in previously irradiated patients is approximately 10%. A tumor complete response rate of approximately 11% and a partial response rate of 20% were noted in 35 patients affected by head and neck recurrent cancers and treated by the University of Torino group (GABRIELE et al. 1990). They also noted that the combination of Lonidamine with heat seemed to increase the complete response rate (GABRIELE et al. 1991). The inability when using hyperthermia to translate early response into long-term local control rates (actuarial probability of complete response at 2 years: <4%) tends to limit the utilization of heat alone to local-regional recurrences not amenable to other treatments (GABRIELE et al. 1990; VALDAGNI 1990). However, when using hyperthermia to treat head and neck tumors with a merely palliative intent, it would seem reasonable to combine it with other therapeutic modalities (VALDAGNI 1990).

Table 4.1. Clinical results with hyperthermia alone in previously irradiated patients with head and neck cancer

Author (s)	No. of patients/lesions	Heating device	Results	Toxicity
MARMOR and HAHN (1978)	14[a]	US	2 CR, 7 PR	Burn (1)
CORRY et al. (1982)	3	US (1–3 MHz)	1 CR, 2 PR	n.a.
MANNING et al. (1982)	n.a.	NW (915–2450 MHz) RF (0.5–3.3 MHz)	2 CR, 1 PR	Minor blistering
JAULERRY et al. (1989)	18[b]	RF (13.56 MHz)	0 CR, 0 PR	n.a.
LELE et al. (1989)	24	US (0.5–5 MHz)	3 CR, 12 PR	2 pts. "Transient (*toxicity*) and related to an atrophic condition of the skin"
GABRIELE et al. (1990)	35	MW (434–915 MHz)	4 CR, 7 PR	Necrosis (1), blistering (3), infection (7)[c]

US, Ultrasound; MW, microwave; RF, radiofrequency; CR, complete response; PR, partial response; n.a. not available; pts., patients
[a] Nine evaluable cases
[b] Primary tumors and nodes
[c] Toxicity evaluable in 31 of the 35 pts. (SANNAZZARI et al. 1989)

4.3 Clinical Experience with Hyperthermia Combined with Irradiation

With the exception of the few clinical trials focused on head and neck tumors, the analysis of clinical studies with hyperthermia and radiation is frequently hampered by the fact that important variables in these phase I–II reports, i.e., histology, status of tumors undergoing the combined treatment (primary or recurrent tumors, metastatic lymph nodes or cutaneous/subcutaneous metastases), primary site of metastatic disease, heating methods and variables, and radiation variables, are often confusingly and/or insufficiently described (OVERGAARD 1989a, 1990).

Clinical studies reporting on thermoradiotherapy of a limited mumber of head and neck tumors among groups of patients with miscellaneous tumors and clinical trials not clearly evaluable for the above-mentioned reasons are excluded from the following analysis.

4.3.1 Primary Tumors

Clinical experience with the combination of hyperthermia and radiation therapy in primary tumors is very limited in the Western world and generally involves the treatment of persistent or recurrent primary cancers located at a depth of less than 3–4 cm, again reflecting our technological inability to heat a nonsuperficial target adequately.

4.3.1.1 Salivary Gland Tumors

Salivary gland tumors represent the most studied superficial or semideep primary neoplasms. Clinical results appear good enough to warrant further studies: a clinical complete response rate of 73% and a partial response rate of 27% have been noted in a bi-institutional study performed in Torino and Trento on 19 advanced or recurrent parotid tumors (GABRIELE et al. 1995).

Reporting on the combined palliative treatment of previously irradiated, persistent or recurrent adenoid cystic carcinomas of the salivary glands, BARNETT et al. (1990) observed excellent local responses in six lesions (two of which were heated with interstitial hyperthermia). All exhibited complete tumor regression and only two showed local failure at 9 and 30 months of follow-up. Excellent results were also noted in Heidelberg by WEISCHEDEL and WIELAND (1987) in the radical treatment of 16 advanced adenoid cystic carcinomas: they observed 100% complete responses compared with 61% in 28 patients treated with irradiation alone in a nonrandomized fashion. A survival difference at 5 years (50% versus 37.5%) favoring the combined treatment was also pointed out.

4.3.1.2 Other Primary Tumors

Sixty-five patients with previously untreated squamous cell carcinoma of the head and neck were managed in a randomized fashion with radical irradiation alone or in combination with 27.12-MHz diathermy by DATTA et al. (1990). Superior tumor control was noted in the combined treatment arm despite the limited number of patients treated; the difference in complete response rates, 73% vs 43%, was statistically significant ($P = 0.02$). Superior 18-month disease-free survival in stage III and IV patients was also reported (25% vs 8%, $P = 0.03$), as shown in Fig. 4.1.

With the exception of the work of KRISHNAMURTHI et al. (1990), discussed in Sect. 4.5, the aforementioned trial represents the only randomized study in patients with head and neck primaries to be published in Western journals. The wide experience in the treatment of head and neck primaries accumulating in Russia is not yet

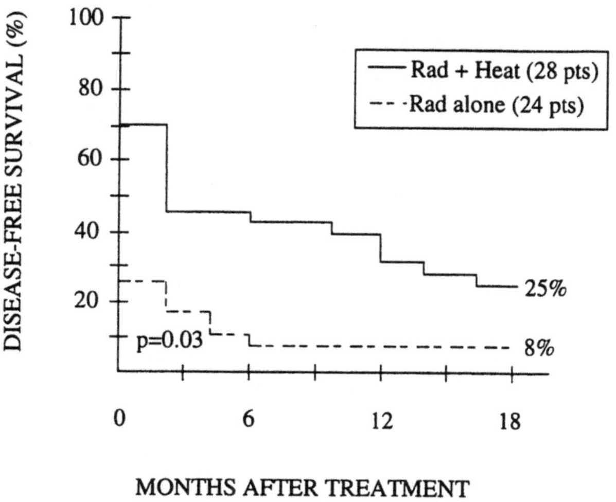

Fig. 4.1. Kaplan-Meier estimate of the probability of disease-free survival as a function of treatment for stage III and IV head and neck patients. (From DATTA et al. 1990)

fully available to the medical community and consequently scientific evaluation is still pending.

Few data are available on the treatment of primary recurrent or persistent malignant melanomas located in the head and neck region. Hypofractionated or conventional irradiation at total doses of 13–66 Gy and at doses per fraction of 2–8 Gy has been used in combination with external hyperthermia. Reported local control rates were in the range of 36% to 59% (EMAMI et al. 1988; ENGIN et al. 1992a).

Other superficial head and neck tumors (basal cell carcinoma, squamous cell carcinoma, Merkel cell carcinoma, and lymphomas) have only rarely been treated (PEREZ et al. 1987; TSUKIYAMA et al. 1987; HOWARD et al. 1987; KNOX and KAPP 1988; ORECCHIA et al. 1989; PETERSEN and KAPP 1990; URBON et al. 1990). Eye tumors will be considered in Chap. 13.

4.3.2 Metastatic Lymph Nodes and Cutaneous/Subcutaneous Metastases

Metastatic squamous cell lymph nodes represent the most frequently treated disease in the head and neck region. The reasons for this appear to be their superficial location (and consequently their potential heatability) and the clinical need to try to increase the response rates achieved with conventional modalities in advanced disease. As a matter of fact, it is well known that fixed, large, widely necrotic nodes are difficult to manage with conventional or interstitial irradiation, surgery, chemotherapy or combinations thereof (FEE et al. 1983; GOFFINET et al. 1984; MENDENHALL et al. 1986; BERNIER and BATAINI 1986; MCCAFFREY 1991; DIMERY and HONG 1993). Failure to achieve regional control in this patient population strongly affects survival and morbidity through the devastating effects of uncontrolled neck disease.

4.3.2.1 Palliative Irradiation and Hyperthermia

Several retrospective and prospective studies have underlined the clinical efficacy of hyperthermia combined with low to moderate doses of conventional or hypofractionated irradiation in previously treated patients. Prescribed total irradiation dose appears to be in the range of 17–60 Gy, with most of the trials utilizing doses of 20–45 Gy. Data from the literature indicate that nodal control can still be considered a realistic goal of the combined therapy and suggest that local control in previously irradiated head and neck metastatic squamous cell lymph nodes is still possible in approximately one-third of patients (VALDAGNI and KAMATA 1989). A review of clinical experience with hyperthermia and low to moderate doses of irradiation in patients with neck lymph nodes is shown in Table 4.2.

The only available randomized phase III study will palliative doses of radiation therapy is RTOG 81-04 with 113 head and neck lesions treated with radiotherapy alone (60 cases) or radiotherapy plus heat (53 cases) (PEREZ et al. 1989b). This report did not show an advantage of the combined treatment over radiotherapy alone. Several possible reasons for the lack of benefit were pointed out by the RTOG (PEREZ et al. 1991) and by others (OLESON 1989; MYERSON et al. 1990). It is advisable to refer to these critical reviews for a better comprehension of this negative study.

Neck disease of histologies other than squamous cell carcinoma, such as melanoma, adenocarcinoma, sarcoma, and Hodgkin's lymphoma, have rarely been the object of clinical experiences and consequently they will not be discussed in this chapter (PEREZ et al. 1987, 1989a; VALDAGNI and AMICHETTI 1987; HOFMAN 1987; SANNAZZARI et al. 1990; PETERSEN and KAPP 1990).

With respect to treatment morbidity, acute toxicity appears acceptable, particularly when hyperthermia is combined with conventionally fractionated radiotherapy. Nonetheless, ARCANGELI et al. (1984) and HOWARD et al. (1987) reported an increased skin reaction when hypofractionated irradiation (4 Gy, twice a week) was used. The most frequently reported events are thermal burn and necrosis or ulceration. They can be caused by the poor vascularization of previously irradiated regions, but it must be underlined that ulceration should also be considered an inevitable consequence of tumor clearance in a widely infiltrating superficial recurrent lesion.

Late sequelae are seldom described due to the poor survival of this patient population. Fibrosis, ulceration, and bone necrosis are the only such toxicities to be mentioned. The type, rate, and severity of chronic cutaneous and subcutaneous side-effects appear similar to those observed with irradiation as the sole modality (PREVOST et al. 1992; PEREZ et al. 1987; AMICHETTI et al. 1987;

Table 4.2. Low/moderate doses of irradiation and hyperthermia: clinical experience in squamous cell lymph nodes

Author(s)	No. of patients/lesions	Previous irradiation		Hyperthermia device	XRT (Gy)		Clinical results (%)	LC (%)	Survival (years)	Notes
		% cases	XRT dose(Gy)		TD	DpF				
NAWALKHA et al. (1979)	10	–	–	RF	30–50	2	CR 50 PR 50	–	–	–
LUK et al. (1984)	37	n.a.	n.a.	MW (915–2450 MHz)	17–44	2.5–4	CR 61.1 PR 13.9	–	–	–
IRISH et al. (1986)	12*	100%	45–65	RF (13.56 MHz)	20–40	HFx	CR 58 PR 17	–	–	* Primary tumors and nodes
PEREZ et al. (1987)	86*	75%	50–65	MW (915 MHz)	20–45	4	CR 39.5 PR 36	84	–	* Only measurable SCC considered
LINDHOLM et al. (1987)	11*	72%	24–70	MW (915–2450 MHz)	30	3	CR 36.3 PR 18.2	–	–	* 2 acinic cell ca.
STEINDORFER et al. (1987)	11*	100%	n.a.	MW (300–350 MHz)	20–32	1.8–2	CR 40 PR 40	–	–	* 10 evaluable cases
LAUCHE et al. (1987)	14	100%	n.a.	RF (13 MHz)	20–40	2	PR 44	–	–	–
EMAMI and PEREZ (1987)	15	n.a.	n.a.	MW (915 MHz)	32–40	4	n.a.	86.5	–	Plus gross surgery
HOFMAN (1987)	15/17*	0%	–	MW (434 MHz)	50	2	CR 36 PR 36	15	60% (2)	* 13/14 evaluable cases
JAULERRY et al. (1989)	83/95*	100%	65–70	RF (13.56 MHz)	24–40	4	CR 20 PR 45	–	10% (3)	* 35 primary tumors and 60 nodes
SIDDIQUI (1989)	33*	100%	≥55	MW (300 MHz)	20	2	CR 7.5 PR 25	–	–	* 27 cases evaluable at 1 month
SANNAZZARI et al. (1990)	51	100%	n.a.	MW (434–915 MHz)	24–40	4	CR 35.3 PR 25.5	20	–	–
TUPCHONG et al. (1990)	56*	~80%	av. 61	n.a.	45	3	CR 42.5 PR 49	85	–	* 47 evaluable cases
PEREZ et al. (1991)	53	~50%	50–60	MW (915 MHz)	32	4	CR 34	–	–	RTOG 81–04
PREVOST et al. (1992)	50	n.a.	n.a.	RF (13.56 MHz)	32–60	4	CR 36 PR 52	66, mean 18.5 months, NED	–	–
AMICHETTI et al. (1992)	29/30	100%	av. 54.9	MW (280–450 MHz)	16–50	2–5	CR 31 PR 48	–	9% (5)	–

TD, Total dose; DpF, dose per fraction; n.a., not available; RF, radiofrequency; MW, microwave; SCC, squamous cell carcinoma; av., average; CR, complete response; PR, partial response; XRT, radiotherapy; HFx, hyperfractionation; NED, not evidence of disease; LC, local control

Ben-Yosef and Kapp 1992). Table 4.3 describes acute and late toxicity when hyperthermia is combined with either low to moderate or radical doses of radiation.

4.3.2.2 Radical Irradiation and Hyperthermia

It is widely recognized that local control of metastatic squamous cell lymph nodes less than 3 cm in diameter frequently can be achieved with radical doses of irradiation as an elective modality (Bataini et al. 1982; Million and Cassisi 1984; Maciejevsky 1987). However, when nodes are bulky and fixed, local failure must be considered a frequent event even with irradiation doses near to normal tissue tolerance (>70 Gy at conventional fractionation) and with surgery used in combination (Fee et al. 1983; Ghossein and Bataini 1984; Peracchia and Salti 1986; Mendenhall et al. 1986; Bernier and Bataini 1986). This background has provided the clinical rationale for utilizing hyperthermia in previously untreated regional disease in head and neck patients in combination with radical irradiation at total doses of 60–70 Gy.

Only limited and nonuniform data on the combination of full-dose conventional irradiation and external hyperthermia in the treatment of neck lymph nodes are available from the literature (Table 4.4), hindering the comparison of clinical trials. These data frequently refer to the results of clinical studies organized in a context of different "pretreatment" variables (significant differences in staging systems, histologies, personal interpretation of nodal fixation, grouping of nodal stages, etc.) and of different "treatment" variables such as variation in irradiation parameters (total dose, dose per fraction, scheduling, split or continuous course, etc.), in hyperthermic parameters [applicator(s) and frequency used, temperature prescription, time prescription, sequencing of the two modalities, total and weekly number of heating sessions, etc.], and finally in both response evaluation times and response criteria.

Only two randomized phase III trials comparing radical doses of irradiation alone or combined with hyperthermia have been published on the treatment of advanced metastatic squamous cell lymph nodes (Valdagni et al. 1988a; Datta et al. 1990); the ESHO protocol 2-85 is currently in progress (Overgaard 1989b).

Valdagni et al.'s report focused on N3 (TNM-UICC 1978) metastatic epidermoid cervical lymph nodes from head and neck tumors: a statistically significant difference in complete response rates at 3 months (Valdagni et al. 1988a) and in local control at 5-year actuarial evaluation (Valdagni and Amichetti 1994) favoring the combined treatment was demonstrated (Fig. 4.2), this in spite of the limited number of cases studied (40 metastatic lymph nodes). This study also showed a statistically significant difference in 5-year actuarial survival (53% vs 0%, $P < 0.02$) in this stage IV group of patients (Fig. 4.3). Better nodal control and a survival benefit in the combined heat and radiation treatment arm was also noted in the already mentioned phase III trial by Datta et al. (1990) on the treatment of both head and neck tumors and metastatic regional disease in stage III and IV patients (Fig. 4.1). With respect to actuarial local control, evidence exists that when conventional irradiation is delivered at total doses of 40–70 Gy, nodal clearance is 58%–83% at 1 year and 68.6% at 5 years (Arcangeli et al. 1985; Perez et al. 1987; Scott et al. 1988; Datta et al. 1990; Valdagni and Amichetti 1994). The analysis of the literature on head and neck patients with metastatic nodes from squamous and nasopharyngeal primaries reveals that few data are evaluable when the considered endpoint is survival (Holt and Nelson 1985; Arcangeli et al. 1985; Wang 1989; Datta et al. 1990; Valdagni and Amichetti 1994). Table 4.5 analyzes local control and survival in head and neck patients treated with thermoradiotherapy.

The above-mentioned randomized studies reported acceptable *acute toxicity*, which was similar in irradiated plus heated or only irradiated neck regions; Valdagni and Amichetti (1994) did not observe thermal enhancement when acute toxicity was considered, the isodose TER being 1.03. Several nonrandomized trials have also underlined that when hyperthermia is combined with conventionally fractionated (1.8–2.0 Gy, five times per week) radical irradiation, acute local toxicity is minimal (Arcangeli et al. 1984, 1985; Luk et al. 1984; Oleson et al. 1984; Valdagni et al. 1986). Recently, Marino and Cividalli (1992), applying several protocols almost identical to those used in the clinic, showed that the dose-response relationships were similar for mouse skin exposed to either quasi-sim-

Table 4.3. Hyperthermia alone or combined with palliative or radical doses of irradiation in head and neck cancer: acute and chronic side-effects

Side-effect	Author(s)	XRT dose	Percentage
Blister/thermal burn	MARMOR and HAHN (1978)	HT alone	11%
	MANNING et al. (1982)	HT alone	"Minor blistering"
	SANNAZZARI et al. (1989)	HT alone	9.5%
	LUK et al. (1984)	Palliative	47% (blister plus ulceration)
	PEREZ et al. (1987)	Palliative	2.7%
	CORRY et al. (1988)	Palliative	18%
	ARCANGELI et al. (1985)	Radical	21%
	PEREZ et al. (1987)	Radical	14%
	SCOTT et al. (1988)	Radical	12%
	VALDAGNI et al. (1988a)	Radical	5%
	VROUVAS et al. (1992)	Radical	5.5%
Necrosis/ulceration	SANNAZZARI et al. (1989)	HT alone	3%
	TUPCHONG et al. (1990)	Palliative	n.a.
	AMICHETTI et al. (1992)	Palliative	6.5%
	LUK et al. (1984)	Palliative	47% (blister plus ulceration)
	PEREZ et al. (1987)	Palliative	24%
	SIDDIQUI (1989)	Palliative	"Some"
	PEREZ et al. (1987)	Radical	14%
	SCOTT et al. (1988)	Radical	7%
	VROUVAS et al. (1992)	Radical	5.5%
Bone necrosis	VALDAGNI and AMICHETTI (1994)	Radical	10%
Carotid rupture	PEREZ et al. (1989a)	Palliative	2.3%
	LINDHOLM et al. (1990)	Palliative	9%
	TUPCHONG et al. (1990)	Palliative	n.a.
	VALDAGNI and AMICHETTI (1994)	Radical	5%
Local pain	IRISH et al. (1986)	Palliative	"Mild discomfort in some patients"
	LINDHOLM et al. (1987)	Palliative	"Some patients"
	CORRY et al. (1988)	Palliative	66%
	JAULERRY et al. (1989)	Palliative	"Frequent"
	AMICHETTI et al. (1992)	Palliative	20%
	VALDAGNI and AMICHETTI (1994)	Radical	15%
Facial edema	DATTA et al. (1990)	Radical	9%
Vertigo	NAWALKHA et al. (1979)	Palliative	50%
Bezold-Jarisch syndrome	SCOTT et al. (1986)	n.a.	1 case
Neurosensory reaction	SCOTT et al. (1985)	n.a.	n.a.
Fibrosis/induration	VALDAGNI et al. (1986)	Palliative and radical	8.8%
	PEREZ et al. (1987)	Palliative	14.2%
	AMICHETTI et al. (1992)	Palliative	6.5%
	SCOTT et al. (1988)	Radical	36% ("minimal")
Telangiectasis	SCOTT et al. (1988)	Radical	7%
Infection	SANNAZZARI et al. (1989)	HT alone	22.5%
	CORRY et al. (1988)	Palliative	3%
	FELDMANN et al. (1993)	n.a.	11.7%
	AMICHETTI and VALDAGNI (1995, unpublished)	Palliative and radical	1.2%
Hemorrhage	GABRIELE et al. (1995)	Palliative and radical	5%

n.a., Not available; HT, hyperthermia

Table 4.4. Radical doses of irradiation and hyperthermia: clinical experience in squamous cell lymph nodes

Author(s)	No. of patients/lesions	XRT (Gy)		Hyperthermia device	Complete response	Local control (years)	Notes
		TD	DpF				
Tan and Li (1984)	50*	>60	n.a.	MW (915–2450 MHz)	66%	–	* 50 pts. (31 nodes) were treated with doses ranging from 30–80 Gy
Arcangeli et al. (1985)	38	40–70	1.5–2 MFD	MW (500–2450 MHz)	79%	58% (2 years)	43 lesions treated with XRT alone in nonrandomized fashion: CR 42%
Valdagni et al. (1986)	19	60–70	2–2.5	MW (280–300 MHz)	68%	–	–
Perez et al. (1987)	48	48–60	2–4	MW (915 MHz)	58%	59% (1 year)	–
Scott et al. (1988)	41	60–70	1.8–2	MW (400–1000 MHz)	51%	–	* Prescribed doses
Kamata et al. (1989)	20	Up to 81	2 or 1.8–2*	RF (13 MHz) MW (433–915 MHz) RF (13.56 MHz)	35%	–	* Plus concomitant boost
Datta et al. (1990)	20	60–65	2	RF (27.12 MHz)	79%	–	Randomized study, XRT alone: 60% CR
Vrouvas et al. (1992)	37	60–70	2	MW (433 MHz)	62%	–	In ESHO 2–85 trial
Valdagni and Amichetti (1994)	21	64–70	2–2.5	MW (280–300 MHz)	83%	68.6% (5 years)	Randomized study, XRT alone: 40.9% CR
Amichetti et al. (1995)	27	69.6–76.8	1.2 b.i.d.	MW (280–300 MHz)	77%	–	–

TD, Total dose; DpF, dose per fraction; n.a., not available; RF, radiofrequency; MW, microwave; CR, complete response; PR, partial response; XRT, radiotherapy; pts., patients; MFD, multiple fraction per day

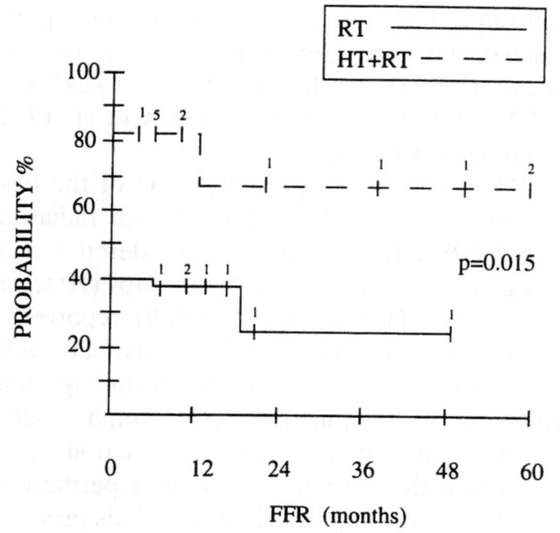

Fig. 4.2. Kaplan-Meier representation of the probability of freedom from local relapse (*FFR*) for only irradiated or heated plus irradiated neck lymph nodes. (From VALDAGNI and AMICHETTI 1994)

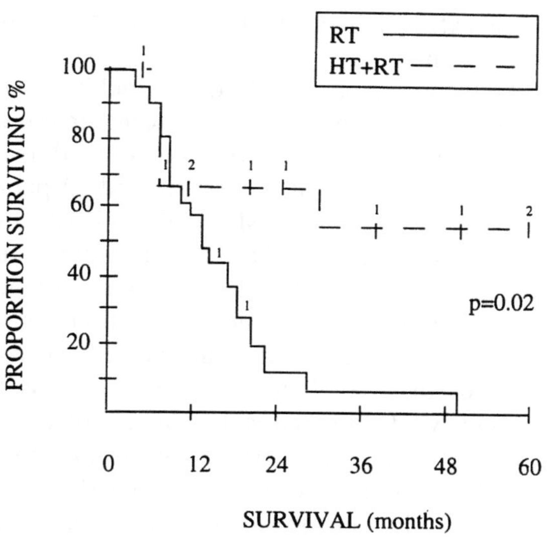

Fig. 4.3. Kaplan-Meier representation of the probability of survival in stage IV patients. (From VALDAGNI and AMICHETTI 1994)

Table 4.5. Local control and survival in patients with head and neck cancer treated with hyperthermia and palliative or radical doses of radiation

Author(s)	% Local control (months)[a]	% Survival (months)	XRT dose
HOFMAN (1987)	15 (24)	60 (24)	Palliative
PEREZ et al. (1987)	84[b]	–	Palliative
EMAMI and PEREZ (1987)	86.5 (12–50, median 18)	33 (12–50, median 18)	Palliative plus gross surgery
JAULERRY et al. (1989)	–	10 (36)	Palliative
TUPCHONG et al. (1990)	85[b]	–	Palliative
AMICHETTI et al. (1992)	5 (60)	9 (60)	Palliative
HOLT and NELSON (1985)	–	68 (36)	Radical
ARCANGELI et al. (1985)	58 (24)	–	Radical
PEREZ et al. (1987)	27 (≥6)	–	Radical
WEISCHEDEL and WIELAND (1987)	–	50 (60)	Radical
WANG (1989)	–	11.6 (60)	Radical
DATTA et al. (1990)			Radical
All patients	–	33 (18)[c]	
Stage III–IV	–	25 (18)[c]	
VALDAGNI and AMICHETTI (1994)	68.6 (60)	53 (60)	Radical

CR, Complete response; XRT, radiotherapy
[a] All patients considered
[b] Percentage of patients who achieved CR
[c] Disease-free survival

ultaneous combined treatments with one or four heating sessions or radiation alone.

Few data are available to evaluate and quantify *late toxicity*: it also appears very limited and only slightly different from that expected as a consequence of a full-dose irradiation alone (OVERGAARD 1989a; BEN-YOSEF and KAPP 1992). The already mentioned 5-year evaluation of VALDAGNI and AMICHETTI's (1994) randomized trial showed an isodose TER for late toxicity of 1.34. Chronic toxicity of hyperthermia treatments is undergoing continued observation; continuous careful surveillance is needed since information is still being accumulated. Besides local and systemic acute side-effects, Table 4.3 also examines late sequelae in the head and neck region cited in the literature when external hyperthermia is added to radical irradiation.

Only preliminary and not yet published data exist on the combined use of external microwave hyperthermia and pure hyperfractionated irradiation. AMICHETTI et al. (1995) treated 22 patients affected by N2–N3 (TNM-UICC 1987) squamous cell lymph nodes in a phase I–II feasibility study. The prescribed total dose was in the range of 69.6–76.8 Gy delivered in two fractions per day of 1.2 Gy at an interval of at least 6 h; heat was applied for a total of two to six sessions at a frequency of 280–300 MHz. Acute toxicity was minimal; complete response rate evaluated at 3 months after the end of the combined treatment was 77%, for an overall response rate of 86%. Further studies are needed to judge clinical results and to evaluate the late toxicity of this combination.

4.4 Clinical Experience with Hyperthermia Combined with Chemotherapy

Hyperthermia shows a positive interaction with several anticancer drugs in experimental studies; however, the clinical experience with thermochemotherapy is very limited (ENGELHARDT 1987; STORM 1989; DAHL and MELLA 1990). There are few clinical data on the use of local-regional hyperthermia and chemotherapy in head and neck cancer, and they have usually been reported in the context of phase I/I–II studies. The true impact of the association of hyperthermia and chemotherapy in patients with head and neck malignancies is therefore difficult to establish: data available in the literature are reviewed in Table 4.6. Phase II studies with selected chemotherapeutic agents specifically active in head and neck cancer are needed before starting controlled studies. This issue is widely discussed in Chap. 2.

4.5 Clinical Experience with Trimodality Therapy

Therapeutic potentiation of cisplatin (CDDP) and radiation by hyperthermia was first reported in a mouse tumor by DOUPLE et al. (1982). The ability of combined hyperthermia, irradiation, and chemotherapy to enhance the treatment effect provides the biological and clinical rationale for applying them in combination (HERMAN et al. 1988). Such a combination has only recently been explored in the clinic. Consequently, few reports on head and neck tumors are available for this review (HERMAN et al. 1989; KRISHNAMURTHI et al. 1990; WUST et al. 1992; PROTSYK et al. 1992; AMICHETTI et al. 1993).

CDDP, widely recognized as one of the best anticancer drugs to be combined with radiation (DEWIT 1987; BEGG 1990), is considered a promising candidate for trimodality therapy (HERMAN et al. 1988). HERMAN et al. (1989) reported a trimodality phase I–II study in patients with locally advanced malignancies, including nine head and neck squamous cell lymph nodes: radical or palliative doses of radiation were delivered with external microwave hyperthermia and 20, 30, or 40 mg/m^2 of CDDP. This protocol proved feasible, effective [50% complete response (CR) in the whole group of lesions entered in the trial], and safe. AMICHETTI et al. (1993) recently published the results of a phase I–II study on 18 squamous cell metastatic neck lymph nodes treated with conventionally fractionated radical radiation, 280- to 300-MHz external hyperthermia and 20 mg/m^2 CDDP weekly. Local toxicity was mild even if greater than in previous experience with irradiation and hyperthermia (VALDAGNI et al. 1986, 1988a); moderate systemic toxicity was also reported (three patients developed WHO grade 3 anemia). Evaluation at 3 months after the end of trimodal therapy showed a CR of 72%. Three-year actuarial nodal control was 53.5%, contributing of 3-year actuarial survival of 50%.

Preliminary clinical experience in head and neck tumors with induction polychemotherapy and subsequent trimodality therapy including CDDP (WUST et al. 1992) or with methotrexate plus irradiation and hyperthermia (PROTSYK et al. 1992) has also been reported.

The only randomized trial available is KRISHNAMURTHI et al.'s (1990) study on radiation, pepleomycin, and hyperthermia in 101 patients affected by oral squamous cell carcinoma. The addition of 8-MHz capacitive hyperthermia to radiation (55–60 Gy, 2.5 Gy three times per week) resulted in 32% CR in comparison with 61% with pepleomycin and radiation, and 69% with the three modalities combined. Acute toxicity was not enhanced by adding hyperthermia to bimodality therapy. The authors concluded that the addition of hyperthermia did not confer any benefit over irradiation plus pepleomycin in patients with oral carcinoma; however, it must be underlined that the number of patients treated in each arm was

Table 4.6. Hyperthermia and chemotherapy: clinical experience in head and neck cancer

Author(s)	No. of patients/lesions	Chemotherapy	Hyperthermia device	Results	Toxicity	Previous therapies (% cases)	Notes
Arcangeli et al. (1979)	A) 8	A) ADM 5 mg i.v. b.i.d. (daily)	MW	A) 3 CR, 5 PR	–	n.a.	CR with ADM alone: 0/8
	B) 7	B) BLM 75 mg i.v. b.i.d. (daily)		B) 3 CR, 4 PR	–		CR with BLM alone: 1/6
Steindorfer et al. (1987)	15	BLM 15 mg/m² i.m. CDDP 25 mg/m² i.v. ± 5FU 750 mg/m² i.v.	MW (300–350 MHz)	0 CR 1 PR 7 MR	–	100%	
Cruciani et al. (1987)	13*	CDDP 20 mg/m² i.v. days 1–5 BlM 10 mg/m² i.v. days 8–12 MTX 100 mg/m² i.v. day 15 + folinic acid	MW (434 MHz)	1 CR 6 PR	No local toxicity	69%	* 10 pts. with head and neck lesions
Pilepich et al. (1989)	12	BLM 15 U/m (1–2 × week)	US (1 GHz)	2 CR	Lung toxicity (3)	100%	* 6 pts. with head and neck lesions
			MW (915 MHz)	3 PR	Necrosis (1)		
Jaulerry et al. (1989)	16	CDDP 20 mg/m² days 1–4 VDS 2 mg/m² days 1 and 4 5FU 500 mg/m² days 1–4 Mito 6 mg/m² day 1	RF (13.56 MHz)	13% CR 19% PR	–	100%	
Formenti et al. (1990)	10	CDDP 100 mg/m² day 1 5FU 100 mg/m² days 1–5	MW	4 CR 5 PR	Burn (1) Severe pain (20%)	50%	Followed by irradiation or chemotherapy

n.a., Not available; VDS, vindesine; MTX, methotrexate; ADM, Adriamycin; BLM, bleomycin; Mito, mitomycin; CDDP, cisplatin; 5FU, 5-fluorouracil; MW, microwave; US, ultrasound; RF, radiofrequency; CR, complete response; PR, partial response; MR, minimal response; pts., patients

limited, that thermometry was not performed "in the later stages of therapy," and finally, that the desired temperature of 42°C in the tumor core might be insufficient to potentiate fully bleomycin cytotoxicity in the periphery of the target volume (DAHL and MELLA 1990). Tumor periphery has been shown to present higher blood flow rates in comparison with tumor core in deep tumors (SAMULSKI et al. 1987; FELDMAN et al. 1990) and in neck nodes (VALDAGNI et al. 1985).

Finally, in the field of radiosensitizing drugs, misonidazole was studied in a trimodality approach showing no benefit over the combination of irradiation and hyperthermia (ARCANGELI et al. 1985). The use of radiation plus hyperthermia and nicotinamide (J. Dragovic, personal communication, April 1993) or Lonidamine (GABRIELE et al. 1991) in patients with head and neck lesions is currently under investigation.

4.6 Clinical and Technical Parameters Influencing Response

A clear knowledge of parameters potentially influencing response is absolutely necessary to standardize, optimize, correctly evaluate, and compare irradiation plus hyperthermia trials. On the other hand, adequate follow-up in heavily pretreated head and neck lesion patients or in patients with advanced local-regional disease is not readily available, since the majority of them (a) will be affected by either systemic disease (MERINO et al. 1977; ZBAEREN et al. 1987; LEIBEL et al. 1991) or metachronous tumors in the upper respiratory/digestive tract (TEPPERMAN and FITZPATRICK 1981; AMICHETTI and SAVINO 1988), (b) will die of nonneoplastic causes mainly related to intercurrent diseases due to concomitant ethanol and tobacco abuse (WYNDER et al. 1969), or (c) will undergo subsequent systemic therapy, thus precluding any further evaluation of the outcome of the combined treatment. Nonetheless, several authors have analyzed pretreatment and treatment variables conditioning results in heated and irradiated neck nodes.

4.6.1 Pretreatment Factors

4.6.1.1 General Patient Status

Several interrelated parameters such as age, previous or concomitant nonneoplastic disease, and the metastatic spread of cancer play an important role in defining and quantifying performance status (PS). This complex variable was found to be statistically related to outcome in a group of palliatively irradiated patients with a variety of superficial lesions including metastatic neck nodes (GABRIELE et al. 1987). An outcome trend favoring high PS was also found in patients with metastatic squamous cell lymph nodes treated with palliative or radical intent (VALDAGNI et al. 1989).

4.6.1.2 Tumor Characteristics

At the present time, the role of histology as a prognostic factor cannot be assessed, since too few tumors of types other than squamous cell carcinoma have been studied. This is also true of tumor morphology (nodular, diffuse, exophytic, ulcerative), metastatic lymph nodes being the most frequently treated lesions. It is reasonable to expect a different outcome depending on whether the lymph node is capsulated or fixed, or when different T and N stages are considered (DATTA et al. 1990). And this because tumor vascularity, amount of necrosis and soft tissue involvement can influence response "per se" and because they may impact differently on our ability to heat the target volume adequately. No data are available to clarify the impact of tumor status, e.g., recurrence versus metastasis, on response (LUK et al. 1984); furthermore, the influence of the radiation dose (palliative or radical), generally delivered in combination, confounds this evaluation. Again, previously irradiated tumor bed and surrounding normal tissue may alter local vascularity and consequently the heating of the lesion.

The influence of site of disease has not been the object of evaluation: it has been reported that submaxillary nodes might have a different response to hyperthermia in comparison with other neck locations because of the possibility of cold spots existing behind bone (VALDAGNI et al. 1989). This also underlines the importance of knowing the properties and limitations of the heating applicator utilized (MYERSON et al. 1990; NISHIMURA et al. 1990).

Finally, among pretreatment variables, tumor dimension currently represents the most significant parameter negatively conditioning response (ARCANGELI et al. 1985; VALDAGNI et al. 1986; PEREZ et al. 1987; VALDAGNI and LIU 1990; PEREZ et al. 1991). Interestingly, it has also been shown that volume effect mainly influences lesions treated with irradiation alone rather than those treated with combined heat and irradiation: this finding implies that the TER increases with increasing tumor dimension (ARCANGELI et al. 1985; VALDAGNI et al. 1988b). Depth of tumor also appears to correlate with complete response (PEREZ et al. 1987). However, note that it is very important to evaluate the heating device utilized, the form of energy chosen, and the frequency of operation when the relation between tumor size and response is to be assessed: all these technical variables may condition heating patterns, and, consequently, tumor heatability (CORRY et al. 1988; MYERSON et al. 1990).

4.6.2 Treatment Factors

4.6.2.1 Radiation Parameters

Total radiation dose has been clearly demonstrated to play a significant role in the local control of heated and irradiated superficial tumors (LUK et al. 1984; VALDAGNI et al. 1988b). This variable has also been noted to influence tumor response in patients with head and neck lesions (TAN and LI 1984; VALDAGNI et al. 1986; PEREZ et al. 1987; VALDAGNI et al. 1989; VALDAGNI and LIU 1990). Nevertheless, the concomitant influence of the nonuniformity of patients in terms of previous radiation exposure, which can determine the subsequent total dose precribed, may confound the true weight of this variable as well as that of the utilized dose per fraction. Analyzing most of the literature on the use of heat in the treatment of advanced neck lymph nodes, OVERGAARD (1989a) showed a composite dose-response curve (Fig. 4.4) for irradiated and irradiated plus heated nodes, from which it is possible to derive an isoeffect TER or 1.6.

4.6.2.2 Thermal Parameters

The only thermal variables proved to be statistically correlated with local control in head and neck trials are: (a) average overall Eq 42.5°C (ARCANGELI et al. 1985), and (b) nodal average thermal gradient (defined as the difference between average maximum and average minimum temperature) (VALDAGNI et al. 1989). In particular, when the thermal gradient was less than 2.5°C, superior CR rates were observed in patients with radically irradiated and heated neck nodes.

The following variables have been found to be statistically correlated with local control of miscellaneous superficial tumors, including neck node lesions: hyperthermia exposure time (LUK et al. 1984), average lesion temperature over all sessions (SCOTT et al. 1988), and iso-SAR (MYERSON et al. 1990). Average minimum temperature and total minimum thermal dose seem to be weakly correlated with nodal control (VALDAGNI et al. 1989). By contrast, the total number and weekly number of heating sessions do not appear to be related with complete response rates (VALDAGNI et al. 1989). It should be noted that, as recently underlined by OLESON et al. (1993), to detect a 5% difference in response rate when comparing the clinical efficacy of two

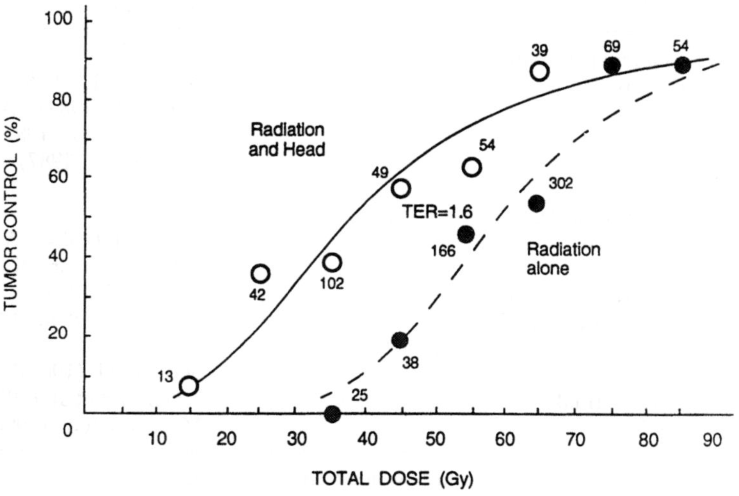

Fig. 4.4. Dose-response relationship for neck lymph nodes treated with irradiation alone or combined irradiation and heat. (From OVERGAARD 1989a)

versus six heating sessions, 1603 patients would be required in each arm of the study.

Finally, no suggestion as to the optimal sequence for the combination of hyperthermia and radiation treatments in patients with head and neck tumors can be derived from the literature; the same holds true when presently available clinical data on thermoradiotherapy for superficial and deep tumors of other sites and histologies are analyzed (Valdagni et al. 1988b).

Statistically significant prognostic factors are summarized in Table 4.7.

4.7 Acute and Late Toxicity

The combination of hyperthermia and radiation does not appear to significantly increase acute or chronic toxicity. This also seems true for the combination of chemotherapy and hyperthermia and for trimodality therapy. For the evaluation of late toxicity it is imperative that efforts be made to analyze morbidity at long-term follow-up because, at present, most patients studied have locally advanced primary or metastatic tumors, which generally limit subsequent long-term observation. As mentioned above, Table 4.3 summarizes acute local/systemic side-effects and chronic sequelae of adding hyperthermia to low to moderate or full-dose irradiation. It should be noted that the reported percentage of acute/chronic side-effects may overestimate the true frequency of events, since they may be related to a specific subset of patients. As an example, we observed two patients with bone necroses (10%) in our randomized study (Valdagni and Amichetti 1994), although they were the only two such cases (1.2%) noted among 173 cases treated in the period 1981–1992.

4.8 Summary

- Head and neck is an anatomical region frequently treated with external and interstitial hyperthermia. In particular, the preferred target is metastatic lymph nodes because of the technological limitations of available heating devices for the treatment of deeper sites.
- Heat alone has only a palliative temporary effect and hyperthermia is consequently usually combined with radiotherapy.
- The clinical experience in primary tumors is generally limited to treating superficial lesions like salivary gland tumors.
- Previously irradiated metastatic lymph nodes can be treated with palliative intent with total doses of 20–45 Gy using hypofractionated schedules with a mean complete response of 35%.
- Previously unirradiated neck nodes can be treated with definitive doses of radiotherapy with local control rates of about 70%.
- Toxicity of both palliative and curative treatments is minimal and substantially comparable to that observed with conventional irradiation alone.

Table 4.7. Hyperthermia and irradiation in head and neck cancer: statistically significant prognostic factors

Prognostic factor	Author(s)
Pretreatment variables	
Stage of disease	Datta et al. (1990)
Size of tumor	Luk et al. (1984)[a], Arcangeli et al. (1985), Valdagni et al. (1986), Perez et al. (1987), Scott et al. (1988)[a], Valdagni and Liu (1990)
Depth of tumor	Perez et al. (1987)
Treatment variables	
Radiation dose	Luk et al. (1984)[a], Valdagni et al. (1986), Perez et al. (1987), Valdagni and Kamata (1989)
Hyperthermia exposure time	Luk et al. (1984)[a]
Average overall Eq. 42.5°C	Arcangeli et al. (1985)
Average lesion temperature (≥43°C) over all sessions	Scott et al. (1988)[a]
Average thermal gradient	Valdagni et al. (1989a)
Iso-SAR	Myerson et al. (1990)[a]

[a] Miscellaneous tumors including head and neck lesions

- Current experience with the combination of hyperthermia and altered fractionation schemes, chemotherapy and chemoradiotherapy should be considered investigative.

Acknowledgements. This work was partly supported by National Research Council (C.N.R.) grant no. 901356. The authors wish to thank Miss T. Magnani and Mr. A. Micheletti for their skill in preparing this manuscript.

References

Amichetti M, Savino M (1988) Second oesophageal cancer in patients with head and neck squamous cell carcinoma. Cancer J 2: 109–111

Amichetti M, Valdagni R, Pani G, Cristoforetti L, Pontalti R (1987) Radioterapia a basse dosi e ipertermia nelle recidive neoplastiche pre-irradiate. In: Convegno Nazionale SARO, Saint Vincent (AO) 1987. Monduzzi Editore, Bologna, pp 443–452

Amichetti M, Graiff C, Bolner A, et al. (1992) Nodal recurrence in patients with previously irradiated head and neck cancer: palliative treatment with external radiotherapy and local hyperthermia. Lyon Chirurgical 88(suppl 1): 68

Amichetti M, Graiff C, Fellin G, Pani G, Bolner A, Maluta S, Valdagni R (1993) Cisplatin, hyperthermia and radiation (trimodal therapy) in patients with locally advanced head and neck tumors: a phase I–II study. Int J Radiat Oncol Biol Phys 26: 801–807

Amichetti M, Bolner A, Busana L, Fellin G, Pani G, Romano M, Valdagni R (1995) Twice a day hyperfractionated radiation therapy and local hyperthermia in squamous cell carcinoma of the head and neck. International Meeting on Progress in Radio-Oncology. ICRO-ÖGRO 5. Kogelnik HD (ed). Monduzzi Editore, pp 527–532

Arcangeli G, Cividalli A, Mauro F, Nervi C, Pavin G (1979) Enhanced effectiveness of adriamycin and bleomycin combined with local hyperthermia in neck node metastases from head and neck cancers. Tumori 65: 481–486

Arcangeli G, Barni E, Cividalli A, et al. (1980a) Effectiveness of microwave hyperthermia combined with ionizing radiation; clinical results on neck node metastases. Int J Radiat Oncol Biol Phys 6: 143–148

Arcangeli G, Barocas A, Mauro F, Nervi C, Spano' M, Tabocchini A (1980b) Multiple daily fractionation (MDF) radiotherapy in association with hyperthermia and/or misonidazole: experimental and clinical results. Cancer 45: 2707–2711

Arcangeli G, Cividalli A, Lovisolo G, Mauro F, Creton G, Nervi F, Pavin G (1980c) Effectiveness of local hyperthermia in association with radiotherapy or chemotherapy: comparison of multimodality treatments on multiple neck node metastases. In: Arcangeli G, Mauro F (eds) Hyperthermia in radiation oncology. Masson, Milan, pp 257–265

Arcangeli G, Nervi C, Cividalli A, Lovisolo GA (1984) Problems of sequence and fractionation in the clinical application of heat and radiation. Cancer Res 44(suppl): 4857s–4863s

Arcangeli G, Arcangeli GC, Guerra A, Lovisolo GA, Cividalli A, Marino C, Mauro F (1985) Tumour response to heat and radiation: prognostic variables in the treatment of neck nodes metastases from head and neck cancer. Int J Hyperthermia 3: 207–217

Barnett TA, Kapp DS, Goffinet DR (1990) Adenoid cystic carcinoma of the salivary glands. Management of recurrent advanced, or persistent disease with hyperthermia and radiation therapy. Cancer 65: 2648–2656

Bataini P, Brugere J, Bernier J, Jaulerry CH, Picot C, Ghossein NA (1982) Results of radiotherapeutic treatment of carcinoma of the pyriform sinus: experience of the Institute Curie. Int J Radiat Oncol Biol Phys 8: 1277–1286

Begg AC (1990) Cisplatin and radiation: interaction probabilities and therapeutic possibilities. Int J Radiat Oncol Biol Phys 19: 1183–1189

Ben-Yosef R, Kapp DS (1992) Persistent and/or late complications of combined radiation therapy and hyperthermia. Int J Hyperthermia 8: 733–745

Bernier J, Bataini JP (1986) Regional outcome in oropharyngeal and pharyngolaryngeal cancer treated with high dose per fraction radiotherapy. Analysis of neck disease response in 1646 cases. Radiother Oncol 6: 87–103

Busch W (1866) Über den Einfluss welchen heftigere Erysipeln zuwerden und organisierte Neubildungen ausueben. Verhandl Natur Preuss Rhein Westfäl 23: 28–30

Caldwell WL (1979) Evaluation of the Perth experience in treating with ionizing radiations and VHF (434 megahertz) radiations. Int J Radiat Oncol Biol Phys 5: 1919–1921

Corry PM, Barlogie B, Tilchen EJ, Armour EP (1982) Ultrasound-induced huperthermia for the treatment of human superficial tumors. Int J Radiat Oncol Biol Phys 8: 1225–1229

Corry PM, Jabboury K, Kong JS, Armour EP, McCraw FJ, Leduc T (1988) Evaluation of equipments for hyperthermic treatment of cancer. Int J Hyperthermia 4: 53–74

Cox JD, Pajak T, Marcial VA, et al. (1990) Dose-response for local control with hyperfractionated radiation therapy in advanced carcinomas of the upper aerodigestive tracts: preliminary report of the Radiation Therapy Oncology Group Protocol 83-13. Int J Radiat Oncol Biol Phys 18: 515–522

Cristoforetti L, Pontalti R, Antolini R, Amichetti M, Valdagni R (1989) Microwave hyperthermia (Ht) treatment planning in metastatic neck lymph-nodes: early results. In: Sugahara T, Saito M (eds) Hyperthermic oncology 1988, vol 1. Taylor and Francis, London, pp 807–808

Cruciani G, Molinari AL, Marangolo M, Morelli M, Gnani G, Mazzotti A, Mauro F (1987) Applicability of local hyperthermia as adjuvant to systemic chemotherapy. Tumori 73: 629–633

Dahl O, Mella O (1990) Hyperthermia and chemotherapeutic aspects. In: Field SB, Hand JW (eds) An introduction to the practical aspects of clinical hyperthermia. Taylor and Francis, London, pp 108–142

Datta NR, Bose AK, Kapoor HK, Gupta S (1990) Head and neck cancers; results of thermoradiotherapy versus radiotherapy. Int J Hyperthermia 6: 479–486

Dewhirst MW, Phillips TL, Samulski TV, et al. (1990) RTOG quality assurance guidelines for clinical trials

using hyperthermia. Int J Radiat Oncol Biol Phys 18: 1249–1259
Dewit L (1987) Combined treatment of radiation and *cis*-diamminedichloroplatinum (II): a review of experimental and clinical data. Int J Radiat Oncol Biol Phys 13: 403–426
Dimery IW, Hong WK (1993) Overview of combined modality therapies for head and neck cancer. J Natl Cancer Inst 85: 95–111
Douple EB, Strohbehn JW, De Sieyes DC, Alborough DP, Trembley BS (1982) Therapeutic potentiation of cisdiaminedichlorplatin (II) and irradiation by interstitial microwave hyperthermia in a mouse tumor. NCI Monogr 61: 259–262
Emami B, Perez CA (1987) Combination of surgery, irradiation, and hyperthermia in treatment of recurrences of malignant tumors. Int J Radiat Oncol Biol Phys 13: 611–613
Emami B, Perez CA, Konefal J, et al. (1988) Thermoradiotherapy of malignant melanoma. Int J Hyperthermia 4: 373–381
Engelhardt E (1987) Hyperthermia and drugs. Recent Results Cancer Res 104: 136–203
Engin K, Tupchong L, Phil D, Waterman FM, Moylan DJ, Nerlinger RE, Leeper DB (1992a) Hyperthermia and radiation in advanced malignant melanoma. Int J Radiat Oncol Biol Phys 25: 87–94
Engin K, Tupchong L, Wasterman FM, Nerlinger RE, Leeper DB (1992b) Optimization of hyperthermia with CT scanning. Int J Hyperthermia 8: 855–864
Fee WE, Goffinet DR, Paryani S, Goode RL, Levine PA, Hopp ML (1983) Intraoperative iodine 125 implants, their use in large tumors in the neck attached to the carotid artery. Arch Otolaryngol 109: 727–730
Feldmann HJ, Molls M, Hoederath A, Krümpelmann S, Romanowski R, Sack H (1990) Correlations between blood flow, thermal clearance and steady state temperatures in pelvic tumors. Strahlenther Onkol 166: 513–514
Feldmann HJ, Hoederath A, Molls M, Sack H (1993) Problems associated with CT-guided catheter insertions. Int J Hyperthermia 9: 219–225
Formenti S, Sapozink MD, Rice D, Grunberg S (1990) Thermochemotherapy in advanced head and neck cancer: preliminary results in ten patients (abstract). Third international head and neck oncology research conference. 26–28b, September 1990, Las Vegas, NV. Soc Head neck Surg A.13.4.
Fowler JF (1992) Intercomparison of new and old schedules in fractionated radiotherapy, Semin Radiat Oncol 2: 67–72
Gabriele P, Orecchia R, Melano A, Tseroni V (1987) Risposta del tumore in funzione della sede, dell'istologia e della distribuzione della temperature. In: Convegon Nazionale SARO, Saint Vincent (AO) 1987. Monduzzi Editore Bologna, pp 425–434
Gabriele P, Orecchia R, Ragona R, Tseroni V, Sannazzari GL (1990) Hyperthermia alone in the treatment of recurrences of malignant tumors. Experience with 60 lesions. Cancer 66: 2191–2195
Gabriele P, Orecchia R, Monetti U, Muñoz F, Ruo Redda MG (1991) Associazione radioterapia, ipertermia e/o lonidamina nel trattamento dei carcinomi del distretto cervico-cefalico. In: 1° Congresso Nazionale AIRO, Assisi 1991. Monduzzi Editore, Bologna, pp 637–644
Gabriele P, Amichetti M, Orecchia R, Valdagni R (1995) Hyperthermia and radiation therapy in inoperable or recurrent parotid carcinoma: a phase I–II study. Cancer 72: 908–915
Ghossein NA, Bataini P (1984) The role of radiotherapy in the treatment of neck metastases from head and neck cancer. In: Wolf GT (ed) Head and neck oncology. Martinus Nijhoff, Amsterdam pp 169–197
Goffinet DR, Fee WE, Goode RL (1984) Combined surgery and postoperative irradiation in the treatment of cervical lymph nodes. Arch Otolaryngol 110: 736–738
Gross EJ, Cetas TC, Stauffer PR, Liu RL, Lumori MLD (1990) Experimental assessment of phased-array heating of neck tumours. Int J Hyperthermia 6: 453–474
Hand JW (1990) quality assurance in hyperthermia. In: Field SB, Hand JW (eds) An introduction to the practical aspects of clinical hyperthermia. Taylor and Francis, London, pp 513–532
Herman TS, Teicher BA, Jochelson M, Clark J, Svensson G, Coleman CN (1988) Rationale for use of local hypertermia with radiation therapy and selected anticancer drugs in locally advanced human malignancies. Int J Hyperthermia 4: 143–58
Herman TS, Jochelson MS, Teicher BA, et al. (1989) A phase I–II trial of cisplatin, hyperthermia and radiation in patients with locally advanced malignancies. Int J Radiat Oncol Biol Phys 17: 1273–1279
Hofman P (1987) Hyperthermia in the head and neck cancer. In: Clinical hyperthermia: medical aspects. Drukkerij Elinkwijk, Utrecht, pp 82–92
Holt JAG (1975) The use of VHF radiowaves in cancer therapy. Australas Radiol 19: 223–241
Holt JAG, Nelson AJM (1985) Combined microwave therapy. Med J Aust 142: 7
Holt JAG, Stanford RW (1986) The synergism between hyperthermia and ionizing radiation. Br J Radiol 59: 795–796
Horiot JC, Le Fur R, N'Guyen T, et al. (1992) Hyperfractionation versus conventional fractionation in oropharyngeal carcinoma: final analysis of a randomized trial of the EORTC cooperative group of radiotherapy. Radiother Oncol 25: 231–241
Howard GCW, Sathiaseelan V, Freedman L, Blehen NM (1987) Hyperthermia and radiation in the treatment of superficial malignancy: an analysis of treatment parameters, response and toxicity. Int J Hyperthermia 3: 1–8
Irish CE, Brown J, Galen WP, et al. (1986) Thermoradiotherapy for persistent cancer in previously irradiated fields. Cancer 57: 2275–2279
Jassem J, Dewit L, Keus R, Bartelink K (1992) Concomitant chemotherapy and radiotherapy. In: Snow GB, Clark JR (eds) Multimodality therapy for head and neck cancer. Thieme Medical, New York, pp 126–146
Jaulerry C, Gaboriaud G, Chevret S, et al. (1989) Hyperthermia and radiotherapy or chemotherapy in the retreatment of primary and nodal head and neck carcinoma. In: Sugahara T, Saito M (eds) Hyperthermic oncology 1988, vol 2. Taylor and Francis, London, pp 454–457
Kamata R, Saito T, Urahashi S, et al. (1989) Hyperthermia and radical dose of radiation therapy in cervical lymph node metastases. In: Sugahara T, Saito M (eds) Hyperthermic oncology 1988, vol 2. Taylor and Francis, London pp 450–453
Knox SJ, Kapp DS (1988) Hyperthermia and radiation therapy in the treatment of recurrent Merkel cell tumors. Cancer 62: 1479–1486

Krishnamurthi S, Shanta V, Vasanthan A, Balakrishnan IS, Jayaraman R (1990) Radiation, pepleomycin and hyperthermia in the therapy of locally advanced squamous cell carcinomas of the buccal mucosa. Clin Oncol 68: 10–13

Lauche HM, El Akoum H, Fischer L, Gautherie M (1987) Capacitive radiofrequency hyperthermia: phase-II therapeutic trials and technological advances. Int J Hyperthermia 3: 547–575

Leibel SA, Scott CB, Mohiuddin M, Marcial VA, Coia LR, Davis LW, Fuks Z (1991) The effect of local-regional control on distant metastatic dissemination in carcinoma of the head and neck: results of an analysis from the RTOG head and neck database. Int J Radiat Oncol Biol Phys 21: 549–556

Lele P (1989) Advanced ultrasonic techniques for local tumor hyperthermia. Radiol Clin North Am 27: 559–575

Leybovich LB, Emami B, Myerson RJ, Straube WL (1990) Hyperthermia device for external heating of deep neck tumors (meeting abstract). Thirty-eighth annual meeting of the Radiation Research Society and tenth annual meeting of the North American Hyperthermia Group. April 7–12, 1990, New Orleans, p 9

Lindholm C-E, Kjellen E, Nilsson P, Hertzman S (1987) Microwave-induced hyperthermia and radiotherapy in human superficial tumours: clinical results with a comparative study of combined treatment versus radiotherapy alone. Int J Hyperthermia 3: 393–411

Lindholm C-E, Andréasson L, Knöös T, Landberg T, Ljungberg O (1990) Arterial rupture after microwave-induced hyperthermia and radiotherapy. Int J Hyperthermia 6: 499–509

Luk KH, Francis ME, Perez CA, Johnson RJ (1984) Combined radiation and hyperthermia: comparison of two treatment schedules based on data from a registry established by the Radiation Therapy Oncology Group (RTOG). Int J Radiat Oncol Biol Phys 10: 801–809

Maciejewsky B (1987) Regression rate of metastatic neck lymph-nodes after radiation treatment as a prognostic factor for local contro. Radiother Oncol 8: 301–308

Manning MR, Cetas TC, Miller RC, Oleson JR, Connor WG, Gerner EW (1982) Clinical hyperthermia: results of a phase I trial employing hyperthermia alone or in combination with external beam or interstitial radiotherapy. Cancer 49: 205–216

Marino C, Cividalli A (1992) Combined radiation and hyperthermia: effects of the number of heat fractions and their interval on normal and tumour tissues. Int J Hyperthermia 8: 771–781

Marmor JB, Hahn GM (1978) Ultrasound heating in previously irradiate sites. Int J Radiat Oncol Biol Phys 4: 1029–1032

McCaffrey TV (1991) Surgical treatment in head and neck cancer. Curr Opin Oncol 3: 519–522

Mendenhall WM, Million RR, Cassisi NJ (1986) Squamous cell carcinoma of the head and neck treated with radiation therapy: the role of neck dissection for clinically positive neck nodes. Int J Radiat Oncol Biol Phys 12: 733–740

Merino OR, Lindberg RD, Fletcher GH (1977) An alaysis of distant metastases from squamous cell carcinoma of the upper respiratory and digestive tract. Cancer 40: 145–151

Million RR, Cassisi NJ (1984) General principles for treatment of cancers of the head and neck: radiation therapy. In: Million RR, Cassisi NJ (eds) Management of head and neck cancer: a multidisciplinary approach. Lippincott, Philadelphia, pp 77–90

Mittal BB, Sathiaseelan V, Kies MS (1990) Simultaneous localized 915 MHz external and interstitial microwave hyperthermia to heat tumors greater than 3 cm in depth. Int J Radiat Oncol Biol Phys 19: 669–675

Myerson RJ, Perez CA, Emami B, Straube W, Kuske RR, Leybovich L, VonGerichten D (1990) Tumor control in long-term survivors following superficial hyperthermia. Int J Radiat Oncol Biol Phys 18: 1123–1129

Nawalkha PL, Jain KC, Punia DP, Singhal NC (1979) Treatment of cervical metastases by combined application of hyperthermia and radiation. Indian J Radiol 33: 321–324

Nishimura Y, Akuta K, Hiraoka M, et al. (1990) Initial clinical results of a 430 MHz microwave hyperthermia system using a lens applicator. Radiother Oncol 17: 219–227

Oleson JR (1989) If we can't define the quality, can we assure it? Int J Radiat Oncol Biol Phys 16: 879

Oleson JR, Sim DA, Manning MR (1984) Analysis of prognostic variables in hyperthermia treatment of 161 patients. Int J Radiat Oncol Biol Phys 10: 2231–2239

Oleson JR, Samulski TV, Leopold KA, Clegg ST, Dewhirst MW, Dodge RK, George SL (1993) Sensitivity of hyperthermia trial outcomes to temperature and time: implications for thermal goals of treatment. Int J Radiat Oncol Biol Phys 25: 289–297

Orecchia R, Gabriele P, Tseroni V, Ragona R, Sannazzari GL (1989) Analysis of prognostic factors in a series of 171 tumors treated by hyperthermia alone or combined with irradiation. In: Sugahara T, Saito M (eds) Hyperthermic oncology 1988, vol 1. Taylor and Francis, London, pp 619–620

Overgaard J (1989a) The current and potential role of hyperthermia in radiotherapy. Int J Radiat Oncol Biol Phys 16: 535–549

Overgaard J (1989b) Clinical trials with hyperthermia and radiotherapy. In: Sugahara T, Saito M (eds) Hyperthermic oncology 1988, vol 2. Taylor and Francis, London, pp 57–62

Overgaard J (1990) The rationale for clinical trials in hyperthermia. In: Field SB, Hand JW (eds) An introduction to the practical aspects of clinical hyperthermia. Taylor and Francis, London, pp 213–241

Peracchia G, Salti C (1986) A method of radiation treatment for advanced neck node metastases. Int J Radiat Oncol Biol Phys 12: 2197–2201

Perez CA, Emami BN (1989) Clinical trials with local (extternal and interstitial) irradiation and hyperthermia. Current and future perspective. Radiol Clin North Am 27: 525–542

Perez CA, Emami B, Scott RS, Hornback NB, Gillespie BW, Hederman MA, VonGerichten D (1987) Irradiation and hyperthermia in the treatment of locally advanced and recurrent head and neck tumors. In: Jacobs JR, Crissman J, Valeriote FA, Al Sarraf M (eds), Head and neck cancer: scientific perspective in management and strategies for cure. Elsewiver, New York, pp 334–347

Perez CA, Emami BN, Straube W, VonGerichten D, Leibovich L, Fox S, Lockett MA (1989a) Irradiation and external hyperthermia in treatment of head and neck cancer. In: Sugahara T, Saito M (eds) Hyperthermic oncology 1988, vol 2. Taylor and Francis, London, pp 446–449

Perez CA, Gillespie B, Pajak T, Hornback NB, Emami B, Rubin P (1989b) Quality assurance problems in clinical hyperthermia and their impact on therapeutic outcome: a report by the radiation therapy oncology group. Int J Radiat Oncol Biol Phys 16: 551–558
Perez CA, Pajak T, Emami B, Hornback NB, Tupchong L, Rubin P (1991) Randomized phase III study comparing irradiation and hyperthermia with irradiation alone in superficial measurable tumors. Am J Clin Oncol 14: 133–141
Peters LJ, Ang KK (1992) The role of altered fractionation in head and neck cancer. Semin Radiat Oncol 2: 180–194
Petersen IA, Kapp DS (1990) Local hyperthermia and radiation therapy in the retreatment of superficially located recurrences in Hodgkin's disease. Int J Radiat Oncol Biol Phys 18: 603–611
Pilepich MV, Jones KG, Emami BN, Perez CA, Fields JN, Myerson RJ (1989) Interaction of blemoycin and hyperthermia – results of a clinical pilot study. Int J Radiat Oncol Biol Phys 16: 211–213
Prévost B, Mirabel X, Moncho V, lévêque C, Chivé M, Fabre JJ (1992) Inoperable recurrent neck nodes in previosuly irradiated fields: results of a combined treatment with radiation and hyperthermia. In: Gerner EW, Cetas TC (eds) Hyperthermic oncology 1992, vol 1. Arizona Board of Regents, Tucson, p 484
Protsyk VS, Osinsky SP, Shimanskaja RB, Bubnovskaja LN (1992) Intratumoral glucose loading in thermoradiochemotherapy of patients with head and neck carcinomas (preliminary results). In: Gerner EW (ed) Hyperthermic oncology 1992, vol 1, addendum. Arizona Board of Regents, Tuscon, p. 491
Samulski TD, Fessenden P, Valdagni R, Kapp DS (1987) Correlations of thermal washout rate, steady state temperatures and tissue type in deep seated recurrent or metastatic tumors. Int J Radiat Oncol Biol Phys 13: 907–916
Sannazzari GL, Gabriele P, Orecchia R, Tseroni V (1989) Head and neck tumours: hyperthermia alone. In: Sugahara T, Saito M (eds) Hyperthermic oncology 1988, vol 2. Taylor and Francis, London, pp 438–441
Sannazzari GL, Gabriele P, Orecchia R (1990) Ipertermia e radioterapia. In: Veronesi U, Molinari R, Banfi A, Santoro A (eds) I tumori della testa e del collo. CEA Casa Editrice Ambrosiana, Milano, pp 61–65
Scott RS, Del Rowe JD (1986) A transient hypotensive episode (Bezold-Jarisch effect) occurring in a patient treated with microwave hyperthermia. Am J Clin Oncol 9: 170–172
Scott RS, Clay L, Storey KV, Johnson RJR (1985) Transient microwave induced neurosensory reactions during superficial hyperthermia treatment. Int J Radiat Oncol Biol Phys 11: 561–566
Scott RS, Gillespie B, Perez CA, et al. (1988) Hyperthermia in combination with definitive radiation therapy: results of a phase I/II RTOG study. Int J Radiat Oncol Biol Phys 15: 711–716
Siddiqui MA (1989) Fractionation of hyperthermia and radiotherapy in recurrent lymph node metastases in head and neck tumors. In: Sugahara T, Saito M (eds) Hyperthermic oncology 1988, vol 2. Taylor and Francis, London, pp 810–812
Steindorfer P, Jakse R, Germann R, Schneider G, Berger A, Mischinger HJ, Rehak P (1987) Hyperthermia as an adjuvant to radiation- and/or chemotherapy in far advanced recurrences of the head and neck region. Strahlenther Onkol 53: 1–4
Storm FK (1989) Clinical hyperthermia and chemotherapy. Radiol Clin North Am 27: 621–627
Tan W, Li Q (1984) Clinical effects of microwave combined with radiation in 50 head-neck malignant tumor patients. In: Overgaard J (ed) Hyperthermic oncology 1984, vol 1. Taylor and Francis, London, pp 357–358
Tepperman BS, Fitzpatrick PJ (1981) Second respiratory and upper digestive tract cancers after oral cancer. Lancet 1: 547–549
Tsukiyama I, Yamashija K, Kajiura Y, Ogino T, Arile Y, Egawa S, Yawagawa S (1987) Results of a noncontrolled trial of hyperthermia combined with radiation for superficial tumors. Int J Hyperthermia 3: 503–512
Tupchong L, Nerlinger RE, Waterman FM (1988) Combined use of external beam radiation and interstitial heat for advanced recurrent head and neck carcinoma. A new approach. 8th annual meeting of the North American Hyperthermia Group, Philadelphia, April 16–21, 1988. Abstract of papers, pp 43
Tupchong L, Waterman FM, McFarlane JD (1990) Hyperthermia and radiation therapy for advanced regional disease due to recurrent head and neck carcinoma. Int J Radiat Oncol Biol Phys 19: 274 (abstr)
Urbon J, Murthy AK, Taylor SG, Hendrickson FR, Lanzl LH (1990) Retrospective analysis of hyperthermia for use in the palliative treatment of cancer: a multimodality evaluation. Int J Radiat Oncol Biol Phys 18: 155–163
Valdagni R (ed) (1990) International consensus meeting on hyperthermia. Final report. Int J Hyperthermia 6: 837–877
Valdagni R, Amichetti M (1987) Clinical hyperthermia: five years experience. Strahlenther Onkol 163: 443–445
Valdagni R, Amichetti M (1994) Report of long-term follow-up in a randomized trial comparing radiation therapy and radiation therapy plus hyperthermia to metastatic lymphnodes in stage IV head and neck patients. Int J Radiat Oncol Biol Phys 28: 163–169
Valdagni R, Kamata R (1989) Hyperthermia of head and neck tumors. In: Sugahara T, Saito M (eds) Hyperthermic oncology 1988, vol 2. Taylor and Francis, London, pp 434–437
Valdagni R, Liu FF (1990) Evaluating radiation in combination with hyperthermia trials: the importance of clinical and technical parameters. Tumori 76: 205–211
Valdagni R, Samulski TV, Cox R, Kapp DS (1985) Local and regional hyperthermia treatment of superficial and deep tumors: analyses of thermal washout. Strahlenther Onkol 161: 552
Valdagni R, Kapp DS, Valdagni C (1986) N_3 (TNM-UICC) metastatic neck nodes managed by combined radiation therapy and hyperthermia: clinical results and analysis of treatment parameters. Int J Hyperthermia 2: 189–200
Valdagni R, Amichetti M, Pani G (1988a) Radical radiation alone versus radiation plus microwave hyperthermia for N_3 (TNM-UICC) neck nodes: a prospective randomized clinical trial. Int J Radiat Oncol Biol Phys 15: 13–24
Valdagni R, Liu FF, Kapp DS (1988b) Important prognostic factors influencing outcome of combined radiation and hyperthermia. Int J Radiat Oncol Biol Phys 15: 959–972
Valdagni R, Amichetti M, Graiff C, Cristoforetti L, Pontalti R, Irler WJ (1989) Parameters influencing outcome of combined radiation therapy (XRT) and hyperthermia (Ht) in neck node metastases. In: Sugahara

T, Saito M (eds) Hyperthermic oncology 1988, vol 2. Taylor and Francis, London, pp 458–461

Vokes EE (1992) Squamous cell carcinoma of the head and ncek. In: Horwich A (ed) Combined radiotherapy and chemotherapy in clinical oncology. Edward Arnold, Hooder and Stoughton London, pp 65–77

Vrouvas J, Dardoufas K, Iordanou I, et al. (1992) Clinical experience in using Ht and RT in treating lymph nodes, relapsed from mastectomy, melanoma and larynx T3 tumors. In: Gerner EW (ed) Hyperthermic oncology 1992, vol 1 addendum. Arizona Board of Regents, Tucson, AZ, p A27

Wang JI (1989) The remote results of hyperthermia combined with radiotherapy in the treatment of NPC and soft tissue sarcomas. In: Sugahara T, Saito M (eds) Hyperthermic oncology 1988, vol 2. Taylor and Francis, London, pp 416–417

Weischedel U, Wieland C (1987) Results in combined hyperthermia/radiotherapy of adenoid cystic carcinomas compared with conventional treatment. Strahlenther Onkol 163: 714–717

Wynder EL, Dodo H, Block DA, Garitt RC, Moore OS (1969) Epidemiologic investigation of multiple primary cancer of the respiratory tract. Cancer 24: 730–739

Wust P, Riess H, Stahl H, Löffel J, Felix R (1992) Local hyperthermia in a trimodal approach for advanced non resectable head and neck tumors: technical/clinical feasibility and response. In: Gerner EW (ed) Hyperthermic oncology 1992. Arizona Board of Regents, Tucson, AZ, p 485

Zbaeren P, Lehmann W (1987) Frequency and sites of distant metastases in head and neck squamous cell carcinoma. Arch Otolaryngol Head Neck Surg 113: 762–764

5 Thermoradiotherapy of Malignant Melanoma

J. OVERGAARD

CONTENTS

5.1 Introduction

The application of hyperthermia as a method of improving radiation response in tumors has been explored for more than 80 years. Probably the first clinical report stemmed from Müller, who described the potential of local diathermy as an adjuvant to radiotherapy (MÜLLER 1910). This was followed by sporadic reports which enthusiastically suggested a likely improvement of the effect of radiation on various superficial tumors. However, it was not until the mid-1970s that the principle of combined heat and radiation was explored in a more scientific manner. This led to the publication of numerous uncontrolled studies, almost all suggesting that adjuvant hyperthermia improves the response to radiation (OVERGAARD 1989a).

Cutaneous malignant melanoma was a prime target in these early studies of combined heat and radiation (OVERGAARD 1979, 1981; KIM et al. 1978, 1982; ARCANGELI et al. 1987; CORRY et al. 1982; EMAMI et al. 1988; GONZALEZ GONZALEZ et al. 1986; JOHNSON et al. 1979; MARCHAL et al. 1986; PEREZ et al. 1981; AMICHETTI et al. 1982; U et al. 1980; SCOTT et al. 1983; HOFMAN et al. 1984; HOWARD and SATHIASEELAN 1987; OVERGAARD and OVERGAARD 1987; SHIDNIA et al. 1990; ENGIN et al. 1992; BEN-YOSEF and KAPP 1993). These publications and several unpublished series together with similar reports on melanomas treated with radiation only (OVERGAARD et al. 1986; OVERGAARD 1986; BENTZEN et al. 1989) have created the database for most of the conclusions drawn in the present chapter.

The interest in cutaneous malignant melanoma has been due to several factors. Firstly, these lesions are mainly superficially located, making the tumors accessible for local heat treatment. Secondly, malignant melanomas have unique radiobiological characteristics to the effect that a beneficial radiotherapy regimen can be given with a few large fractions (OVERGAARD and BENTZEN 1990; BENTZEN et al. 1989; OVERGAARD et al. 1986), which allows a better combination with hyperthermia. In addition, many patients with metastatic malignant melanoma have multiple lesions, which make possible a comparison of different treatment schedules within the same patient.

Despite the radiocurability of malignant melanoma, surgery is the prime treatment of this disease and the indication for radiotherapy in cutaneous malignant melanoma is in general limited to recurrent or metastatic disease (OVERGAARD et al. 1990). The present chapter will therefore address the place of thermoradiotherapy

---

J. OVERGAARD, MD, Danish Cancer Society, Department of Experimental Clinical Oncology, Radiumstationen, Nørrebrogade 44, DK-8000 Aarhus C, Denmark

in the treatment of advanced malignant melanoma and will especially deal with recurrent or metastatic lesions with special emphasis on local treatment of metastases. Both endpoints of local control and palliation will be considered.

5.2 Role of Radiotherapy in the Treatment of Malignant Melanoma

The role of hyperthermia will be to enhance the effect of local radiotherapy. This implies that the indication for thermoradiotherapy must be similar to the indication for radiation alone. Consequently, the biological basis and clinical role of radiotherapy will be briefly summarized.

In 1903, the first published report of radiation treatment of melanoma appeared (MARSH 1903). Following this a strange controversy developed which gradually led to the establishment of the dogma found in most textbooks: that malignant melanoma is an extremely radioresistant tumor. At the same time, however, radiotherapy was increasingly applied in the primary treatment of melanoma, especially in German-speaking countries (OVERGAARD et al. 1990; TROTT 1993). Although large doses were required, it was evident that the 5-year survival following radiotherapy equalled that obtained by excision. This did not place radiotherapy as the primary modality in the treatment of early melanoma, since surgery continues to be the treatment of choice; however, it illustrates that malignant melanoma is far from a radioresistant tumor, and that the textbook dogma has no scientific basis. In more recent years there are indications to support the view that the so-called radioresistance may be due to unique radiobiological properties of malignant melanoma. The in vitro radiation survival curve for malignant melanoma is in general characterized by being very "curvy," which means that these tumors are relatively resistant to treatment with conventional fractionation schedules, whereas they appear to be sensitive to radiation applied with large doses per fraction (OVERGAARD et al. 1990; OVERGAARD and BENTZEN 1990). By applying properly designed fractionation schedules, tumor control can be achieved at doses that yield no greater late normal tissue damage than is seen after treatment of tumors which are considered sensitive to radiation (OVERGAARD et al. 1990; OVERGAARD and BENTZEN 1990; BENTZEN et al. 1989). Although surgery is not challenged as the treatment of choice for most cutaneous melanomas, situations may occur (tumors located in delicate anatomical regions, such as the eye, certain areas of the head and neck, or at mucosal surfaces) where primary radiotherapy is indicated, and the latter has indeed been shown to be capable of achieving tumor control. In fact radiotherapy may be considered the treatment of choice for ocular melanoma, and the thermoradiotherapy of this disease has been described elsewhere in this series (RIEDEL 1993).

The main indication for radiotherapy is, however, advanced malignant disease, i.e., inoperable, recurrent, or metastatic disease, and there is strong evidence that radiation treatment has a place in the palliative therapy of such patients, and may even be curative in situations where patients only have a single or a few lesions that are all accessible for treatment.

In palliative therapy, radiotherapy may be preferable to surgery from the patient's point of view, and especially in advanced cases it has been demonstrated that there is a high probability of palliation when a few large radiation fractions are given (OVERGAARD et al. 1986; OVERGAARD 1986). This option can thereby contribute significantly to the quality of life of patients with advanced and progressive disease.

5.3 Clinical Radiobiology of Malignant Melanoma

Cells derived from different histopathological tumor types have shown substantial differences in their in vitro radiosensitivity (PETERS 1990). Although there are significant variations within tumors with a specific histopathology, some types can be considered radiosensitive and others more resistant. Malignant melanomas have constantly been found to belong to the radioresistant tumors although different malignant melanoma cell lines have shown substantial heterogeneity in their in vitro sensitivity (ROFSTAD 1986; PETERS 1990). This resistance is especially expressed by the so-called SF2 value in primary biopsies, i.e., the survival fraction after a dose of 2 Gy, equivalent to the dose of a conventional fraction. However, if the sensitivity to larger fractions is estimated, malignant melanomas are seen to be more sensitive due to the curvy shape of the radiation survival curve (OVERGAARD et al. 1990).

This is in agreement with the clinical data, which have demonstrated an extremely strong fractionation sensitivity characterized by an α/β ratio at 2.5 Gy or below, whereas α/β ratios in most other tumors are in the range of 10–25 Gy (BENTZEN et al. 1989; OVERGAARD 1986). A high fractionation sensitivity does not in itself mean that treatment with large doses per fraction will be a superior strategy because it is normally associated with an increased risk of late normal tissue morbidity. However, it has been established that the fractionation sensitivity of malignant melanoma is so pronounced that an increased dose per fraction tends to increase the therapeutic gain between tumor response and late radiation-induced fibrosis (BENTZEN et al. 1989). Another respect in which malignant melanomas deviate from other tumors is in the apparent lack of influence of overall treatment time. As long as the treatment time is below 5–6 weeks, no significant influence on the probability of achieving local control has been demonstrated (BENTZEN et al. 1989).

TROTT (1993) has disputed the described radiobiological properties of malignant melanoma and a randomized clinical trial by the RTOG (SAUSE et al. 1991) could not demonstrate a significant benefit of a high dose per fraction schedule as compared with a conventional schedule. This was not, however, to be expected since the biological dose in the two schedules must be considered almost equivalent. Neither did the trial have a size which allowed it to eliminate the risk of a type 2 error. It illustrates, however, that a few large dose fractions may yield results no different from those of a more protracted conventional fractionation schedule with more discomfort for patients.

5.4 Biological Rationale for Thermoradiotherapy

The biological rationale for combining hyperthermia and radiation has been described in detail elsewhere (HORSMAN and OVERGAARD 1992; HORSMAN and OVERGAARD 1989; OVERGAARD 1989a; OVERGAARD et al. 1987; OVERGAARD and BACH ANDERSEN 1995). Briefly, it consists of two different mechanisms, namely hyperthermic radiosensitization and direct hyperthermic cytotoxicity.

Hyperthermic radiosensitization is expressed as increased damage from radiation when hyperthermia and radiation are applied concomitantly. This effect does not qualitatively alter the radiation response; rather it provides only a quantitative enhancement. Hyperthermic radiosensitization occurs to an equal extent in normal tissues and in tumors and is clearly most pronounced when there is truly simultaneous application of the modalities.

Hyperthermic cytotoxicity is seen as direct heat killing of cells in a deprived microenvironment characterized by insufficient blood supply with subsequent poor nutrition and increased acidity due to anaerobic metabolism and accumulation of lactic acid and other waste products. Cells situated in such an area are highly sensitive to hyperthermia and can be destroyed by a heat treatment which does not cause significant damage to cells in a "normal" environment. Furthermore, the environmental parameters which enhance the hyperthermic damage are typically those which reduce the radiation response (i.e., hypoxia). Thus, the areas of a tumor which, due to insufficient vascularization, are resistant to radiation are likely to be precisely those which are sensitive to hyperthermia. On the other hand, the well-vascularized tumor areas (characterized by a normal physiological environment) are sensitive to radiotherapy but relatively resistant to hyperthermia.

On this basis two strategies can be applied in respect of combined heat and irradiation (OVERGAARD 1989a; OVERGAARD and BACH ANDERSEN 1995; OVERGAARD 1993). One is to use hyperthermia as a radiosensitizing agent, enhancing the effect of ionizing radiation in heated tissues. This strategy is only valid if hyperthermia and radiation are applied simultaneously. The other strategy utilized the specific cytotoxic effect of heat against radioresistant cells, which results in damage to radioresistant areas of the tumors and is achieved by sequential treatment. Although hyperthermic radiosensitization with simultaneous treatment is able to yield the highest thermal enhancement ratio (TER), the clinical applicability of this protocol is dubious due to technical problems and it is likely that the dominant effect is due to the hyperthermic cytotoxicity.

This biological rationale has been documented in a clinical trial comparing the effects of simultaneous and sequential treatments in malignant melanoma and its surrounding skin (OVERGAARD 1981; OVERGAARD and OVERGAARD 1987) (see below).

5.5 Endpoint and Tumor Response

The intention of treatment in patients with malignant melanoma depends on the extent and dissemination of the disease. In patients with only a single or a few known lesions accessible to treatment, there exists the probability of obtaining persistent control and consequently prolonged survival (see below). The treatment should therefore aim towards obtaining such local control, i.e., a complete and persistent disappearance of all tumors. It is characteristic for malignant melanoma that once complete response has been achieved, there is a high probability of maintaining local control. This is seen in Fig. 5.1, which shows the probability of obtaining persistent local control in a series of 598 patients in whom initial complete response was achieved. This indicates that complete response may be an acceptable endpoint in clinical studies and that the information obtained in patients during a relatively short observation time may have credibility in scientific evaluation. It also implies that clinical trials in malignant melanoma can be performed on patients in whom the life expectancy is fairly short.

Despite the low probability of failure after complete response, it has been noted (MEYER et al. 1989; PEREZ et al. 1989, 1991) that tumors treated with thermoradiotherapy may have a lower subsequent recurrence rate than is seen after radiation alone. A similar observation was made in our case material, where the 5-year actuarial control probability was 87% for 202 tumors subjected to combined treatment as compared with 76% for 396 tumors treated with radiation alone. This implies that the benefit of hyperthermia tends to increase with duration of the observation period (MEYER et al. 1989). Biologically this may be explained by the fact that most radioresistant cells are in a kind of dormant state and after some time will give rise to recurrence if not properly destroyed. With combined treatment such cells are likely to be destroyed by heat alone and therefore a tumor disappearing completely after combined treatment may have a very low probability of containing viable cells.

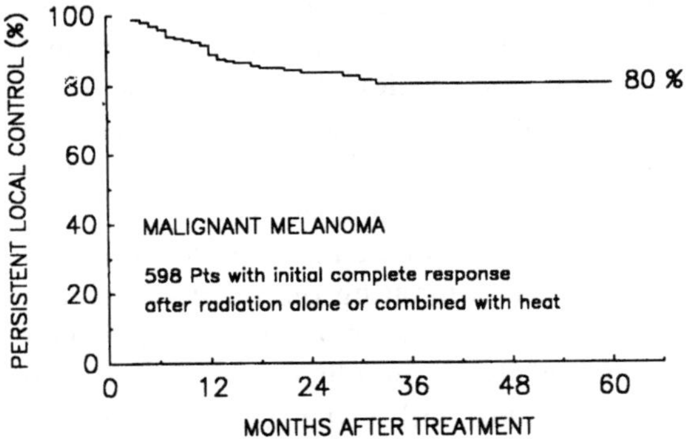

Fig. 5.1. Probability of persistent local control in patients with malignant melanoma showing an initial complete response. Data collected from literature and unpublished observations

The use of *partial response* has no implication and should be avoided since it may be misleading. It should be noted that a special phenomenon has been described following thermoradiotherapy of malignant melanoma, namely so-called *persistent regression* (OVERGAARD and OVERGAARD 1987; ENGIN et al. 1992; BEN-YOSEF and KAPP 1993). This indicates a slow, but continuous regression of the treated lesions, which often may leave a small residue of the tumor for months. On surgical excision the remaining part normally appears to be without viable cells but is reminiscent of fat necrosis. In some situations proper evaluation of thermoradiotherapy in this disease may therefore be based on the *time to progression* rather than complete clearance of tumors since some tumors may show persistent regression without achieving a complete response, although the therapy must be considered successful.

In patients with disseminated or advanced disease, the aim of treatment is to obtain *alleviation of symptoms*, especially pain. Both radiation alone and radiation combined with hyperthermia have been shown to be very useful in this regard, and in clinical trials a significant palliative effect has been described in more than 80% of the treated cases (OVERGAARD et al. 1986; OVERGAARD 1986). In clinical studies dealing with palliation the endpoint is completely different, and must be directed towards symptoms rather than objective findings. A detailed description of the problems of evaluating palliative treatment has recently been provided by NIELSEN et al. (1992).

5.6 Clinical Thermoradiotherapy of Malignant Melanoma

The clinical evaluation of thermoradiotherapy has almost solely been limited to superficial tumors due to the problem of sufficient delivery of the hyperthermia.

There have been several reports describing the benefit of thermoradiotherapy in these lesions, and Table 5.1 shows a series of uncontrolled studies where comparable lesions were treated with either radiation alone or the same kind of radiation given in combination with hyperthermia. In all studies, the complete response rate was substantially higher for the combined therapy, indicating that thermoradiotherapy indeed may be beneficial in malignant melanoma. Table 5.1 also indicates the thermal enhancement ratio estimated as the isodose TER (response to thermoradiotherapy relative to the response to radiation alone). The isodose TER gives the impression that the combined treatment is superior to radiation alone, but should otherwise not be considered of numerical importance.

The various studies described in Table 5.1 used different fractionation schedules and comparison between the series therefore cannot be performed. However, while the use of different fractionation schedules makes it generally difficult to compare published material, in a previous study analyzing the clinical radiobiology of malignant melanoma it was possible to derive a formalism based on the described fractionation sensitivity (α/β ratio: 2.5 Gy) which allows the use of a common dose denominator by employing the concept of equivalent total dose (ETD) (OVERGAARD et al. 1986, 1990). Figure 5.2 shows a detailed analysis of almost a thousand tumors from various published and unpublished studies (including the data in Table 5.1) and noncomparative reports of treatment with either radiation alone or thermoradiotherapy. In Fig. 5.2, the total doses have been normalized according to WITHERS et al. (1983), assuming daily fractionation of 2 Gy and an α/β ratio of 2.5 Gy. Furthermore, correction has been made for variation in tumor volume according to the principle previously described (OVERGAARD et al. 1986; OVERGAARD 1986), so the dose-response curves represent the expected response of a 1-cm tumor.

Figure 5.2 demonstrates a well-described dose-response relationship for both radiation alone and thermoradiotherapy. As is seen, the dose-response curve for thermoradiotherapy is shifted to the left, indicating greater sensitivity to such treatment. Based on the dose-response data, the probability of obtaining tumor control in half of the treated lesions (TCD_{50}) could be estimated for the two curves and was found to be 32.9 Gy and 49.1 Gy, respectively, for thermoradiotherapy and radiation alone. The ratio between these two

Table 5.1. Complete response rates in studies of radiotherapy alone and radiotherapy combined with heat. In each study the tumors have been treated with comparable radiation doses but with different fractionation schedules

Reference	No. of tumors	Rad. alone	Rad. + heat	Isodose TER[a]
OVERGAARD and OVERGAARD (1987)	63	57%	90%	1.58
CORRY et al. (1982)	20	0%	64%	≫1
GONZALEZ et al. (1986)	24	17%	83%	4.88
KIM et al. (1982, 1984)	149	43%	67%	1.56
ARCANGELI et al. (1987)	38	53%	76%	1.43
AMICHETTI et al. (unpublished)	74	29%	75%	2.59
MARCHAL et al. (1986)	24	0%	42%	≫1
EMAMI et al. (1988)	116	24%	59%	2.45
SHIDNIA et al. (1990)	181	52%	75%	1.44
ESHO 3-85[b]	128	35%	62%	1.77

[a] TER (isodose): frequency of response after radiation with heat/frequency of response after the same radiation dose alone

[b] Randomized trial, included in table for comparison

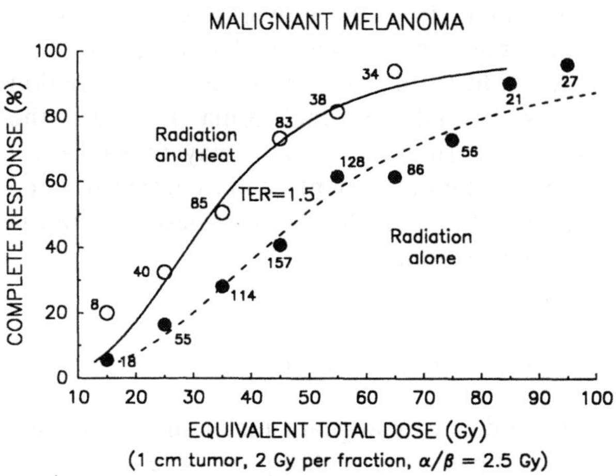

Fig. 5.2. Dose-response relationship for malignant melanoma treated with radiation alone or combined radiation and hyperthermia. The curves are based on data from unpublished observations and the literature. The different fractionation schedules have been converted into an "equivalent" total dose from an assumption of 2 Gy per fraction and an α/β ratio of 2.5 Gy, and have been corrected for volume in such a way that the curve demonstrates the dose-response relationship for a tumor with a diameter of 1 cm. The isoeffective TER is defined as: radiation dose alone to achieve endpoint/radiation dose with heat to achieve endpoint

values indicates the isoeffective TER and this was found to be 1.50 (95% confidence limits: 1.33–1.69).

Whereas this isoeffective TER may be the biologically important parameter, the clinically important figure is the isodose TER, provided that the normal tissue morbidity is of the same magnitude in the two schedules. Since this appears to be the case, it is obvious that a very low or a very high radiation dose does not result in major separation between the two schedules; rather the highest separation is at doses in the order of 40–50 Gy (see below).

In addition to the described treatment of advanced malignant melanoma, there are some indications that hyperthermia may play a role in primary therapy. In a Russian study (Savchenko et al. 1987) preoperative thermoradiotherapy resulted in a significantly higher 5-year survival rate than when preoperative radiation was given without hyperthermia (5-year survival 73% vs 48%, respectively). Detailed information on this study has not, however, been obtained.

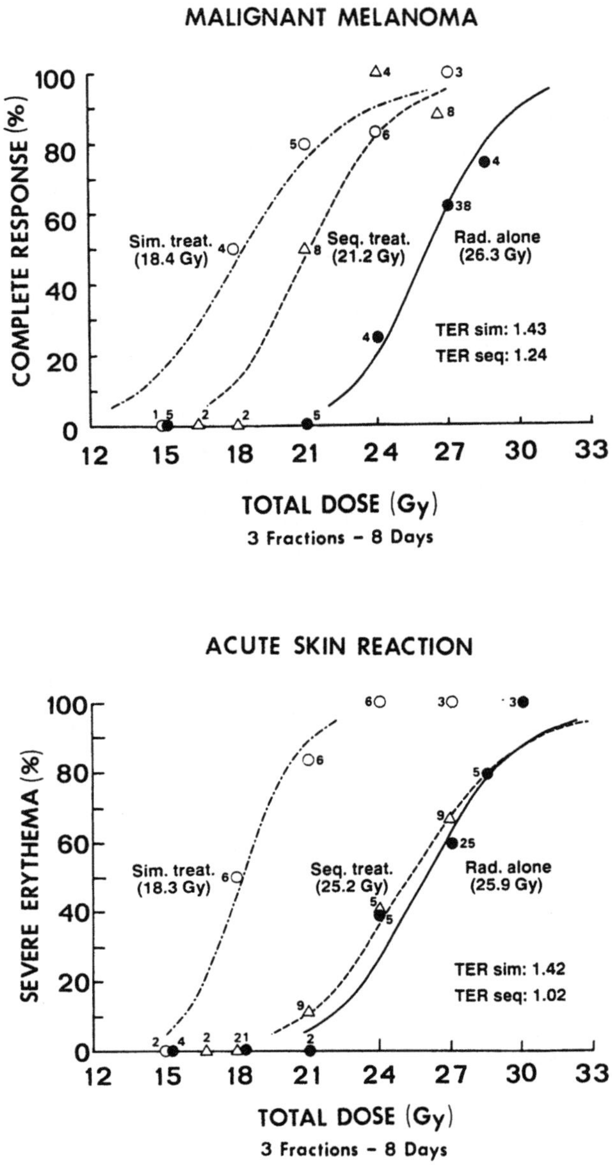

Fig. 5.3. Dose-response relationship for radiation alone or combined radiation and hyperthermia in malignant melanomas (*top*) and surrounding skin (*bottom*). One hundred and fifteen cutaneous or lymph node metastases or recurrent primary tumors were treated with three fractions of radiation in 8 days given either alone or with heat given less than 30 min after each radiation fraction (simultaneous) or 3–4 h after each fraction (sequential). The TER was calculated as the ratio between the radiation doses necessary to produce tumor control or severe erythema in 50% of the treated fields when using (a) radiation alone and (b) radiation in combination with heat. (Modified from Overgaard and Overgaard 1987)

5.7 Prognostic Parameters and Other Factors of Importance for the Outcome of Thermoradiotherapy

As is evident from the previous section, clinical studies have as a whole demonstrated that adjuvant hyperthermia improves the radiation response of malignant melanoma. However, the effect of thermoradiotherapy may depend on a number of tumor-, patient-, and treatment-related prognostic factors, which will be described in the following section.

5.7.1 Sequence and Interval

Early studies of malignant melanoma were used to investigate the validity of the biological rationale for combining hyperthermia and radiation, consideration being given to both the simultaneous and the sequential principle (Overgaard and Overgaard 1987; Overgaard 1979, 1981; Arcangeli et al. 1985). In general, a striking qualitative similarity has been found between the experience obtained with animal tumors and the clinical treatment. Figure 5.3 shows the results of our previous study with 115 tumors treated with three fractions of radiation alone or followed by heat either immediately (simultaneous treatment) or after an interval of 3–4 h (sequential treatment). The radiation dose varied between 5 and 10 Gy per fraction, allowing a dose-response analysis. An evaluation of the acute radiation response in the skin was also possible, because no attempt was made to obtain skin cooling and consequently the surrounding skin and the tumors were heated to a similar extent.

An isoeffective TER of 1.4 was observed after so-called simultaneous treatment, but a similar enhancement occurred with respect to the acute radiation damage in the surrounding skin, resulting in *no therapeutic gain* if tumor and normal tissue were heated to the same extent. An interval of 3–4h between radiation and hyperthermia (sequential treatment) produced a smaller TER of 1.2 in tumor, but caused no enhancement in the normal tissue, resulting in a *significant therapeutic gain*.

In the aforementioned clinical study the "simultaneous" treatment was different from that applied in the animal studies, since it was not given truly concomitantly; rather for practical reasons up to a 30-min interval was allowed between radiation and hyperthermia. Studies in animal tumors have clearly indicated that even an interval of a few minutes is crucial and that maximal sensitization undoubtedly is obtained by a *truly simultaneous approach* (OVERGAARD et al. 1987; HORSMAN and OVERGAARD 1992; OVERGAARD 1993). The enhancement seen with the clinical "simultaneous" schedule is therefore most likely considerably less than that which might be biologically achievable if a truly simultaneous application were to be performed. It can be anticipated that the most powerful effect of thermoradiotherapy will derive from a truly simultaneous application of the two modalities. TERs in the order of 4–5 may be easily achievable and early studies have indicated that in the situation of boost treatment a combination of interstitial hyperthermia and external beam radiotherapy may be feasible. A detailed description of the strategies and rationale for such treatment has been given elsewhere (HORSMAN and OVERGAARD 1992; OVERGAARD et al. 1987).

Whereas the results described above have provided clinical confirmation of the biological rationale, they not necessarily illustrate the typical clinical treatment. In practice normal tissue heating is avoided and at least the maximal tumor temperature will normally be substantially higher than that in the surrounding normal tissue (KIM et al. 1982). This means that the risk of enhanced radiation damage in normal tissue is smaller. A short interval between the two modalities does not normally result in significantly increased normal tissue response (ENGIN et al. 1992; OVERGAARD et al. 1994; OVERGAARD and BACH ANDERSEN 1995; BEN-YOSEF and KAPP 1992). It should, however, be recognized that this is not due to a biological phenomenon but is a consequence of differential temperature between the tumor and normal tissue, and if this cannot be obtained one must be aware of the risk of enhanced normal tissue damage.

5.7.2 Number of Heat Treatments

In general, a strong relationship between the number of heat treatments and response has not been demonstrated (OVERGAARD 1989a). KAPP et al. (1990) have addressed this issue in the treatment of malignant melanoma and did not find a significant difference between treatments given with two and with six heat fractions.

The effect of combined treatment may theoretically depend on the interval between the two modalities. If hyperthermia is applied simultaneously with all radiation fractions in order to obtain hyperthermic radiosensitization, the interval between each of the combined treatment sessions must be sufficiently long to avoid thermal tolerance (OVERGAARD and NIELSEN 1983; OVERGAARD 1989a). This implies a long interval between radiation fractions which may be less than optimal. In fact, an optimal hyperthermia treatment schedule may demand that radiation is only given once or twice per week, or, alternatively, that the radiation is given as a conventional schedule and hyperthermia is only given in conjunction with some of the radiation fractions. If a high dose per fraction schedule is applied in malignant melanoma, this problem is of less importance since the few treatment fractions can be spaced due to the apparent lack of a strong overall treatment time effect in this tumor type (BENTZEN et al. 1989).

In addition to the biological problems related to thermotolerance and heat radiosensitization versus direct heat kill, the technical problems may be of importance for the number of heat fractions. The inability to provide sufficient heating in most sessions will obviously increase the likelihood of sufficient heating with increasing number of heat treatments, and consequently multiple heatings may be superior. Until well-described homogeneous heating can be clinically applied, the issue of how many heat treatments are required probably cannot be answered in a relevant fashion.

5.7.3 Radiation Dose

Both total dose and dose per fraction are highly significant parameters for the response to thermoradiotherapy of malignant melanoma (OVERGAARD et al. 1990; OVERGAARD and OVERGAARD 1987; ENGIN et al. 1992; EMAMI et al. 1988). This is illustrated in Fig. 5.2, which shows the steep dose-response relationship for both radiation alone and radiation combined with hyperthermia. A similar dose-response relationship has been found in clinical radiobiological studies of malignant melanoma, but characteristically the dose-response curves are less steep than would be expected from in vitro survival curves, and it has been suggested that a "hidden" parameter may be associated with this tumor type (BENTZEN et al. 1990). This could be related to various individual characteristics of a given patient, such as immunological status or inherent radiosensitivity. That the latter expresses substantial heterogeneity when estimated in vitro has previously been demonstrated (TROTT 1993; ROFSTAD 1986; BENTZEN et al. 1990).

The importance of the total dose for the outcome can also be inferred from the data in Fig. 5.2. If the intention of the combined treatment is to improve the response to radiation, it is obvious that significant room for improvement must exist. This means that the tumor control with radiation alone must not be too high, neither should it be very small, since adding hyperthermia then may still not be sufficient to reach the threshold for tumor control. Figure 5.4 shows that in absolute terms the highest gain is obtained using treatment schedules where the radiation effect yields approximately 50% complete response. A decrease or increase in dose level will tend to diminish the gain that can be obtained by adding hyperthermia. This implies that the major indication for thermoradiotherapy may lie in palliative settings or in larger tumors where the probability of achieving control by means of radiation is limited.

The importance of radiation dose per fraction has been discussed by several authors. There is some confusion over the issue since a high dose per fraction will result in a lower overall total dose, and no straightforward conclusion can be derived (EMAMI et al. 1988; ARCANGELI et al. 1985; BEN-YOSEF and KAPP 1993). The evaluation of these studies is also hampered by the non-optimal heating of the tumors. However, from a theoretical point of view large doses per fraction may have an advantage, and in most of the clinical studies where a benefit of thermoradiotherapy has been seen, such fractionation schedules have been applied (EMAMI et al. 1988; GONZALEZ GONZALEZ et al. 1986; OVERGAARD and OVERGAARD 1987; ARCANGELI et al. 1987). The theoretical benefit of using hyperthermia with large doses per fraction may be seen in the attempt to apply a simultaneous treatment utilizing hyperthermic radiosensitization. In this situation only sensitization to the radiation dose applied close to hyperthermia will be achieved, and it is only in a schedule with a few large dose fractions that thermoradiotherapy can be applied in close association with the entire or most of the radiation applied. Thus, a schedule with high doses per fraction is, for practical reasons, likely to result in greater radiosensitization. That such a schedule is also more beneficial for the patients and less labor intensive may further support its use.

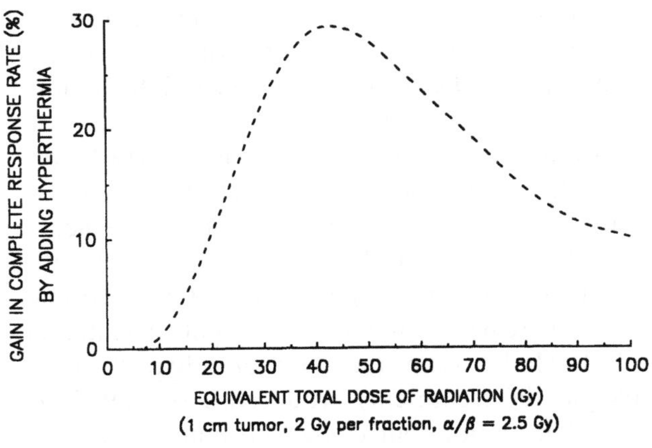

Fig. 5.4. Optimization of treatment benefit by thermoradiotherapy. The figure shows the gain in the complete response rate achieved by adding hyperthermia to radiation. The curve is based on the data in Fig. 5.2 and expresses the vertical displacement between the two dose-response curves as a function of equivalent total dose of radiation

5.7.4 Tumor Volume

Tumor volume is one of the most important parameters for the outcome of radiation given alone or combined with heat (OVERGAARD and OVERGAARD 1987; KIM et al. 1982; ARCANGELI et al. 1987; HERMAN et al. 1988). However, adding hyperthermia to the radiation therapy tends to diminish the volume effect. If properly heated, larger tumors have been found to be relatively more sensitive to thermoradiotherapy, i.e., the TER increases with increasing volume (OVERGAARD and OVERGAARD 1987; ARCANGELI et al. 1987; OVERGAARD 1989b). This is seen in Fig. 5.5 (upper panel), which shows our experience with the three-fraction schedule. With radiation alone the complete response rate is strongly correlated with tumor size. A similar observation is found for the combined treatment, although tumors given such treatment do better than after radiation alone. However, the two curves tend to separate, and the TER, estimated as the ratio between the two curves, shows an increase as a function of tumor size (Fig. 5.5, lower panel). In other words, there is a relative benefit of thermoradiotherapy with increasing tumor size. The biological rationale for an improved effect of thermoradiotherapy in larger tumors is probably to be found in the change in the microvascular tumor environment as larger tumors are more characterized by insufficient nutrition and blood supply causing hypoxia and acidity.

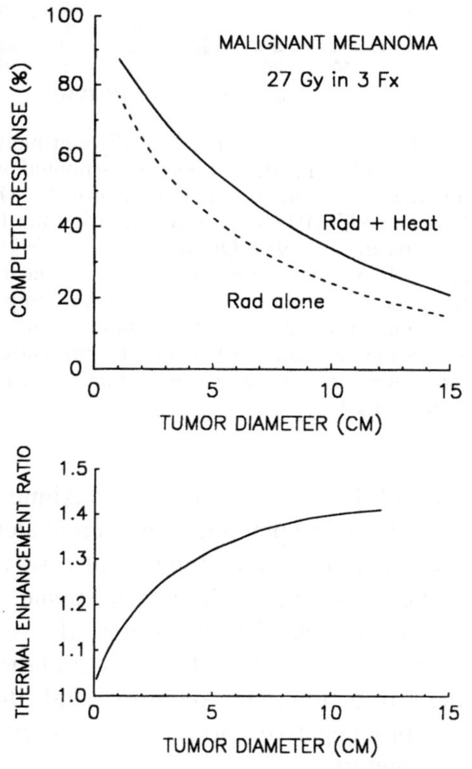

Fig. 5.5. *Upper panel*: Volume effect. Tumor control following 27 Gy in three fractions given as radiotherapy alone or combined with hyperthermia, and plotted as a function of average tumor diameter. Calculation performed as described by BENTZEN et al. (1989); OVERGAARD and BENTZEN (1990). *Lower panel*: TER, estimated as the ratio between the tumor response to combined treatment relative to that to radiation alone (see Table 5.1), as a function of tumor diameter. The TER is calculated from the data shown in the *upper panel*

One should, however, be careful not to confuse absolute and relative gains, and with respect to tumor size, the following is obvious:

1. The tumor control probability rapidly decreases as a function of increasing tumor size, in such a way that small tumors always do better than larger tumors, irrespective of whether radiation is given alone or combined with hyperthermia.
2. The effect of thermoradiotherapy relative to radiation alone does, however, increase with tumor size, i.e., the detrimental effect of size is less pronounced for tumors receiving combined treatment. This results in an increased TER with increasing tumor volume, but the gain obtained with thermoradiotherapy is less than the loss suffered from the increased size, and a large tumor given combined treatment will do worse than a small tumor given radiation alone.
3. The apparent relative benefit of combined treatment in large tumors is counteracted by the technical difficulties in heating such tumors sufficiently. Clinical trials such as the RTOG 81-04 (PEREZ et al. 1991; ENGIN et al. 1992) have therefore shown that larger tumors generally benefit less from combined treatment, not because they are less sensitive biologically but simply due to insufficient heating.
4. The clinical implications of the volume effect are that treatment should not be delayed, since both the probability of tumor control and, consequently, palliation are greatest if tumors are treated at a small size.

5.7.5 Heat Dose

From biological studies it must be anticipated that an increasing thermal dose will yield a better response to thermoradiotherapy (OVERGAARD 1984). This is also the clinical experience, and tumors not receiving significant heating do worse than when the treatment has resulted in high temperatures. It has, however, been difficult to evaluate clinically the importance of the various temperatures due to the heterogeneity of the heating, and because most tumors are not treated using standardized thermometry. The issue has been discussed in detail and several quality assurance protocols have been initiated, but experience is still very sparse, especially with malignant melanoma.

Numerous thermal parameters influence the outcome. These are associated both with individual heat treatments and with the sum of several heat treatments (VALDAGNI et al. 1988; Cox and KAPP 1992; BEN-YOSEF and KAPP 1993). It is not the intention to go into detail with regard to these parameters in the present chapter. Here only the following should be mentioned:

The outcome of thermal radiotherapy of malignant melanoma has been found to correlate with minimum tumor temperature (ENGIN et al. 1992; BEN-YOSEF and KAPP 1993) and maximum tumor temperature (EMAMI et al. 1988; OVERGAARD et al. 1995).

The overall *quality of heating* tends to decrease with increasing tumor volume simply due to insufficient penetration of hyperthermia in most larger tumors: although the highest maximal temperatures are in fact frequently observed in large tumors, they are obtained in necrotic areas without blood flow.

The conclusion regarding heat dose and thermoradiotherapy of malignant melanoma is therefore that there are insufficient data to permit detailed correlation with the various thermal parameters, but without doubt it has been shown that the quality of heating is correlated with the outcome (OLESON et al. 1989) and that poor hyperthermia may not yield better results than radiation alone. The risk of obtaining poor heating is especially associated with deep-seated tumors and one should not overestimate the capacity of external heating equipment. However, the results reported in the literature have been obtained with relatively poor heating equipment and the experience described in this chapter therefore demonstrates what may be achieved with nonoptimal hyperthermia. An improvement in the heating quality is likely to yield significantly better results.

The problem of insufficient heating is also evident from some of our early experience with superficial heating of lymph nodes or cutaneous malignant melanomas (Fig. 5.6). The upper panel shows the cumulative maximum and minimum measured tumor temperatures as well as the maximum normal tissue temperature. Although

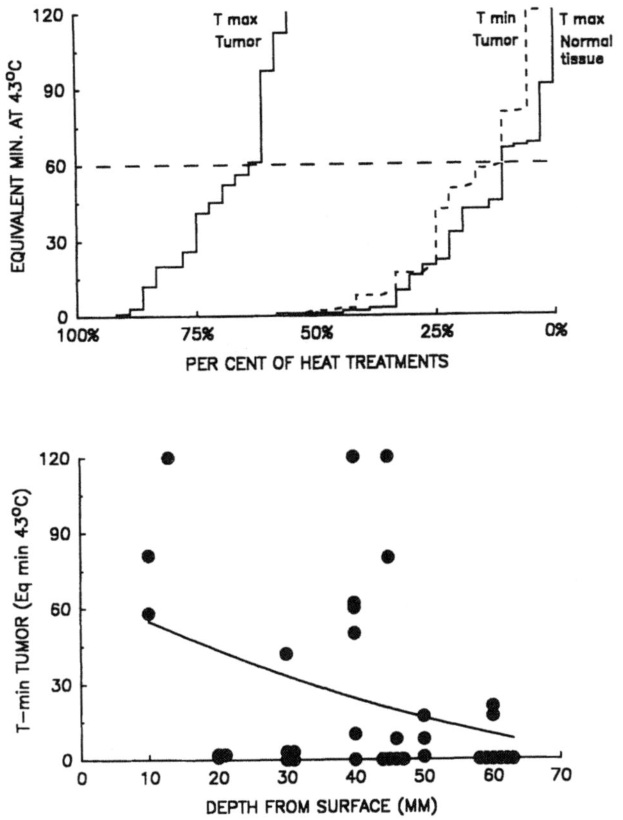

Fig. 5.6. Quality assurance in malignant melanoma. The ability to obtain sufficient heating estimated as equivalent minutes at 43°C in 36 tumors treated with 144-MHz, 432-MHz, or 915-MHz superficial hyperthermia (OVERGAARD and OVERGAARD 1987; OVERGAARD et al. 1994). The *upper panel* shows the cumulative maximum measured tumor temperature, minimum measured tumor temperature, and maximum normal tissue temperature. The *lower panel* shows the relationship between the measured minimum tumor temperature and tumor thickness measured as depth from surface

most of the tumors received a maximum temperature above the planned 60 min equivalent at 43°C, the minimum tumor temperature was not much higher than that of the normal tissue. The lower panel of Fig. 5.6 illustrates the relationship between the depth of the tumor and the minimum measured tumor temperature, and illustrates an obvious negative correlation between these two parameters.

5.7.6 Other Prognostic Parameters

Several other factors have been shown to influence the response. These include site of the tumor, primary or recurrent lesion, sex, time span since primary lesion, and whether lesions are single or multiple (OVERGAARD et al. 1995; MEYER et al. 1989; BEN-YOSEF and KAPP 1993). In addition, BENTZEN et al. found a correlation between the outcomes of differently treated multiple lesions in individual patients (BENTZEN et al. 1990). Although at present one can only speculate as to the mechanisms behind such a correlation, this finding indicates that a host factor is involved in determining the radiotherapeutic response of melanomas.

5.8 Quality Assurance

The quality of the treatment is of the utmost importance. A careful recording of relevant parameters is a fundamental prerequisite for a proper therapy evaluation. However, this quality control should include all important parameters (hyperthermia, radiotherapy, chemotherapy, patient data, endpoint evaluation, etc.) and should not be concerned only with the heating (OVERGAARD 1990; OVERGAARD and BACH ANDERSEN 1995).

Efforts have been made to create *international guidelines* and to stimulate multi-institutional cooperation, including visits by a quality assurance committee that, on standard reference phantoms, will compare the applied equipment and offer advice to institutions in order to secure the most uniform and best available heating technique (OVERGAARD and BACH ANDERSEN 1995; HAND et al. 1989; SHRIVASTAVA et al. 1989; SHRIVASTAVA et al. 1988).

5.9 The European Multicenter Randomized Clinical Trial with Thermoradiotherapy in Malignant Melanoma (ESHO 3-85)

The fact that malignant melanoma has been found to respond well to radiotherapy given in large doses per fraction, and that the response apparently can be significantly improved by adding hyperthermia, makes this tumor type one of the most suitable clinical models for investigations of the interaction of radiotherapy and hyperthermia. The small number of fractions, which can be spaced at relatively long intervals (several days) apparently without influencing the probability of tumor control, allow treatment with hyperthermia in association with each radiation fraction without having the treatment compromised by problems of thermotolerance (OVERGAARD and NIELSEN 1993; SAPARETO 1987). A pilot study clearly indicated the feasibility of such a strategy and several studies have indicated that a three-fraction radiation schedule using a dose of 8–9 Gy per fraction appears to be one of the most suitable radiotherapy schemes for this disease (OVERGAARD and OVERGAARD 1987).

On this basis in January 1986 the European Society for Hyperthermic Oncology initiated a prospective multicenter randomized clinical trial (ESHO protocol 3-85). The aim was to assess the efficacy of local hyperthermia given as an adjuvant to radiotherapy in the treatment of advanced malignant melanoma lesions, to evaluate tumor response and probability of local control, to assess early and late tolerance in normal tissues, and to evaluate the feasibility of various heating techniques (OVERGAARD 1987; OVERGAARD et al. 1995).

A total of 134 metastatic or recurrent malignant melanoma lesions in 70 patients were randomized to receive radiotherapy alone (three fractions in 8 days) or radiotherapy plus hyperthermia (aiming for 43°C for 60 min) after each fraction. Radiation was given with high-voltage photons or electrons. Criteria for inclusion were superficial tumors suitable for heating, a life expectancy >3 months, evaluable tumors, and no other concurrent treatment. Tumors were stratified according to size (above or below 4 cm) and randomly assigned to a total radiation dose of either 24 or 27 Gy to be given with or without hyperthermia. The endpoint was persistent complete response in the treated area. The trial was closed in April 1992, and 128 tumors were evaluable, with an observation time between 3 and 72 months. Sixty-five tumors were randomized to radiation alone and 63 to radiation + heat. Sixty received 24 Gy and 68 received 27 Gy. Size was <4 cm in 81 and ≥4 cm in 47 tumors.

The ESHO 3-85 protocol confirmed that hyperthermia significantly enhances the effect of radiation, evaluated both as complete response (Table 5.1) and as persistent local control. Overall the 2-year actuarial local tumor control was 37%, and univariate analysis showed a prognostic influence of hyperthermia (radiation alone 28% vs radiation + heat 46%, $P = 0.008$) and radiation dose (24 Gy 25% vs 27 Gy 56%, $P = 0.02$) but not of tumor size (small 42% vs large 29%, $P = 0.21$). The benefit of the combined treatment was in the same order as that previously described in uncontrolled studies (Table 5.1). A multivariate logistic

Table 5.2. Results from the European multicenter randomized trial ESHO 3-85. Multivariate stepwise logistic regression analysis using complete response as the endpoint

Variable	*P* value	Relative risk
Hyperthermia (rad. + heat vs rad. alone)	0.0015	4.01 (1.77–9.08)*
Tumor size (largest diameter in cm)	0.0048	0.77 (0.65–0.91)
Radiation dose (27 vs 24 Gy)	0.049	2.31 (1.03–5.16)
Sex (female)	0.018	2.81 (1.23–6.41)
Time to recurrence (months)	0.41	Not estimated
Tumor localization (Node vs cutaneous)	0.56	Not estimated
Number of tumors (multiple vs single)	0.65	Not estimated
Age (years)	0.65	Not estimated

* 95% confidence limits

regression analysis (Table 5.2) also showed that female sex was beneficial for complete response, whereas the number of tumors in each patient and the type of lesions appeared to be unimportant. The complications of treatment were acceptable and, with the exception of a few heat-induced burns or ulcerations, there was no significant difference between the early damage seen in the fields treated with radiation and that seen when radiation was combined with hyperthermia, in agreement with the experience of others (Ben-Yosef and Kapp 1992). Although most heat treatments were given within half an hour after radiation, this did not result in any substantial enhancement of radiation damage, probably due to the use of active skin cooling in most cases.

5.10 Impact of Local Control on Survival

Although most cases in which (thermo)radiotherapy has been applied in advanced malignant melanoma have involved patients with disseminated disease (where local treatment will have no influence on survival), there are frequently situations where only a single or a few metastatic or recurrent lesions are known. In our collected case material, all known disease was included in the irradiated fields in 349 patients. Overall the 5-year actuarial survival was found to be 32%. However, the patients in whom persistent local control was obtained showed a 5-year actuarial survival probability which was significantly better than that in patients in whom the treatment was unsuccessful (Fig. 5.7). The fact that patients in whom persistent local control of all known disease is achieved at the time of treatment have relatively good survival is in accordance with previous observations (Overgaard and Bentzen 1990; Overgaard 1986; Overgaard et al. 1986; Lee 1980; Overett and Shiu 1985) where similar lesions have been treated with either radiation or surgical excision. Thus, between one-third and one-half of such patients may be expected to be alive after 5 years. This implies that an aggressive approach should be taken in patients in whom only a single or a few metastatic lesions are known. Thus, one should attempt to achieve local control of these lesions, even if this may be associated with a certain risk of late sequelae due to, for example, radiation-induced fibrosis. Furthermore, the patients subjected to thermoradiotherapy have normally been those found to be unfit for surgical treatment and therefore represent a poor prognositc group. Nevertheless, their results are at least as good as those that can be obtained by local surgery, and with considerably lower morbidity. In addition, a number of other parameters may influence survival, as indicated in Table 5.3.

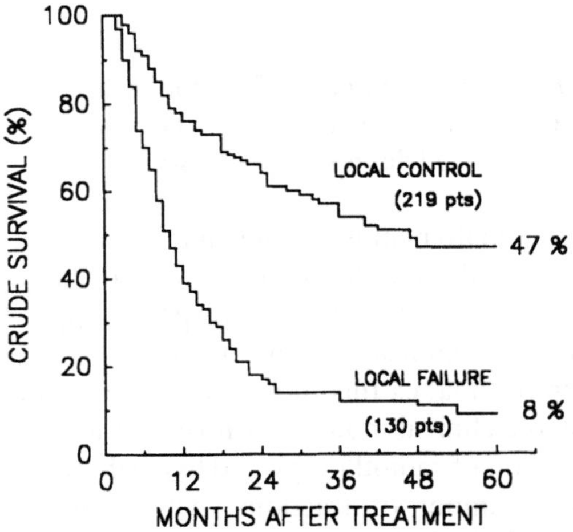

Fig. 5.7. Survival as a function of persistent tumor control in patients in whom all known disease was included in the irradiated field. Data from literature and unpublished studies, including treatment with both radiation alone and thermoradiotherapy

Table 5.3. Prognostic factors for survival after treatment of recurrent or metastatic malignant melanoma

Parameter	Reference
Local control of all lesions	ENGIN et al. (1992), OVERETT and SHIU (1985), OVERGAARD et al. (1995), MARKOWITZ et al. (1991)
Sex (female)	OVERGAARD et al. (1995), PRESANT and BARTOLUCCI (1982), MORTON et al. (1991)
Multiplicity of tumors	OVERGAARD et al. (1995), KARAKOUSIS et al. (1983), OVERETT and SHIU (1985), LEE (1980), BERDEAUX et al. (1985)
Tumor site (visceral vs nonvisceral)	BERDEAUX et al. (1985), MARKOWITZ et al. (1991)
Time to recurrence	KARAKOUSIS et al. (1983), LEE (1980), REINTGEN et al. (1987)

5.11 Concluding Remarks

After 90 years, it has finally been established that radiotherapy is an effective modality in malignant melanoma. Provided lesions are only local, the treatment can be curative and in many patients results in a substantial probability of long-term survival.

It has been demonstrated beyond doubt from noncontrolled trials and a randomized clinical trial that the effect of radiotherapy can be significantly enhanced by combining it with hyperthermia and that such treatment is likely to yield substantial tumor control and pallative effect. Other parameters of importance are the tumor volume and radiation dose.

5.12 Summary

The aforementioned knowledge establishes the following indications for thermoradiotherapy of cutaneous malignant melanomas:

- As *palliative therapy* for cutaneous or lymph node metastases that are easily accessible with radiation and hyperthermia and where no critical structures will be included in the radiation field.
- As aggressive adjuvant therapy in patients with a single or a few local recurrent or metastatic lesions. Such patients should be treated with the aim of cure if there is no evidence of disseminated disease. Since tumor volume is an important parameter, the treatment should be instituted without delay.
- As primary therapy in special cases where surgery is difficult to perform or is contraindicated (e.g., in the head and neck region).
- Treatment can beneficially be given with a few large dose fractions (e.g., 9 Gy ×3), with one or two fractions per week. In order to avoid enhanced radiation morbidity the use of multiple radiation portals may be advised, e.g., if sensitive tissues are at risk, such as during treatment of lymph nodes in the groin. The outcome of such treatment will depend on the tumor volume but is likely to yield significant palliation in up to 80% of the treated patients.
- Hyperthermia should be applied shortly after radiation, and by means of a large dose per fraction schedule it may be feasible to give it in association with each radiation fraction. In such cases one should be careful to avoid heating of normal tissues since this may enhance radiation damage.
- Thermoradiotherapy can today be considered a modality with an established indication in the treatment of recurrent or metastatic cutaneous malignant melanoma, but there are substantial technical shortcomings, and numerous biological questions still need to be answered. It is therefore advisable that the continued use of this modality takes place within the framework of multicenter clinical trials in order to accelerate progress in the treatment. Anyone who looks back and realizes how little has in fact been achieved over the last 90 years can but support this conclusion.

References

Amichetti M, Valdagni R, Pani G (1982) Metastatic melanoma: new prospects with the combination of local hyperthermia and radiotherapy: preliminary notes. Rays 7: 113–117

Arcangeli G, Nervi C, Cividalli A, Lovisolo GA, Mauro F (1985) The clinical use of experimental parameters to evaluate the response to combined heat (HT) and radiation (RT). In: Overgaard J (ed) Hyperthermic oncology 1984, vol 1. Taylor & Francis, London, pp 329–332

Arcangeli G, Benassi M, Cividalli A, Lovisolo GA, Mauro F (1987) Radiotherapy and hyperthermia. Analysis of clinical results and identification of prognostic variables. Cancer 60: 950–956

Ben-Yosef R, Kapp DS (1992) Persistent and/or late complications of combined radiation therapy and hyperthermia. Int J Hyperthermia 8: 733–745

Ben-Yosef R, Kapp DS (1993) Prognostic factors in metastatic malignant melanoma treated with combined radiation therapy and hyperthermia. Int J Hyperthermia 9: 767–781

Bentzen SM, Overgaard J, Thames HD, Overgaard M, Hansen PV, von der Maase H, Meder J (1989) Clinical radiobiology of malignant melanoma. Radiother Oncol 16: 169–182

Bentzen SM, Thames HD, Overgaard J (1990) Does variation in the in vitro cellular radiosensitivity explain the shallow clinical dose-control curve for malignant melanoma? Int J Radiat Biol 57: 117–126

Berdeaux DH, Moon TE, Meyskens FL (1985) Clinical-biologic pattern of metastatic melanoma and their effect on treatment. Cancer Treatment Reports 69: 397–401

Corry PM, Spanos WJ, Tilchen EJ, Barlogie B, Barkley HT, Armour EP (1982) Combined ultrasound and radiation therapy treatment of human superficial tumors. Radiology 145: 165–169

Cox RS, Kapp DS (1992) Correlation of thermal parameters with outcome in combined radiation therapy-hyperthermia trials. Int J Hyperthermia 8: 719–732

Emami B, Perez CA, Konefal J, et al. (1988) Thermoradiotherapy of malignant melanoma. Int J Hyperthermia 4: 373–381

Engin K, Tupchong L, Phil D, Waterman FM, Moylan DJ, Nerlinger RE, Leeper DB (1992) Hyperthermia and radiation in advanced malignant melanoma. Int J Radiat Oncol Biol Phys 25: 87–94

Gonzalez Gonzalez D, van Dijk JDP, Blank LECM, Rümke P (1986) Combined treatment with radiation and hyperthermia in metastatic malignant melanoma. Radiother Oncol 6: 105–113

Hand JW, Lagendijk JJW, Bach Andersen J, Bolomey JC (1989) Quality assurance guidelines for ESHO protocols. Int J Hyperthermia 5: 421–428

Herman TS, Teicher BA, Jochelson M, Clark J, Svensson G, Coleman CN (1988) Rationale for use of local hyperthermia with radiation therapy and selected anticancer drugs in locally advanced human malignancies. Int J Hyperthermia 4: 143–158

Hofman P, Lagendijk JJW, Schipper J (1984) The combination of radiotherapy with hyperthermia in protocolized clinical studies. In: Overgaard J (ed) Hyperthermic oncology 1984, vol 1. Taylor & Francis, London, pp 379–382

Horsman MR, Overgaard J (1989) Thermal radiosensitization in animal tumors: the potential for therapeutic gain. In: Urano M (ed) Hyperthermia and oncology, vol 2. VNU Scientific Publishers, The Netherlands, pp 113–145

Horsman MR, Overgaard J (1992) Simultaneous and sequential treatment with radiation and hyperthermia: a comparative assessment. In: Handl-Zeller L (ed) Interstitial hyperthermia. Springer, Berlin Heidelberg New York, pp 11–33

Howard GCW, Sathiaseelan V (1987) Hyperthermia and radiation in the treatment of superficial malignancy: an analysis of treatment parameters, response and toxicity. Int J Hyperthermia 3: 1–8

Johnson RJR, Sandhu TS, Hetzel FW, Song S-Y, Bicher HI, Subjeck JR, Kowal HS (1979) A pilot study to investigate skin and tumor thermal ratios of 41.5–42.0 degrees centigrade hyperthermia with radiation. Int J Radiat Oncol Biol Phys 5: 947–953

Kapp DS, Petersen IA, Cox RS, et al. (1990) Two or six hyperthermia treatments as an adjunct to radiation therapy yield similar tumor responses: results of a randomized trial. Int J Radiat Oncol Biol Phys 19: 1481–1495

Karakousis CP, Moore R, Holyoke ED (1983) Surgery in recurrent malignant melanoma. Cancer 52: 1342–1345

Kim JH, Hahn EW, Tokita N (1978) Combination hyperthermia and radiation therapy for cutaneous malignant melanoma. Cancer 41: 2143–2148

Kim JH, Hahn EW, Ahmed SA (1982) Combination hyperthermia and radiation therapy for malignant melanoma. Cancer 50: 478–482

Kim JH, Hahn EW, Ahmed SA, Kim YS (1984) Clinical study of the sequence of combined hyperthermia and radiation therapy of malignant melanoma. In: Overgaard J (ed) Hyperthermic oncology 1984. Taylor & Francis, London, pp 387–390

Lee Y-TN (1980) Loco-regional recurrent melanoma. I. Natural history. Cancer Treat Rev 7: 59–72

Marchal C, Bey P, Hoffstetter S, Robert J (1986) Ultrasound and microwave hyperthermia in the treatment of superficial human cancerous tumors. In: Anghileri LJ, Robert J (eds) Hyperthermia in cancer treatment, vol II. CRC Press, Boca Raton, Fl, pp 211–265

Markowitz JS, Cosimi LA, Carey RW, Kang S, Padyk C, Sober AJ, Cosimi AB (1991) Prognosis after initial recurrence of cutaneous melanoma. Arch Surg 126: 703–708

Marsh (1903) A case of multiple melanotic sarcoma unsuccessfully treated by X-rays. Am J Med Sci

Meyer JL, Kapp DS, Fessenden P, Hahn GH (1989) Hyperthermic oncology: current biology, physics and clinical results. Pharmacol Ther 42: 251–288

Morton DL, Wanek L, Nizze JA, Elashoff RM, Wong JH (1991) Improved long-term survival after lymphadenectomy of melanoma metastatic to regional nodes. Ann Surg: 491–501

Müller C (1910) Eine neue Behandlungsmethode bösartiger Geschwülste. Munch Med Wochenschr 28: 1490–1493

Nielsen OS, Munro AJ, Warde PR (1992) Assessment of palliative response in hyperthermia. Int J Hyperthermia 8: 1–10

Oleson JR, Dewhirst MW, Harrelson JM, Leopold KA, Samulski TV, Tso CY (1989) Tumor temperature distributions predict hyperthermia effect. Int J Radiat Oncol Biol Phys 16: 559–570

Overett TK, Shiu MH (1985) Surgical treatment of distant metastatic melanoma. Indications and results. Cancer 56: 1222–1230

Overgaard J (1979) Hyperthermia and radiotherapy. In: Moore M (ed) Advances in medical oncology, research and education. Pergamon Press, Oxford, pp 235–245

Overgaard J (1981) Fractionated radiation and hyperthermia. Experimental and clinical studies. Cancer 48: 1116–1123

Overgaard J (1984) Formula to estimate the thermal enhancement ratio of a single simultaneous hyperthermia and radiation treatment. Acta Radiol Oncol 23: 135–139

Overgaard J (1986) The role of radiotherapy in recurrent and metastatic malignant melanoma: a clinical radiobiological study. Int J Radiat Oncol Biol Phys 12: 867–872

Overgaard J (1987) Hyperthermia as an adjuvant to radiotherapy. Review of the randomized multicenter studies of the European Society for Hyperthermic Oncology. Strahlenther Onkol 163: 453–457

Overgaard J (1989a) The current and potential role of hyperthermia in radiotherapy. Int J Radiat Oncol Biol Phys 16: 535–549

Overgaard J (1989b) Combined hyperthermia and radiation treatment of malignant melanoma. In: Sugahara T, Saito M (eds) Hyperthermic Oncology 1988. Taylor & Francis, London, pp 464–467

Overgaard J (1990) The rationale for clinical trials. In: Field SB, Hand JW (eds) Practical aspects of clinical hyperthermia. Taylor & Francis, London, pp 213–241

Overgaard J (1993) The future of hyperthermic therapy. In: Gerner EW, Cetas TC (eds) Hyperthermic oncology 1992, vol 2, plenary and symposia lectures. Arizona Board of Regents, Tucson, AZ, pp 87–92

Overgaard J, Bach Andersen J (1995) Hyperthermia. In: Peckham M (ed) Textbook of oncology. Oxford University Press, Oxford

Overgaard J, Bentzen SM (1990) Radiotherapy alone or combined with hyperthermia in the treatment of advanced malignant melanoma. In: Rümke P (ed) Pigment cell, vol 10, Therapy of advanced melanoma. Karger, Basel, pp 14–35

Overgaard J, Nielsen OS (1983) The importance of thermotolerance for the clinical treatment with hyperthermia. Radiother Oncol 1: 167–178

Overgaard J, Overgaard M (1987) Hyperthermia as an adjuvant to radiotherapy in the treatment of malignant melanoma. Int J Hyperthermia 3: 483–501

Overgaard J, Overgaard M, Hansen PV, von der Maase H (1986) Some factors of importance in the irradiation treatment of malignant melanoma. Radiother Oncol 5: 183–192

Overgaard J, Nielsen OS, Lindegaard JC (1987) Biological basis for rational design of clinical treatment with combined hyperthermia and radiation. In: Field SB, Franconi C (eds) Physics and technology of hyperthermia. NATO ASI Series E: Applied Sciences No. 127. Martinus Nijhoff, Amsterdam, pp 54–79

Overgaard J, Zucali R, Bentzen SM, Kenda R (1990) The role of radiotherapy in the treatment of melanoma. In: Cascinelli N, Santinami M, Veronesi U (eds) Cutaneous melanoma biology and management. Masson, Milan, pp 257–272

Overgaard J, Gonzalez Gonzalez D, Hulshof MCCM, Arcangeli G, Dahl O, Mella O, Bentzen SM (1995) Randomized trial of hyperthermia as adjuvant to radiotherapy for recurrent or metastatic malignant melanoma. Lancet 345: 540–543

Perez CA, Kopecky W, Rao DV, Baglan R, Mann J (1981) Local microwave hyperthermia and irradiation in cancer therapy: preliminary observations and directions for future clinical trials. Int J Radiat Oncol Biol Phys 7: 765–772

Perez CA, Gillespie B, Pajak T, Hornback NB, Emami BN, Rubin P (1989) Quality assurance problems in clinical hyperthermia and their impact on therapeutic outcome: a report by the Radiation Therapy Oncology Group. Int J Radiat Oncol Biol Phys 16: 551–558

Perez CA, Pajak T, Emami B, Hornback NB, Tupchong L, Rubin P (1991) Randomized phase III study comparing irradiation and hyperthermia with irradiation alone in superficial measurable tumors. Am J Clin Oncol 14: 133–141

Peters LJ (1990) Inherent radiosentitivity of tumour and normal tissue cells as a predictor of human tumor response. Radiother Oncol 17: 177–190

Presant CA, Bartolucci AA (1982) Prognostic factors in metastatic malignant melanoma. The Southeastern Cancer Study Group experience. Cancer 49: 2192–2196

Reintgen DS, Vollmer R, Tso CY, Seigler HF (1987) Prognosis for recurrent stage I malignant melanoma. Arch Surg 122: 1338–1342

Riedel KG (1993) Thermoradiotherapy for malignant choroidal melanoma: the development of a new microwave hyperthermia system. In: Alberti WE, Sagerman RH (eds) Radiotherapy of intraocular and orbital tumors. Springer, Berlin Heidelberg New York, pp 79–97

Rofstad EK (1986) Radiation biology of malignant melanoma. Acta Radiol Oncol 25: 1–10

Sapareto SA (1987) Thermal isoeffect dose: addressing the problem of thermotolerance. Int J Hyperthermia 3: 297–305

Sause WT, Cooper JS, Rush S, et al. (1991) Fraction size in external beam radiation therapy in the treatment of malignant melanoma. Int J Radiat Oncol Biol Phys 20: 429–432

Savchenko NE, Zhakov IG, Fradkin SZ, Zhavrid EA (1987) The use of hyperthermia in oncology. Med Radiol (Mosk) 32: 19–24

Scott RS, Johnson RJR, Kowal H, Krishnamsetty RM, Story K, Clay L (1983) Hyperthermia in combination with radiotherapy: a review of five years experience in the treatment of superficial tumours. Int J Radiat Oncol Biol Phys 9: 1327–1333

Shidnia H, Hornback NB, Shen RN, Shupe RE, Yune M (1990) An overview of the role of radiation therapy and hyperthermia in treatment of malignant melanoma. Adv Exp Med Biol 267: 531–545

Shrivastava PN, Saylor TK, Matloubieh AY, Paliwal BR (1988) Hyperthermia thermometry evaluation: criteria and guidelines. Int J Radiat Oncol Biol Phys 14: 327–335

Shrivastava P, Luk K, Oleson J, et al. (1989) Hyperthermia quality assurance guidelines. Int J Radiat Oncol Biol Phys 16: 571–587

Trott KR (1993) The fractionation sensitivity of malignant melanomas. In: Beck-Bornholdt H-P (ed) Current topics in clinical radiobiology of tumours, Springer, Berlin, Heidelberg New York, pp 75–85

U R, Noell T, Woodward KT, Worde BT, Fishburn RI, Miller LS (1980) Microwave-induced local hyperthermia in combination with radiotherapy of human malignant tumors. Cancer 45: 638–646

Valdagni R, Liu F-F, Kapp DS (1988) Important prognostic factors influencing outcome of combined radiation and hyperthermia. Int J Radiat Oncol Biol Phys 15: 959–972

Withers HR, Thames HD, Peters LJ (1983) A new isoeffect curve for change in dose per fraction. Radiother Oncol 1: 187–191

6 Thermoradiotherapy combined with Chemotherapy for Esophageal Tumors

K. KITAMURA and K. SUGIMACHI

CONTENTS

6.1 Introduction

Esophageal carcinoma is known usually to have a poor prognosis even when the lesion is removed by surgery. Many clinical trials on adjuvant therapy have been attempted, and such therapy has been reported to improve the prognosis (KELSEN et al. 1983; SUGIMACHI et al. 1986). In general, there have been four alternative treatment modalities for esophageal cancer: radiotherapy, chemotherapy, hyperthermia, and immunotherapy. Nowadays, immunotherapy is little used, whereas the other three modalities remain popular. In particular, hyperthermia has recently become well established and is widely used in combination with chemotherapy and/or irradiation (LI and HOU 1987; SUGIMACHI et al. 1988).

In this chapter, we discuss the principles and technique of RF (radio-frequency wave) heating for esophageal tumors. Clinical results of retrospective and prospective studies on combined hyperthermia, chemotherapy, and radiotherapy are presented, and the results of other group studies are also mentioned.

K. KITAMURA, MD, Department of Surgery II, Kyushu University, 3-1-1, Maidashi, Higashi-ku, Fukuoka 812, Japan

K. SUGIMACHI, MD, FACS, Professor, Department of Surgery II, Kyushu University, 3-1-1, Maidashi, Higashi-ku, Fukuoka 812, Japan

6.2 The Experience of Kyushu University

6.2.1 Materials and Methods

6.2.1.1 Retrospective Study

Between January 1965 and December 1989, 737 Japanese patients were admitted to the Department of Surgery II, Kyushu University, with a diagnosis of esophageal carcinoma. Of these patients, we excluded 338 patients with (a) cervical esophageal cancer, (b) adenocarcinoma, (c) early stage carcinoma confined up to submucosa (SUGIMACHI et al. 1991), or (d) multiple primary cancer from this study. The remaining 399 patients were divided into two groups according to operative status. Group 1 included 259 patients who underwent subtotal esophagectomy, while group 2 included 140 patients who were not treated with surgical resection of the carcinoma. We further divided each of these two groups into two subgroups according to treatment modalities. The treatment arms included combined hyperthermia, chemotherapy, and radiotherapy (HCR) and chemoradiotherapy (CR). In group 1, 114 patients treated with HCR composed group 1a, and 145 patients treated with CR formed group 1b. In group 2, 46 patients treated with HCR composed group 2a, and 94 patients treated with CR made up group 2b (Table 6.1). The reasons for nonresection are shown in Table 6.2.

6.2.1.2 Prospective Study

From January 1988 to December 1991, 169 patients underwent subtotal esophagectomy. In accordance with the described indications, 66 patients with resectable primary squamous cell carcinoma of the thoracic esophagus were included in this study. Randomization utilized the coin-flip method for the first of each pair of patients. Thirty-two patients were included in the HCR

Table 6.1. Details of patients, treatment, and results in the retrospective study

	Group 1 (n = 259)[a]		Group 2 (n = 140)[a]	
	1a (n = 114)	1b (n = 145)	2a (n = 46)	2b (n = 94)
Age (yrs)				
Mean	63.3 ± 39.9	63.3 ± 7.8	67.3 ± 9.0	63.3 ± 8.9
Range	38–81	42–80	49–80	35–86
Sex				
Male	97 (85.1)[b]	121 (83.4)	42 (91.3)	79 (84.0)
Female	17 (14.9)	24 (16.6)	4 (8.7)	15 (16.0)
Site of lesion				
Upper	17 (14.9)	30 (20.7)	7 (15.2)	23 (24.5)
Middle	76 (66.7)	87 (60.0)	30 (65.2)	58 (61.7)
Lower	21 (18.4)	28 (19.3)	9 (19.6)	13 (13.8)
TNM stage[c]				
I/II	49 (43.0)	44 (30.3)	19 (41.3)	32 (34.0)
III/IV	65 (57.0)	101 (69.7)	27 (58.7)	62 (66.0)
Mean doses				
Hyperthermia (times)	5.6 ± 1.6	–	7.4 ± 5.2	–
BLM (mg)	30.3 ± 7.6	28.4 ± 13.3	30.6 ± 8.8	36.1 ± 75.0
CDDP (mg)	150	150	150	150
Radiation (Gy)	31.2 ± 3.6	35.6 ± 6.0	47.6 ± 21.8	47.8 ± 23.6
Assessment of treatment				
Markedly effective	25 (21.9)	17 (11.7)	–	–
Moderately effective	54 (47.4)	52 (35.9)	–	–
Imeffective	35 (30.7)	76 (52.4)	–	–

[a] Groups as defined in the text
[b] Percentages are shown within parentheses throughout the table
[c] All patients were classified into TNM stage I through IV according to preprocedural findings

Table 6.2. Reasons for nonresection in group 2

Reasons	No. of patients (%)
Infiltration of surrounding tissue	47 (33.6)
Distant metastatic disease	42 (30.0)
Poor general physical condition	35 (25.0)
Refusal of patient	16 (11.4)
Total	140 (100.0)

group, and 34 patients were included in the CR group (Table 6.3).

6.2.1.3 Technique of Hyperthermia and Heating Equipment

The Endoradiotherm 100A (Olympus Optical Co. LTD., Japan) is an apparatus for delivering intraluminal hyperthermia using 13.56-MHz RF (Fig. 6.1). The output power up to 250 W, temperature and heating time were controlled by means of an automatic on-off system within the ranges set in advance. At the same time as the heating apparatus was developed, we also design-

Table 6.3. Patients in controlled prospective study

	HCR (n = 32)	CR (n = 34)
Age (yrs)		
Mean	61.1 ± 9.7	64.8 ± 7.1
Range	43–82	48–76
Sex		
Male	28 (87.5)[a]	34
Female	4 (12.5)	0
Site of lesion		
Upper	3 (9.4)	10 (29.4)
Middle	24 (75.0)	18 (52.9)
Lower	5 (15.6)	6 (17.7)
Length (cm)		
Mean	5.7 ± 2.2	5.2 ± 2.0
Range	3.0 – 11.0	3.0 – 11.0
TNM stage		
I/II	12 (37.5)	12 (35.3)
III/IV	20 (62.5)	22 (64.7)
Mean doses		
Hyperthermia (times)	5.6 ± 0.8	–
BLM (mg)	26.7 ± 8.0	21.8 ± 13.6
CDDP (mg)	150	150
Radiation (Gy)	29.1 ± 5.3	31.4 ± 5.0
Assessment of treatment		
Markedly effective	8 (25.0)	2 (5.9)
Moderately effective	14 (43.8)	13 (38.2)
Ineffective	10 (31.2)	19 (55.9)

[a] Percentages are shown within parentheses throughout the table

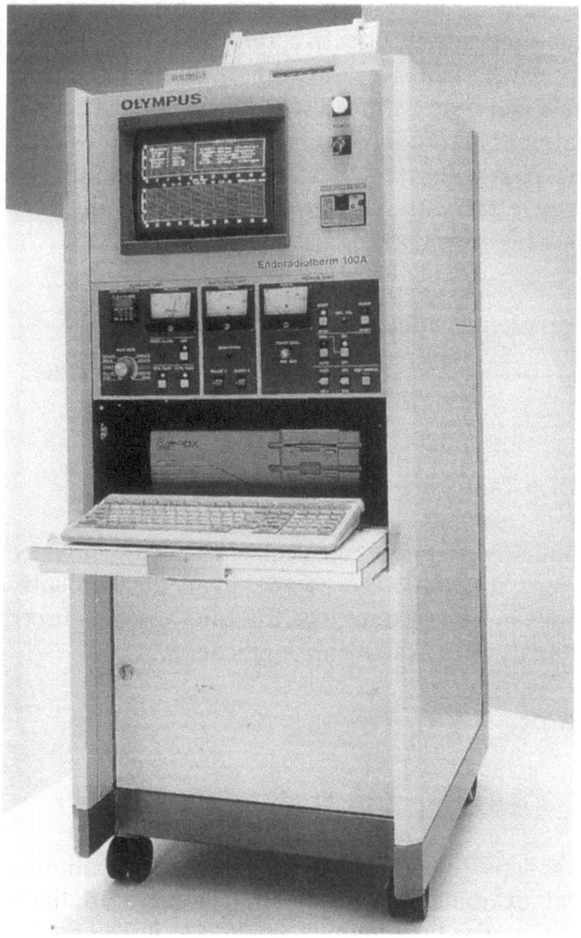

Fig. 6.1. 13.56-RF heating apparatus, Endoradiotherm 100A (Olympus Optical Co. Ltd., Japan)

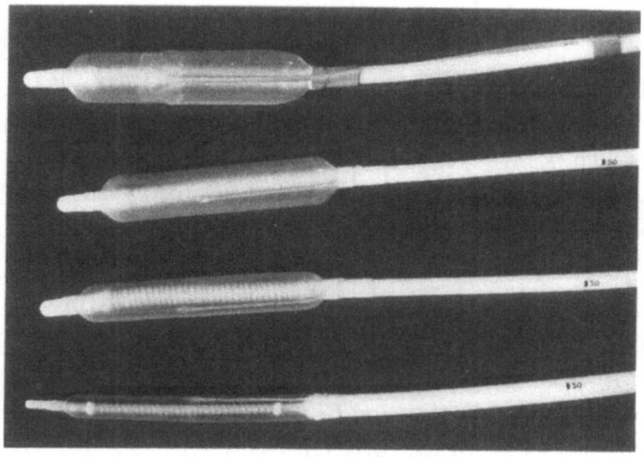

Fig. 6.2. Intraluminal electrodes for intraluminal hyperthermia; different applicator diameters are shown

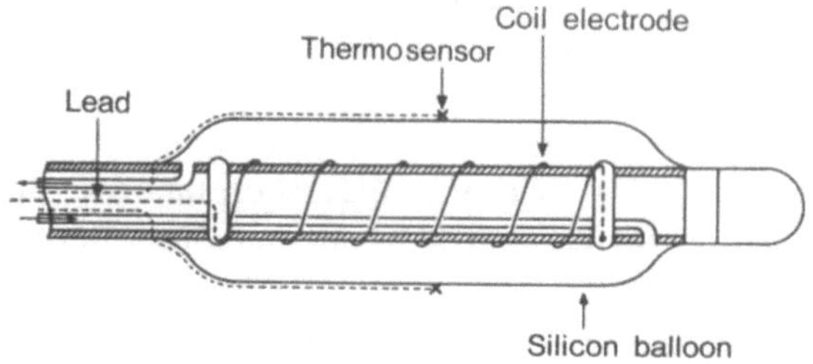

Fig. 6.3. Basic design of the intraluminal electrode

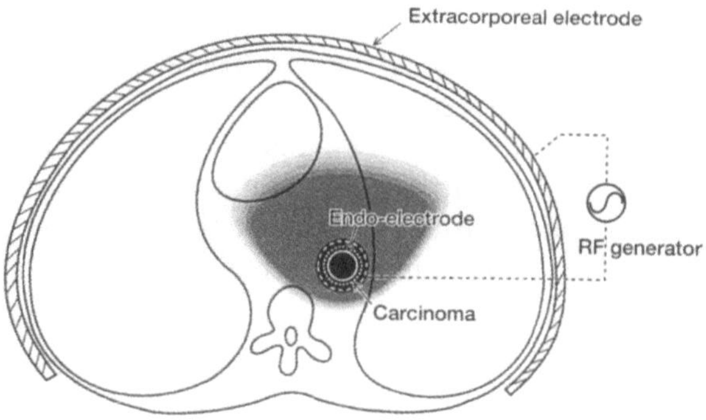

Fig. 6.4. Area heated with RF hyperthermia. Previous applicators could not avoid the diffusion of the electromagnetic field; however, the new endotract electrode is capable of concentrating the electromagnetic field around the esophageal lesion

ed a special intraluminal electrode (SUGIMACHI et al. 1983), which has a flexible applicator, for esophageal heating using RF (Fig. 6.2). Three kinds of applicators are available: 20 mm, 15 mm, and 10 mm in diameter; the choice as to which applicator is used is made according to the severity of the esophageal stenosis. The applicator consists of a microelectrode, a silicon balloon in which water circulates for cooling of the surrounding tissue and two thermosensors for monitoring the temperature at the tumor surface (Fig. 6.3). Since the the effective temperature (over 42.5°C) can reach up to 2 cm in depth, tumors are usually heated adequately. The applicator is inserted into the esophagus and attached to the lesion. A large extracorporeal electrode is placed on the anterior chest. The difference of squares (cm^2) of these two electrodes focuses the electromagnetic field at the smaller electrode (Fig. 6.4). Hence, only the area around the lesion is properly heated.

The preparation for heating is as easy as that for endoscopic examination. The patients are advised only to fast for 2 or 3 h prior to the treatment.

6.2.1.4 HCR Treatment Schedule

The applied HCR treatment regimen is shown in Fig. 6.5. Irradiation (1.5–2.0 Gy) given for 5 days per week was combined with two fractions of hyperthermia (42.5°–45.0°C for 30 min). Chemotherapy comprised bleomycin (BLM, 5 mg i.v.) or cisplatin (CDDP, 50 mg div.; not shown on Fig. 6.5), given simultaneously with heating within an hour. One schedule of HCR lasts 3 weeks, and total doses are six fractions of hyperthermia, 30 Gy of irradiation, and 30 mg BLM or 150 mg CDDP as chemotherapy (Sugimachi et al. 1988).

For patients with resectable carcinoma, one schedule of HCR is given preoperatively. Approximately a week after termination of HCR, subtotal esophagectomy with lymph node dissection is performed. For patients without surgical resection, we try to repeat the HCR therapy as often as possible, depending upon each patient's condition. Data on patients treated with chemoradiotherapy (CR), without hyperthermia, are also presented for comparison. All patients tolerated both HCR and CR well. Averages of all doses for each treatment modality are shown in Tables 6.1 and 6.3.

6.2.1.5 Histopathological Evaluation

All resected specimens, including dissected lymph nodes, were investigated histopathologically in order to evaluate the effectiveness of preoperative treatment modalities. Treatment results wese categorized according to microscopic findings as follows: (a) treatment ineffective (grades 0, 1) – most cancer cells were intact (Fig. 6.6A); (b) treatment moderately effective (grade 2) – although most cancer cells were extremely damaged, a few viable cells were still present (Fig. 6.6B), and (c) treatment markedly effective (grade 3) – all viable cancerous cells were destroyed (Fig. 6.6C). The effective response rates were calculated with the following formula:

$$\frac{\text{No. of patients with (markedly effective + moderately effective) response}}{\text{No. of all patients}} \times 100(\%).$$

6.2.1.6 Statistics

Cumulative survival rates calculated with Kaplan-Meier's method were compared in the two subgroups in each group. The log-rank test was used for analysis of statistical significance.

6.2.2 Results

6.2.2.1 Retrospective Study

In groups 1a and 1b, respectively, histopathological examinations revealed treatment to have been markedly effective in 25 (21.9%) and 17 (11.7%) specimens, moderately effective in 54 (47.4%) and 52 (35.9%), and ineffective in 35 (30.7%) and 76 (52.4%) (Table 6.1). The effective response rates were 69.3% in group 1a and 47.6% in group 1b ($P < 0.05$).

The survival curves of 259 patients with surgical resection are shown in Fig. 6.7. The overall

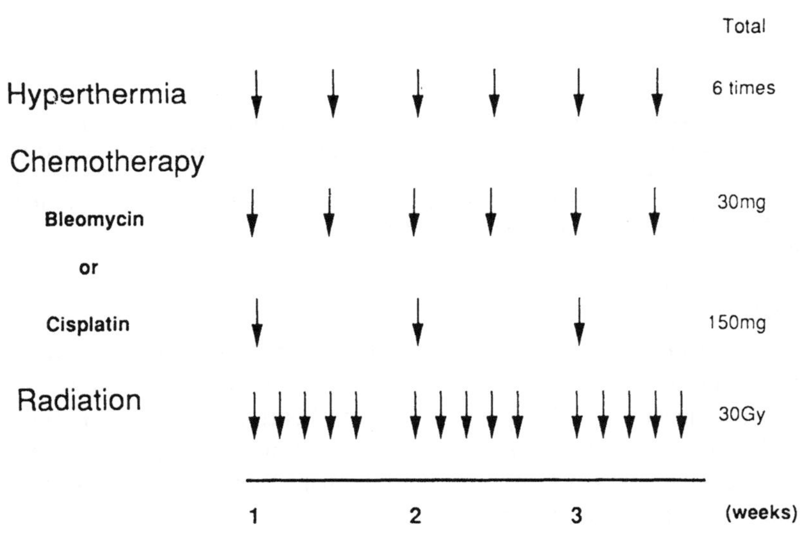

Fig. 6.5. HCR treatment regimen

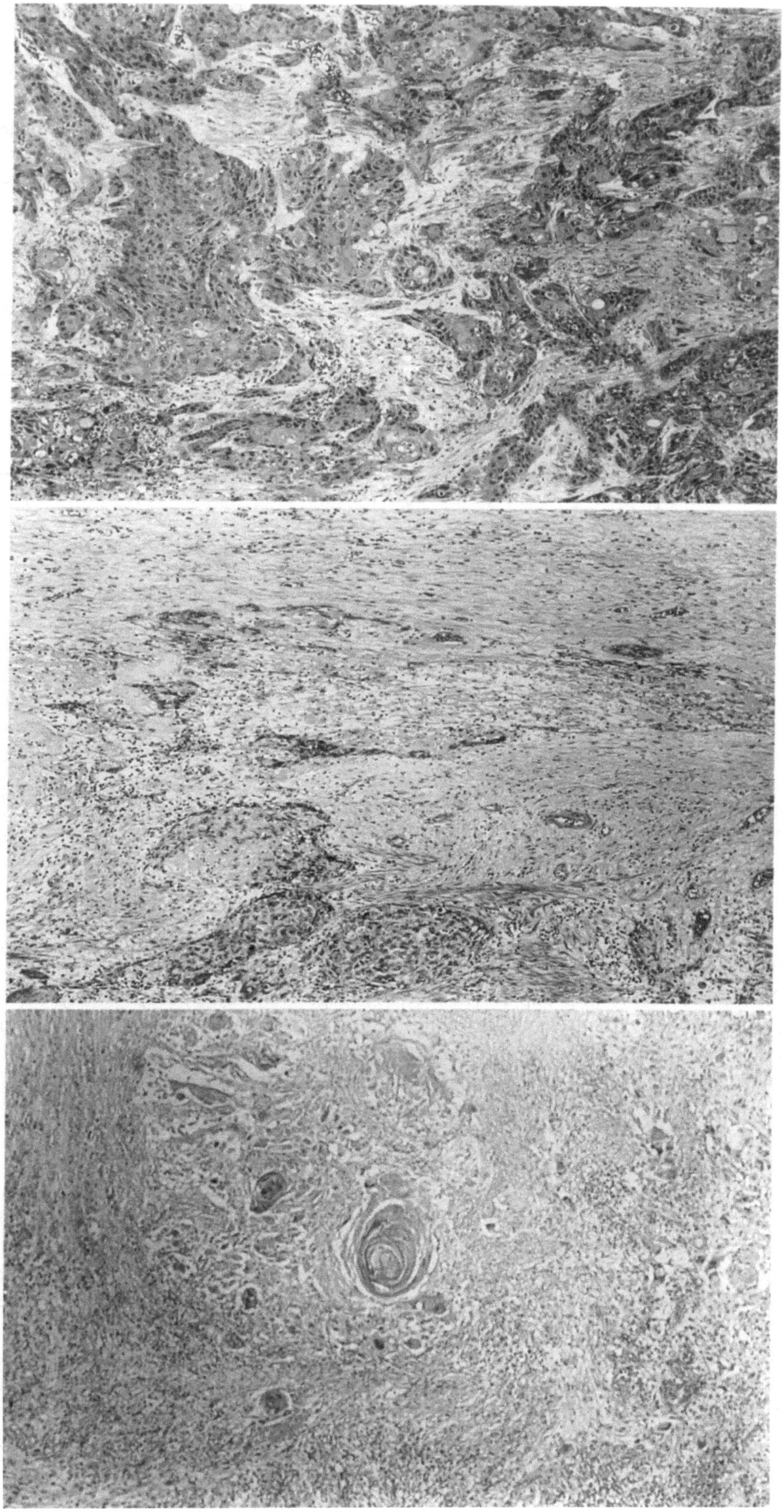

A

B

C

Fig. 6.6A–C. Examples of the three histopathological grades, illustrating treatment effect. **A** Ineffective treatment, grade 0/1. H&E, ×4. **B** Moderately effective treatment, grade 2. H&E, ×4. **C** Markedly effective treatment, grade 3. H&E, ×4

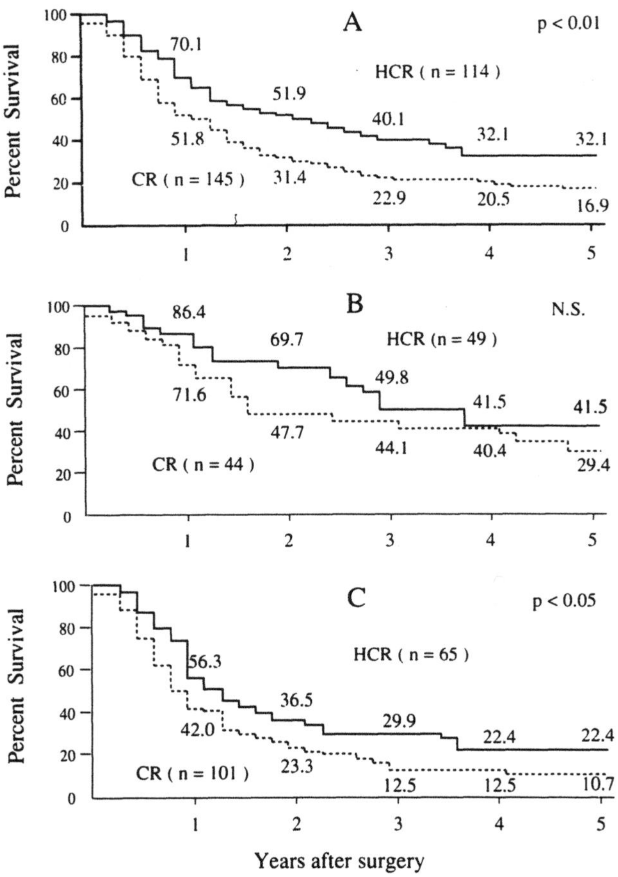

Fig. 6.7A–C. Survival of patients who underwent surgery (*solid line*, group 1a; *broken line*, group 1b). **A** Overall results; **B** patients with TNM stage I/II; **C** patients with TNM stage III/IV

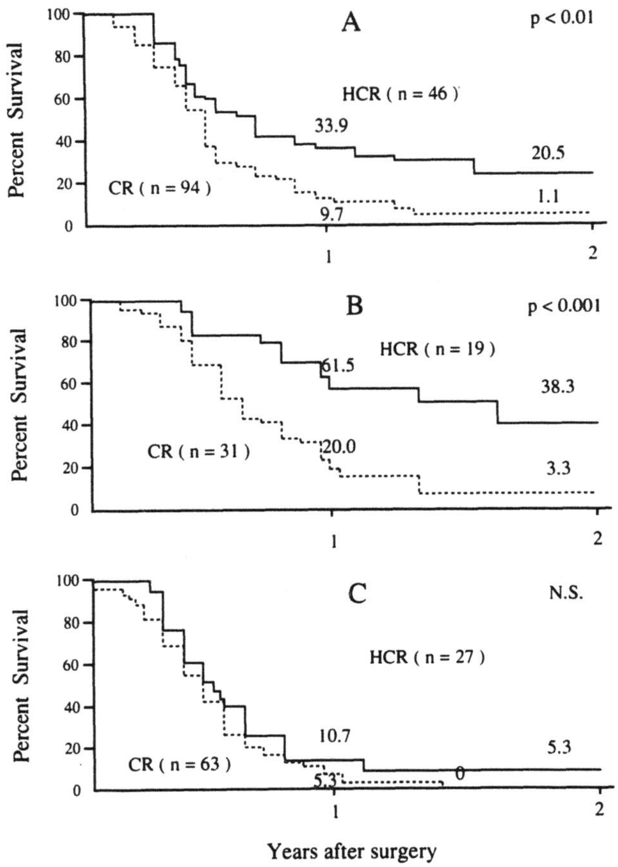

Fig. 6.8A–C. The survival curves of patients without surgical resection (*solid line*: group 2a; *broken line*: group 2b). **A** Overall resullts; **B** patients with TNM stage I/II; **C** patients with TNM stage III/IV

1-, 3-, and 5-year survival rates were 70.1%, 40.1%, and 32.1% in group 1a, and 51.8%, 22.9%, and 16.9% in group 1b ($P < 0.001$) (Fig. 6.7A). With regard to the TNM stage (Harmer and Sobin 1987), the 5-year survival rates of patients with stage I/II disease were 41.5% in group 1a and 29.4% in group 1b (nonsignificant difference) (Fig. 6.7B), while those of patients with stage III/IV disease were 22.4% in group 1a and 10.7% in group 1b ($P < 0.05$) (Fig. 6.7C).

The survival curves of 140 patients who did not undergo surgical resection are shown in Fig. 6.8. The overall 1- and 2-year survival rates were, respectively, 33.9% and 20.5% in group 2a, and 9.7% and 1.1% in group 2b ($P < 0.01$) (Fig. 6.8A). The 2-year survival rates of patients with TNM stage I/II were 38.3% in group 2a and 3.3% in group 2b ($P < 0.001$) (Fig. 6.8B), while those of patients with TNM stage III/IV were 5.3% in group 2a and 0% in group 2b (nonsignificant difference) (Fig. 6.8C).

Esophagram and endoscopic studies before and after HCR therapy are shown in Figs. 6.9A and 6.9B, respectively. A Borrmann type II carcinoma disappeared after one schedule of HCR therapy, with no cancer cells being detected in the resected specimens.

6.2.2.2 Prospective Study

Treatment results as assessed on the basis of histopathological examination of the resected specimens in each group were as follows: In the HCR group eight specimens (25%) indicated markedly effective treatment, 14 (43.8%), moderately effective treatment, and 10 (31.2%), ineffective treatment. On the other hand, in the CR group two specimens (5.9%) indicated markedly effective treatment, 13 (38.2%) moderately effective treatment, and 19 (55.9%), ineffective treatment (Table 6.3). The effective response rates

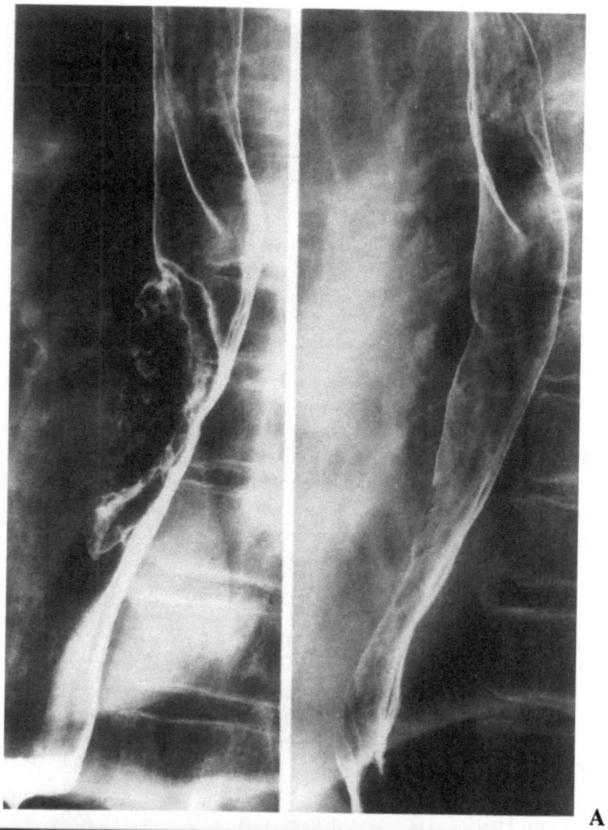

A

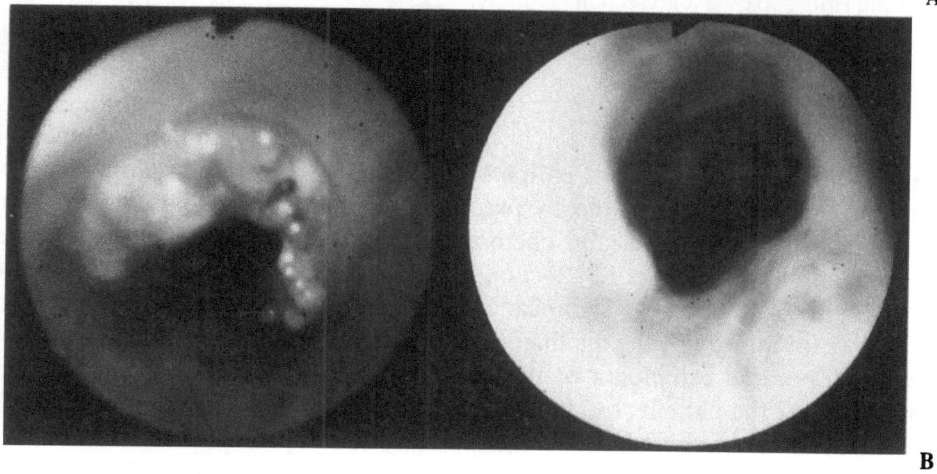

B

Fig. 6.9. **A** Esophagrams before and after treatment. An 8-cm mass with ulceration exists in the middle esophagus (*left*). After one schedule of HCR therapy, the lesion has disappeared completely (*right*). **B** An initial endoscopic examination shows a Borrmann II type carcinoma (*left*). The tumor has disappeared and a shallow ulceration still remains after treatment (*right*)

were 68.8% in the HCR group and 44.1% in the CR group ($P < 0.05$). The 1- and 3-year survival rates were, respectively, 68.1% and 56.5% in the HCR group and 60.3% and 27.5% in the CR group ($P < 0.05$) (Fig. 6.10).

6.3 Results of Other Trials

Several studies applying hyperthermia with chemo(radio)therapy have been reported (Li and Hou 1987; Sugimachi et al. 1988, 1992, 1994; Shimizu et al. 1994). Table 6.4 includes one preoperative study and two trials for non-resected cases. In addition to the favorable results of the HCR studies presented herein, the prospective group study of preoperative combined hyperthermia and chemotherapy by Sugimachi et al. also revealed improvement in both clinical and pathological findings compared with patients treated with chemotherapy alone (Sugimachi et al. 1994). The efficiency rate was 50% with no severe side-effects. With regard to results in patients who did not undergo resection, Li and Hou reported that

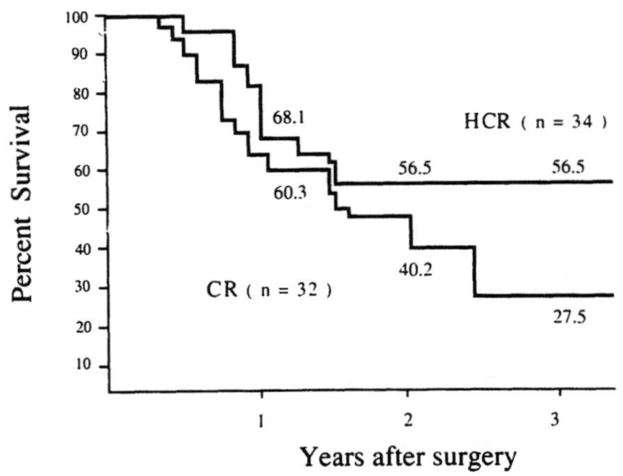

Fig. 6.10. The survival rates were 68.1% at 1 year and 56.5% at 2 and 3 years in the HCR group. The survival rates were 60.3%, 40.2% and 27.5% at 1, 2 and 3 years, respectively, in the CR group

Table 6.4. Results of other trials

Author (year)	No.	Treatment sequence	Treatment	Efficiency rate
Sugimachi et al. (1994)	40	Preop.	HC	50%
Li and Hou (1987)	32	Nonresection	HC	25%
Shimizu et al. (1994)	42	Nonreseciton	HCR	53.3%

the mean survival period of patients with a complete response when treated by preoperative intraluminal hyperthermia and chemotherapy was more than 1 year (range: 12–26 months). Shimizu et al. (1994) stressed the significance of adjuvant therapy for improving the quality of life of patients with inoperable carcinoma of the esophagus. In their series, the patients treated with intraluminal hyperthermia combined with chemotherapy survived 262.2 days on average, while those treated with chemoradiotherapy without hyperthermia survived an average of only 112.6 days. The mean periods of effective oral intake and home stay, which were 211 days and 167 days respectively in the heating group, were much longer than those in the other treatment groups.

6.4 Discussion

Early diagnosis is the key to improving upon the poor results achieved in the surgical treatment of esophageal cancer. About 95% of patients, however, already have advanced carcinoma at the initial diagnosis (Sugimachi et al. 1991). Froelicher and Miller (1986) reported the incidence of early esophageal carcinoma, which is localized within the submucosal layer, to be 0.75% in European countries. Even after curative surgery the 5-year survival rate is reported to be as low as approximately 20% (Müller et al. 1990). Numerous clinical trials, using radiotherapy, chemotherapy and hyperthermia in various combinations and schedules have therefore been carried out in an attempt to improve the treatment results in esophageal cancer. Thus far, radiation and chemotherapy have become well-accepted treatment modalities, sometimes being used alone, sometimes in combination (Kelsen et al. 1983; Sugimachi et al. 1986; Leichmann et al. 1984). However, high-dose applications of radiotherapy or anticancer drugs are often associated with a higher incidence of postoperative morbidity and mortality since surrounding normal tissues also may be damaged (Leichmann et al. 1984). We have therefore prescribed additional heating in order to reduce the doses of radiotherapy and chemotherapeutic agents. There is much controversy as to (a) the time interval between these treatment modalities and (b) when they should be given in relation to surgery (Oleson et al. 1988). Maximum cytotoxicity is usually obtained when the treatments are combined simultaneously. We chose the preoperative phase since (a) the condition of patients following surgery may make it more difficult to complete the whole treatment schedule, and (b) micrometastasis through the vascular system in the early postoperative period may be related to intraoperative manipulation of cancer cells (Sugimachi et al. 1988). Radiotherapy and hyperthermia are both treatments for improvement of regional control; chemotherapy is expected to have a systemic effect. As chemotherapeutic agents, we chose BLM and CDDP, both of which have been proven to provide intensive synergism with hyperthermia and irradiation (Kelsen et al. 1983; Leichmann et al. 1984; Teicher et al. 1988).

In general, the essential problems facing clinical application of hyperthermia to the esophagus are: (a) how to heat properly a tumor located deeply in the body, and (b) how to measure the exact temperature of the tumor during noninvasive heating. We conquered the first problem by designing an endotract electrode for RF heating, based on the fact that an electromagnetic field concentrates on the smaller electrode when there are two electrodes of different squares (cm^2). Esophageal tumors accordingly can be heated selectively. With regard to the second problem, we have measured the heating temperature intraoperatively. When the temperature of esophageal mucosa at the heated side reached 44.5°C, we found that on the adventitia side the temperature exceeded 42.5°C (SUGIMACHI et al. 1988). This preliminary study demonstrated that the thermal power could reach a maximum depth of 2 cm from the applicator surface. During clinical use, tumor temperature is monitored by two thermometers built into the applicator surface.

Our data reported herein, and the data in the literature shown in Table 6.4, reveal that adding hyperthermia to the treatment regimen does not result in an increased frequency of side-effects. Our preoperative treatment schedule, involving lower doses of each treatment modality and a reasonable interval from adjuvant therapy to surgery (7–10 days) may have contributed to the lack of severe postoperative complications. In the retrospective series of patients with and without surgical resection, long-term results have been improved with HCR, depending on the TNM stage. In addition, the presented results in the prospective randomized study again disclose that preoperative HCR is of great benefit in the treatment of esophageal cancer. It is difficult to compare the significance of the effectiveness of each treatment modality since the treatment conditions of the studies are quite different, including the initial background of patients; however, the fact that adding hyperthermia improves treatment result should be paid much attention.

Hence, much progress has been made in clinical hyperthermia. Nevertheless, approximately 30% of the patients still have no response to HCR, and the survival rates of these patients are far from ideal. In view of this fact, further work is recommended in the following areas:

1. Development of an effective assay which is capable of predicting the response to adjuvant therapy
2. Conduct of new and completion of ongoing prospective studies
3. Definition of "thermal dose" as well as provision of further specific details on radiation therapy and chemotherapeutic drugs
4. Improvement of present heating equipment and applicators
5. Exploration of the technique of noninvasive and accurate measurement of temperature.

6.5 Summary

- Esophageal cancer is one of the most difficult malignancies to control by resection alone. To improve the unfavorable prognosis, RF hyperthermia can be applied combined with chemotherapy and irradiation.
- In both retrospective and prospective studies, hyperthermia combined with chemoradiotherapy showed significantly better results in respect of not only local control but also long-term effects without serious complications.
- In 1990, we started another prospective trial of combined hyperthermia and chemotherapy, and this has revealed favorable results in terms of both clinical and pathological findings. Furthermore, adjuvant therapy with hyperthermia has been applied with excellent results for the treatment of patients without surgical resection.
- Hyperthermia can be regarded as a reliable option for treatment of carcinoma of the esophagus.
- Detailed research on the mechanisms of thermal cytotoxicity and thermal sensitization of malignant tumors is required.

References

Earlam R, Cunha-Melo JR (1980) Oesophageal squamous cell carcinoma: a critical review of surgery. Br J Surg 67: 381–390

Froelicher P, Miller G (1986) The European experience with esophageal cancer limited to the mucosa and submucosa. Gastrointest Endosc 32: 88–90

Harmer MH, Sobin LH (1987) TNM classification of malignant tumors. UICC, 4th edn. Springer, Berlin Heidelberg New York

Kelsen DP, Hilaris B, Cooley C, Chapman R, Lesser M, Dukeman M, Heelan R, Bains M (1983) Cisplatin, Vindesine and bleomycin chemotherapy of local regional and advanced esophageal carcinoma. Am J Med 75: 639–652

Leichmann L, Steiger Z, Seydel HG, Vaitkevicius VK (1984) Combined preoperative chemotherapy and radiation therapy for cancer of the esophagus: The Wayne State University, Southwest Oncology Group and Radiation Therapy Oncology Group Experience. Semin Oncol 11: 178–185

Li DJ, Hou BS (1987) Preliminary report in the treatment of esophageal cancer by intraluminal microwave hyperthermia and chemotherapy. Cancer Treat Rep 71: 1013–1019

Müller JM, Erasmi H, Stelzen M, Stelzner M, Zieren U, Pichlmaier H (1990) Surgical therapy of oesophageal carcinoma. Br J Surg 77: 845–857

Oleson JR, Calderwood SK, Coughlin CT, Dewhirst MW, Gerweck LE, Gibbs FA, Kapp DS (1988) Biological and clinical aspects of hyperthermia in cancer therapy. Am J Clin Oncol 11: 368–380

Shimizu T, Sakamoto T, Takemori S, Masuko Y, Karaki Y, Tazawa K, Fujimaki M (1994) Quality of life of patients treated by radiochemotherapy combined with hyperthermia for inoperable advanced cancer od the thoracic esophagus Jpn J Hyperthermia 10: 309–315

Sugimachi K, Inokuchi K, Kai H, Sogawa A, Kawai Y (1983) Endotract antenna for application of hyperthermia to malignant lesion. Gan To Kagaku Ryoho 74: 622–624

Sugimachi K, Matsufuji H, Kai H, Mauda H, Ueo H, Inokuchi K, Jingu K (1986) Preoperative irradiation for carcinoma of the esophagus. Surg Gynecol Obstet 162: 174–176

Sugimachi K, Matsufuji H, Ohno S, Fukuda A, Matsuoka H, Mori M, Kuwano H (1988) Long term effects of hyperthermia combined with chemotherapy and irradiation for the treatment of patients with carcinoma of the esophagus. Surg Gynecol Obstet 167: 319–323

Sugimachi K, Kitamura K, Matsuda H, Mori M, Kuwano H, Ide H (1991) Proposed new criteria for early carcinoma of the esophagus. Surg Gynecol Obstet 173: 303–308

Sugimachi K, Kuwano H, IdeH, Saku M, Oshiumi Y (1994) Chemotherapy combined with or without hyperthermia for patients with oesophageal carcinoma: a prospective randomized trial. Int J Hyperthermia 10: 485–493

Teicher BA, Herman TS and Holden SD (1988) Combination modality therapy with bleomycin, radiation and hyperthermia. Cancer Res 48: 6291–6297

7 Thermoradiotherapy for Upper Abdominal Tumors

M. Hiraoka and M. Abe

CONTENTS

7.1 Introduction

Upper abdominal tumors such as liver cancer, pancreatic cancer, and gastric cancer are very often detected at an advanced stage. In this situation the local control rate achieved with conventional radiation therapy and/or surgery plus chemotherapy is usually very low. It is highly probable that an improvement in local control would result in a higher cure rate. Therefore, patients with advanced upper abdominal tumors are considered to be good candidates for new treatment approaches like locoregional hyperthermia provided that the tumor can be adequately heated and the tumor temperature can be well monitored.

7.2 Technical Options

Methods of locoregional hyperthermia reported for upper abdominal tumors include external heating with ultrasound or electromagnetic waves using microwave and radiofrequency (RF) devices. External heating administers heat to the tumor through various body structures and the ideal heating device should be capable of raising the temperature of the whole tumor volume to a therapeutic level without overheating adjacent normal tissues. One possible method for the selective heating of deep-seated tumors is focused ultrasound. Major problems of ultrasound applications are that ultrasound is reflected at the soft tissue/air and bone/soft tissue interfaces and is attenuated rapidly in bone; both these factors make ultrasound difficult to apply to tumors adjacent to air or bone. However, preliminary experience with scanned focused ultrasound has indicated some promise for the treatment of abdominal tumors (Hynynen et al. 1990).

The most commonly used deep heating method is so-called regional heating. Since regional heating techniques apply energy to the adjacent deep-seated tumors in an unfocused manner, energy is also delivered to the adjacent normal tissues. Under such conditions, selective heating of tumors over the normal tissue is only possible when heat dissipation by blood flow is more predominant in the normal tissue.

An annular phased array system delivering 60- to 80-MHz electromagnetic waves and RF capacitive heating apparatus are examples of regional heating devices. The former system has the advantage in that subcutaneous fat is not excessively heated and it is thus suitable for obese patients. However, this method causes systemic symptoms such as tachycardia and malaise which result from the use of large applicators. Systemic stress is reported to be more severe in patients with abdominal tumors than in those with pelvic tumors or tumors of the extremities (Sapozink et al. 1984), suggesting the limited usefulness of this heatimg modality for tumors in the upper abdomen.

M. Hiraoka, MD, Department of Radiology, Faculty of Medicine, Kyoto University, 54 Shogoin Kawaharacho, Sakyo-ku, Kyoto 606, Japan

M, Abe, MD, Director, Kyoto National Hospital 1-1, Fukakusa Mukohatacho, Fushimi-ku, Kyoto 612, Japan

RF capacitive heating is the most widely used method for the external hyperthermia of upper abdominal tumors. Figure 7.1 shows an 8-MHz RF capacitive heating device (Thermotron RF8, Yamamoto Vinita Co., Osaka, Japan) which we have developed with a grant from Research Development Corporation of Japan (ABE et al. 1986). The size of the electrodes to be used is determined according to the size and location of the tumor, and a pair of equal-sized electrodes 20–28 cm in diameter are usually employed. When the tumor is eccentrically located, a pair of different-sized electrodes are employed, with the smaller one being placed on the skin close to the tumor so that the high temperature area is shifted toward the lesion. Each electrode is covered with a water pad and a temperature-controlled salt solution is perfused into the water pad to avoid excessive heating of the skin and the subcutaneous fat. The advantages of RF capacitive heating are its wide applicability to various anatomical sites and the relatively minor systemic stress it causes. Its main disadvantage is the excessive heating of subcutaneous fat and the fact that patients with a subcutaneous fat thickness of more than 1.5–2 cm are difficult to treat with this modality (HIRAOKA et al. 1987).

More invasive heating methods, including intraoperative external heating or interstitial heating for pancreatic cancer and isolated hyperthermic liver perfusion for liver cancer, have also been investigated by some authors. Table 7.1 shows the technical options by treatment sites.

7.3 Thermoradiotherapy for Liver Tumors

7.3.1 *Heating Methods and Effectiveness*

Most recent studies have employed an 8-MHz RF capacitive heating device. In a trial involving nine patients with hepatocellular carcinoma, the maximum tumor temperature ranged from 40.1° to 42.1°C with a mean of 41.5°C (KONDO et al. 1993). In another study of patients with metastatic liver tumors, the maximum tumor temperature exceeded 42°C in six out of nine cases (HAMAZOE et al. 1991b). We have also obtained thermal data

Table 7.1. Technical options by treatment sites

Treatment sites/ Heating methods	Non-invasive methods	Invasive methods
Liver	RF capacitive APAS	Isolated hyperthermic liver perfusion
Pancreas	RF capacitive APAS	Intraoperative US, RF Interstitial microwave
Stomach	RF capacitive APAS	Peritoneal perfusion with hot water

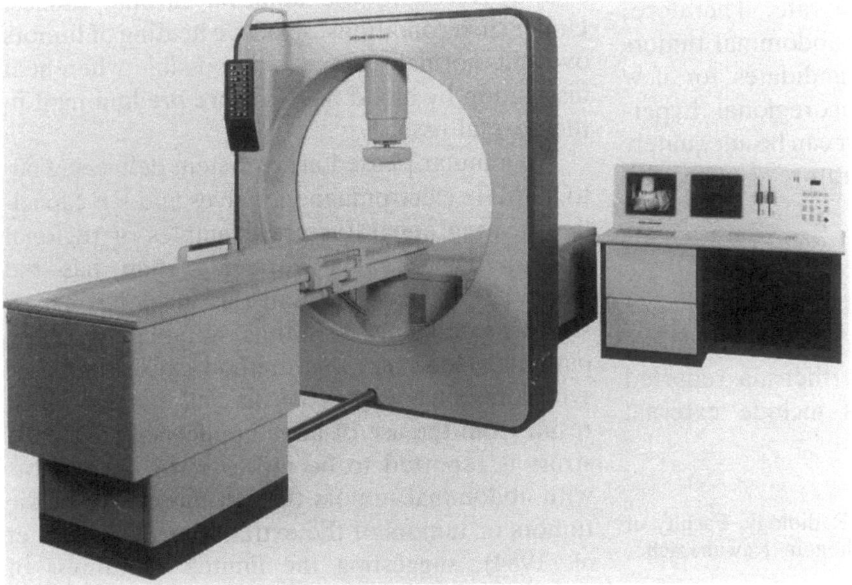

Fig. 7.1. An 8 MHz RF capacitive heating device

during the treatment of liver tumors. Regional hyperthermia was given using a pair of electrodes 25 cm in diameter. A Teflon-coated microthermocouple was inserted into the tumor through an angiocatheter which was inserted into the tumor under ultrasonic guidance. The distribution of temperatures in the tumor and the surrounding liver tissue was then obtained by withdrawing the thermal probe in 1-cm steps immediately after termination of hyperthermic treatment. Figure 7.2 displays a thermal distribution profile and a CT scan showing the location of the angiocatheter inserted into a metastatic liver tumor. The heating capability of the 8-MHz RF capacitive heating device was evaluated for 67 liver tumors including 41 hepatocellular carcinomas, 6 cholangiocarcinomas, and 20 metastatic tumors. The average maximum temperatures achieved for the hepatocellular carcinomas, cholangiocarcinomas, and metastatic tumors were 41.5°, 42.8°, and 42.7°C, respectively, and the average minimum temperatures were 40.0°, 40.4°, and 41.0°, respectively. Among the three subtypes of hepatocellular carcinoma, the diffuse type showed higher tumor temperatures than the massive or nodular types. The temperatures of the liver tumors, the adjacent liver tissue, and the subcutaneous fat were compared in 20 patients with hepatocellular carcinoma. The normal liver tissue temperature was always less than 41.4°C and the mean was 39.8°C. The maximum and minimum tumor temperatures were higher than the normal liver tissue temperature in 17 and 12 cases, respectively (NAGATA et al. 1990). A poorer heating efficiency of hepatocellular carcinoma compared with metastatic liver tumors has been confirmed in another study (TANAKA et al. 1992). This difference is probably attributable to differences in the blood flow pattern, since hepatocellular carcinoma is considered to have a higher blood flow than other tumors.

Regional hyperthermia with an annular phased array has been assessed in a multicenter study enrolling 49 patients with hepatic metastases (PETROVICH et al. 1989). The target was a tumor temperature of 42.5°C maintained for 30 min, but this proved difficult to achieve and therefore equivalent heating at a temperature from 40° to 42°C was used instead. The thermal dose was defined as the number of minutes at 42.5°C or its equivalent. In 21 (43%) patients, a temperature less than 40°C was obtained. The thermal dose was less than or equal to 50 min in 17 (35%) patients, above 50 min and less than or equal to 100 min in seven (14%) patients, and greater than 100 in four (8%) patients.

A number of strategies have been proposed for the selective heating of tumors. One of these is the manipulation of regional blood flow with degradable starch microspheres (DSMs). DSMs are cross-linked starch microspheres with a mean diameter of 45 μm, which are dissolved by α-amylase in the serum and have a biological half-life of 15–30 min. Tumor blood flow is decreased transiently, leading to an increase in heating, when DSMs are administered into a feeding artery during hyperthermia. An accelerated increase in the liver temperature after infusion of DSMs into the common hepatic artery during regional hyper-

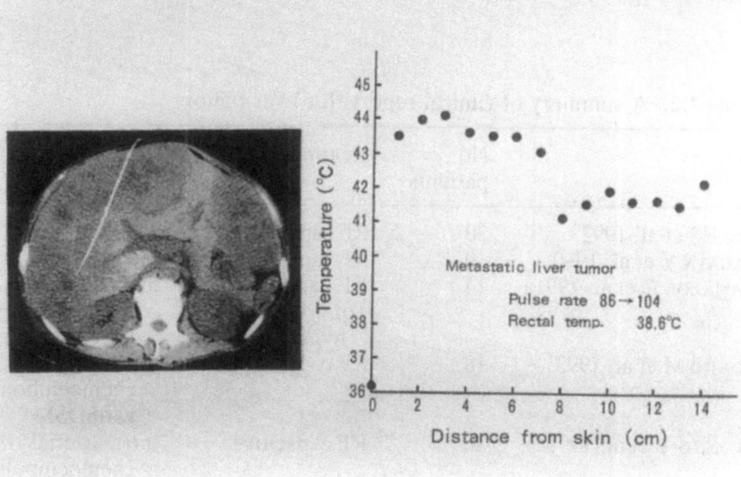

Fig. 7.2. A thermal distribution profile obtained after regional hyperthermia in a patient with liver metastases. The accompanying CT scan shows the location of the angiocatheter

thermia was demonstrated in an experiment using pigs (AKUTA et al. 1987). A subsequent clinical trial showed that transarterial embolization (TAE) with DSMs achieved a 0.9°C increase in the maximum tumor temperature (KONDO et al. 1993). More commonly used embolic agent are Lipiodol and Gelfoam particles, which have a more durable effect than DSMs. Increased elevation of tumor temperature and improvement of the temperature distribution profile for hepatocellular carcinoma have been demonstrated with the use of TAE plus regional hyperthermia when compared with regional hyperthermia alone (SHIMADA et al. 1986). Another study demonstrated that all ten hepatocellular carcinomas treated by TAE could be heated to more than 42.5°C (YUMOTO et al. 1991).

The above thermometry results indicate that an 8-MHz RF capacitive heating device is applicable to various kinds of liver tumors. The heating capability is not satisfactory in that not all of the tumor volume can be heated to the therapeutic range, but combination with TAE will increase the efficacy of regional hyperthermia.

Isolated hyperthermic liver perfusion is also being investigated as a method of heating the whole liver (SKIBBA and QUEBBEMAN 1986).

7.3.2 Clinical Response and Complications

There are few reports concerning thermoradiotherapy for liver cancer. Table 7.2 shows a summary of clinical reports for liver tumors. A phase II trial of combined external radiotherapy and hyperthermia was performed in 30 patients with unresectable hepatocellular carcinoma. External radiotherapy was delivered to a total dose of 30.6 Gy over 3.5 weeks, and hyperthermia was applied twice a week for a total of six treatment sessions using an 8-MHz RF capacitive heating device. A partial response was obtained in 40% of the patients and improvement of abdominal pain was observed in 78.6%. The 1-year survival rates for all patients and for partial responders were 34% and 50%, respectively. A mild sensation of heat, fever, first-degree skin burns, and nausea were the treatment-related side-effects (KIM et al. 1992). We have treated 11 liver tumors (eight hepatocellular carcinomas and three metastatic tumors) by regional hyperthermia in combination with radiotherapy. All tumors were located in the lateral segment of the left lobe or the posterior segment of the right lobe so that irradiation with a total dose of 50–60 Gy was acceptable. Of the 11 tumors, ten (91%) showed a partial response (NAGATA et al. 1990, 1992a). These preliminary results suggest the usefulness of thermoradiotherapy for liver cancer. Figure 7.3 shows a patient with unoperable liver tumor which responded well to thermoradiotherapy.

The usefulness of combined intra-arterial chemotherapy and hyperthermia has also been suggested by several clinical studies. In a trial involving 14 patients with unresectable liver metastases from colorectal cancer or gastric cancer, ten patients were treated by regional hyperthermia using RF capacitive equipment and the remaining four were treated by total-body hyperthermia. The chemotherapy agents given were cisplatin and 5-fluorouracil. The clinical effects and side-effects of this thermochemotherapy were compared with those of intra-arterial chemotherapy in 31 patients given the same regimen. The response rates for thermochemotherapy and chemotherapy alone were 57% and

Table 7.2. A summary of clinical reports for liver tumors

Authors	No. patients	Heating methods	Combined reatment	Response rate (CR + PR)	Complications
KIM BS et al. 1992	30	RF capacitive	radiotherapy	40%	minimal
NAGATA Y et al. 1990	10	RF capacitive	radiotherapy	70%	minimal
HAMAZOE R et al. 1991a	14	RF capacitive, Total-body hyperthermia	intra-arterial chemotherapy	57%	minimal
KONDO M et al. 1993	18	RF capacitive	intra-arterial chemoembolization with DSM	56%	pain, fever
YUMOTO Y et al. 1991	20	RF capacitive	intra-arterial chemoembolization	40%	mostly related to embolization

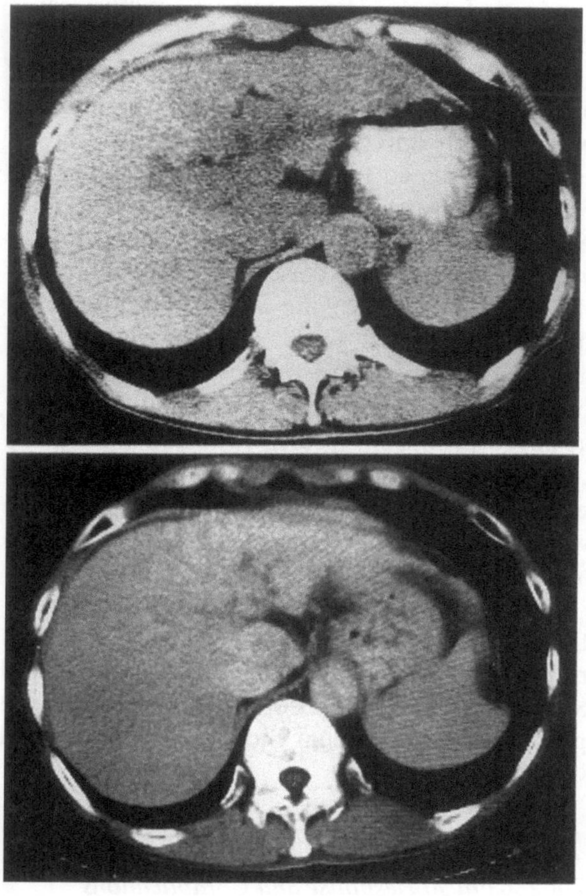

a

b

Fig. 7.3. A patient with unoperable hepatocellular carcinoma treated by hyperthermia and radiation therapy. **a** A large tumor with 8 × 8 cm in the diameter was shown in a CT scan before treatment **b** A total of 5 sessions of RF capacitive hyperthermia and a total of 50.4 Gy of external irradiation were given to this tumor. A CT scan after treatment showed marked tumor regression

33%, respectively. Furthermore, three of the six patients who failed to respond to intra-arterial chemotherapy alone showed a response to thermochemotherapy. Among the patients with liver metastases from colorectal cancer, the mean 50% survival time was 11 months in the chemotherapy group and 23 months in the thermochemotherapy group. The complication rate associated with hyperthermia was minimal, and the toxicity of chemotherapy was not potentiated by combination with hyperthermia (HAMAZOE et al. 1991a). Improvement of both the response rate and the survival time in patients with liver metastases from colorectal cancer has also been demonstrated following combined treatment with regional hyperthermia and systemic or intra-arterial chemotherapy (MOFFAT et al. 1985).

The effects of combination therapy using regional hyperthermia and intra-arterial chemoembolization with DSMs were investigated in 18 patients with unresectable hepatocellular carcinoma, and the results were compared with those of chemoembolization alone in another 30 patients. The response rate was not different between hyperthermia plus chemoembolization and chemoembolization alone when the whole patient population was analyzed. However, when only tumors larger than 7 cm in diameter were assessed, combined treatment of hyperthermia and chemoembolization demonstrated a far higher response rate than chemoembolization alone (5/9 vs 0/11). Most of the complications were related to chemoembolization and the major problems included fever and epigastric pain (KONDO et al. 1993).

The clinical benefit of combined hyperthermia and TAE has also been demonstrated in a randomized trial in which 20 patients were randomly assigned to either hyperthermia plus TAE or TAE alone. Regional hyperthermia was administered (with the tumor temperature being raised above 42.5°C for 40 min) twice a week for a total of 10–38 sessions. The response rate was 40% in the ten patients treated by hyperthermia plus TAE and 20% in the ten patients treated by TAE alone. The median survival period for patients receiving hyperthermia plus TAE was 20 months and that for patients receiving TAE alone was 10.6 months. This difference in survival period, however, was not significant ($P < 0.1$). The main side-effects of TAE plus hyperthermia were low-grade fever, localized pain, myelosuppression, and liver dysfunction, but these were transient and eventually resolved (YUMOTO et al. 1991).

A clinical study of thermochemotherapy using isolated hyperthermic liver perfusion indicated a high response rate in terms of tumor regression. However, some patients died of complications associated with the hyperthermic procedure so the technique needs to be improved before it can be applied more widely (SKIBBA and QUEBBEMAN 1986).

It has been demonstrated that the effect of hyperthermia is potentiated by combination with biological response modifiers (BRMs), including tumor necrosis factor, and there have been several reports on the clinical use of this combination therapy (WATANABE et al. 1988; HIRAOKA et al. 1992).

7.4 Thermoradiotherapy for Pancreatic Tumors

7.4.1 *Heating Methods and Effectiveness*

An 8-MHz RF capacitive heating device is usually used for external heating. The tumors treated are locally advanced unresectable cancer and thermal probes are often inserted into the lesions at operation. A large external electrode of 25–28 cm in diameter is usually paired with an electrode of the same size. However, the limited clinical thermometry data currently available suggest that the heating capability of this device is not satisfactory for treating pancreatic cancer. The percentage of tumors in which the maximum tumor temperature could be raised above 42°C has been variously reported as 13%, 20%, and 29% (Hiraoka et al. 1987; Yamamoto et al. 1991; Hamazoe et al. 1991b). A study employing a 13.56-MHz RF capacitive heating device gave similar results (Yamada et al. 1992). The most common factor limiting power elevation was unacceptable heat sensation or pain affecting the skin around the electrode. These thermometry results are markedly inferior to those for tumors at other anatomical sites. Possible reasons for the relatively poor heating of pancreatic cancer include the deeper location of the tumors, the presence of gastrointestinal gas or bone in front of or behind the pancreas (which might prevent the RF current from entering the tumor), the cooling effect of large vessels located close to the pancreas, and the relatively small tumor volume which also restricts temperature elevation.

Invasive heating methods have recently been applied to pancreatic cancer, and intraoperative hyperthermia utilizing either ultrasound, RF, or microwave is currently being investigated. Nineteen patients with deep-seated tumors, including seven with pancreatic cancer, were treated with ultrasound in the operating room during surgical resection (Ryan et al. 1992). Immediately following intraoperative radiation therapy, thermocouples were inserted into the tumors and adjacent normal tissues and the patients were then given heat treatment for 60 min with an intraoperative ultrasound applicator. The average maximum temperature attained was 46.6°C. In addition, the temperature which 90% of all measured points equalled or exceeded (T_{90}) was 39.2°C and the T_{50} (equalled or exceeded by 50% of measured points) was 42.9°C. These thermometry data are far superior to those obtained for superficial tumors at the same institute.

Yamashita et al. (1993) have also reported on intraoperative RF capacitive hyperthermia for patients with unresectable pancreatic cancer. A specially designed applicator 8 cm in diameter was placed directly on the pancreatic tumor at operation and an opposing applicator 25 cm in diameter was placed under the back of the patient so that the high temperature zone was shifted close to the tumor. The initial trials using a conventional applicator were not satisfactory but subsequent trials with the specially developed applicator achieved promising results. Intratumor temperatures reached more than 44°C in four of the five patients treated with this system and only 5–11 min was required to raise the tumor temperature to above 42.5°C.

In addition to the above methods, intraoperative interstitial microwave hyperthermia has been reported by several researchers (Coughlin and Strohbehn 1989; Goldson et al. 1987) and the preliminary results seem encouraging with regard to feasibility.

7.4.2 *Clinical Response and Complications*

A summary of clinical reports for liver tumors is shown in Table 7.3. A multicenter study was undertaken in 34 patients with locally advanced pancreatic cancer (Kakehi et al. 1990). Six patients were in stage III and 28 in stage IV. Hyperthermia was administered twice a week to a total of eight to ten sessions using an 8-MHz RF capacitive heating device. Twelve of the 34 patients also received radiotherapy (1.8–2.0 Gy per fraction, and five fractions per week to a total dose of 50–60 Gy). One patient showed a complete response and three exhibited a partial response. All of the 12 patients complained of severe pain before treatment and marked pain relief was achieved in 11 of them (92%). The remaining 22 patients received thermochemotherapy using Mitomycin C (MMC) and 5-fluorouracil (5-FU) derivatives. A complete response was achieved in three patients (14%) and a partial response in five (23%). Pain relief was obtained in 17 of these 22 patients (77%). The complications associated with the treatment were not described. Figure 7.4 shows a patient with unoperable pancreatic tumor which responded well to thermoradiotherapy.

Table 7.3. A summary of clinical reports for pancreatic tumors

Authors	No. patients	Heating methods	Treatment methods	Response rate	Complications
KAKEHI et al. 1990	34	RF capacitive	radiotherapy chemotherapy	33% in thermoradiotherapy 36% in thermochemotherapy	not stated
YAMADA S et al. 1992	14	RF capacitive	intraoperative radiotherapy	63% in thermoradiotherapy 38% in radiotherapy	not stated
GOLDSON A et al. 1991	13	Interstitial microwave	intraoperative radiotherapy		gastrointestinal bleeding

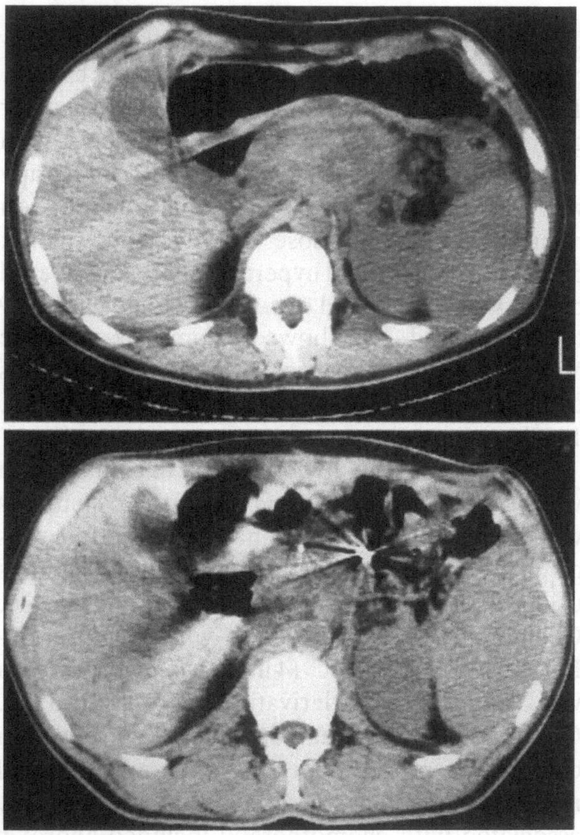
a
b

Fig. 7.4. A patient with unoperable pancreatic cancer treated by hyperthermia and radiation therapy **a** A CT scan before treatment showed a large mass which occupied the body and tail of the pancreas. **b** After external irradiation with a total dose of 30 Gy, this patient received intraoperative irradiation with a single dose of 30 Gy. During the operation, thermal probes were inserted in the tumor, and thereafer 4 sessions of hyperthermia were combined by 25.2 Gy of external irradiation. A CT scan taken 10 months after the treatment showed complete regression of the tumor. This patient is living without evidence of recurrence 8 years after the treatment

The effect of combined intraoperative radiotherapy and regional hyperthermia was investigated in 14 patients an the results were compared with those obtained in 55 patients treated without hyperthermia. Some of the patients in both treatment groups received additional external radiotherapy and chemotherapy. A slight improvement in local response rate and the survival rate was shown in the patients receiving hyperthermia. The response rate was 63% in the hyperthermia group and 38% in the control group. As regards the survival rate, the former group showed 21.4% survival at 1 year and 7.1% at 2 years, whereas the latter group showed 12.7% survival at 1 year and 1.8% at 2 years (YAMADA et al. 1992).

In another study, intraoperative interstitial microwave hyperthermia combined with intraoperative radiotherapy was applied to 13 patients with unresectable pancreatic cancer. Interstitial hyperthermia was applied to the pancreas for 40 min at a steady-state temperature of 42.5°C–44°C. Twenty minutes into steady-state hyperthermia, 20–25 Gy of high-energy electrons was delivered to the pancreatic tumor mass without interrupting the intraoperative hyperthermia procedure. In addition, 40 Gy of external irradiation was given to the tumor postoperatively. The mean and median survival times for the five patients who completed the entire protocol were 17.7 months and 19 months, respectively; these results were superior to those achieved by intraoperative radiotherapy with or without external radiotherapy at the same institution. The main problem encountered was trauma from the hyperthermia implant, which induced gastrointestinal bleeding (GOLDSON and ASHAYERI 1991).

Although it is too early to draw any conclusions about the clinical benefit of thermoradiotherapy for unresectable pancreatic cancer, the preliminary results seem encouraging. A major effort should be made in the future to develop techniques which allow more efficient and uniform tumor heating.

7.5 Thermoradiotherapy for Gastric Tumors

7.5.1 Heating Methods and Effectiveness

The heating methods reported for the treatment of gastric cancer are regional RF capacitive heating and peritoneal perfusion with hot water. There are very few reports concerning the heating achieved with the RF capacitive device, largely because of the difficulties involved in intratumoral temperature measurement. We measured intratumoral temperatures in 13 patients with locally advanced gastric cancer. These tumors were in contact with the abdominal wall so that percutaneous insertion of a thermal probe into the tumor under ultrasonic guidance was possible. The number of intratumoral points measured ranged from 1 to 4, with a mean of 2.5. An 8-MHz RF heating device was used, generally with two opposing 25-cm-sized electrodes. The maximum, average, and minimum tumor temperatures, respectively, were 41.0°–45.0°C (mean: 43.5°C), 40.2°–43.0°C (mean: 42.1°C), and 39.3°–43.0°C (mean: 41.3°C) (Nagata et al. 1992b). The effectiveness of the same device for heating peritoneally disseminated lesions arising from gastric or colorectal tumors was also investigated. Intratumoral temperatures were measured with thin Teflon-coated microthermocouples implanted into the center of each tumor at laparotomy or inserted transcutaneously under ultrasonic guidance. Among the six tumors treated, the tumor temperature could be raised to above 43°C in one, to 42°–43°C in one, and to less than 42°C in the remaining four (Hamazoe et al. 1991b).

A method of intraperitoneal hyperthermic perfusion has also been reported (Hamazoe et al. 1993). Shortly before closing the abdominal wall after surgical treatment, tubes are placed into the pelvic and abdominal cavities for the infusion and drainage of heated saline containing anticancer drugs. After closing the abdomen, the infusate is heated in a thermostatically regulated waterbath and infused into the peritoneal cavity through the intrapelvic tube attached to a pump. The inflow and outflow temperatures are maintained at 44°–45°C and 40°–42°C, respectively. Modified methods of peritoneal perfusion have also been reported by other researchers (Fujimoto et al. 1990; Yonemura et al. 1991).

7.5.2 Clinical Response and Complications

Unfortunately, few reports are available concerning thermoradiotherapy for gastric cancer. Table 7.4 shows a summary of clinical report for gastric tumors. We have treated patients with locally advanced gastric cancer. Radiotherapy was administered by a conventional fractionation regimen to a total dose of 40–72 Gy (mean: 52.6 Gy), and regional hyperthermia was delivered once a week for a total of 4–11 sessions. Of the 19 tumors treated, two showed a complete response and 11 showed a partial response. No serious complications were observed (Nagata et al. 1992b).

In another study, hyperthermia in combination with chemotherapy was applied to 33 patients with gastric cancer. Regional hyperthermia was given twice a week for a total of 6–40 sessions using an 8-MHz RH capacitive heating device. Chemotherapy was also given with MMC and 5-FU derivatives. MMC (4 mg) was given twice a week and the 5-FU derivatives were given daily. Of the 33 patients treated, three (9%) showed a complete response and ten (30%) showed a partial response. Transient side-effects that were possibly associated with chemotherapy included anorexia and abdominal discomfort, while the only complication attributable to hyperthermia was fat necrosis in one patient (Kakehi et al. 1990).

The efficacy of intraperitoneal hyperthermic perfusion with chemotherapy agents has been demonstrated for the prevention of peritoneal

Table 7.4. A summary of clinical reports for gastric tumors

Authors	No. patients	Heating methods	Treatment methods	Response rate	Complications
Nagata Y et al. 1992	19	RF capacitive	radiotherapy	68%	minimal
Kakehi M et al. 1990	33	RF capacitive	chemotherapy	39%	fat necrosis

dissemination (HAMAZOE et al. 1991a) and for the treatment of peritoneally disseminated disease (FUJIMOTO et al. 1990; YONEMURA et al. 1991). However, the combination of intraperitoneal hyperthermic perfusion with radiotherapy has not yet been investigated.

7.6 Summary

- Because of the difficulties in obtaining complete thermometry data for upper abdominal tumors, the heating effectiveness of the current heating techniques have not been fully evaluated and optimized. The limited number of reports available, however, indicate that all of the implemented heating devices are unsatisfactory in that not all of the tumor volume is raised to therapeutic temperatures. Thus, a major effort is needed to develop more efficient heating devices.
- Among the various heating devices available, the RF capacitive technique is most commonly used and is probably most applicable to upper abdominal tumors. The heating effectiveness of RF capacitive devices depend on the anatomical location and tumor type.
- Metastatic liver tumors and gastric tumors are more readily heated than pancreatic tumors and hepatocellular carcinomas.
- New technigques are under investigations: Invasive hyperthermia methods have shown some promise for treating pancreatic cancer and need to be investigated in further clinical trials. Transarterial embolization has been shown to increase the heating of hepatocellular carcinoma, and in addition such biological methods manipulating blood flow may be expected to improve further the heating of various tumors.
- At present it is too early to assess the clinical response of upper abdominal tumors to hyperthermia in combination with radiotherapy; rather, further accumulation of clinical data is required. However, most of the preliminary results suggest an increase in the response rate without any substantial increase in serious complications. Thus, at the present stage of clinical research a well-designed phase III trial would seem to be strongly warranted in this field.

References

Abe M, Hiraoka M, Takahashi M, et al. (1986) Multi-institutional studies on hyperthermia using an 8 MHz radiofrequency capacitive heating device (Thermotron RF8) in combination with radiation for cancer therapy. Cancer 58: 1589–1595

Akuta K, Hiraoka M, Jo S, et al. (1987) Regional hyperthermia combined with blockade of the hepatic arterial blood flow by degradable starch microspheres in pigs. Int J Radiat Oncol Biol Phys 13: 239–242

Coughlin CT, Strohbehn JW (1989) Interstitial thermoradiotherapy. Radiol Clin North Am 27: 577–588

Fujimoto S, Shrestha RD, Kokubun M, et al. (1990) Positive results of combined therapy of surgery and intraperitoneal hyperthermic perfusion for far-udvanced gastric cancer. Ann Surg 212: 592–596

Goldson AL, Ashayeri E (1991) Update on intraoperative interstitial hyperthermia (IOIHT) and intraoperative radiotherapy (IORT) for pancreatic cancer at Howard University Hospital. In: Abe M, Takahashi M (eds) Intraoperative radiation therapy. Pergamon Press, Oxford, p 260

Goldson AL, Smyles J, Ashayeri E (1987) Simultaneous intraoperative radiation therapy and intraoperative interstitial hyperthermia for unresectable adenocarcinoma of the pancreas. Endocurietherapy/Hyperthermia Oncology 3: 201–208

Hamazoe R, Murakami A, Hirooka Y, Maeta M, Kaibara N (1991a) A phase II pilot study of the combined application of hyperthermia and intra-hepato-arterial chemotherapy using cisplatinum and 5-fluorouracil. J Surg Oncol 48: 127–132

Hamazoe R, Maeta M, Murakami A, Yamashiro H, Kaibara N (1991b) Heating efficiency of radiofrequency capacitive hyperthermia for treatment of deep-seated tumors in the peritoneal cavity. J Surg Oncol 48: 176–179

Hiraoka M, Takahashi M, Abe M (1986) Hyperthermia for pancreatic cancer. Semin Gastrointest 25: 271–288 (In Japanese)

Hiraoka M, Jo S, Akuta K, Nishimura Y, Takahashi M, Abe M (1987) Radiofrequency capacitive hyperthermia for deep-seated tumors. I. Studies on thermometry. Cancer 60: 121–127

Hiraoka M, Li YP, Tsutsui K, Abe M, Miyachi Y (1992) Effects of tumor necrosis factor and hyperthermia on Meth-A tumors. Jpn J Cancer Res 82: 1171–1174

Hynynen K, Shimm D, Anhalt B, Stea B, Sykes H, Cassady JR, Roemer RB (1990) Temperature distributions during clinical scanned, focused ultrasound hyperthermia treatments. Int J Hyperthermia 6: 891–908

Kakehi M, Ueda K, Mukojima T, Hiraoka M, Seto O, Akanuma A, Natatsugawa S (1990) Multi-institutional clinical studies on hyperthermia combined with radiotherapy or the chemotherapy in advanced of deep-seated organs. Int J Hyperthermia 6: 719–740

Kim BS, Chung HC, Seong JS, Suh CO, Kim GE (1992) Phase II trial for combined external radiotherapy and hyperthermia for unresectable hepatoma. Cancer Chemother Pharmacol 31(suppl I): s119–s127

Koga S, Hamazoe R, Maeta M, Shimizu N, Murakami A, Wakatsuki T (1988) Prophylactic therapy for peritoneal recurrence of gastric cancer by continuous hyperthermic peritoneal perfusion with a solution that contains an anticancer drug. Cancer 61: 232–237

Kondo M, Oyamada H, Yoshikawa T (1993) Therapeutic effects of chemoembolization using degradable starch microspheres and regional hyperthermia on unresectable hepatocellular carcinoma. In: Matsuda T (ed) Cancer treatment by hyperthermia, radiation and drugs. Taylor & Francis, London, p 317

Moffat FL, Gilas, T, Calhoun K, et al. (1985) Further experience with regional radiofrequency hyperthermia and cytotoxic chemotherapy for unresectable hepatic neoplasia. Cancer 55: 1291–1295

Nagata Y, Hiraoka M, Akuta K, et al. (1990) Radiofrequency thermotherapy for malignant liver tumors. Cancer 65: 1730–1736

Nagata Y, Abe M, Hiraoka M, et al. (1992a) Radiofrequency hyperthermia and radiotherapy for hepatocellular carcinoma. In: Tobe T (ed) Primary liver cancer in Japan. Springer, Berlin Heidelberg New York, p 315

Nagata Y, Hiraoka M, Nishimura Y, et al. (1992b) Radiofrequency hyperthermia for advanced gastric cancer. In: Gerner EW (ed) Hyperthermic oncology 1992. Arizona Board of Regents, Tucson, A2, p 407

Petrovich Z, Langholz B, Kapp DS, Emami B, Oleson JR, Luxton G, Astrahan M (1989) Deep regional hyperthermia of the liver. A clinical study of 49 patients. Am J Clin Oncol 12: 378–383

Ryan TP, Colacchio TA, Douple EB, Strohbehn JW, Coughlin CT (1992) Techniques for intraoperative hyperthermia with ultrasound: the Dartmouth experience with 19 patients. Int J Hyperthermia 4: 407–421

Sapozink MD, Gibbs FA, Gates KS, Stewart JR (1984) Regional hyperthermia in the treatment of clinically advanced, deep seated malignancy: results of a pilot study employing an annular applicator. Int J Radiat Oncol Biol Phys 10: 775–786

Shimada T, Nakao N, Miura T (1986) Hyperthermia in the treatment of digestive tract tumor. Dig Med 4: 348–355 (In Japanese)

Skibba JL, Quebbeman EJ (1986) Tumoricidal effects and patient survival after hyperthermic liver perfusion. Arch Surg 121: 1266–1271

Tanaka Y, Yamamoto K, Murata T, Nagata K (1992) Effects of multimodal treatment and hyperthermia on hepatic tumors. Cancer Chemother Pharmacol 31(suppl I): s111–s114

Watanabe N, Niitsu Y, Umeno H, et al. (1988) Synergistic cytotoxic and antitumor effects of recombinant human tumor necrosis factor and hyperthermia. Cancer Res 48: 650–653

Yamada S, Takai Y, Nemoto K, et al. (1992) Intraoperative radiation therapy combined with hyperthermia against pancreatic carcinoma. Tohoku J Exp Med 166: 395–401

Yamamoto K, Nakatsugawa S, Shiga T, Ishii Y, Kojima Y, Katayama K, Nakagawara G (1991) Intraoperative radiotherapy and external beam radiotherapy in combination with hyperthermia for the unresectable pancreatic cancer. Jpn J Hyperthermic Oncol 7: 204–207 (In Japanese)

Yamashita T, Hashida I, Nakazawa M, et al. (1993) Intraoperative radiotherapy and hyperthermia for unresectable pancreatic cancer. In: Matsuda T (ed) Cancer treatment by hyperthermia, radiation and drugs. Taylor & Francis, London, p 60

Yonemura Y, Fujimura T, Fushida S, et al. (1991) Hyperthermo-chemotherapy combined with cytoreductive surgery for the treatment of gastric cancer with peritoneal dissemination. World J Surg 15: 503–536

Yumoto Y, Jinno K, Tokuyama K, et al. (1991) Transcatheter hepatic arterial injection of lipiodol soluble anti-cancer agent SMANCS and ADR suspension in lipiodol combined with arterial embolization and local hyperthermia for treatment of hepatocellular carcinoma. Int J Hyperthermia 7: 7–17

8 Thermoradiotherapy for Tumors of the Lower Gastrointestinal Tract

D. González González

CONTENTS

8.1 Introduction

Colorectal cancer is the second most common malignancy in the United States following lung cancer, and it was responsible for 61 000 deaths in 1990 (American Cancer Society 1990). Males and females are equally affected, and the mean age of incidence is 62 years. At present, 38% of cases occur proximally and 62% distally; compared with the incidence several years ago this represents a tendency toward an increasing incidence of colon cancer as compared with rectal cancer (Beart et al. 1983). Surgery remains the treatment of choice with either curative or palliative intent. About 15% of the patients are inoperable at presentation for medical reasons or have tumors that are technically unresectable during laparotomy or are only resectable for palliation (Cameron et al. 1979; Sugarbaker 1986). The best prognostic indicator after curative resection is the staging of the disease. Whereas tumors within the bowel wall with negative lymph nodes (Astler-Coller stages A, B1) have a good prognosis, tumors beyond the bowel wall with or without lymph node involvement (stages B2, C1, C2) have a high risk of local relapse, i.e., between 22% and 70% for rectal cancer and between 14% and 41% for colon cancer (Cass et al. 1976; Gilbert 1978; Gunderson et al. 1987; Mendenhall et al. 1983; Rich et al. 1983; Walz et al. 1981; Willet et al. 1983; Gunderson et al. 1985b). In general, local failure rates are higher in reoperation series than in series where the diagnosis of relapse has been made only on a clinical basis. The risk of distant metastases is between 25% and 35% in reoperation series (Gunderson et al. 1985a). Both preoperative and postoperative irradiation are frequently used in subgroups of patients with rectal cancer as an adjuvant to curative resection and with the aim of diminishing local recurrence and ultimately improving survival. The efficacy of adjuvant radiation therapy in rectal cancer in decreasing local relapse and improving survival has been demonstrated in several prospective randomized studies (Douglass and Moertel 1986; Fisher et al. 1988; Gastrointestinal Study Group 1985; Gerard et al. 1988; Mendenhall et al. 1985; National Cancer Institute 1991; Stockholm Rectal Cancer Study Group 1987). No randomized studies have been performed in patients with colon cancer, but several studies of selected groups of patients have indicated that postoperative irradiation improves local control in the tumor bed area and, potentially, survival (Brenner et al. 1983; Duttenhaver et al. 1986).

During recent years results from prospective studies have confirmed that adjuvant chemotherapy improves disease-free survival and overall survival in Astler-Coller stage C colon cancer (NIH Consensus Conference 1990; Moertel et al. 1990). In rectal cancer, adjuvant treatment combining pelvic irradiation and chemotherapy has been shown to improve local control and survival as compared with pelvic irradiation alone

D. González González, MD, Department of Radiation Oncology Academisch Medisch Centrum, University of Amsterdam, Meibergdreef 9, NL-1105 AZ Amsterdam, The Netherlands

(Gastrointestinal Study Group 1985; DOUGLASS and MOERTEL 1986; KROOK et al. 1991; National Cancer Institute 1991). However, if local recurrence occurs or the tumor is unresectable, curative therapy will not be available for the majority of the patients, and the only aim is long-term palliation. In patients with isolated locoregional relapse of rectal cancer treated with radiotherapy the overall survival at 3 years is 10%–13% (LYBEERT et al. 1992; CIATTO and PACINI 1982). Duration of palliation has been reported to be about 3–6 months (JAMES and SCHOFIELD 1985; VILLALON and GREEN 1981). In several studies combined radiation and chemotherapy has been reported to improve symptomatic control and mean survival in patients with unresectable large bowel cancer (MOERTEL et al. 1975; BOELIS-WASSIF 1983), but results from prospective studies have been negative (ROMINGER et al. 1985; DANJOUX et al. 1985).

The prognosis of *carcinoma of the anal canal* is primarily related to the size of the tumor. In general, locoregional recurrences following abdominoperineal resection can be expected to occur in 27%–35% of patients (HARDCASTLE and BUSSEY 1968; GREENALL et al. 1985a,b; BOMAN et al. 1984). However, if only a local excision is performed, the risk of locoregional relapse is 39%–47% (HARDCASTLE and BUSSEY 1968; GREENALL et al. 1985a,b).

External beam irradiation or brachytherapy or a combination thereof is a good alternative to surgery, with anal function being preserved in a large proportion of patients. Among patients with tumors less than 4 cm in diameter, control and preservation of anal function are obtained in 76%–90% of cases (PAPILLON 1982; CUMMINGS et al. 1982, 1984; LEICHMAN et al. 1985; SCHLIENGER et al. 1989). This rate decreases to 38%–84% for tumors equal to or larger than 4 cm. Chemotherapy (mitomycin C and 5-fluorouracil) combined with radiation has been used in large tumors as neoadjuvant treatment preceding surgery. High complete remission rates (48%–100%), both clinically and histologically, have been reported (NIGRO 1984; MICHAELSON et al. 1983; SISCHY 1985; JOHN et al. 1985; CUMMINGS et al. 1984). Several ongoing prospective studies are testing the value of combined chemotherapy and radiotherapy and focusing on the preservation of anal function.

8.2 Rationale of Thermoradiotherapy for Lower Gastrointestinal Tract Carcinomas

It is obvious from the above data that in spite of the considerable advances achieved in the curative treatment of colorectal and anal carcinoma, there is still a need to improve both locoregional control and overall survival. The need for new therapeutic strategies for either cure or palliation is even more urgent in patients with unresectable tumors at presentation or relapsing after failure of standard treatment.

The radiation doses used in the adjuvant treatment, namely 40–50 Gy, produce a complication rate which is at the limit of what is considered acceptable. In unresectable or recurrent tumors the results are very poor, even with doses as high as 60–70 Gy. The biological rationale for using hyperthermia in oncology is well known (see Chap. 1 this volume) and will not be discussed here. The combination of hyperthermia and radiation used either pre- or postoperatively in the curative treatment of colorectal and anal cancer is attractive because the local control rates could be improved. Further, in unresectable tumors this combined treatment could render more tumors resectable than has been the case to date with radiation alone. Finally, local palliative treatment of colorectal tumors remains difficult, and the results with radiation alone, although well recognized, are far from being optimal and of long-term effect.

8.3 Clinical Data on Thermoradiotherapy for Colorectal Carcinoma

The majority of the reported results on thermoradiotherapy in colorectal carcinomas concern phase I/II studies in patients with recurrent tumors. Further, the number of reports dealing specifically with colorectal cancer is very small: usually the reports describe the results of hyperthermia treatment in deep-seated tumors in general. Variations in treatment techniques, apparatus for hyperthermia delivery, thermometry, selection of patients, and radiation doses, as well as the combination with chemotherapy in some series, make it difficult to analyze the reported results. Only a few prospective phase III studies have been published. With these limitations in mind a review of the relevant clinical results is presented.

8.3.1 Nonrandomized Studies

From 1980 through 1986, 353 patients were treated with deep regional hyperthermia in 14 medical centers in the United States (PETROVICH et al. 1989). Within this group, 146 patients (41%) had adenocarcinoma of the gastrointestinal tract. Unfortunately this group of patients was not reviewed separately, and consequently only some general data are discussed. A large proportion of patients (71%) had recurrent or persistent tumors. One-third had a poor general condition (Karnofsky performance status lower than 50), and pain was present in 55%. Hyperthermia was administered with an annular phased array system (BSD Medical Corporation). Hyperthermia alone was administered in 47 patients (including 16 with pelvic and 12 with abdominal tumors), hyperthermia and radiation in 245 patients (including 152 with pelvic and 52 with abdominal tumors) hyperthermia and chemotherapy in 42 patients (including 18 with pelvic and seven with abdominal tumors), and hyperthermia combined with radiation and chemotherapy in 15 patients (including six with pelvic and two with abdominal tumors); in four patients the treatment was unknown. Due to their poor general condition, 65 patients received only one hyperthermia session. Temperatures were monitored by placing one or more catheters into the tumor. Thermal dose (TD) was defined as the number of minutes at 42.5°C or its equivalent. The mean number of hyperthermia treatments was four (range 1–17). In 150 patients (42%) temperatures were low and no TD was accumulated. In the other 203 patients (57%) the TD was <50 min in 29% of patients, >50–<100 min in 11% of patients, >100–<200 min in 7% of patients, and <200 min in 10% of patients. Complete response (CR) was observed in 10% of patients, the rate being 12% in patients receiving radiotherapy versus 2% in those in whom radiotherapy was not given. For patients receiving radiation doses higher than 45 Gy the CR rate was 29% and the combined CR and PR (partial response) rate, 61%. No correlation was found between TD and response. Twelve of the 35 patients achieving a CR had a gastrointestinal tumor and all received radiotherapy (20–62 Gy). Median survival in the whole group was 42 weeks and the overall survival at 2 years was 13%. The average duration of CR was 8 months. Complete relief of pain was obtained in 23% of patients (n = 195) and partial relief in 39%, no pain relief was achieved in the remaining 38%. Treatment tolerance was good in 42% of patients, fair in 32%, poor in 18%, and not registered in 8%. Pain during hyperthermia treatment was observed in 35% of the patients. Other toxicities were infrequent. From this experience the authors concluded that (a) the majority of the patients tolerated four hyperthermia treatments with acute toxicity that was acceptable but at the limit of tolerance, (b) 25% of the patients experienced substantial tumor regression (CR + PR), (c) radiation dose was important in achieving response, and (d) no TD – response relationship could be observed.

KAKEHI et al. (1990) reviewed the experience of seven institutions in Japan during the period 1985–1988. Hyperthermia combined with radiotherapy or chemotherapy was administered to 177 patients with deep-seated tumors. In this series 34 patients had a recurrent rectal cancer. Hyperthermia was given using a RF capacitive device (Thermotron RF-8, Yamamoto Vinyter Co.), with two sessions a week and eight to ten sessions in total. The aim of the treatment was to achieve temperatures above 42°C for 40–50 min. Temperatures were measured intrarectally near the tumor (not in the tumor). The average temperature was 41°C, the maximum, 43.8°C. Radiation doses were 50–60 Gy in fractions of 1.8–2 Gy. CR was observed in two patients (5.9%) and PR in 14 patients (41.2%). Pain relief was obtained in 19 cases (55.9%).

EMAMI et al. (1991) reported the results of a phase I/II study activated by the Radiation Therapy Oncology Group combining radiotherapy and hyperthermia in the treatment of deep-seated malignant tumors. A total of 53 patients with locally advanced abdominal (25% of patients) or pelvic malignancies (75% of patients) were accrued. In 44 patients the histology was adenocarcinoma. Hyperthermia was delivered with an annular phased array system (BSD Medical Corporation) in 35 patients and with an RF capacitive device (Thermotron, Yamamoto Corporation) in 18 patients. Intratumoral temperatures were monitored with probes inserted directly into the tumor through closed-end Teflon catheters. The aim of treatment was to achieve minimum tumor temperatures of 42°C for a minimum of 40 min. The average number of sessions per patient was 4.8 (range 1–13). The median radiation dose was 35 Gy (range 1.8–60 Gy). In 44 patients available for response there were 17 CRs (39%) and six PRs (14%). In 72 out of 256 sessions (28%) the temperature was at or above 42°C for more than 20 min. The CR rate was not correlated with the number of hyperthermia sessions at or above 42°C and was similar for the two used heating devices. Patient refusal (26%) and unacceptable toxicity (11%) were the most common reasons for permanent interruption of the treatment.

NISHIMURA et al. (1992) have published one of the few papers specifically concerned with unresectable and recurrent colorectal cancer treated with combined hyperthermia and radiotherapy. They compared the results of thermoradiotherapy in 36 patients (group I) with the results achieved in 35 patients treated during the same period with radiation alone (group II). Patients in the latter group were unsuitable for hyperthermia mainly because of difficulaties with the insertion of temperature probes or the thickness of the patients. For deep-seated tumors hyperthermia was administered with an 8-MHz RF capacitive device, while a 434-MHz microwave system was used for more superficial, abdominal wall recurrences. Hyperthermia was given 10–30 min following radiotherapy, aiming for tumor temperatures above 42°C for 30–40 min. The mean number of number of hyperthermia sessions was 5.7 (range 2–14) and the majority of patients received one session a week. Intratumoral temperatures were monitored by inserting one or more probes into the tumor. the mean radiation dose was 58 Gy in group I (hyperthermia and radiotherapy) and 57 Gy in group II (radiotherapy alone). The overall objective response rate (CR + PR) was 54% in group I versus 36% in group II. In particular the objective response rates for primary tumors (unresectable) and recurrences in previously irradiated cases were considerably higher in group I than in group II, (71% vs 0% and 50% vs 0%, respectively). Absence of local tumor progression at 12 months was 31% and 22% in groups I and II, respectively. Three tumors in the hyperthermia plus radiotherapy group became resectable versus no tumors in the radiation alone group. The objective response rate was 47% in patients treated with 8-MHz RF (deep tumors) and 100% in patients treated with 430 MHz (superficial tumors). For the 27 deep-seated tumors the T_{min}, T_{av} (average), and T_{max} were 40.3°C, 41.3°C, and 42.2°C, respectively. For the five superficial relapses the corresponding T values were higher, namely 40.6°C, 43.3°C, and 45.4°C, respectively. Optimal treatments defined as a $T_{min} > 42°C$ for >30 min were achieved in only 13% of the 115 hyperthermia sessions, and any intratumoral point exceeding 42°C for >20 min in 53% of the sessions. The response rate for 15 tumors with a T_{av} of more than 42°C was 67% as compared to 47% when the T_{av} was lower, but this difference was not statistically significant. Within the group treated with combined hyperthermia and radiotherapy there was no clear correlation between the administered radiation dose and the objective response rate. Approximately 50% of the patients treated with RF complained of pain at the field edge or under the electrodes. Local infection caused by insertion of thermal probes and chronic bowel damage appeared to be increased by the application of hyperthermia.

In a recent report, FELDMANN et al. (1993b) described the results in 37 patients with locally advanced deep-seated tumors treated with thermoradiotherapy. Eighteen patients in this group had a recurrent and one an advanced rectal cancer. The authors paid special attention to the thermal parameters. Hyperthermia was administered with the annular phased array or Sigma-60 applicator (BSD Medical Corporation). Under computed tomography (CT) scan guidance, one to three thermometry catheters were inserted into the tumor. Other catheters were placed in the vagina, bladder, and rectum. Two hyperthermia sessions a week were given, in each case 1 h after radiotherapy, aiming for temperatures of 42°C or above for at least 60 min. The mean number of hyperthermic treatments per patient was seven. Radiotherapy was administered five times a week, 1.8–2 Gy per fraction, to a nominal tumor dose of 30–62 Gy with a mean of 46.5 Gy. The overall objective response rate (CR + PR) was 31%, including two CRs and nine PRs. The objective response rate was higher in the group of patients receiving radiation doses above 40 Gy. The authors did not mention possible correlations between temperatures and tumor response. Complete pain relief was obtained in 47% of the patients, partial pain relief in 31%, and no pain relief in 22%. The whole group of patients with rectal cancer received 84 hyperthermic treatments. The minimum, mean, and maximum intratumoral temperatures were 39.3°C, 40.8°C, and 42.4°C, respectively. Values for time-averaged temperatures T_{90}, T_{50}, and T_{20} were 39.8°C, 40.7°C, and 41.5°C, respectively. In 60% of the treatments acute toxicity was a limiting factor for the duration of hyperthermia and the achieved temperature elevation. Pain inside the applicator field and general discomfort were recorded in 37% and 32% of the treatments, respectively. The authors concluded that with the available heating equipment it is very difficult to heat substantial parts of the tumors to cytotoxic levels (>42.0°C) and that acute toxicity continues to limit the duration of treatment and the magnitude of power deposition. The variations in blood flow in deep fat and muscle tissue related to the blood flow in the periphery and center of the tumors were discussed in this paper, as well as in other papers published by the same group (FELDMANN et al. 1991, 1992a, 1992b). As in the report by PETROVICH et al. (1989), objective response was higher in patients receiving radiation doses above 40 Gy.

MARCHAL and BEY (1992) reported on a nonrandomized study in patients with pelvic recurrences of rectal carcinoma. Radiation doses were 30–40 Gy in 3–4 weeks in previously irradiated cases and 60 Gy in 6 weeks if no radiation had been given in the past. Hyperthermia was delivered with a large ridged waveguide system operating at 27 MHz (Sairem Co.). Comparing three groups of patients treated with radiation alone (20 patients), radiation and hyperthermia (33 patients), and radiation, hyperthermia, and 5-fluorouracil (11 patients), the authors did not detect any improvement in either local control or survival in the latter two groups.

In a review article by OVERGAARD (1989), one Russian study by SAVCHENKO et al. (1987) was cited in which a group of 56 patients with rectal cancer who received radiotherapy alone was compared with a group who received combined radiotherapy and hyperthermia. Unfortunately no data on patient and treatment characteristics were provided, except that a preoperative radiation dose of 20 Gy in five fractions was given. The survival for patients receiving radiation alone and patients receiving radiation combined with hyperthermia was 55% and 71%, respectively.

In a recent publication, TAKESHITA et al. (1993) reported on the changes on CT images and their prognostic value when thermoradiotherapy was applied in deep-seated tumors. Low-density areas appeared or expanded over time in 24 out of 41 patients, and this correlated with histologically confirmed coagulative necrosis. The probability of survival of patients showing an increase in low-density areas on CT scan was significantly higher than in those without any CT changes.

Heating techniques other than electromagnetic external heating are under study. SEEGENSCHMIEDT et al. (1992) have treated localized implantable recurrent pelvic tumors, including six rectal tumors, with interstitial thermoradiotherapy. Complete remission at 3 months was achieved in 67% (16/24) of the patients. Interstitial hyperthermia has also been used by COUGHLIN et al. (1989) in selected patients with deep-seated tumors. LEWIS et al. (1992) used intracavitary ultrasound hyperthermia and standard radiotherapy in four patients with locally advanced pelvic malignancies, including one with rectal cancer. The average T_{max} and T_{min} were 45°C and 40.8°, respectively. The clinical results were encouraging: two CRs, one PR. The patient with a recurrent rectal cancer was treated preoperatively; resection was carried out and the patient was alive and free of disease at 5 months. Scanned focused ultrasound hyperthermia has also been tested in pelvic tumors (CORRY 1989). HAND et al. (1992a,b) treated nine patients with pelvic tumors, six of whom had rectal cancer. Time-averaged temperatures were 42.4°C and 39.9°C for the highest and lowest sensors, respectively.

Table 8.1 summarizes the objective response rates reported by different authors. Series not specifically dealing with colorectal carcinomas but including a considerable proportion of patients with pelvic adenocarcinomas have been included. Objective regression rates varied between 25% and 70%. In comparative series, the objective regression rate for thermoradiotherapy was higher than that for radiation alone by a factor of about 2. The palliative effect in recurrent tumors is summarized in Table 8.2. In general, complete or partial pain relief was obtained in more than 60% of the patients.

8.3.2 Randomized Studies

In the series reported by KAKEHI et al. (1990) 14 patients were randomly assigned to receive preoperative radiation alone or radiation combined with hyperthermia. Hyperthermia was administered in a similar way as in recurrent cases (see above). The radiation dose was 40 Gy. The staging of the nine patients treated with the combined treatment was one Dukes A, seven Dukes B1, and one Dukes B2. No data were

Table 8.1. Objective response rate in colorectal cancer treated with thermoradiotherapy

Author (year)	No. of pts.	CR		PR		CR + PR		Remarks
		RT	RT + HT	RT	RT + HT	RT	RT + HT	
Feldmann et al. (1993)	36	–	2	–	9	–	11 (31%)	Colorectal = 18 rec., 1 adv.
Nishimura et al. (1992)	71	2	4	8	15	10 (36%)	19 (54%)	62 rec., 9 adv.
Wust et al. (1992)	25	–	–	–	–	–	(30%)	Rec. rectal or cervix
Emami et al. (1991)	44	–	17	–	6	–	23 (52%)	Pelvis, abdomen, 44% adenocarcinomas
Berdov et al. (1990)	115	1	9	20	30	21 (36%)	39 (70%)	Rectal, randomized study
Kakehi et al. (1990)	43	–	2	–	23	–	25 (58%)	Rectal, 34 rec., 9 preoperative
Petrovich et al. (1989)	196	–	18	–	33	–	51 (26%)	Pelvic tumors
Menteshavili et al. (1989)	117	–	–	–	–	–	(69%)	See. Overgaard (1989)
Goldobenko et al. (1989)	40	0	11	–	–	–	–	See. Overgaard (1989)
Matsuda (1989)	38	–	3	–	18	–	21 (55%)	Colorectal
Shimm et al. (1988)	32	–	5	–	3	–	8 (25%)	Pelvic tumors
Gonzalez Gonzalez[a]	73	–	3	–	8	–	11 (15%)	Colorectal, 36% SD

adv., advanced; rec., recurrent
[a] See text

Table 8.2. Pain relief with thermoradiotherpy in pelvic tumors

Author	No. of pts.	Pain relief		
		CP	PP	CP + PP
Feldmann et al. (1993)	32	47%	31%	78%
Wust et al. (1992)	25	–	–	70%
Mittal et al. (1992)	16	–	–	75%
Kakehi et al. (1990)	34	–	–	56%
Berdov et al. (1990)	48	–	–	86%
Petrovich et al. (1989)	195	23%	39%	62%
González González[a]	69	42%	37%	79%

CP, complete palliation of pain; pp, partial palliation of pain
[a] See text

provided on the staging of the five patients treated with radiation alone. Further, the authors compared these two groups of patients with a third historical group of seven patients treated preoperatively with a radiation dose of 60 Gy. The overall response rate (CR + PR) was 100% in the patients treated with radiation and hyperthermia, 20% in the group receiving 40 Gy, and 57% in the historical group receiving 60 Gy. According to the authors these differences in response were statistically significant. An improvement in subjective symptoms was observed in all the cases in which hyperthermia was administered, in only one case in the 40-Gy group, and in four cases in the 60-Gy historical group.

Berdov and Menteshashvili (1990) reported on a prospective study comparing radiation alone with thermoradiotherapy in locally advanced carcinoma of the rectum. Patients with stage T4N0M0 (78% had a tumor length above 5 cm) were randomized to receive either radiation alone (59 patients) or radiation combined with local hyperthermia (56 patients). The patient and treatment parameters of the two arms were well balanced with regard to sex, age, anatomical type, length of the lesion, and histological type. The delivered radiation dose was 40 Gy in 10 fractions, three times a week. Local hyperthermia was delivered with an endocavitary antenna in four or five sessions, aiming for temperatures of 42°C–43°C over 1 h. Intratumoral temperature measurements were made in only seven patients. The data on heat distribution in these patients were used for optimization of the temperature regimens in all the following patients. Hyperthermia was given 10 min preceding radiation and the first session was applied from the third fraction of radiation in order to reduce the risk of induction of metastases. The strategy was to wait 4 weeks after the assigned treatment and, depending on the therapeutic effect, to consider surgery (in the case of good regression) or to continue radiotherapy up to 80 Gy. Apart from a slightly higher incidence of proctitis in patients receiving thermoradiotherapy, the acute reactions were similar in both arms. The objective tumor response rate (CR + PR) was 69.7% and 35.6% for thermoradiotherapy and radiation alone, respectively. The proportion of patients who underwent radical surgery was 55.4% (31 patients) in the arm with local hyperthermia, as compared to 27.1% (16 patients) if only radiotherapy was given. Postoperative mortality and postoperative complications did not differ significantly between the arms. Survival rates at 3 and 5 years were 44% and 36%, respectively, in the thermoradiotherapy arm and 7% and 7% in the radiation alone arm. This is one of the first well-described prospective studies showing the advantage of thermoradiotherapy as *neoadjuvant treatment* in locally advanced rectal cancer.

You et al. (1992, 1993) from the Harbin Medical University in China performed a three-arm prospective study in patients with rectal cancer, comparing preoperative radiotherapy and intracavitary hyperthermia, preoperative radiotherapy alone, and surgery alone. A total of 146 patients were entered in the study and 122 patients underwent radical surgery. Radiation doses were 30 Gy in eight fractions, twice a week, or 40 Gy in 20 fractions five times a week. Intracavitary hyperthermia was delivered with a 915-MHz microwave applicator 30 min following radiation. Intratumoral temperatures were not measured. The temperature of the probe attached to the tumor surface was maintained at 45°C–50°C for 45 min. Two sessions a week were given, to a total of six to eight sessions. The post-treatment percentages of stages 0 and A were 45% (20/44) in the thermoradiotherapy arm, 23.7% (9/38) in the radiation alone arm, and 12.5% (5/40) in the surgery alone arm. The authors concluded that a significant downstaging was achieved with the combination of radiation and intracavitary hyperthermia. Histopathological analysis of the surgical specimens showed significantly more tumor cell degeneration and more cases with total disappearance of cancer cells in the thermoradiotherapy arm than in the other two arms. The 5-year actuarial survival rates was 67%, 50%, and 41% for thermoradiotherapy, radiation alone, and surgery alone, respectively. The corresponding local failure rates in the three arms were 15%, 23%, and 41%.

8.4 The Amsterdam (AMC) Data on Colorectal Carcinoma

Between 1985 and 1992, 72 patients with pelvic recurrences of colorectal cancer were treated with combined radiotherapy and hyperthermia. All patients had deep-seated tumors. Seven patients with recurrences in the abdominal wall or perineum are not included in the present analysis. In 27 patients the relapse occurred following surgery without postoperative radiotherapy; 27 other patients had received irradiation either postoperatively or at the time of first relapse, and 18 patients had unresectable disease at first presentation. The disease was locoregional in 49 patients and locoregional with distant metastases in 23 patients. Radiotherapy was administered with megavoltage equipment and a four-field box radiation technique was generally used. In patients previously irradiated or in poor general condition the radiation schedule consisted of six to eight fractions of 4 Gy twice a week up to a total dose of 24–32 Gy (mean 31 Gy). In the group without previous irradiation the planned dose was 50 Gy, five fractions per week (mean 49 Gy). Patients with unresectable tumors received 60–66 Gy in 6–7 weeks, five fractions per week (mean 59 Gy). The irradiation fields were reduced after 40–45 Gy. Hyperthermia was applied using a four-antennae array (matched phased array) operating at 70 MHz (Van Dijk et al. 1989) (Fig. 8.1). One or two intratumoral closed-end catheters were placed for thermometry purposes. Thermocouple multisensor probes with seven sensors per probe were introduced inside the catheters for monitoring temperatures during the treatment (Fig. 8.2). Additional probes were placed in the bladder, vagina, rectum lumen (in the case of low anterior resection), and skin for estimation of the temperatures in normal tissues. The aim was to give four to six hyperthermia sessions, one or twice a week, with the intention of achieving temperatures above 41°C for at least 30 min during each session. Hyperthermia was given within 30 min after irradiation. The major endpoints of this phase I/II study were analysis of the heating capability of the hyperthermia machine, the tolerance during hyperthermia, the toxicity, and the palliative effect of the treatment. Objective response and survival rates were of secondary relevance.

A total of 292 hyperthermia treatments were applied with a mean of four sessions per patient.

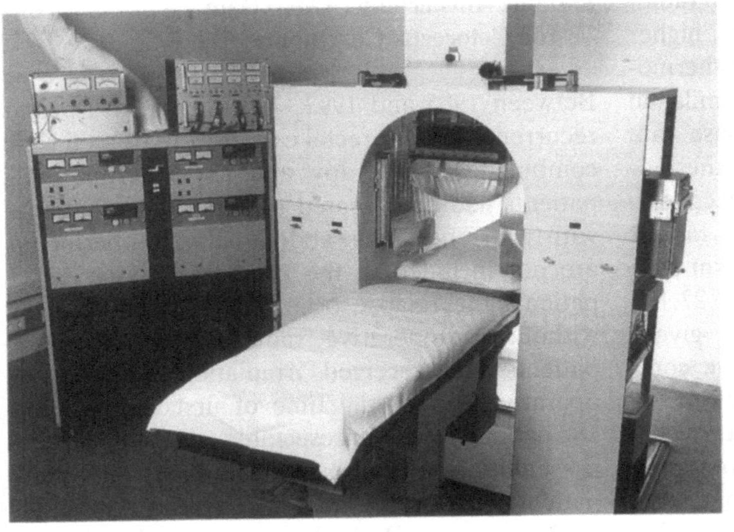

Fig. 8.1. The Amsterdam Multiple Phased Array system (MPA). The 4 applicators with water bolus on the right and the 4 generators operating at 70 MHz on the left

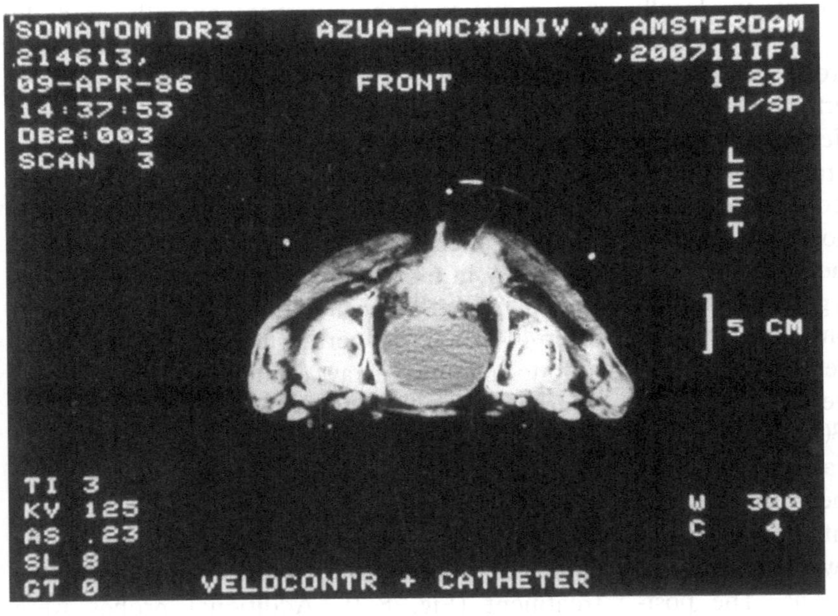

Fig. 8.2. Computer Tomography scan of a large presacral recurrence of rectal cancer, 2 years after surgery. For thermometry purposes an invasive catheter has been placed into the tumor

A detailed summary of the thermal parameters is shown in Table 8.3. The means of all the minimum (T_{min}), median (T_{med}), and maximum (T_{max}) temperatures were 39.6°C, 40.2°C, and 41.2°C, respectively. It is clear from these results that only a relatively small proportion of patients reached intratumoral temperatures above what is considered the therapeutic range. This also held true when the percentage of sensors (20%, 50%, 90%) at a given index temperature was estimated, i.e., in only 17% of the sessions were 90% of the temperature sensors above 40°C. The number of minutes per session at a minimum temperature of 42°C was 1.1 and at a maximum temperature of 42°C, 15.9. As the mean number of sessions per patient was four, the cumulative number of minutes at a maximum temperature of 42°C within the tumor was 80. A comparison of our results with other reported thermal parameters in pelvic tumors is presented in Table 8.4. In general, our results are in agreement with these other series.

The palliative effect as well as the duration of palliation is presented in Table 8.5. As reported in the literature, good palliation was achieved in about 75% of the patients, with a mean duration of 12 months. The percentage of palliated patients was higher when high radiation doses were

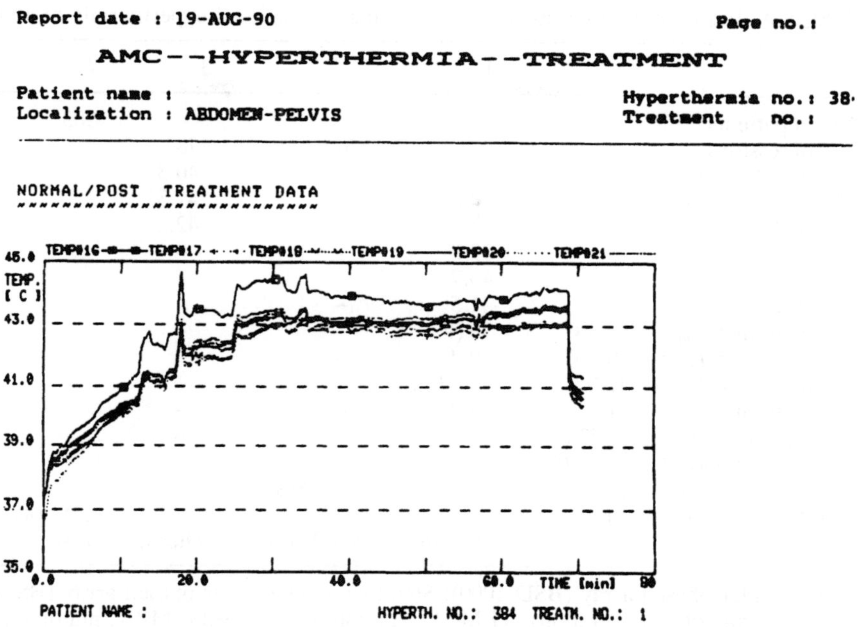

Fig. 8.3. Register of intratumoral temperatures. In this particular case all 6 sensors were at 43°C for 40 min. Note that it took 20 min to reach the plateau temperature

Table 8.3. Thermal parameters in 72 patients with colorectal recurrences

	Range (°C)	No. of pts.	Mean ± SD
T_{min}	38.0–39.0	23 (32%)	
	39.1–40.0	31 (43%)	
	40.1–41.0	16 (22%)	
	>41.0	2 (3%)	39.6 ± 0.92
T_{max}	38.0–39.0	6 (8%)	
	39.1–40.0	11 (15%)	
	40.1–41.0	20 (28%)	
	41.1–42.0	21 (29%)	
	>42.0	14 (19%)	41.1 ± 1.57
T_{med}	38.0–39.0	30 (43%)	
	39.1–40.0	18 (26%)	
	40.1–41.0	11 (16%)	
	41.1–42.0	11 (16%)	
	Unknown	2 (3%)	40.2 ± 1.02
T_{20}[a]	38.6–39.0	3 (7%)	
	39.1–40.0	9 (22%)	
	40.1–41.0	15 (37%)	
	41.1–42.0	9 (22%)	
	>42.0	5 (12%)	40.6 ± 1.11
T_{50}[a]	38.4–39.0	6 (15%)	
	39.1–40.0	19 (46%)	
	40.1–41.0	10 (24%)	
	41.1–42.0	6 (15%)	40.0 ± 0.96
T_{90}[a]	37.8–39.0	17 (41%)	
	39.1–40.0	17 (41%)	
	40.1–41.0	7 (17%)	39.2 ± 0.84
Av. T_{min} 42°C[a]	0–5	35 (86%)	
(min)	>5	6 (14%)	1.1 ± 2.55 (min)
Av. T_{max} 42°C[a]	0–20	23 (56%)	
(min)	21–30	14 (35%)	
	>30	4 (9%)	15.9 ± 11.78 (min)

[a] estimated in only 41 patients

Table 8.4. Intratumoral thermometry data during locoregional hyperthermia of abdominopelvic tumors

	1	2	3	4	5	6	7	8[a]
No. of patients	–	–	–	203	32	16	17	72
No. of sessions	84	256	178	–	–	52	40	292
Mean of T_{min} (°C)	39.3	–	40.3	–	40.6	40.5	39.5	39.6
Mean of T_{mean} (°C)	40.8	–	41.3	–	41.3	41.7	40.6	40.2
Mean of T_{max} (°C)	42.4	–	42.2	–	41.9	42.6	41.6	41.1
T_{90} (°C)	39.8	–	–	–	–	40.5	–	39.2
T_{50} (°C)	40.7	–	–	–	–	41.8	–	40.0
T_{20} (°C)	41.5	–	–	–	–	–	–	40.6
Cumulat. min T_{90} >= 40.0°C	76 (97)	–	–	–	–	–	–	–
Cumulat. min T_{90} >= 40.5°C	49 (94)	–	–	–	–	–	–	–
Cumulat. min T_{50} >= 41.0°C	73 (103)	–	–	–	–	–	–	–
Cumulat. min T_{50} >= 41.5°C	44 (88)	–	–	–	–	–	–	–
Cumulat. min av. T_{min} = 42.0°C	–	–	–	–	–	–	–	4.1
Cumulat. min av. T_{max} = 42.0°C	–	–	–	–	–	–	–	80.0
No. of sessions >40°C 20 min	–	35 (15%)	–	–	–	–	–	–
TD (50–100 min at 42.5)	–	–	–	11% pts[a]	–	27%	–	–
Device	AA/S60	AA/Therm.	Therm.	AA	AA	S60	TEM	MPA

AA, annular phased array (BSD 1000); S60, Sigma 60 annular phased array (BSD 2000); Therm., Thermotron RF-8 MHz (Yamamoto Corporation); TEM, TEM applicator, Utrecht; MPA, multiple phased array system
1, Feldmann et al. 1993; 2, Emami et al. 1991; 3, Nishimura et al. 1992; 4, Petrovich et al. 1989; 5, Shimm et al. 1988; 6, Mattal et al. 1992; 7, Van Es et al. 1992; 8, Gonzalez Gonzalez, see test
[a] Of 203 patients with finite TD, 150 did not reach 42.5°C or the equivalent

Table 8.5. Palliative effect of thermoradiotherapy in 72 colorectal recurrences

	Before	At 3 months
Pain character		
No pain/sporadic	29%	69%
Moderate	20%	16%
Severe	51%	15%
Pain medication		
No/sporadic	29%	65%
Non-narcotics	33%	19%
Narcotics	38%	26%
Medication frequency		
No/sporadic	22%	62%
4–6 h	32%	17%
1–3 h	46%	21%
Tenesmus		
No	63%	82%
Yes	37%	18%
Discharges		
No	64%	93%
Yes	36%	7%
Bleeding		
No	72%	94%
Yes	28%	6%

Mean duration of palliation: 12.1 ± 11.5 months

administered. No correlation was found between palliative effect and thermal parameters. Confirmed objective remission was obtained in 11 patients (15%), three CRs and eight PRs. The three CRs were also confirmed pathologically. We could not demonstrate any correlation of objective remission with thermal parameters. Median survival (actuarial) was 11 months and 17% of the patients were alive at 3 years.

8.5 Toxicity

A summary of the more relevant toxicities observed by different authors (including the present author) following locoregional hyperthermia for deep-seated abdominopelvic tumors is presented on Table 8.6. During the course of the hyperthermia treatment, local pain inside or around the heated field is relatively frequent and is the most important limiting factor in delivering hyperthermia. Most authors report that pain leads to power reduction and not infrequently a definitive cessation or patient refusal of the hyperthermia treatment. General discomfort, anxiety, and malaise are also frequently found. Systemic hyperthermia effects such as tachycardia, hypertension, and rise in the core temperature above 39°C occur, but in general are not a major cause for treatment interruption. However, most authors agree in not selecting patients with severe cardiovascular disease and deficits for locoregional hyperthermia. Van der Zee et al. (1992) described a patient with a large recurrent rectal cancer who

Table 8.6. Toxicity of locoregional thermoradiotherapy for abdominopelvic tumors (the majority colorectal) in various clinical studies

	1	2	3	4	5
Local pain in heated field	68%	37%[a]	50%	35%	33%
General discomfort	23%	32%[a]	–	3%	17%
Tachycardia	13%	35%[a]	–	3%	29%
Thermal blister	2%	5%	0%	3%	0%
Infection due to catheter	7%	8%	16%	1%	10%
% treatments stopped	68%	–	–	–	17%
Systemic temperature >39°C	–	3%[a]	–	–	–
Fat/muscle necrosis	–	5%	6%	–	0%
Obstructive ileus	–	–	23%	–	0%
Intestinal fistula	–	–	10%	–	0%
Intestinal perforation	–	–	6%	–	0%
Bladder bleeding	–	–	0%	–	0%
Hydronephrosis	–	–	–	–	3%
Lost catheter	–	–	–	–	1%

1, Emami et al. 1991; 2, Feldmann et al. 1993; 3, Nishimura et al. 1992; 4, Petrovich et al. 1989; 5, Gonzalez Gonzalez, see test

[a] Percentage of sessions where a given toxicity was registered

developed acute hypotension following epidural analgesia during deep regional hyperthermia. Infection at the place of insertion of the thermometry catheters varied from 1% to 16%, and sometimes necessitated removal of the catheters and cessation of treatment (Feldmann et al. 1993). Thermal blisters were not a major problem, probably reflecting good functioning of the cooling systems with the available hyperthermia devices. Fat/muscle necrosis was observed in 5%–6% of the patients. Sapozink et al. (1988) described a case of severe myonecrosis following deep pelvic hyperthermia and Ben-Yosef et al. (1992) reported on two cases of myonecrosis and peripheral neuropathy following deep regional hyperthermia for recurrent prostatic cancer. We did not observe fatty necrosis in our study on colorectal cancer, but in a series of 15 patients with cervical carcinoma three cases of fat necrosis occurred, one requiring surgery for removal of the necrotic tissue. These three patients were extremely obese. From the reviewed reports, it appears that the addition of locoregional hyperthermia in the treatment of abdominopelvic tumors does not clearly enhance the known acute toxicity caused by radiation alone.

Late toxicity was reported by Nishimura et al. (1992). These authors observed a relatively high percentage of obstructive ileus and intestinal fistula. However, in their series the mean radiation dose was 58 Gy (range 40–70 Gy), four patients had received previous irradiation (59–78 Gy) and a further three patients received chemotherapy. The high radiation dose per se could easily explain the observed complications, i.e., they need not be attributed to hyperthermia. Two of our patients who had a rectal cancer considered unresectable at laparotomy were treated with 66 Gy and 68 Gy plus hyperthermia. Five weeks after treatment a second laparotomy was performed and the tumor could be radically removed in both cases. About 6 months after treatment these two patients developed bilateral hydronephrosis which was solved by means of nephrostomy drainage. A third patient with a rectal recurrence received 66 Gy and 8 months after treatment developed an ulceration of the rectal wall and bleeding which required the performance of a colostomy. The condition of the patient deteriorated, leading to death 20 months after treatment. At autopsy massive necrosis of the small bowel and rectum was observed without any signs of vital tumor. The role of hyperthermia in these complications is not clear but it may have contributed to them in conjunction with surgery (two laparotomies) and the high radiation doses.

Coltart et al. (1988) performed a prospective study in patients receiving pelvic radiotherapy alone or combined pelvic radiotherapy and deep hyperthermia. Also a control group receiving radiation outside the pelvis was studied. The authors investigated possible changes in the permeability of the small bowel by estimating the absorption of ^{51}Cr-EDTA, [^{14}C]mannitol, and lactulose. They found no additive effect of heat in increasing permeability of the small bowel.

It is noteworthy that in the series reporting on the results of endocavitary hyperthermia in rectal cancer, no or few complications were observed (Berdov et al. 1990; You et al. 1992). Finally, Van der Zee et al. (1992b) draw attention to the possible risk of tumor growth along the thermometry catheter track by reporting on one case in which this complication was observed. They advised placement of the track of the thermometry catheters within the radiation field.

8.6 Thermoradiotherapy in Anal Carcinoma

Clinical data on thermoradiotherapy in anal carcinoma are very scanty. However, anal carcinoma represents a very good clinical situation for the use of external, endocavitary, and interstitial heating. These tumors are relatively superficial and thermometry is rather easy. In the series by SEEGENSCHMIEDT et al. (1992), two localized anal carcinomas were treated with interstitial thermoradiotherapy but the results were not specified for tumor localization. We have treated three patients with extensive recurrences following radiotherapy and chemotherapy. All the patients received a second course of radiation (8 × 4 Gy twice a week) plus 434-MHz microwave hyperthermia. In one patient considerable regression was obtained and radical surgery was then possible. This patient is alive and free of disease 3 years after treatment. In the other two patients regression of less than 50% was achieved and the tumors developed progression after 5 and 7 months respectively.

8.7 Conclusions

From the reviewed data it is not possible to derive definitive conclusions on the value of hyperthermia in the treatment of colorectal and anal cancer. In the preoperative setting, two randomized studies showed that thermoradiotherapy was superior to radiation alone, improving tumor response rate and patient survival. The results of several phase I/II studies seem to indicate that thermoradiotherapy is feasible and acute and late toxicity is not a major problem. However, in practically all the studies, in a large proportion of patients pain and discomfort during hyperthermia hampered optimal power deposition and forced the inclusion of treatment breaks and, not infrequently, definitive treatment cessation or the acceptance of patient refusal. The objective remission rate was about 45% (range 15%–70%) and palliation was achieved in more than 60% of the patients. Currently the most disappointing fact is that with the available hyperthermia equipment the increase in intratumoral temperature did not in general reach the therapeutic range, i.e., >42°C for at least 30 min. However, it is possible that temperatures in the range of 40°C–41°C can have some direct cytotoxic effect and also can homogenize blood flow in the tumor, which could increase radiosensitivity. Prospective randomized studies must be performed before we shall be able to definitively establish the role of hyperthermia in the management of cancer in general and of cancer of the lower gastrointestinal tract in particular.

8.8 Summary

- Treatment of unresectable or recurrent rectal cancer with radiation and/or chemotherapy achieves poor results. The same is true for locally advanced carcinoma of the anal canal.
- Combination of radiation and Hyperthermia can improve local control and survival in operable patients (neoadjuvant treatment). In unresectable or recurrent tumors, the combined treatment can increase resectability and, prolong palliation.
- With the presently available hyperthermia equipment it is practically impossible to heat homogeneously deep-seated tumors at temperatures of 43°C during 60 min.
- Local pain inside the heated field and at the edge at the applicator and general discomfort occur frequently, cause treatment interruptions and limit optimal power deposition in the tumor.
- Acute and late radiation toxicity does not seem to be increased by the addition of hyperthermia.
- Randomized clinical trials are needed to demonstrate the superiority of radiation combined with hyperthermia as compared to radiation alone.

References

American Cancer Society (1990) Cancer facts and figures – 1990, vol 40. American Cancer Society, Atlanta, pp 9–26

Beart RW, Melton LJ, Maueta M, et al. (1983) Trends in right- and left-sided colon cancer. Dis Colon Rectum 26: 393–398

Ben-Yosef R, Sullivan DM, Kapp DS (1992) Peripheral neuropathy and myonecrosis following hyperthermia and radiation therapy for recurrent prostatic cancer: correlation of damage with predicted SAR pattern. Int J Hyperthermia 8: 173–185

Berdov BA, Menteshashvili GZ (1990) Thermoradiotherapy of patients with locally advanced carcinoma of the rectum. Int J Hyperthermia 6: 881–890

Boman BM, Moertel CG, O'Connell MJ, et al. (1984) Carcinoma of the anal canal: a clinical and pathologic study of 188 cases. Cancer 54: 114

Boulis-Wassif S (1983) Ten years experience with a multimodality treatment of advanced stages of rectal cancer. Cancer 52: 2017–2024

Brenner HJ, Bibi C, Chaitchik S (1983) Adjuvant therapy for Dukes C adenocarcinoma of colon. Int J Radiat Oncol Biol Phys 9: 1789–1792

Cameron MC, Verdenheimer MC, Callan JA (1979) Colorectal carcinoma: a decade's experience at the Lahey Clinic. Am Colon Rectum 22: 4777–4779

Cass AW, Million RR, Pfaff WW (1976) Patterns of recurrence following surgery alone for adenocarcinoma of the colon and rectum. Cancer 37: 2861–2865

Ciatto S, Pacini P (1982) Radiation therapy of recurrences of carcinoma of the rectum and sigmoid after surgery. Acta Radiol Oncol 21: 105–109

Coltart RS, Howard GCW, Wraight EP, Bleehen NM (1988) The effect of hyperthermia and radiation on small bowel permeability using ^{51}Cr EDTA and ^{14}C mannitol in man. Int J Hyperthermia 4: 467–477

Corry PM (1989) Overview of ultrasonic hyperthermia. In: Sugahara T, Saito M (eds) Hyperthermic oncology, vol II. Taylor and Francis, London, pp 528–531

Coughlin CT, Strohbehn JW, Ryan TP, Roberts DW, Colacchio TA, Douple EB (1989) Interstitial hyperthermia for deep seated malignancies. In: Sugahara T, Saito M (eds) Hyperthermic oncology, vol I, summary papers. Taylor and Francis, London, pp 496–597

Cummings BJ, Thomas GM, Keane TJ, et al. (1982) Primary radiation therapy in the treatment of anal canal carcinoma. Dis Colon Rectum 25: 778–782

Cummings BJ, Keane TJ, Thomas GM, et al. (1984) Results and toxicity of the treatment of anal canal carcinoma by radiation therapy and chemotherapy. Cancer 54: 2062–2068

Danjoux CE, Gelber RD, Catton GE, Klaassen DJ (1985) Combination chemo-radiotherapy for residual recurrent or inoperable carcinoma of the tectum. ECOG Study (EST 3276). Int J Radiat Oncol Biol Phys 11: 765–771

Douglass HO Jr, Moertel CG (1986) Survival after postoperative combination treatment of rectal cancer. The N Engl J Med 315: 1294–1295

Duttenhaver J, Hoskins RB, Gunderson LL, Tepper JE (1986) Adjuvant postoperative radiation therapy in the management of adenocarcinoma of the colon. Cancer 57: 955–963

Emami B, Myerson RJ, Scott C, Gibbs F, Lee C, Perez CA (1991) Phase I/II study, combination of radiotherapy and hyperthermia in patients with deep-seated malignant tumors: report of a pilot study by the radiation therapy oncology group. Int J Radiat Oncol Biol Phys 20: 73–79

Feldmann HJ, Molls M, Adler S, Meyer-Schwickerath M, Sack H (1991) Hyperthermia in eccentrically located pelvic tumors: excessive heating of the perineal fat and normal tissue temperatures. Int J Radiat Oncol Biol Phys 20: 1017–1022

Feldmann HJ, Molls M, Hoederath H, Krümpelmann S, Sack H (1992a) Blood flow and steady state temperatures in deep seated tumors and normal tissues. Int J Radiat Oncol Biol Phys 23: 1003–1008

Feldmann HJ, Molls M, Romanowski R, Sievers K, Fuller J, Sack H (1992b) Regional Hyperthermia in combination with radiation therapy in pelvic tumors: determinants for temperature elevation and tumor response. In: Gerner EW (ed) Hyperthermic oncology 1992, vol 1, summary papers. Arizona Board of Regents, Tucson, AZ, p 414

Feldmann HJ, Hoederath A, Molls M, Sack H (1993a) Problems associated with CT-guided catheter insertions. Int J Hyperthermia 9: 219–225

Feldmann HJ, Molls M, Heinemann H-G, Romanowski R, Stuschke M, Sack H (1993b) Thermoradiotherapy in locally advanced deep seated tumours – thermal parameters and treatment results. Radiother Oncol 26: 38–44

Fisher B, Wolmark N, Rockette H, Redmond C, et al. (1988) Postoperative adjuvant chemotherapy or radiation therapy for rectal cancer: results from NSABP Protocol R-01. J Natl Cancer Inst 80: 21–29

Gastrointestinal Tumor Study Group (1985) Prolongation of the disease-free interval in surgically treated rectal carcinoma. – Engl J Med 312: 1465–1472

Gerard A, Berrod JL, Pene F, et al. (1988) Preoperative radiotherapy and radical surgery as combined treatment in rectal cancer. Recent Results Cancer Res 110: 130–133

Gilbert SG (1978) Symptomatic local tumor failure following abdominoperineal resection. Int J Radiat Oncol Biol Phys 4: 801–807

Greenall MJ, Quan HQ, DeCosse JJ (1985a) Epidermoid cancer of the anus. Br J Surg (suppl) 72: s97

Greenall MJ, Quan SHQ, Stearns MW, et al. (1985b) Epidermoid cancer of the anal margin. Pathologic features, treatment, and clinical results. Am J Surg 149: 95–101

Gunderson LL, Russell AH, Llewellyn HJ, Doppke KP, Tepper JE (1985a) Treatment planning for colorectal cancer: radiation and surgical techniques and value of small-bowel films. Int J Radiat Oncol Biol Phys 11: 1379–1393

Gunderson LL, Sosin H, Levitt S (1985b) Extrapelvic colon areas of failure in a reoperation series: implications for adjuvant therapy. Int J Radiat Oncol Biol Phys 11: 731–741

Gunderson LL, Beart RW, O'Connell MJ (1987) Current issues in the treatment of colorectal cancer. Curr Res Oncol Hematol 6: 223–259

Hand JW, Vernon CC, Prior MV (1992a) Initial experience of the sonotherm 6500 scanned focused ultrasound hyperthermia system. In: Gerner EW (ed) Hyperthermic oncology 1992, vol 1, summary papers. Arizona Board of Regents, Tucson, AZ, p 332

Hand JW, Vernon CC, Prior MV (1992b) Early experience of a commercial scanned focused ultrasound hyperthermia system. Int J Hyperthermia 8: 587–607

Hardcastle JD, Bussey HJR (1968) Results of surgical treatment of squamous cell carcinoma of the anal canal and anal margin seen at St Mark's Hospital 1928–1966. Proc R Soc Med 61: 629

James RD, Schofield PF (1985) Resection of "inoperable" rectal cancer following radiotherapy. Br J Surg 72: 279–281

John M, Flam M, Podolsky W, et al. (1985) Feasibility of non-surgical definitive management of anal canal carcinoma. Int J Radiat Oncol Biol Phys 11(suppl): 109

Kakehi M, Ueda K, Mukojimas T, Hiraoka M, Seto O, Akanuma A, Nakatsugawa S (1990) Multi-institutional clinical studies on hyperthermia combined with radiotherapy or chemotherapy in advanced cancer of deep-seated organs. Int J Hyperthermia 6: 719–740

Krook JE, Moertel CG, Gunderson LL, et al. (1991) Effective surgical adjuvant therapy for high-risk rectal carcinoma. – Engl J Med 324: 709–715

Leichman L, Nigro N, Vaitkevicius VK, et al. (1985) Cancer of the anal canal: model for preoperative adjuvant combined modality therapy. Am J Med 78: 211

Lewis LJ, Stea B, Hynynen K, Hatch K, Fosmire H, Villar H (1992) In: Gerner EW (ed) Hyperthermic oncology 1992, vol 1, summary papers. Arizona Board of Regents, Tucson, AZ, p 474

Lybeert MLM, Martijn H, De Neve W, Crommelin MA, Ribot JG (1992) Radiotherapy for locoregional relapses of rectal carcinoma after initial radical surgery: definite but limited influence on relapse-free survival and survival Int J Radiat Oncol Biol Phys 24: 241–246

Marchal C, Bey P (1992) Clinical studies comparing radiation therapy alone to radiation combined with hyperthermia with or without prolonged intravenous 5 FU for pelvic recurrences of rectal carcinomas. In: Gerner EW (ed) Hyperthermic oncology 1992, vol 1, summary papers. Arizona Board of Regents, Tucson, AZ, p 432

Matsuda T (1989) Present status of clinical hyperthermic oncology in Japan – on the basis of joint research. In: Sugahara T, Saito M (eds) Hyperthermic oncology, vol II. Taylor and Francis, London, pp 14–19

Mendenhall WM, Million RP, Pfaff WW (1983) Patterns of recurrence in adenocarcinoma of the rectum and rectosigmoid treated with surgery alone: implications in treatment planning with adjuvant radiation therapy. Int J Radiat Oncol Biol Phys 9: 977

Mendenhall WM, Million RP, Bland KL, Pfaff WW, Copeland EM (1985) Preoperative radiation therapy for clinically resectable carcinoma of the rectum. Ann Surg 202: 215–222

Michaelson RA, Magill GB, Quan SHQ, et al. (1983) Preoperative chemotherapy and radiation therapy in the management of anal epidermoid carcinoma. Cancer 51: 390

Mittal BB, Sathiaseelan V, Brand WN, et al. (1992) Regional hyperthermia using BSD-2000 system with sigma-60 applicator for advanced malignant tumors. In: Gerner EW (ed) Hyperthermic oncology 1992, vol 1, summary papers. Arizona Board of Regents, Tucson, AZ, p 411

Moertel CG, Schmitt AJ, Hahn RG, Reitemeier RJ (1975) Therapy of advanced gastrointestinal cancer with a combination of 5-FU, methyl-CCNU and vincristine. J Natl Cancer Inst 54: 69–71

Moertel CG, Fleming TR, MacDonald JS, et al. (1990) Levamisole and fluorouracil for adjuvant therapy of resected colon cancer. N Engl J Med 322: 352–358

National Cancer Institute (1991) Adjuvant therapy of rectal cancer. U.S. Dept of Health and Human Service, public health service clinical announcement, March, 1991, pp 144–150

Nigro ND (1984) An evaluation of combined therapy for squamous cell cancer of the anal canal. Dis Colon Rectum 27: 763–766

NIH Consensus Conference (1990) Adjuvant therapy for patients with colon and rectal cancer. JAMA 264: 1444–1450

Nishimura Y, Hiraoka M, Akuta K, Jo S, Nagata Y, Masunagra SI, Takahashi M, Abe M (1992) Hyperthermia combined with radiation therapy for primarily unresectable and recurrent colorectal cancer. Int J Radiat Oncol Biol Phys 23: 759–768

Overgaard J (1989) The current and potential role of hyperthermia in radiotherapy. Int J Radiat Oncol Biol Phys 16: 535–549

Papillon J (1982) Rectal and anal cancers. Conservative treatment by irradiation. An alternative to radical surgery. Springer, Berlin Heidelberg New York

Petrovich Z, Langholz B, Gibbs FA, et al. (1989) Regional hyperthermia for advanced tumors: a clinical study of 353 patients. Int J Radiat Oncol Phys 16: 601–607

Rich T, Gunderson LL, Lew R, Galdabini JJ, Cohen AM, Donaldson G (1983) Patterns of recurrence of rectal cancer after potentially curative surgery. Cancer 52: 1317–1329

Rominger CJ, Gunderson LL, Gelber RD, Conner N (1985) Radiation therapy alone or in combination with chemotherapy in the treatment of residual or inoperable carcinoma of the rectum or rectosigmoid or pelvic recurrence following colorectal surgery. Radiation therapy oncology group study (76-16). Am J Clin Oncol 8: 118–127

Sapozink M, Gibbs P, Gibbs FA, Jolles C (1988) Myonecrosis following deep pelvic hyperthermia. Int J Hyperthermia 4: 251–258

Schlienger M, Krzisch C, Pene F, et al. (1989) Epidermoid carcinoma of the anal canal. Treatment results and prognostic variables in a series of 242 cases. Int J Radiat Oncol Biol Phys 17: 1141–1151

Seegenschmiedt MH, Seydel R, Klautke G, Brady LW, Sauer R (1992) Interstitial thermal radiation therapy for advanced and recurrent pelvic tumors: initial and long-term results. In: Gerner EW (ed) Hyperthermic oncology 1992, vol 1, summary papers. Arizona Board of Regents, Tucson, AZ, p 476

Shimm DS, Cetas TC, Oleson JR, Gross ER, Buechler DN, Fletcher AM, Dean SE (1988) Regional hyperthermia for deep-seated malignancies using the BSD annular array. Int J Hyperthermia 4: 159–170

Shimm D, Stea B, Cetas T, et al. (1989) Clinical results of interstitial hyperthermia using thermally regulating ferromagnetic seeds. In: Sugahara T, Saito M (eds) Hyperthermic oncology, vol II. Taylor and Francis, London, pp 536–539

Sischy B (1985) The use of radiation therapy combined with chemotherapy in the management of squamous cell carcinoma of the anus and marginally resectable adenocarcinoma of the rectum. Int J Radiat Oncol Biol Phys 11: 1587–1593

Stockholm Rectal Cancer Study Group (1987) Short-term preoperative radiotherapy for adenocarcinoma of the rectum: an interim analysis of a randomized multicenter trial. Am J Clin Oncol 10: 369–375

Sugarbaker PH (1986) Colorectal tumor. In: Cameron JL (ed) Current surgical therapy, vol 2. Mosby, St. Louis, pp 121–122

Takeshita N, Tanaka Y, Matsuda T (1993) Evaluation of CT images, tumour response and prognosis after thermoradiotherapy for deep-seated tumours. Int J Hyperthermia 9: 1–17

Van Es CA, Wyrdeman HK, De Leeuw AAC, Lagendijk JJW, Battermann JJ (1992) Pilot study: regional hyperthermia with the "coaxial tem" system in advanced pelvic disease. In: Gerner EW (ed) Hyperthermic oncology 1992, vol 1, summary papers. Arizona Board of Regents, Tucson, AZ, p 415

Van der Zee J, Hoff AM, Oudkerk M, de Kock W, van de Merwe SA, de Jong PC (1992a) Risk of acute hypotension following epidural analgesia during deep regional hyperthermia: a case report. Int J Hyperthermia 8: 625–629

Van der Zee J, Veeze-Kuijpers B, Wiggers T, van de Merwe SA, Treurniet-Donker AD (1992b) Short communication: risk of tumour growth along ther-

mometry catheter track: a case report. Int J Hyperthermia 8: 621–624
Van Dijk JDP, González González D, Blank LECM (1989) Deep local hyperthermia with a four aperture array system of large waveguide radiators. Results of simulation and clinical application. In: Sugahara T, Saito M (eds) Hyperthermic oncology, vol I, summary papers. Taylor and Francis, London, pp 573–575
Villalon AH, Green D (1981) The use of radiotherapy for pelvic recurrence following abdominoperineal resection for carcinoma of the rectum: a 10-year experience. Aust N Z J Surg 51: 149–151
Walz BJ, Green MR, Linstrom ER, et al. (1981) Anatomic prognostic factors after abdominal perineal resection. Int J Radiat Oncol Biol Phys 7: 477–484
Willet C, Tepper JE, Cohen A, Orlow E, Welch C, Donaldson G (1983) Local failure following curative resection of colonic adenocarcinoma. Int J Radiat Oncol Biol Phys 10: 645–651
Wust P, Nadobny J, Felix R, Deuffhard P, Louis A, John W (1991) Strategies for optimized application of annular phased array systems in clinical hyperthermia. Int J Hyperthermia 7: 157–173
Wust P, Stahl H, Löffel J, Riess H, Felix R (1992) A phase I study with regional hyperthermia (sigma-60 applicator) of recurrent pelvic tumors: feasibility, in vivo-measurements and response. In: Gerner EW (ed) Hyperthermic oncology, vol 1, summary papers. Arizona Board of Regents, Tucson, AZ, p 402
You QS, Wang RZ, Yan FC, Zhao JH, Cui SR (1992) Clinicopathological study and results of combined preoperative radiation with intracavitary hyperthermia in rectal cancer. In: Gerner EW (ed) Hyperthermic oncology 1992, vol 1, summary papers. Arizona Board of Regents, Tucson, AZ, pp 481–481b
You QS, Wang RZ, Suen G-Q, et al. (1993) Combination preoperative radiation and endocavitary hyperthermia for rectal cancer: long-term results of 44 patients. Int J Hyperthermia 9: 19–24

9 Thermoradiotherapy for Genitourinary and Gynecological Tumors

F.A. GIBBS, JR.

CONTENTS

9.1 Introduction

Advances in the clinical application of thermoradiotherapy in the treatment of genitourinary and gynecological malignancies have been hampered by the same limitations as in most other sites: (a) methods are inadequate for sufficiently heating the entire tumor without exceeding normal tissue or patient tolerance; (b) documentation of tumor heating with adequate invasive thermometry is difficult, hazardous, and uncomfortable; (c) tumor responses in an individual patient may be attributable to the conventional treatment modality alone rather than the adjunctive hyperthermia.

The major sites worthy of specific discussion in this chapter are bladder, prostate, cervix, and ovary. Due to limitations of space, not all references can be cited and discussed; anecdotal reports of tumors of the penis (e.g., BEN-YOSEF and KAPP 1992), vagina (e.g., SORBE et al. 1993; VALDAGNI et al. 1988), and vulva (e.g., SEEGENSCHMIEDT et al. 1993a,b) are mentioned only in passing. There is little experience specifically relating to corpus uteri and renal carcinomas.

A potentially very important recent study that has thus far been reported only at meetings is a randomized prospective deep regional heating trial in patients with advanced bladder, cervical, and rectal tumors conducted in The Netherlands. This trial is currently being reported as showing a significant benefit form the addition of hyperthermia to conventional radiotherapy. The reader is directed to author lists including Dr. J. van der Zee to search for future publications concerning this trial.

9.2 General and Technological Considerations

Clinical reports must be viewed with the enlightenment form the Radiation Therapy Oncology Group (RTOG) studies 8104 (PEREZ et al. 1991) and 8419 (EMAMI et al. 1993) in which adjunctive superficial and interstitial (respectively) hyperthermia were prospectively compared with radiotherapy alone. Both these studies showed no advantage to hyperthermia (except in subgroup analysis of small tumors in 8104). There is ample reason to believe that these studies failed because hyperthermia *was neither adequately delivered nor documented*. Therefore, there is little reason for enthusiasm over anecdotal clinical results where the heating technology and/or thermometric documentation are suspect and observed results may have been unrelated to the administration, or effective *lack* of administration, of hyperthermia. Unfortunately, the work that has been

F.A. GIBBS, JR., MD, Department of Radiation Oncology, University of Utah, 50 North Medical Drive, Salt Lake City, UT 84132, USA

performed thus far in deep pelvic sites is so suspect.

Although specific heating techniques will be discussed in connection with the specific sites, scanned-focused ultrasound (SFUS) will be mentioned now. SFUS is a method with considerable promise for heating genitourinary and gynecological sites but specific applications to such have not been reported thus far. Results of this method in heating pelvic tumors in general (Hand et al. 1992; Harari et al. 1991; Hynynen et al. 1990) appear to be better than those reported with other noninvasive techniques and further reports should be awaited with interest.

9.3 Bladder

9.3.1 Introduction

Patients with bladder cancers that regress well with moderate doses of radiotherapy can often be spared cystectomy by definitive irradiation; cystectomy can be reserved for the possibility of tumor recurrence. A technique such as hyperthermia, which could perhaps improve local tumor regression and downstaging, might offer significant benefit.

9.3.2 Technical Considerations

Microwave (MW) devices placed in the bladder would be expected to produce focal, Superficial, nonhomogeneous, and probably poorly reproducible heating patterns due to the sensitivity of power deposition to the antenna's proximity and orientation with respect to tumor and mucosa. This approach has been reported (Colombo et al. 1995; Rigatti et al. 1991) but the SAR patterns and potential thermometry artifacts have not been characterized.

The use of a saline-filled balloon catheter serving as an internal radiofrequency (RF) electrode has been advocated to improve power deposition in the region of the prostate, bladder, and uterus (Inatomi et al. 1992) but there are no reports of clinical implementation. RF heating of the bladder by means of a cystoscopic electrode and saline filling of the bladder has also been alluded to (Bichler et al. 1984, 1989). The use of hyperthermic bladder perfusion along with regional heating would seem attractive as a means of stabilizing the wall of the distended bladder at a fixed temperature relative to the externally heated surrounding tissues. This approach has been anecdotally reported (Kubota et al. 1984b) but apparently not persistently used, and thermal dosimetric studies to measure its advantages have not been reported.

Uchibayashi et al. (1992) performed thermometry in 30 patients during RF hyperthermia treatments for bladder cancer and found that intravesical urine temperature measurements correlated ($P = 0.01$) with measurements from the tumor center and periphery. Mean tumor center temperatures were 44.2°C, tumor periphery, 43.4°C, and intravesical, 42.9°C. However, the minimum average absolute error, after addition of a correction factor to the urine temperature, was still 1.3°C for the tumor center (range −3.6°C to +2.9°C) and 0.7°C for the tumor periphery (range −2.7°C to +1.4°C). Therefore, measurement of the urine temperature would not appear to be a very good control parameter in the individual patient. These same authors also noted that tumors of the bladder base seemed to be less well heated than those of the lateral or posterior walls (they surmised that higher electrical impedance due to the pubic symphysis and other anatomical factors interfered with power deposition near the bladder base) and that subcutaneous fat thicknesses ≥3 cm resulted in excessive subcutaneous heating (even with surface cooling) and intravesical temperatures <42°C. The study did not address the temporal stability or the achievable duration of the reported temperatures.

9.3.3 Clinical Results

Intravesical bladder perfusion of mitomycin C under hyperthermic conditions (intravesical microwave and controlled perfusate temperature) has been reported to give a 70% CR rate in a Phase I trial in superficial bladder cancers (Colombo et al. 1995) but the significance of the hypethermia and its mode of application (microwave or perfusion) will require further study.

Treatment of bladder cancer with regional hyperthermia using annular array applicators has been alluded to in an analysis of multi-institutionally derived data (Petrovich et al. 1991). Fifty-three patients with locoregionally advanced tumors (81% pelvic, 41% bladder) were analyzed and only half of these had tumor temperature elevations greater than 40°C for long enough to accumulate any significant thermal dose. Twelve had ⩾0 and ⩽50 equivalent min at 42.5°C, six had >50 and ⩽100 eq. min, and ten had >100 eq. min (no analysis of the spatial uniformity of heating was presented). Most were treated with radiotherapy and hyperthermia. Among 14 patients with evaluable transitional cell carcinomas, there were no complete responses (CRs) and two partial responses (PRs). There was no overall correlation of response with thermal dose.

Matsui et al. (1991) reported the experience from Yokohama University using radiotherapy (1.5–2.0 Gy/fraction; 35–40 Gy in 4 weeks) followed twice weekly by bladder perfusion with bleomycin in saline, 30 μg/ml, at 42°–43°C for 1 h. Eight to twelve hyperthermia sessions were administered. Degree of bladder distention was unspecified (this should be an important thermal-dosimetric consideration). There were 38 cases of T2–3 tumors. Sixteen similar cases were "randomly selected" (selection methodology not otherwise discussed) to be treated with aggressive radiotherapy alone (50–70 Gy). Response assessment was by CT, cystoscopy, and biopsy and bimanual examination 4–5 weeks post-treatment. There were 15 CRs in the hyperthermia group and none in the radiotherapy alone group despite the more aggressive radiation treatment ($P < 0.001$). The astonishing lack of CRs in the radiotherapy alone group was not discussed by the authors. This series, without the benefit of follow-up data, was previously reported in 1984 (Kubota 1984; Kubota et al. 1984a). Evidently, since 1984 the Yokohama group has focused their attention on RF hyperthermia.

Noguchi et al. (1992) tried adding a cycle of M-VAC chemotherapy along with a similar course of radiation/hyperthermia and compared this with a group of patients treated with radiation and hyperthermia alone. Fewer than half the cases were T3–4. Bladder temperatures monitored by thermometers placed on balloon catheters in the bladder ranged from 40°C to 47°C with means of 43.9°C (nonchemotherapy) and 42.5°C (chemotherapy). The target temperature was 42°C. They found 4/17 CRs in the nonchemotherapy group and 4/18 in the chemotherapy group and concluded that the chemotherapy was of no apparent value.

Kakehi et al. (1990) reported a series of 24 cases, 16 treated with radiation and RF hyperthermia and eight with thermochemotherapy. There were two CRs in each group. Intravesical temperatures >42°C were obtained in 20 cases; the "maximum heating temperature was 44°C and average heating temperature was 42°C" (not otherwise defined). Half the cases experienced side-effects such as burns, fatty induration, pain and pollakiuria.

Strotsky et al. (1991) reported a randomized trial of 102 patients with T1–T3 tumors treated with preoperative radiotherapy, half of which were also treated with adjunctive hyperthermia. They purported to have found a significant improvement in both survival and local tumor control in the heated group. Unfortunately, this was only an abstract and a trial of this size suggesting an improvement in survival in patients who had all undergone cystectomy raises the question of statistical bias due to case selection or some other confounding factor.

In a study by Masunaga et al. (1994), 21 patients with bladder tumors received preoperative radiotherapy alone and 29 got radiotherapy plus RF hyperthermia. Selection for the latter was not randomized but was based on patients' willingness to undergo hyperthermia and/or a subcutaneous fat thickness <2 cm. Radiotherapy was in 4-Gy fractions, three fradctions per week to a total of 24 Gy. Ten of 12 patients who achieved an average intravesical temperature ⩾14.5°C were downstaged as compared with 6 of 16 with ⩽41.5°C and 10 of 21 with radiotherapy alone ($P < 0.05$). The ⩾41.5°C tumors also showed a significantly greater frequency of histological degeneration. However, there were 3/12, 4/12, and 4/12 CRs in each group respectively and the ratios of T1–2/T3–4 were 2.2, 0.71, and 0.75 respectively. There was only one local recurrence, a nonsignificant increase in distant metastases in the ⩾41.5°C group, and there were no significant differences in survival. The study was inconclusive due to confounding factors but, once again, it suggests the importance of effective heating.

9.3.4 *Discussion*

Pathologically negative cystectomy specimens in 25%–35% of preoperatively irradiated (40–50 Gy/4–5 weeks) patients with invasive bladder tumors have been reported in more than 500 cases (Batata et al. 1980; Bloom et al. 1982; Hall and Heath 1981; Miller 1977; Van der Werf-Messing 1979). Therefore, the results noted above cannot be regarded as evidence of benefit from hyperthermia. Adequate Phase I–II studies demonstrating in the neighborhood of 50% relatively uncomplicated CRs at planned cystectomy or evidence of a thermal dose-response suggesting optimal target thermal parameters should first be conducted. The previously noted RTOG experience exemplifies why Phase III trials should not be done unless a negative result can be attributed to the ineffectiveness of a definable heat exposure rather than an uncertainty as to whether the intended hyperthermic exposure was even delivered.

9.4 Prostate

9.4.1 Introduction

Patients who fail to achieve local control of their prostatic disease by radiotherapy sometimes experience unfortunate symptoms resulting from locally progressive local-regional tumor and also have been noted to have a shorter survival than those whose prostatic disease is controlled. It remains uncertain whether the latter observation is directly attributable to failure to achieve local control or, instead, is because of a systemically aggressive nature of tumors with a propensity to recur locally. Indeed, this question is probably moot without improved means of achieving local control. Hence the rationale is well provided for the addition of hyperthermia to stage B2 and C prostatic carcinomas, which have a fairly high probability of persistence following radiotherapy.

9.4.2 Technical Considerations

Methods for achieving prostatic hyperthermia have concentrated on interstitial methods using MW antennas, RF electrodes, "hot-source" needles or seeds, or noninvasive regional heating with annular array applicators. Regional RF heating has not been reported much for this treatment site although the bladder electrode technique discussed previously might be applicable (Inatomi et al. 1992). Intracavitary urethral MW devices generally heat too superficially with a 6°C fall in temperature within 1 cm of the applicator and no significant heating beyond this depth (Astrahan et al. 1991). Surface-cooled rectal MW applicators can heat up to 2 cm depth but the combination of phase-synchronous antennas operated simultaneously in the prostatic urethra and rectum shows promise of improving the uniformity of prostatic heating over either technique alone (Debicki et al. 1992).

Transrectal ultrasound would be expected on physical grounds to be able to heat the prostatic region with greater uniformity than MW. Preliminary experience with a rectal ultrasound probe having a multielement crystal array, radially and anteriorly directed through a water-cooled membrane, was reported in a Phase I trial by Fosmire et al. (1993). The study was composed of 22 treatments in 14 patients with C2–D1 disease or prostatic bed recurrences eligible for radiotherapy. All but one patient had three transperineal catheters placed for temperature mapping. Best-treatment analysis demonstrated that 60% of the time-averaged temperatures within the target volume exceeded 42°C. In general, 78% of the sensors measured ≥42.5°C at some point during the treatments. There was only a 0.5°C difference (43°C to 42.5°C) between temperatures measured at 0.5–1 cm from the rectum as compared to those at 2–2.5 cm depth. Tolerance during the 30-min treatment was considered good in 17/22, fair in 3/22, and treatment limiting in 2/22.

A refinement of the intraluminal rectal US applicator using a 64 element phased-array has been reported and studied in phantoms (Buchanan and Hynynen 1994) and may offer promise for achieving an electrically steered power deposition pattern.

Anscher et al. (1992) at Duke University used the Sigma-60 annular-dipole-array system (BSD Corp., Salt Lake City, Utah) to induce regional and prostatic hyperthermia in 12 patients. Mild sedation and analgesia were used. They found that patient tolerance and prostatic temperatures were poor and distal rectal temperatures somewhat higher than prostate temperatures. Only one patient reached 42.5°C and the maximum T_{90} (highest index temperature achieved in 90% of the measured intraprostatic points) was only 40.6°C. Adjustment of the electromagnetic phase of the power supplying the diodes was of no apparent benefit. The authors stated that increased sedation and/or analgesia might have permitted somewhat higher temperatures but they were skeptical of the value of such due to the observed preferential rectal heating. In a more limited study from Stanford using the annular array predecessor to the Sigma-60 (Kaplan et al. 1991), four patients with recurrent prostatic tumors were treated with adjunctive hyperthermia and in one case the prostatic urethral temperature reached the 42°–43°C target. The treatments in the other three casses were limited by patient tolerance. Treatments with these devices have been generally fairly taxing for patients, and significant tissue injury, though transient, has been described (BEN-YOSEF et al. 1992; SAPOZINK et al. 1988), thereby giving pause to the idea of increasing prostatic heating by merely increasing administered power by increasing sedation or analgesia.

9.4.3 Clinical Results

The palliative benefit of prostatic hyperthermia for prostatic carcinoma using a surface-cooled transrectal 915-MHz MW applicator was reported by MONTORSI et al. (1992). A total of 46 patients with severe prostatism were treated with only hyperthermia, all of whom were said to have progressive disease despite hormonal measures. They received ten 1-h heating sessions at 3-day intervals at temperatures believed to be 43.5° ± 0.5°C (an unspecified algorithm was employed for predicting prostatic temperatures based on urethral and rectal surface measurements but no confirmation of the validity of the algorithm was cited or is evident in the literature and there was no discussion regarding electromagnetic perturbations of thermistor readings). Patients were reevaluated at 1, 12, and 24 months, with 26 evaluable at the latter time. Ninety percent of the patients had significant reductions in prostatic volume ($P < 0.05$), 50% (12) of those in pretreatment urinary retention were decatheterized and nine were still catheter-free at 2 years. Post-treatment prostate-specific antigen levels did not change. Those able to void prior to treatment experienced significantly reduced residual urine volumes ($P < 0.05$). There were no CRs (presumably referring to prostatic disease only); 12 PRs lasted 7–18 months, 30 cases stabilized for at least 7 months, and four cases immediately progressed. Quality of life was considered definitely improved in 80%, with reductions in pelvic pain and discomfort considered much improved in 50%. One patient with infiltration of the rectal wall developed a transient fistula but the treatment was otherwise well tolerated. The authors commented that, "Large prostates and glands with a prominent middle lobe should not undergo hyperthermia, since a uniform and effective distribution of heat cannot be achieved . . . " but no relevant data were provided.

Studies from Tel Aviv (SERVADIO and LIEB 1991) and Warsaw (STAWARZ et al. 1993; SZMIGIELSKI et al. 1988) reported similar benefits with the same or a similar device. Eight patients with local disease only in the former study also received definitive radiotherapy to 70 Gy with no complications. There were no conclusions to be drawn concerning the adjunctive benefit of the hyperthermia in these patients. In each study there were two patients with disseminated disease demonstrating not only improvement in the prostatic disease but in their bone scans as well. In the latter study, there were two cases of complete regression of the prostatic disease and in the former there was at least one case treated with heat alone that had a negative post-treatment prostatic biopsy. There was no specific analysis to rule out a possible effect of some other form of therapy in the Tel Aviv cases but the authors stated that in general the patients were not thought to be likely to benefit further from whatever hormonal measures had been instituted. In the Warsaw cases, all patients were said to have progressive disease with failed hormonal therapy having been stopped for 6 months and prostatic hyperthermia having been the sole intervention. In both series, the authors postulated a possible beneficial immunological effect of the hyperthermia to explain the negative scans.

Effects on cell-mediated immunity were addressed in a subsequent study (STAWARZ et al. 1993; SZMIGIELSKI et al. 1991) which demonstrated that hyperthermic treatment of 15 patients with prostatic carcinoma resulted in a significant increase in depressed levels of natural killer cell activity, OKT4/OKT8 ratio, and mitogenic response of peripheral blood mononuclear cells. The immune response peaked at 2 months post-treatment and decreased to near pretreatmment levels at 6 months. These effects were not seen in 15 patients treated with hyperthermia for benign prostatic hypertrophy or in 30 normal control cases. However, there was no apparent correlation between immune response and tumor response.

Intracavitary MW with radiotherapy in the definitive treatment of prostatic carcinoma has been preliminarily reported (VALDAGNI et al. 1991; YERUSHALMI 1988) and appears to be tolerable but meaningful data concerning benefit and effectiveness of tumor heating are lacking.

Bagshaw et al. (1993) reported the Stanford preliminary experience with external beam irradiation, temporary iridium brachytherapy implant, and RF interstitial hyperthermia. Thirteen patients with locally advanced lesions and pathologically negative nodes were treated at initial presentation and three patients were treated with thermobrachytherapy for recurrent disease. Responses were considered encouraging and morbidity was not reported to be a significant factor but results were too preliminary to be meaningful. Prionas et al. (1994) recently updated the thermometric analysis of the Stanford experience in 36 patients. The percentage of mapped temperatures exceeding 41°C, 42°C, and 43°C were 67%, 46%, and 27%, respectively in tumor and 26%, 11%, and 4%, respectively in normal tissue. The relative tumor specificity was considered encouraging but the lack of effective heating in a third of the measured intratumor points emphasizes the problem. Drs. Puthawala and Syed have also used this technique in a good many patients but have not reported their results with hyperthermia in the literature. Their local control rates without hyperthermia (Marinelli et al. 1992) have been 90%–95% in biopsied patients with the exception of Stage C lesions, 55% of which they reported to have no histological evidence of persistence. Stromberg et al. (1993) report a biopsy-negative result in 80% of predominantly stage C tumors with combined external beam and brachytherapy without hyperthermia.

9.4.4 Discussion

The palliative benefit of transrectal prostatic hyperthermia as a sole modality of treatment seems to be real and the observations concerning disappearance of prostatic disease and abscopal systemic effects with normalization of once positive bone scans in a few patients bear further study. Whether or not the described effects on cell-mediated immunity are therapeutically significant and have any bearing on tumor response remains debatable and also requires further study.

There remains a significant gulf between locally curative adjunctive hyperthermia and mere palliation. Narrowing this gulf will almost certainly depend on improved delivery of heating and adequate thermal dosimetry. It seems doubtful whether transrectal MW will provide sufficient dose uniformity but in-phase operation of urethral and rectal antennas would appear to offer a significant improvement, as does transrectal ultrasound. SFUS may also be a promising approach.

With respect to interstitial methods, one must remember that a good interstitial implant is a very effective means of local tumor control; one must not underestimate its potential, even in recurrent tumors, and assume, in the absence of evidence from a randomized clinical trial, that any good result is attributable to attempted administration of adjunctive interstitial hyperthermia. Multi-institutional trials with brachytherapy represent a tremendous quality control problem. Even within a single institution, substantial case-to-case variation in dose uniformity may exist and rigorous target-dose analyses and dose optimization with differential-source loading are only beginning to be adopted. The associated problems of thermal dosimetry are even more complex and indeterminate. Unfortunately, if one cannot optimize implant geometry, the relative *thermo*biologically effective dose uniformity will be even worse than the *radio*biologically effective dose uniformity. Furthermore, the gradient of cell lethality is the same for both methods, i.e., highest nearest the sources, whereas, ideally, it should be reversed in order for the methods to be complementary. The result may be enhanced supralethality near the sources and no benefit in the interstices with no overall improvement in tumor control. The difficulty of adequately performing such treatments is exemplified by the RTOG 8419 experience (Emami et al. 1993; Emami, personal communication, 1993) which demonstrated that few if any of the accessioned cases met the RTOG quality assurance guidelines (Emami et al. 1991) for minimally acceptable heating. Cooling or thermal stabilization of the probes and the tissue in their immediate vicinity by air-flow or water cooling has been numerically modelled and studied in animals for both RF (Eppert et al. 1991; Prior 1991) and MW (Yeh et al. 1994). This would appear to be a very attractive way to significantly improve temperature uniformity and patient tolerance. Hynynen (1992) has also reported on the feasibility of interstitial ultrasound needles which may offer further improvements in heating uniformity. There is also a growing interest in continuous low-temperature hyperthermia with simultaneous low-dose-rate or multifraction high-dose-rate brachytherapy (Armour et al. 1993; Wang et al. 1992).

9.5 Uterine Cervix

9.5.1 Introduction

Cervix cancer is a major focus for hyperthermia research because of its relative anatomical accessibility, the fact that it is generally treated nonsurgically, and because the disease can frequently be cured by control of local-regional tumor. Even when it is not curable, a maximum effort at regional control is generally justified because of the extreme morbidity of uncontrolled pelvic disease.

9.5.2 Technical Considerations

Most efforts at heating cervix cancers have focused on intracavitary and interstitial methods. Regional MW and RF methods have also been employed to a lesser extent.

Intracavitary techniques would appear to be inherently deficient for all but small central lesions due to their inability to heat more than a centimeter in depth. Surface cooling should improve the penetration depth but probably not sufficiently. ZIMMERMAN et al. (1993) recently studied a 27-MHz capacitively coupled, surface-cooled intracavitary device specifically designed for the treatment of cervix cancer that would probably be expected to heat at depth about as well as can be done with such an instrument. Without surface cooling they demonstrated only a 50% specific absorption rate at only a few millimeters from the applicator. In nonperfused phantom, this depth could be extended to about 1.5 cm with surface cooling. The device was studied in pigs but no measurements of effective heating depths were made.

Problems with interstitial and regional methods are similar to those described in the preceding section on prostate. Problems with preferential vaginal heating with annular array methods have been described, making intratumor temperature measurements mandatory over vaginal measurements in monitoring treatments (SAPOZINK et al. 1990).

9.5.3 Clinical Results

Hyperthermia in the treatment of cervix cancer was initially performed at the University of Arizona (SURWIT et al. 1983). Twenty-one patients with advanced or recurrent tumors were treated with RF interstitial thermobrachytherapy of whom eight showed a sustained CR. There were four serious complications (fistulas). The Arizona experience with interstitial hyperthermia was subsequently analyzed by SHIMM et al. (SHIMM et al. 1990). This latter report did not specifically analyze the experience with cervical carcinoma (49/72 were pelvic tumors) but was encouraging in that it demonstrated a significant correlation between effectiveness of heating and CR with minimum temperatures <42.5°C associated with a 28% probability of CR and ≥42.5°C, a 69% probability ($P < 0.003$). A relationship between increased complications and maximum temperatures ≥43°C (9% incidence vs 31%, $P < 0.045$) was also noted.

VORA and LUK (1993) reported on 40 patients with pelvic tumors (32 had cervical carcinomas) treated with RF interstitial or ferromagnetic seed implants and brachytherapy. They observed 19 CRs. The only evaluable thermal parameter was that of heating duration (30 vs 60 min) and there was no correlation between it and tumor response.

GRIGSBY and EMAMI (1993) treated 14 pelvic tumors with RF interstitial thermobrachytherapy of which five were cervix cancers. They observed no correlation between thermal parameters and tumor response.

SEEGENSCHMIEDT et al. (1993a,b) treated 26 pelvic tumors with MW interstitial thermobrachytherapy, of which eight were cervix cancers. CRs were observed in 17 cases, of which one relapsed within the treated volume and four relapsed regionally outside the treated volume. Seven patients had complications with ulcers or fistulas with delayed healing. There was a suggestion of increased complications with high maximum temperatures and improved response with quality of heating but there was no statistical significance with the small numbers involved.

SAPOZINK et al. (1990) reported on 26 cases of advanced cervix cancer treated with annular-array type devices. Acute toxicity was power limiting in 43%, pain within the device aperture being the dominant problem. The mean overall average intratumor temperature was 41° ± 1.1°C for 30 min; 5% and 35% of the measured intratumor loci exceeded 43°C and 42°C, respectively. Temperatures in the cervical os and proximal vagina appeared lower relative to the monitored normal structures in the region and corresponded to lower electric field measurements in the proximal than in the distal vagina. Subacute toxicity such as protracted pain and superficial second degree burns occurred in five patients. Temperatures were slightly higher with the older generation annular array system than with the newer Sigma-60 device, possibly because of slightly greater systemic heating with the former and because the power-steering capability of the latter would not be expected to be of any advantage in heating a centrally located site such as the cervix. The authors considered the results disappointing.

9.5.4 Discussion

The only techniques which have thus far consistently achieved potentially therapeutic temperatures in the treatment of cervix cancer have been the *interstitial methods*. The noninvasive electromagnetic techniques have been disappointing and, although SFUS is promising, data are too limited. The intracavitary electromagnetic techniques are probably incapable of heating to a sufficient depth and no clinical work on intracavitary ultrasound has been reported.

As regards the interstitial methods, the same caveats apply here as in the case of prostatic carcinoma. CR rates in advanced or recurrent cervical carcinoma with interstitial brachytherapy alone have been reported in the 40%–85% range depending on stage (Aristizabal et al. 1983; Puthawala et al. 1982); these rates appear to compete favorably with those noted above for thermobrachytherapy. With the suggestion of increased complications associated with high maximum temperatures, no assumptions are currently warranted as to the value of adjunctive hyperthermia in the treatment of this site.

9.6 Ovary

9.6.1 Introduction

The major attraction of the use of hyperthermia in the therapy of ovarian cancer is the promise of an improvement in the therapeutic index of treatment of Stage III disease. Significant improvements in treatment have resulted from combined surgical debulking and chemotherapy yet patients may still fail with recurrent abdominal disease. Therefore, a method that would improve the control of the abdominal disease is desirable.

9.6.2 Technical Considerations

Since the entire peritoneal cavity may contain tumor seeding, it would be desirable to uniformly heat the entire abdominal cavity, including sizable tumor deposits. Regional heating techniques can directly heat tumors but cannot deposit power uniformly over such a large volume. Even high-flow intraperitoneal (IP) lavage with systemic cooling to prevent excessive systemic hyperthermia would be unlikely to achieve uniform heating in all peritoneal recesses and will have little effect on significant tumor masses.

Leopold et al. (1993) at Duke University reported the use of an EM annular phased array in patients treated with IP cisplatin. The target temperature was 41.5°C at 50% of the monitored IP points (T_{50} = 41.5°C) for 60 min. This was achieved in only five of 51 treatments to 15 patients. The median T_{90} and T_{10} were 39.7°C and 41.6°C, respectively, for IP measurements, and 38.8°C and 41°C, respectively, for vaginal measurements. The highest IP temperature was 44.2°C. The IP temperature range is certain to be an underestimate as the temperatures recorded were obtained from various positions along a single IP catheter. Temperatures of important areas such as the surface of the diaphragm and dome of the liver were certain to be lower. The power-limiting factor in those patients where it could be identified was patient discomfort. Four of the 15 patients had some evidence of minor thermal injury (blisters, erythema, or thigh fat necrosis).

9.6.3 Clinical Results

In the Duke study (Leopold et al. 1993), there was no difference in the pharmacokinetics of cisplatin as a result of the hyperthermia; the ratios of plasma to IP concentration times time were the same with or without heat. The maximally tolerated dose of cisplatin (80–120 mg/m^2) was also similar to that without hyperthermia. Ten of the 15 patients had a decline in CA-125 level but in only two patients did this persist beyond the course of treatment. The authors felt that renal protective methods such as IV thiosulfate would be required and technically improved heating would be necessary to achieve temperatures more likely to be therapeutic.

GILLY et al. (1992) have treated 32 patients with peritoneal carcinomatosis (both gastrointestinal and ovarian) using hyperthermic peritoneal lavage. In 18 patients, the primary tumor could be resected. Immediately after abdominal exploration and optimization of peritoneal fluid distribution, the abdomen was closed and the peritoneal cavity perfused in a closed circuit through three sites with mitomycin C or cisplatin in 6 l of peritoneal dialysate at an inflow temperature of 46°–49°C while maintaining core temperature at 32°C. There was only one treatment-related death and minimal morbidity. Median survival was 11.2 months and malignant ascites was controlled in 11 of 12 patients.

Using a somewhat similar approach, HUERTAS et al. reported in an abstract (1994) treating 29 patients with various stages of ovarian cancer with IP hyperthermic lavage with cisplatin or carbo-

Table 9.1. Clinical hyperthermia trials in genitourinary and gynecological tumors

Author	?Rx[a] + Heat	Heat method	N[b]	CRs	% CR	Comment
Bladder (superficial)						
COLOMBO et al. (1995)	MMC[c]	MW/perfusion	44		70	
Bladder (mostly invasive)						
PETROVICH et al. (1991)	XRT	AA/Sigma-60	14	0	0	
MATSUI et al. (1991)	XRT/Bleo[d]	RF	38	15	39	e
NOGUCHI et al. (1992)	XRT ± M-VAC	RF	35	8	23	
KAKEHI et al. (1990)	XRT or chemo.	RF	24	4	17	
MASUNAGA et al. (1994)	XRT	RF	24	7	29	f
		Total:	135	34	25	
Nonheat trials (invasive)		Total:	>500		25–35	
Prostate (symptomatic palliation)						
MONTORSI et al. (1992)	None	Rectal MW	46	0		g
SERVADIO and LIEB (1991)	None; XRT	Rectal MW				c, h
STAWARZ et al. (1993)	None	Rectal MW				c, d
SZMIGIELSKI et al. (1988)	None	Rectal MW				c, d
Cervix						
SURWIT et al. (1983)	Brachyther.	RFI[i]	21	8	38	
SHIMM et al. (1990)	Brachyther.	RFI	49[j]		28–69	k
VORA and LUK (1993)	Brachyther.	RFI/ferro[l]	32	19	59	
GRIGSBY and EMAMI (1993)	Brachyther.	RFI	14			
SEEGENSCHMIEDT et al. (1993)	Brachyther.	RFI	7			
Nonheat trials					40–85	
Ovary						
LEOPOLD et al. (1993)	Cisplatin	AA/Sigma-60	15	0	0	
GILLY et al. (1992)	MMC/cisplatin	IP lavage	32	0	0	
HUERTAS et al. (1994)	Cis-/carboplatin	IP lavage	29	NS[m]	NS	

[a] Column specifies principal therapy to which hyperthermia was added
[b] Number of cases
[c] Mitomycin C
[d] Bleomycin
[e] Radiotherapy alone resulted in no CRs
[f] Correlation of intravesical temp. ≥41.5°C with downstaging
[g] Palliation of pain and obstruction
[h] Possible systemic tumor control in a few cases resulting from local prostatic hyperthermia (question of immunotherapeutic benefit)
[i] RF interstitial
[j] Pelvic tumors (not all cervix cancers)
[k] Correlation of thermal dose with response ($P < 0.003$)
[l] Ferromagnetic seeds
[m] Not stated

platin at 41°–42°C without systemic cooling. Complications occurred in 30% and there was one death. Median control of ascites was only 3 months but none of the seven patients treated in complete pathologic response had relapsed, with a median response time of 7 months (range 3–24).

9.6.4 Discussion

Thermochemotherapeutic lavage with cisplatin-containing dialysate in patients with minimal peritoneal disease that has been responsive to IV cisplatin appears to be feasible and worthy of further investigation. The rationale would appear to be strongest in circumstances where tumor nodules would be small enough to be well heated by conduction and affected by drug through surface contact. Such an approach might be useful in the treatment of patients who have undergone a negative second-look operation but are still at substantial risk of eventual abdominal relapse, or as initial treatment in patients with minimal residual Stage III disease or those at significant risk of abdominal dissemination. Since complete peritoneal distribution would be critical, the method would appear to be optimally applied only immediately postoperatively with very high flow rates of dialysate.

Regional heating in the abdomen has had significant technical limitations and would seem inherently incapable of adequately heating the entire peritoneal cavity. Limited clinical trials have not been promising to date.

Local-regional hyperthermia with radiotherapy or chemotherapy might eventually play a role if directed at debulking of surgically unresectable masses so that the masses might be rendered surgically resectable or the patients might be more effectively treated with methods addressing the entire peritoneal surface.

9.7 Summary

- Adequate methods for heating pelvic tumors and documenting the temperatures achieved require further study and development.
- Heating patterns in tumors are generally heterogeneous with temperatures lower than desirable; excessive normal tissue heating can be limiting in the case of regional heating methods.
- There is a palliative effect of hyperthermia alone on prostatism due to prostatic cancer or benign prostatic hypertrophy.
- Improved tumor response from adjunctive hyperthermia for genitourinary and gynecological neoplasms is suggested by some studies.
- Thermochemotherapeutic IP lavage may prove to be beneficial in the treatment of ovarian cancer patients, especially those with chemo-responsive minimal or subclinical IP disease; further study is warranted.
- As with all anatomical sites, the major emphasis belongs on improved methods of hyperthermia induction and Phase II studies designed to optimize the treatment and determine the relationship between time-temperature parameters, tumor response, and complications.
- A tabular summary of major clinical hyperthermia trials in genitourinary and gynecological tumors is given in Table 9.1.

References

Anscher MS, Samulski TV, Leopold KA, Oleson JR (1992) Phase I/II study of external radiofrequency phased array hyperthermia and external beam radiotherapy in the treatment of prostate cancer: technique and results of intraprostatic temperature measurements. Int J Radiat Oncol Biol Phys 24: 489–495

Aristizabal SA, Surwit E, Valencia A, Hevezi J (1983) Treatment of locally advanced cancer of the cervix with transperineal interstitial irradiation. Report on 106 cases. Am J Clin Oncol 6: 645–650

Armour EP, McEachern D, Wang Z, Corry PM, Martinez A (1993) Sensitivity of human cells to mild hyperthermia. Cancer Res 53: 2740–2744

Astrahan MA, Ameye F, Oyen R, Willemen P, Baert L, Petrovich Z (1991) Interstitial temperature measurements during transurethral microwave hyperthermia. J Urol 145: 304–308

Bagshaw MA, Kaplan ID, Cox RC (1993) Prostate cancer. Radiation therapy for localized disease. Cancer 71: 939–952

Batata MA, Whitmore WF, Chu FC, Hilaris BS, Unal A, Chung S (1980) Patterns of recurrence in bladder cancer treated by irradiation and/or cystectomy. Int J Radiat Oncol Biol Phys 6: 155–159

Ben-Yoset R, Kapp DS (1992) Cancer metastatic to the penis: treatment with hyperthermia and radiation therapy and review of the literature. J Urol 148: 67–71

Ben-Yosef R, Sullivan DM, Kapp DS (1992) Peripheral neuropathy and myonecrosis following hyperthermia and radiation therapy for recurrent prostatic cancer: correlation of damage with predicted SAR pattern. Int J Hyperthermia 8: 173–185

Bichler KH, Harzmann R, Fluchter ST, Erdmann W (1984) Results of local transurethral high frequency hyperthermia in bladder carcinoma. In: Overgaard J (ed) Hyperthermic oncology, vol 1. Taylor and Francis, London, pp 775–778

Bichler KH, Flüchter SH, Steimann J, Strohmaier WL (1989) Combination of hyperthermia and cytostatics in the treatment of bladder cancer. Urol Int 44: 10–14

Bloom HJ, Hendry WF, Wallace DM, Skeet RG (1982) Treatment of T3 bladder cancer: controlled trial of preoperative radiotherapy and radical cystectomy versus radical radiotherapy. Second report and review (for the Clinical Trials Group, Institute of Urology). Br J Urol 54: 136–151

Buchanan MT, Hynynen K (1994) Design and experimental evaluation of an intracavitary ultrasound phased array system for hyperthermia. IEEE Trans Biomed Eng 41: 1178–1187

Colombo R, Lev A, Da Pozzo LF, Freschi, M, Gallus G, Rigatti P (1995) A new approach using local combined microwave hyperthermia and chemotherapy in superficial transitional bladder carcinoma treatment. J Urol 153: 959–963

Debicki P, Astrahan MA, Ameye F, Oyen R, Baert L, Haczewski A, Petrovich Z (1992) Temperature steering in prostate by simultaneous transurethral and transrectal hyperthermia. Urology 40: 300–307

Emami B, Stauffer P, Dewhirst MW, et al. (1991) RTOG quality assurance guidelines for interstitial hyperthermia. Int J Radiat Oncol Biol Phys 20: 1117–1124

Emami B, Scott C, Perez C, et al. (1993) Phase III study of interstitial thermoradiotherapy compared with interstitial radiotherapy alone in the treatment of recurrent or persistent human tumors: a prospectively controlled randomized study by the Radiation Therapy Oncology Group (abstract). Int J Radiat Oncol Biol Phys 27(S1): 155

Eppert V, Trembly BS, Richter HJ (1991) Air cooling for an interstitial microwave hyperthermia antenna: theory and experiment. IEEE Trans Biomed Eng 38: 450–460

Fosmire H, Hynynen K, Drach GW, Stea B, Swift P, Cassady JR (1993) Feasibility and toxicity of transrectal ultrasound hyperthermia in the treatment of locally advanced adenocarcinoma of the prostate. Int J Radiat Oncol Biol Phys 26: 253–259

Gibbs FA, Jr-, Buechler, DN, Gibbs PF (1990) Nonhomogeneous pelvic power deposition using an annular array applicator: clinical/phantom studies (meeting abstract). In: Thirty-eighth Annual Meeting of the Radiation Research Society and Tenth Annual Meeting of the North American Hyperthermia Group, Gilly et al. 1992: p 91

Gilly FN, Carry PY, et al. (1992) Treatment of malignant peritoneal effusion in digestive and ovarian oancer. Med Oncol Tumor Pharmacother 9: 177–181

Grigsby PW, Emami B (1993) Interstitial thermoradiotherapy for pelvic tumors: the Washington University experience. In: Seegenschmiedt MH, Sauer R (eds) Interstitial and intracavitary thermoradiotherapy. Springer, Berlin Heidelberg New York, pp 265–270

Hall RR, Heath AB (1981) Radiotherapy and cystectomy for T3 bladder carcinoma. Br J Urol 53: 598–601

Hand JW, Vernon CC, Prior MV (1992) Early experience of a commercial scanned focused ultrasound hyperthermia system. Int J Hyperthermia 8: 587–607

Harari PM, Hynynen KH, Roemer RB, Anhalt DP, Shimm DS, Stea B, Cassady JR (1991) Development of scanned focussed ultrasound hyperthermia: clinical response evaluation. Int J Radiat Oncol Biol Phys 21: 831–840

Huertas E, Chacon RD, Colagiovanni F, Nadal J, Vilanova M, Zylberman M, Orlando M (1994) Pilot study of intraoperative intraperitoneal hyperthermia combined with chemotherapy (IIHC) in ovarian cancer (meeting abstract). Proc Annu Meet Am Soc Clin Oncol 13: A840

Hynynen K (1992) The feasibility of interstitial ultrasound hyperthermia. Med Phys 19: 979–987

Hynynen K, Shimm D, Anhalt D, Stea B, Sykes H, Cassady JR, Roemer RB (1990) Temperature distributions during clinical scanned, focused ultrasound hyperthermia treatments. Int J Hyperthermia 6: 891–908

Inatomi H, Sugita A, Terashima H, Yoshiura T, Kunugita N, Norimura T, Tsuchiya T (1992) Thermal distribution in the agar phantom by a new intracavitary RF applicator for prostate gland. Sangyo lka Daigaku Zasshi 14: 39–45

Kakehi M, Ueda K, Mukojima T, Hiraoka M, Seto O, Akanuma A, Nakatsugawa S (1990) Multiinstitutional clinical studies on hyperthermla combined with radiotherapy or chemotherapy in advanced cancer of deep-seated organs. Int J Hyperthermia 6: 719–740

Kaplan I, Kapp DS, Bagshaw MA (1991) Secondary external-beam radiotherapy and hyperthermia for local recurrence after 125-iodine implantation in adenocarcinoma of the prostate. Int J Radiat Oncol Biol Phys 20: 551–554

Kubota, Y (1984) Hyperthermic therapy of the urinary bladder cancer: combination therapy with hyperthermia, radiation and bleomycin. In: Overgaard J (ed) Hyperthermic oncology, vol 1. Taylor and Francis. London, pp 779–782

Kubota Y, Shuin T, Miura T, Nishimura R, Fukushima S, Takai S (1984a) Treatment of bladder cancer with a combination of hyperthermia, radiation and bleomycin. Cancer 53: 199–202

Kubota Y, Takebayashi S, Oshima H (1984b) Application of shortwave radiofrequency (RF) on urogenital malignancies. In: Overgaard J (ed) Hyperthermic oncology, vol 1. Taylor and Francis, London, pp 771–774

Leopold KA, Oleson JR, et al. (1993) Intraperitoneal cisplatin and regional hyperthermia for ovarian carcinoma. Int J Radiat Oncol Biol Phys 27: 1245–1251

Marinelli D, Shanberg AM, Tansey LA, Sawyer DE, Syed N, Puthawala A (1992) Follow-up prostate biopsy in patients with carcinoma of the prostate treated by 192-iridium template irradiation plus supplemental external beam radiation. J Urol 147: 922–925

Masunaga SI, Hiraoka M, Akuta K, et al. (1994) Phase I/II trial of preoperative thermoradiotherapy in the treatment of urinary bladder cancer. Int J Hyperthermia 10: 31–40

Matsui K, Takebayashi S, Watai K, Kakehi M, Kubota Y, Yao M, Shuin T (1991) Combination radiotherapy of urinary bladder carcinoma with chemohyperthermia. Int J Hyperthermia 7: 19–26

Miller LS (1977) Bladder cancer. Superiority of preoperative irradiation and cystectomy in clinical stages B2 and C. Cancer 39: 973–980

Montorsi F, Guazzoni G, Colombo R, Galli L, Bergamaschi F, Rigatti P (1992) Transrectal microwave hyperthermia for advanced prostate cancer: long-term clinical results. J Urol 148: 342–345

Noguchi S, Kubota Y, Miura T, Shuin T, Hosaka M (1992) Use of methotrexate, vinblastine, adriamycin, and cisplatin in combination with radiation and hyperthermia as neo-adjuvant therapy for bladder cancer. Cancer Chemother Pharmacol 30(Suppl): 63–5

Perez CA, Pajak T, Emami B, Hornback NB, Tupchong L, Rubin P (1991) Randomized phase III study comparing irradiation and hyperthermia with irradiation alone in superficial measurable tumors. Final report by the Radiation Therapy Oncology Group. Am J Clin Oncol 14: 133–141

Petrovich Z, Emami B, Kapp D, et al. (1991) Regional hyperthermia in patients with recurrent genitourinary cancer. Am J Clin Oncol 14: 472–477

Prionas SD, Kapp DS, Goffinet DR, Ben-Yosef R, Fessenden P, Bagshaw MA (1994) Thermometry of interstitial hyperthermia given as an adjuvant to brachytherapy for the treatment of carcinoma of the prostate. Int J Radiat Oncol Biol Phys 28: 151–162

Prior MV (1991) A comparative study of RF-LCF and hot-source interstitial hyperthermia techniques. Int J Hyperthermia 7: 131–140

Puthawala AA, Syed AM, Fleming PA, Disaia PJ (1982) Re-irradiation with interstitial implant for recurrent pelvic malignancies. Cancer 50: 2810–2814

Rigatti P, Lev A, Colombo R (1991) Combined intravesical chemotherapy with mitomycin C and local bladder microwave-induced hyperthermia as a preoperative therapy for superficial bladder tumors. A preliminary clinical study. Eur Urol 20: 204–10

Sapozink MD, Gibbs P, Gibbs FA Jr, Jolles C (1988) Myonecrosis following deep pelvic hyperthermia. Int J Hyperthermia 4: 251–258

Sapozink MD, Joszef G, Astrahan MA, Gibbs Fa, Jr., Petrovich Z, Stewart JR (1990) Adjuvant pelvic hyperthermia in advanced cervical carcinoma. I. Feasibility, thermometry and device comparison. Int J Hyperthermia 6: 985–996

Seegenschmiedt MH, Sauer R, Miyamoto C, Brady LW (1993a) Interstitial thermoradiotherapy for pelvic tumors: a cooperative Phase I–II study. In: Seegenschmiedt MH, Sauer R (eds) Interstitial and intracavitary thermoradiotherapy. Springer, Berlln Heidelberg New York, pp 271–288

Seegenschmiedt MH, Sauer R, Miyamoto C, Chalal JA, Brady LW (1993b) Clinical experience with interstitial thermoradiotherapy for localized implantable pelvic tumors. Am J Clin Oncol 16: 210–222

Servadio C, Leib Z (1991) Local hyperthermia for prostate cancer. Urology 38: 307–309

Shimm DS, Klttelson JM, Oleson JR, Aristizabal SA, Barlow LC, Cetas TC (1990) Interstitial thermoradiotherapy: thermal dosimetry and clinicla results. Int J Radiat Oncol Biol Phys 18: 383–387

Sorbe B, Roos D, Smed-Sörensen C, Frankendahl B (1993) Intracavitary thermoradiotherapy for vaginal carcinoma. In: Seegenschmiedt MH, Sauer R (eds) Interstitial and intracavitary thermoradiotherapy. Springer, Berlin Heidelberg New York, pp 305–310

Stawarz B, Zielinski H, Szmigielski S, Rappaport E, Debicki, P Petrovich Z (1993) Transrectal hyperthermia as palliative treatment for advanced adenocarcinoma of prostate and studies of cell-mediated immunity. Urology 41: 548–553

Stromberg J, Martinez A, Benson R, et al. (1993) Improved local control and survival for surgically staged patients with locally advanced prostate cancer treated with up-front low dose rate iridium-192 prostate implantation and external beam irradiation. Int J Radiat Oncol Biol Phys 28: 67–75

Strotsky AV, Fradkin SZ, Zhavrid EA, Karpovich UA (1991) Combined therapy of bladder cancer with the use of hyperthermia (meeting abstract). Strahlenther Onkol 167

Surwit EA, Manning MR, Aristizabal SA, Oleson JR, Cetas TC (1983) Interstitial thermoradiotherapy in recurrent gynecologic malignancies. Gynecol Oncol 15: 95–102

Szmigielski S, Zielinski H, Stawarz B, et al. (1988) Local microwave hyperthermia in treatment of advanced prostatic adenocarcinoma. Urol Res 16: 1–7

Szmigielski S, Sobczynski J, Sokolska G, Stawarz B, Zielinski H, Petrovich Z (1991) Effects of local prostatic hyperthermia on human NK and T cell function. Int J Hyperthermia 7: 869–880

Uchibayashi T, Nakajima K, Hisazumi H, Mihara S, Yamamoto H, Koshida K (1992) Studies of temperature rise in bladder cancer and surrounding tissues during radiofrequency hyperthermia. Eur Urol 21: 298–303

Valdagni R, Amichetti M, Cristoforetti L (1988) Intracavitary hyperthermia: construction and heat patterns of individualized vaginal prototype applicators. Int J Hyperthermia 4: 457–466

Valdagni R, Montanaro P, Italia C, Bosisio G (1991) Radical radiation (XRT) combined with endocavitary hyperthermia (HT) for prostate cancer: preliminary report of a Phase I–II study (meeting abstract). Strahlenther Onkol 167: 348–349

Van der Werf-Messing B (1979) Preoperative irradiation followed by cystectomy to treat carcinorma of the urinary bladder category T3NX, 0-4M0. Int J Radiat Oncol Biol Phys 5: 395–401

Vora NL, Luk KH (1993) Interstitial thermoradiotherapy for pelvic tumors: the City of Hope experience. In: Seegenschmiedt MH, Sauer R (eds) Interstitial and intracavitary thermoradiotherapy. Springer, Berlin Heidelberg New York, pp 257–264

YeH MM, Trembly BS, Douple EB, Ryan TP, Hoopes PJ, Jonsson E, Heaney JA (1994) Theoretical and experimental analysis of air cooling for intracavitary microwave hyperthermia applicators. IEEE Trans Biomed Eng 41: 874–882

Yerushalmi A (1988) Localized, non-invasive deep microwave hyperthermia for the treatment of prostatic tumros: the first 5 years. Recent Results Cancer Res 107: 141–146

Zimmermann M, Schorcht J, Andree W (1993) Theoretical and experimental investigations of a newly developed intracavitary applicator system for the radiothermotherapy of gynaecological tumours. Int J Hyperthermia 9: 463–477

10 Thermoradiotherapy of Uterine Carcinoma

J. Schorcht, M.H. Seegenschmiedt, and M. Zimmermann

CONTENTS

10.1 Introduction

In 1993, about 48 000 new cases of invasive uterine carcinoma were observed, comprising 14 000 cases of cervical and 34 000 of endometrial cancer. The mortality is disproportionate to the incidence, with an estimated 6000 deaths from cervical and 4000 from endometrial cancer. Overall, the incidence and mortality have steadily decreased over the years due to early detection and screening programs including Pap tests and physical examinations (American Cancer Society 1993).

The overall 5-year survival rate for the cervical cancer population is 67%; for patients diagnosed early it reaches 88%, but it is only about 50% for advanced tumor stages with regional spread of disease. The Annual Report (Kottmeier 1988) reported a 5-year survival rate of 58% among patients with stage II and III cervical carcinomas. For endometrial cancer the overall 5-year survival rate (85%) is better, but the rate for early stage disease (92%) is almost the same. Overall, during recent decades there has been a moderate improvement in the survival rates for both tumor entities.

Usually precancerous (in situ) lesions and early tumor stages are treated by local cryotherapy, electrocoagulation, or surgery, while precancerous endometrial lesions may receive progesterone. Advanced uterine cancers often require aggressive surgery including hysterectomy, salpingectomy, ovariectomy, and pelvic lymph node dissection. Especially at advanced tumor stages at higher risk for local relapse, adjunctive external beam and/or interstitial radiotherapy or both are applied. However, no "gold standard" has yet been developed for this situation (Aristizabal 1985; Martinez et al. 1985; Brenner et al. 1991; Gaddis 1983).

Unfortunately, a relatively large proportion of uterine cancers (about 30% of cervical and 20% of endometrial cancers) are inoperable at first diagnosis because of overt regional or metastatic spread. Moreover, even in early tumor stages, a considerable proportion of patients may develop local recurrences within the small pelvis, which are usually difficult to manage. These advanced and recurrent cervical or endometrial cancers constitute a group which has a poor prognosis.

In the Washington University series (Perez 1980) involving 203 patients with stage III cervical carcinoma there was a 25% incidence of central

Johannes Schorcht, MD, Klinik und Poliklinik für Strahlentherapie, Universitätsklinikum Carl Gustav Carus der TU Dresden, Fetscherstraße 74, D-01307 Dresden, FRG

M. Heinrich Seegenschmiedt, MD, Department of Radiation Oncology, University of Erlangen-Nürnberg, Universitätsstraße 27, D-91054 Erlangen, FRG

Michael Zimmermann, PhD, Isotopen-Technik, Dr. Sauerwein GmbH, Bergische Straße 16, D-42781 Han, FRG

relapses without concurrent distant metastases. This implies that insufficient brachytherapy and/ or teletherapy may have contributed to the development of local failures. Thus, inadequate results of surgery, radiotherapy, or combined treatment of advanced, inoperable, or recurrent uterine cancer make it essential to reconsider the "standard treatment concepts," analyze possible failures, and evaluate other adjuvant modalities.

10.2 Historical Remarks

Cautery was well developed and widely applied in the nineteenth century. Various cautery techniques and electrical heating elements became available at the beginning of the twentieth century, and nowadays cautery is still a useful tool in surgery. In 1830, the French gynecologist and surgeon Recamier implemented *galvanocautery* in the treatment of uterine cancer. Over a period of some decades this technique came to be adopted in many other countries of Europe and North America (MEYER 1984a).

The first use of a localized, temperature-controlled heat applicator without cautery was reported by the Swedish gynecologist WESTERMARK in 1898. For ulcerated inoperable cancers of the cervix, a spiral hollow metal tube was positioned in the vagina against the tumor and perfused with hot water. However, at that time heat was considered not to be of value for cancer therapy, but rather to be a useful method of treating infections after cauterization. In 1919, THEILHABER started to treat uterine and vaginal cancers with high-frequency electrical currents, but even at that time the observed antitumor effect was thought to be the effect of, and to provide evidence for, stimulation of the host's immune system. In 1912, MÜLLER was one of the first to report on the effects of combined irradiation and heat by means of *diathermy*. In his study, more than 100 tumors were successfully treated; however, only a few of them were located in the uterus. More details on historical aspects of hyperthermia have been published by MEYER (1984a) and in the first volume of this book (vol. 1, Chap 1: SEEGENSCHMIEDT and VERNON).

10.3 Rationale for Hyperthermia Treatment

10.3.1 Biological Rationale

Radioresistance is probably one of the main obstacles to the effective application of radiotherapy. It is often encountered with bulky solid tumors like advanced uterine carcinomas. Some of the major reasons for radioresistance are: (a) large tumors contain many *clonogenic tumor stem cells*; (b) bulky tumors are poorly vascularized and contain *hypoxic tumor regions*; (c) some tumors have an *inherent radioresistance* which is associated with their high differentiation grade, low mitotic index, or cell division rate; (d) *insufficient radiation dose distribution* may be achieved within the target volume, usually due to the dose-limiting conditions of the surrounding normal tissue. On the basis of cytotoxic and radiosensitizing effects, heat has a great potential to overcome these adverse tumor-related conditions (OVERGAARD 1989; SEEGENSCHMIEDT AND SAUER 1992).

10.3.2 Clinical Rationale

Heat can be applied as a *palliative* or *adjuvant modality* in combination with radiotherapy; interstitial/endocavitary or percutaneous regional heating techniques may be utilized, but the role of heat in the management of uterine carcinoma is closely related to the general role of external radiotherapy or brachytherapy in this tumor site. The use of heat also depends on availability, interdisciplinary cooperation, and the importance of brachytherapy within the treatment regimen. At least in stage IIB/III uterine carcinoma, brachytherapy is essential for curative radiotherapy, either to fill the radiation gap in the central shielded part or as a boost within the externally irradiated pelvis. When using radiotherapy with high-(HDR) or low-dose-rate (LDR) afterloading techniques, 5-year survival rates of 54%–84% in stage II and 36%–74% in stage III cancers have been reported (HERRMANN et al. 1993). SHARMA et al. (1991a,b) observed central relapses in 17% of cases. Similarly, as already mentioned, in their series of 203 stage III patients, PEREZ (1980) found central relapses without concurrent distant metastases in 25% of cases. This indicates that insufficient radiotherapy may have contributed to the limited life expectancy.

Recently, TOUBOL et al. (1992) emphasized the importance of tumor size (besides nodal involvement) for treatment outcome. In a multivariate analysis, LOWREY et al. (1992) confirmed that tumor size, but not stage, was the best prognostic parameter for tumor control. The prevalent cause of failure after radiation therapy of progressing uterine cancer has been assumed to be the large tumor burden and the amount of radioresistant hypoxic cells (DISCHE et al. 1983; VAUPEL 1990). As early as 1965, Kolstadt found that patients with an intercapillary distance of tumor vessels of >350 μm had a higher local failure rate than others with a smaller intercapillary distance. Changes in tumor perfusion during radiotherapy were detected in 12 patients with cervical carcinoma by means of T2-weighted MR imaging (HIETSCHOLD et al. 1993). The biological and clinical rationale for combined heat and radiotherapy is outlined in Table 10.1.

10.3.3 Treatment Objectives

The major objective of thermoradiotherapy is the achievement of therapeutic gain by the addition of hyperthermia to radiotherapy. This can be quantified by comparison of the effectiveness of radiotherapy with or without hyperthermia in respect of specific treatment endpoints such as local tumor control (in case of a palliative and adjuvant treatment) or tumor operability (in case of a neoadjuvant treatment) but also treatment toxicity (thermal- versus radiation-related acute and late treatment sequelae) in a randomized protocol.

Patients with inoperable tumors in the pelvis, in whom there is a relatively small chance that standard treatments will achieve local control, are very eligible for clinical studies. Patients may be included in such studies when: (a) a malignant tumor with measurable dimensions is present; (b) adequate radiotherapy is planned as part of the standard treatment, (c) patient performance status is adequate (Karnofsky score ≥70; life expectancy >3 months), (d) placement of invasive probes for thermometry control is possible; (e) the patient gives informed consent; (f) patient compliance allowing long-term follow-up assured. Specific exclusion criteria are related to the applied heating technique and may include metal implants in the treated region and pacemakers; additional severe internal disorders (cardiac, pulmonary, hepatic, or renal dysfunction) should not be present.

Table 10.1. Rationale for combined heat treatment and radiotherapy in cervical carcinoma

Biological and clinical findings	Study
Large numbers of radioresistant hypoxic cells are present and persist in rapidly progressing malignancies	DISCHE et al. (1983), VAUPEL (1900)
Tumors with a large intercapillary distance (>350 μm) have a high incidence of local failure	KOLSTADT (1965), AWWAD et al. (1986)
Low vascular density of tumor stroma correlates with a short survival	SIRACKY et al. (1988)
Low intratumoral pO_2 < 10 mmHg is associated with poor prognosis (low tumor control probability)	HÖCKEL et al. (1993)
Tumor perfusion does not improve during the radiation therapy course	SCHORCHT (1994)
Tumor volume is a decisive prognostic factor for the outcome of patients with cervical cancer	TOUBOUL et al. (1992), LOWREY et al. (1992), PEREZ et al. (1992)
A considerable percentage of local failures (17%–25%) occur only in the central portion of the pelvis)	SHARMA et al. (1991b), PEREZ (1980)

10.4 Hyperthermia Techniques

Many heating methods have been developed and clinically utilized for tumors of the uterus. They fall into two categories: (a) *endocavitary/interstitial heating* for local therapy in combination with brachytherapy; (b) *percutaneous regional heating* for regional therapy in combination with external beam radiotherapy to the pelvis. The clinical results which have been achieved when utilizing these techniques have been quite different, as different patient populations with different tumor types and tumor volumes have been selected for these therapies, which have also been quite differently prescribed and clinically applied (single versus fractionated application in combination with either brachytherapy or fractionated radiotherapy).

10.4.1 Endocavitary and Interstitial Techniques

Table 10.2 lists the presently applied endocavitary and interstitial heating techniques. In accordance with their limited range of energy deposition within tissue they are commonly combined not only with afterloading radiation techniques such as HDR or LDR iridium-192 brachytherapy, but also with external beam radiotherapy to match the appropriate tumor or target volume. Thus, the induced heating effect is confined to the tumor-bearing region; it may not fully cover peripheral extension of bulky primary or recurrent tumors of the uterus.

The presently available endocavitary/interstitial techniques can be divided into two categories: (a) *electromagnetic techniques* including resistive and capacitive radiofrequency, radiative microwave, and inductive ferromagnetic implant heating methods; (b) *ultrasound techniques* involving the use of tubular radiators or acoustic antennas. The latter heating technique holds great promise, as it has been shown to produce not only a very large radial but also an almost unlimited longitudinal power deposition pattern (DIEDERICH and HYNYNEN 1993). Further technical developments for endocavitary heating are in progress, including the implementation of thermal modelling (LAGENDIJK et al. 1993).

Table 10.2. Techniques for endocavitary and interstitial hyperthermia

Treatment technique	Study
Ultrasound techniques	
Tubular radiators/ acoustic antennas	DIEDERICH and HYNYNEN (1993)
Electromagnetic techniques	
Radiofrequency techniques (0.5–27 MHz)	
Capacitive radiofrequency technique (8 or 27 MHz)	AKUTA et al. (1989); MARCHAL et al. (1989); DEURLOO et al. (1989); SCHORCHT et al. (1989
Resistive local current field technique (0.5–1.0 MHz)	EMAMI et al. (1987); GAUTHERIE et al. (1989); VORA and LUK
Microwave technique (300–2450 MHz) 9.15-MHz dipole antema systems	COUGHLIN et al. (1991); HAND et al. (1982); LI et al. (1991); PARISI et al. (1990); PETROVICH et al. (1989); PUTHAWALA et al. (1985); ROOS (1993); SEEGENSCHMIEDT et al. (1993)
Ferromagnetic implant techniques	VORA and LUK (1993); STEA et al. (1993)

10.4.2 Clinical Results of Endocavitary and Interstitial Techniques

Unfortunately the clinical results reported over the past 10 years have mostly been derived from relatively small intra-institutional phase I–II pilot studies designed for testing newly developed hyperthermia applicators or other hyperthermia system components. In these early studies, treatment toxicity and feasibility have been the primary study goals.

When reviewing clinical hyperthermia studies, MARTINEZ et al. (1993) summarized the conclusions as follows: When used as a single agent, locoregional hyperthermia is of limited short-term palliative benefit, but when combined with suboptimal radiotherapy, hyperthermia may double the complete response rate from about 25% to 50% and increase the duration of tumor response and long-term control. Interestingly, the improvement appears to be independent of the specific tumor cell type. Further improvements may be possible with better heating techniques and optimized treatment schedules. Nevertheless, it remains unclear whether or not heat improves local control and cure rates when used in conjunction with definitive radiation therapy. So far it has not been shown that locoregional hyperthermia increases acute and chronic toxicity when combined with irradiation or chemotherapy.

Generally, heating as a single agent has no impact on tumor response and should only be applied, if at all, as a last attempt to palliate tumor-related symptoms when no other alternatives are available. However, if heat is combined with radiotherapy, both modalities should be applied at their best level and with an optimized treatment schedule. Therefore the treatment prescription has to define not only the radiation dose but also all "thermal dose" parameters, including the total number of heating sessions, the overall treatment time per session, the thermal level to be considered therapeutic, and the sequence of radiation and hyperthermia application. To optimize thermoradiotherapy, possible prognostic parameters have to be determined such as thermal variables or factors indicating the quality of heating (e.g., minimum and maximum average temperatures or treatment time exceeding an average temperature of 41°C); in addition, the impact of tumor volume and stage has to be taken into account, along with the applied external beam or brachytherapy dose, either retrospectively as a confounding factor in the data analysis or prospectively as a stratification criterion.

Table 10.3 shows the clinical results achieved when utilizing endocavitary and interstitial thermoradiotherapy. In most of the cited trials, uterine carcinoma was just one of many treated tumor entities. Consequently it is rare for all the relevant details on treatment performance and site-specific outcome to have been reported. For some studies the table therefore contains only figures relating to whole series, and this makes it difficult to draw further conclusions. The mentioned prognostic tumor and treatment parameters, including the thermal parameters, were rarely exactly registered and properly analyzed for their possible impact on treatment outcome. In conclusion, further technical improvements and controlled multicenter trials are essential to establish the final role of localized hyperthermia in the palliative and adjuvant therapy of uterine carcinomas.

10.4.3 Percutaneous Regional Techniques

In contrast to localized endocavitary/interstitial heating, which produces a relatively small but

Table 10.3. Clinical results of endocavitary and intersitial thermoradiotherapy

Study	No. of Pts.	Treatment prescription and treatment schedule	CR n (%)	PR *n* (%)	Toxicity *n* (%)	Special remarks
ARISTIZABAL and OLESON (1984)	36 (I)	1 × 42°C, 30 min; 30 Gy LDR IRT	14 (39)	NA	NA (13)	Grade 3 toxicity
COUGHLIN et al. (1991)	12 (I)	1–2 × 42.5°–43°C, 60 min; 20–60 LDR IRT	8 (67)	4 (33)	NA	–
GAUTHERIE et al. (1989)	23 (I)	1–2 × 42°–43.5°C, 45–60 mn; 15–60 Gy LDR IRT	11 (48)	NR	NR (16)	Deep necrosis, fistulas
GRIGSBY and EMAMI (1993)	8 (I)	2 × 42.5°–43°C, 60 min; 30–50 Gy LDR IRT	5 (63)	NR	3 (38)	3 fistulas
HANDL-ZELLER (1993)	7 (I)	1–2 × 43°–45°C, 45–60 min; various LDR/HDR IRT	NR (60)	NR	NR (3)	Grade 1–3 toxicity
MARTINEZ et al. (1993)	25 (I)	1 × 41°–43°C, 2–4 h; 15–40 Gy LDR IRT	11 (44)	9 (36)	NA; "well tolerated"	Tumor type: 80% relapses
PARISI et al. (1993)	3 (E)	1–3 × 41°–45°C, 45–60 min; 40–45 Gy ERT + 3 × 7 Gy HDR IRT	2 (67)	1 (33)	NR	–
PETROVICH et al. (1989)	4 (I)	1–2 × 42.5°C, 45–60 min; 25–50 Gy LDR IRT	3 (75)	1 (25)	1 (25)	Ulcer
PUTHAWALA et al. (1985)	9 (I)	2 × 41.5°–43°C, 45–60 min; 2 × 20–25 Gy LDR IRT	7 (78)	2 (22)	3 (33)	Fistula formation
SEEGENSCHMIEDT et al. (1993, 1994)	15 (I)	1–2 × 41°–44°C, 45–60 min; 20–40 Gy LDR IRT	9 (60)	4 (13)	4 (27)	Deep ulceration; fistulas
SHARMA et al. (1989, 1990)	25 (E)	3/wk × 42°–43°C, 30 min; 45 Gy ERT + 35 Gy IRT	14 (56)	NR	7 (28)	Radiation cystitis and proctitis
STEA et al. (1993)	11 (I)	1–2 × 42°C, 60 min; 10–75 Gy ERT plus 10–50 Gy LDR IRT	7 (64)	NA	NA (7)	Grade 3 toxicity
SURWIT et al. (1983), SHIMM et al. (1990)	21 (I)	1 × 42°C, 30–60 min; 20–50 Gy LDR IRT	8 (38)	9 (43)	4 (19)	4 fistulas
VORA and LUK (1993)	32 (I)	1–2 × 43°C, 60 min; 45–50 Gy ERT plus 30–45 Gy LDR IRT	15 (47)	NA	3 (11)	3 fistulas

I, interstitial heating technique; E, endocavitary heating techinque; CR, complete remission; PR, partial remission; ERT, external beam radiotherapy; IRT, interstitial radiotherapy; HDR, high-dose-rate afterloading therapy; LDR, low-dose-rate afterloading therapy

well-circumscribed power deposition pattern in the tissue, percutaneous heating techniques are much less collimated and are rarely able to precisely focus the energy deposition to a confined target volume. Instead, in most clinical situations a large body region containing the tumor volume has to be heated to induce more or less effective tumor heating. This approach and the utilized heating systems are sometimes optimistically described as "regional heating" (Table 10.4). With regard to advanced or recurrent uterine carcinomas, these heating devices may be able to overcome some shortcomings of endocavitary and interstitial heating techniques, as they are theoretically able to encompass not only the primary tumor site but also the regional lymph nodes or parametrial tissues.

The available heating methods fall into two groups: (a) *electromagnetic techniques* including the annular phased array systems (BSD 1000 and BSD 2000, BSD Medical Corporation, Salt Lake City) and the capacitive 8-MHz radiofrequency system (Thermotron RF-8, Yamamoto Vinyter, Osaka), and (b) *deep ultrasound techniques* including single-source and multiple focused array systems. In Western European countries and North America the annular phased array systems BSD 1000 and BSD 2000 have been preferred, while the capacitive systems have mostly been applied in Japan, where people tend to be less obese and better suited for the capacitive heating technique, which is characterized by relatively high power deposition within the subcutaneous tissues beneath the opposing electrodes. In contrast, the annular phased array system consists of several large dipole microwave applicators (50–110 MHz) which are positioned cylindrically or elliptically around the body region. While this technique is well suited to the treatment of tumors in the pelvis and the extremities, it is less frequently used for thoracic and upper abdominal lesions. New developments promise dynamic, electronic, and three-dimensional power steering within the heating zone by the use of pretreatment planning and thermal modelling (TURNER 1993). By combining and focusing several single-source ultrasound applicators, a focused multiapplicator ultrasound heating system can be composed which has many interesting possibilities for clinical implementations (MEYER 1984b).

Table 10.4. Percutaneous regional heating techniques

Treatment technique	Study
Electromagnetic techniques	
Annular phased array systems	
BSD 1000 (50–110 MHz)	SAPOZINK et al. (1990)
BSD 2000 (Sigma 60) (60–110 MHz)	FELDMANN and SACK (1992), NOTTER and SCHWEGLER (1992), TURNER (1993), VAN DER ZEE et al. (1991,1993), WUST et al. (1992)
Capacitive radiofrequency system	
Thermotron RF-8 (8 MHz)	NAGATA et al. (1993)
Dep ultrasound techniques	
Single-source system	MEYER (1984b)
Focused array system	VERNON (1992)

10.4.4 Clinical Results of Percutaneous Regional Techniques

Table 10.5 summarizes the results of clinical series in which percutaneous regional hyperthermia has been applied. Again, most of the studies lack reporting details with regard to the specific radiation and heating parameters and the treatment outcome. OVERGAARD and HORSMANN (1992) compiled the results of randomized studies performed to test the value of combined thermoradiotherapy versus radiotherapy alone for the treatment of cervical carcinoma. The clinical data are quite impressive and the calculated TER values have exceeded 2 (Fig. 10.1).

10.4.5 Treatment Complications

In many reports side-effects are not mentioned at all or only some general comments or percentage ranks are provided. However, it would not be good practice to assume that no problems were encountered during the treatment. In their clinical series of 26 pelvic tumors treated with combined interstitial thermoradiotherapy, SEEGENSCHMIEDT et al. (1993) found more complications when maximum temperatures exceeded 44°–45°C. Thus, in accordance with the literature, it was recommended that only a "narrow thermal treatment window" of at least 41°C minimum tumor temperature but less than 45°C maximum temperature should be allowed in clinical practice. In several studies, severe complications such as fistulas were observed (Table 10.3), but it was

Table 10.5. Clinical results of percutaneous regional thermoradiotherapy

Study	No. of pts.	Treatment prescription	CR	PR	Toxicity	Special remarks
FELDMANN et al. (1993)	6	1–2 × HT/wk: 42.5°C, 60 min; range: 41.8°–39.9°C observed	NA	NA	Pain	CR + PR: 31% recurrent tumors
LÖFFEL et al. (1993)	14	1–2 × HT/wk: 42°C, 60 min	14%	3		Locally advanced
NAGANO et al. (1993)	10	1–2 × HT/wk: >40°C, 40–60 min; 50–62 Gy + Al IRT: 20–24 Gy	NA	NA		Stage III–IV disease
NAGA et al. (1993)	6	4–10 × HT total; 42°C, 60 min; 20–50 Gy	NA	NA		CR + PR: 39%
SAPOZINK et al. (1990)		1–2 × HT/wk: 42°C, 60 min; range: 40.2°–41°C observed; 50 Gy ERT	NA	NA	39%–63% pain	
SHIGA et al. (1993)	6	1–2 × HT/wk: 42°C, 45–60 min	NA	NA		CR + PR: 40%
VAN DER ZEE et al. (1991, 1993)	52	5 × HT total; 42°C, 60 min	78%	NA	Catheter related	Stage IIB, IIIB, IV; HT well tolerated

HT, hyperthermia; ERT, external beam radiotherapy; IRT, interstitial radiotherapy; AL, afterloading; CR, complete remission; PR, partial remission

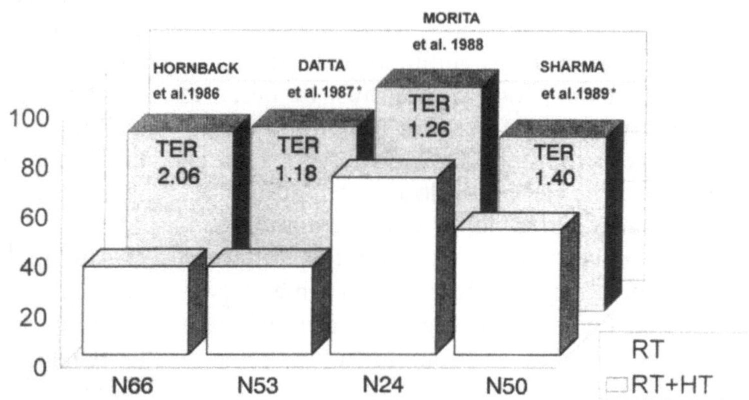

Fig. 10.1. TER values obtained in studies comparing thermoradiotherapy with radiotherapy alone. *, randomized study; *N*, no. of patients

also pointed out that the rate of complications was acceptable considering the advanced stage of disease and the pretreatment conditions. Generally, acute thermal reactions like sensations of local heating or pain and second-degree burns are frequently observed and may occasionally limit the individual treatment session as well as the total treatment course.

In conclusion, the results of combined regional heating and radiotherapy appear disappointing, but this is probably due to technical insufficiencies and inadequate tumor selection. Again, it is emphasized that controlled multicenter trials are essential to establish the role of combined thermoradiotherapy in the palliative and adjuvant management of uterine carcinomas (OVERGAARD 1989).

10.5 The Dresden 27-MHz Endocavitary Heating Technique

10.5.1 The Applicator System

At the University Hospital, Dresden a 27-MHz radiofrequency heating method has been developed and clinically applied for cervical carcinoma (SCHORCHT et al. 1989). The intracavitary thermoradiotherapy applicator has been devised to combine both HDR-IRT afterloading brachytherapy and endocavitary hyperthermia. The applicator combines various technical features and facilitates clinical application:

1. The applicator consists of components which allow delivery of hyperthermia and radiation without any intervening component replacement.
2. The system can be quickly set up and does not require long intervals for switching between the treatment modalities.
3. From radiobiological experiments it has been suggested that a short interval between the two treatments is more advantageous.
4. The applicator offers the option of individually shaping the radiation isodose and thermal isotherm contours to the desired target volume, which usually should encompass the whole tumor region.
5. The warm-up of the target region can be achieved in two different ways: either by means of a hot-water circuit or by energy absorption from the electromagnetic 27-MHz radiofrequency applicators.

When HDR-IRT is combined with endocavitary hyperthermia, special care must be taken to avoid superposition of possible radiation or thermal damage in nontarget regions. As the radial symmetry of the radiation dose distribution does not necessarily correspond with the tumor configuration, it is important to adapt the thermal distribution to the specific tumor volume. Histopathological findings may suggest additional areas at risk to be included, and complex tumor volumes should be taken into consideration.

At the University Hospital Dresden a thermoradiotherapy system was designed which consisted of three components: a rectum applicator, an applicator for the uterus, an applicator for the bladder. The uterine applicator was constructed such that selective cervical and endometrical heating or both together with endocavitary radiotherapy is feasible. moreover, the thermal performance of each of the three applicators can be affected by internal countercurrent water circuits which are individually controlled by thermostats. Thus, additional heating and cooling can be provided to the tumor region, which allows individual shapping of the thermal distribution. A scheme of the heating system and the treatment setup is illustrated in Fig. 10.2.

Figure 10.3b shows the details of the intrauterine applicator. It combines the capacitive 27-MHz radiofrequency-induced hyperthermia applicator and the radiotherapy afterloading device. For this reason it was called the "RF gamma applicator." It consists of three parts: (a) the *electrode heating system* with electrodes I and II and their coupling elements 1 and 2, isolation and dielectrical components, and the ground contact; (b) the *cooling system*, which contains a thermally controlled coolant for countercurrent flow, special seals, and a perforated spacing cap (the direction of the coolant flow is symbolized by arrows); (c) the *radiation system* with special connectors to afterloading tubes, insulation sheat, guide sleeve, and the inner component of the rod-shaped electrode I.

The radiation isodose contour is adapted to the specific anatomical and histopathological tumor situation. The radiation is delivered as usual by a numerically controlled oscillation of a gamma source which is positioned inside the rod-shaped electrode I. The interaction between this applicator and a given surrounding tumor situation is affected by the shape and physical material properties of some elements of this applicator. The induction of different RF energy deposition patterns along the electrodes is possible and is controlled by the electrical coupling elements 1 and 2. They provide the electrical contact to the HF voltage which is applied at the guide sleeve (Fig. 10.3b).

The interactions between he applicator system and the surrounding tissue were investigated by applying theoretical finite-element modelling (ZIMMERMANN et al. 1993). Complex two-dimensional calculations of the specific absorption rate (SAR) and three-dimensional thermal distribution calculations were performed and analyzed. Thermographic experiments were also performed. It was shown in these experiments that the theoretical models proved to be correct. Figure 10.3 demonstrates the theoretical three-dimensional thermal distribution and the SAR function in a tissue model.

10.5.2 Animal Experiments

Experiments in adult miniature pigs were described by SULLIVAN et al. (1980). As the pelvic anatomy of these animals is similar to the human pelvis, it seemed appropriate for the assessment of thermal effects and possible damage in the locally heated pelvis (PROBERT et al. 1977). Simi-

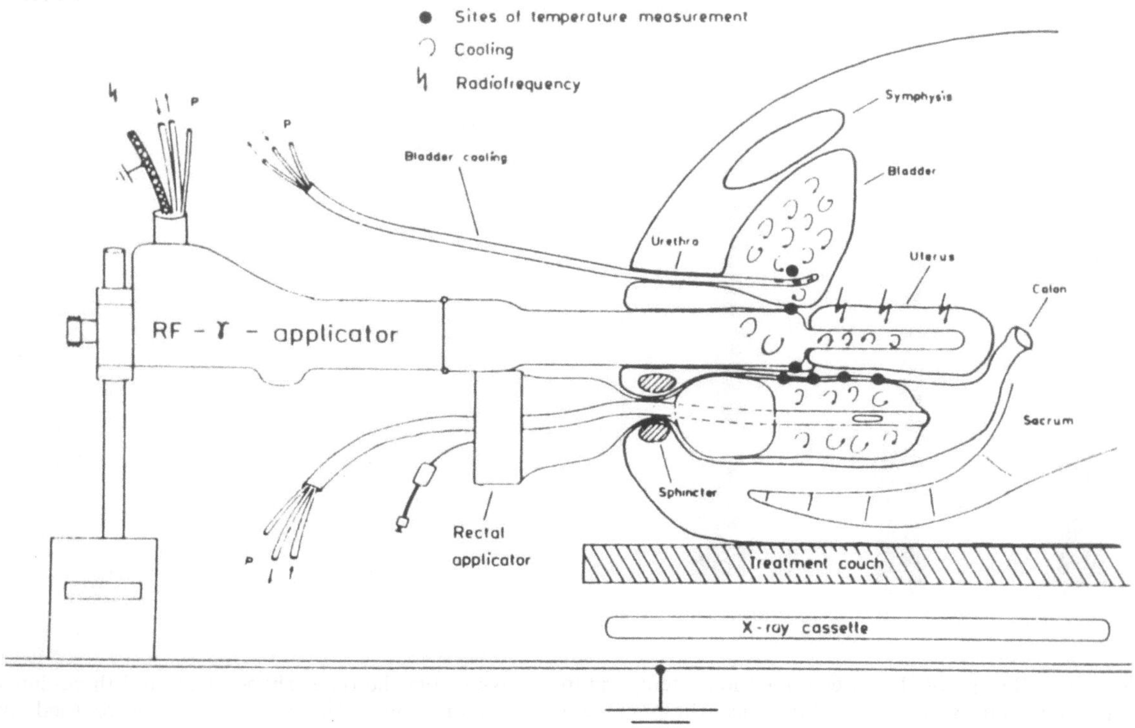

a

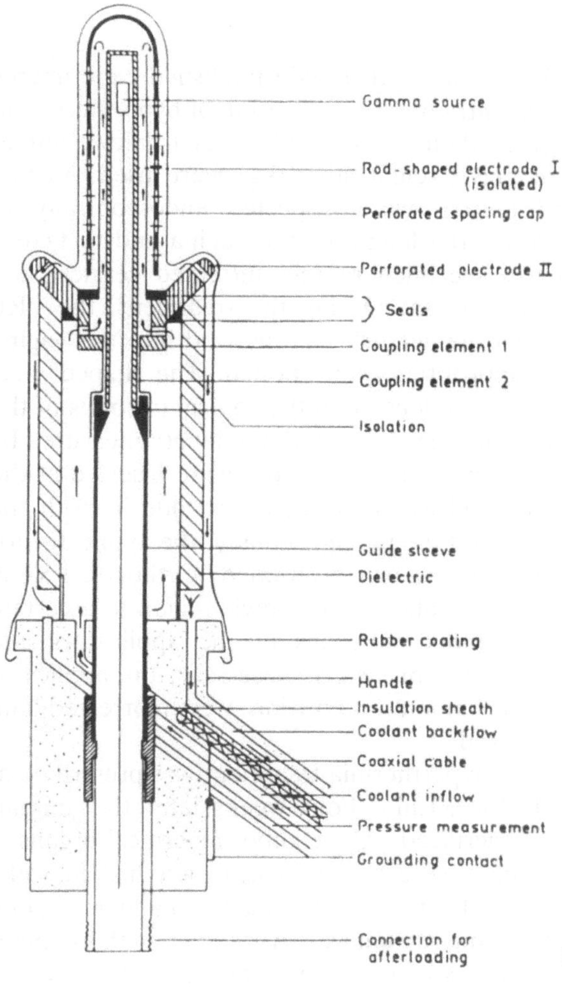

b

Fig. 10.2. a Schematic presentation of the applicator system for local radiothermotherapy of the cervical region. The *black points* symbolize areas of temperature measurement; the *circular arrows* show the thermostated regions in the bladder, rectum, and the inner part of the RF gamma applicator. **b** Schematic presentation of the RF gamma applicator. It consists of three internal systems: (a) an electrode system (electrodes I and II, coupling elements 1 and 2, isolation, dielectric and grounding contact); (b) a cooling system (coolant in- and backflow, seals, perforating spacing cap); and (c) a radiation system (connection for afterloading, isolation sheath, guide sleeve, inner part of the rod-shaped electrode I)

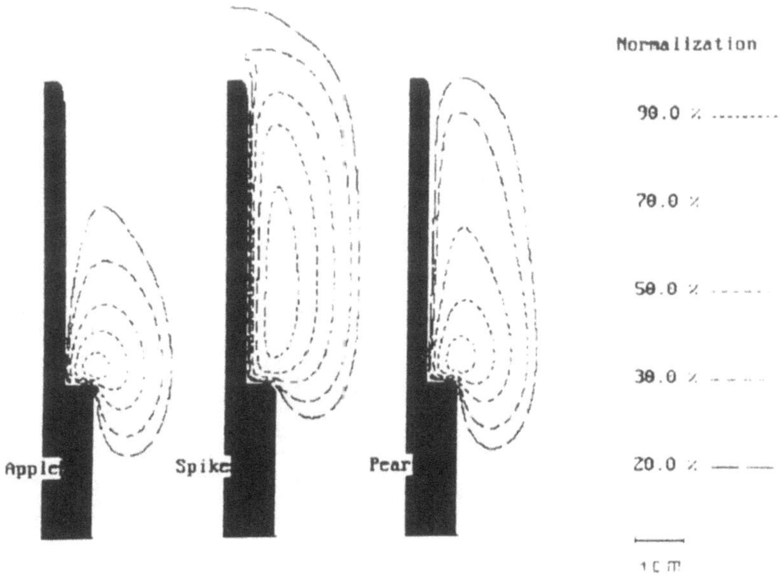

Fig. 10.3. Results of the three-dimensional temperature field calculations with the SAR functions. These temperature curves are expected with the application of the cooled RF gamma applicator in a homogeneous nonperfused model tissue. The terms "apple," "spike," and "pear" were taken from the outer shape of the full three-dimensional rotation figure. These calculations were used for comparison with experiments, as well as for controlling the accuracy of the program system

larly, HAND et al. (1982) published experiments on the intrauterine application of hyperthermia in pigs. In their animal study, four Minlewe miniature pigs (weight 40–70 kg) were used. Vagina and rectum were inspected endoscopically to measure the length of the vagina and to take a biopsy specimen of the untreated cervical and rectal mucosa. During the treatment, the "RF gamma applicator" was inserted into the vagina and appropriately positioned. The shaped electrodes were located in the conical introitus of the cervix in accordance with the length measured by endoscopy. Thermal probes were inserted at the same level as the shaped electrode in both the vagina and the rectum. Finally, the applicator for rectal cooling was positioned. Orthogonal x-ray films were taken of the pelvic region to ascertain the intended positions of the applicators and the thermal probes. If necessary, the applicator and thermometry position were corrected and optimized.

The hyperthermia treatment was prescribed at 42°C for 30 min. Four weeks later the animals were sacrificed. All neighboring critical organs in the pelvis were macroscopically and histologically examined for thermal damage. Bladder, vagina, cervix, and rectum were worked up in this manner and effects of steep thermal gradients were observed. This was assumed to express either the cooling effects of the coolant or the effects of locoregional blood flow. In the histological investigations three animals were found to demonstrate no specific thermal effects such as edema, vascular ectasia, hypercellularity or repair mechanisms, necrosis, or fibrosis. Only one pig developed moderate necrosis and hypercellularity. In this case, the temperature level had been increased during the heating to 45.5°C for 15 min.

10.5.3 Preliminary Results

In a pilot study, eight patients with advanced inoperable carcinomas of the cervix were treated. All treatments were well tolerated. Figure 10.4 displays a typical temperature curve. We now intend to conduct a randomized study comparing the effects of endocavitary thermoradiotherapy versus radiotherapy only. Figure 10.5 shows the individual treatment prescription for each arm.

10.5.4 Future Research

Concomitant experimental investigations are required to elucidate the pathophysiological effects

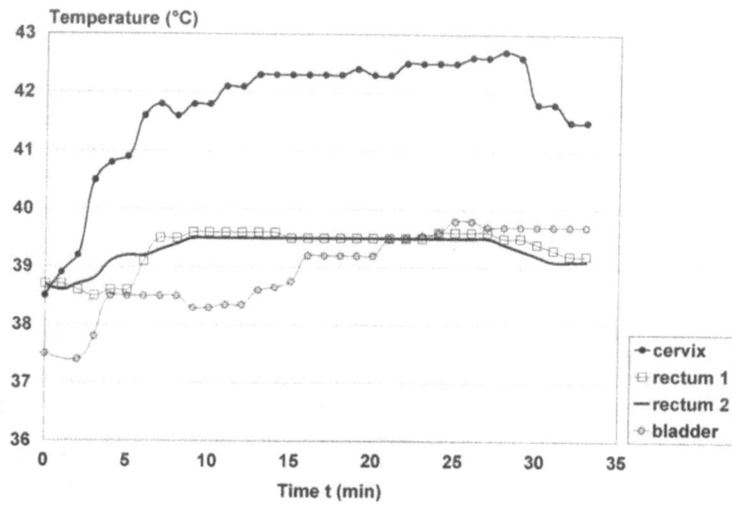

Fig. 10.4. Typical temperature curve for thermoradiotherapy of a patient with cervix carcinoma

Percutaneous Radiotherapy

40 Gy small pelvis / 60 Gy parametrium

↓

↓——— plus **Afterloading IRT** ———↓

Arm A :	*Arm B:*
5 x 10 Gy / 1 cm tissue	2 x 10 Gy/1cm; 3 x 10 Gy/1cm tissue
without additional hyperthermia	plus 45 min hyperthermia at 42.5° C

Fig. 10.5. Treatment prescription for each arm of a planned randomized study of endocavitary thermoradiotherapy versus radiotherapy alone

of adjuvant hyperthermia in the tumor and adjacent normal tissues. Therefore the following aspects will be included in the future clinical research project:

1. Better adaptation of the radiation and thermal distribution to the tumor configuration by means of careful clinical and radiological investigations
2. Measurements of tumor blood flow characteristics by use of magnetic resonance imaging before and after heating
3. Measurements of tumor oxygen by using invasive pO_2 measurements with the Eppendorf pO_2 meter (Eppendorf Corp., Hamburg) before and after heating
4. Registration of side-effects in the urethra, bladder, and rectal mucosa by endoscopic examination
5. Improved assessment of tumor response by means of careful clinical and radiological investigations

10.6 Summary

- Neither palliative nor adjuvant hyperthermia is an established routine modality in the treatment of advanced or recurrent carcinoma of the uterus. Combined thermoradiotherapy may be a useful modality to overcome the dismal results of conventional therapies, but it is still experimental. Overall, there is a meaningful biological and clinical rationale for implementation.
- Retrospective studies and a prospective randomized trial indicate a thermal enhancement ratio of 1.18–2.06 when hyperthermia is added to radiotherapy for cervical cancer. However, further studies with improved heating techniques are required to prove the clinical value of adjuvant hyperthermia within a defined treatment plan for uterine carcinomas.
- Careful patient selection should be undertaken, with due regard to biological parameters, pathophysiological conditions, and clinical as-

pects such as unfavorable radiotherapy options. Only those patients who might derive a clear benefit from adjunctive hyperthermia treatment should be included in future controlled clinical trials.

References

Akuta K, Hiraoka M, Jo S, et al. (1989) A newly developed interstitial applicator for RF current heating. In: Sugahara T, Saito M (eds) Hyperthermic oncology 1988, vol 1. Taylor & Francis, London, pp 878–880

American Cancer Society (1993) Cancer facts and figures 1993. American Cancer Society, Atlanta

Aristizabal SA (1985) Interstitial parametrial irradiation in cancer of the cervix stages IIB-IIIB: analysis of pelvic control and complications. Int J Endocurie/Hyperthermia Oncol 1: 41–48

Aristizabal SA, Oleson JR (1984) Combined interstitial irradiation and localized current field hyperthermia: results and conclusions from clinical studies. Cancer Res 44(suppl): 4757s–4760s

Awwad HK, Naggar ME, Mocktar N, Barsoum M (1986) Intercapillary distance measurement as an indicator of hypoxia in carcinoma of the cervix uteri. Int J Radat Oncol Biol Phys 12: 1329–1333

Brenner DI, Huang Y, Hall EJ (1991) Fractionated high-dose-rate versus low-dose-rate regimens for intracavitary brachytherapy of the cervix: equivalent regimens for combined brachytherapy and external irradiation. Int J Radiat Oncol Biol Phys 21: 1415–1423

Coughlin CT, Ryan TP, Stafford JH (1991) Interstitial thermoradiotherapy: the Dartmouth experience 1981–1990. In: Chapman JD, Dewey WC, Whitmore GF (eds) Radiation research – a twentieth-century perspective, vol 1. Academic Press, San Diego, p 386 [P 31 02 WP] (abstract)

Datta NR, Rose AK, Kapoor HK (1987) Thermoradiotherapy in the management of carcinoma of the cervix IIIB: a controlled clinical study. Indian Med Gazette 121: 68–71

Deurloo IIK, Visser AG, Ruifrok ACC, Lakeman RF, van Rhoon GC, Levendag PC (1989) Radiofrequency interstitial hyperthermia: a multicentric program of quality assessment and clinical trials. In: Sugahara T, Saito M (eds) Hyperthermic Oncology 1988, vol 1. Taylor & Francis, London, pp 864–875

Diederich CJ, Hynynen KH (1983) Ultrasound technology for interstitial hyperthermia. In: Seegenschmiedt MH, Sauer R (eds) Interstitial & intracavitary thermoradiotherapy. Springer, Berlin Heidelberg New York, pp 55–62

Dische S, Anderson PJ, Sedly R, Watson ER (1983) Carcinoma of the cervix – anaemia, radiotherapy and hyperbaric oxygen. Br J Radiol 56: 251–255

Emami B, Perez CA, Konefal J, et al. (1987) Interstitial thermoradiotherapy in treatment of malignant tumors. Int J Hyperthermia 3: 107–118

Feldmann JH, Sack H (1992) Achieved temperature distributions in dependency on applicator technique and/or perfusions values. Strahlenther Onkol 168: 657–659

Feldmann HJ, Molls M, Heinemann H-G, Romanowski R, Stuchke M, Sack H (1993) Thermoradiotherapy in locally advanced deep seated tumors – thermal parameters and treatment results. Radiother Oncol 26: 38–44

Gaddis O (1983) Treatment of cervical carcinoma employing a template for transperineal interstitial 192 iridium brachytherapy. Int J Radiat Oncol Biol Phys 9: 819–824

Gautherie M, Cosset JM, Gerard JP, et al. (1989) Radiofrequency interstitial hyperthermia: a multi-centric program of quality assessment and clinical trials. In: Sugahara T, Saito M (eds) Hyperthermic oncology 1988, vol 2. Taylor & Francis, London, pp 711–714

Grigsby PW, Emami B (1993) Interstitial thermoradiotherapy for pelvic tumors: the Washington University experience. In: Seegenschmiedt MH, Sauer R (eds) Interstitial and intracavitary thermoradiotherapy. Springer, Berlin Heidelberg New York, pp 265–270

Hand JW, Blake PR, Hopewell JW, Lambert HW, Field SB (1982) A coaxial applicator for intra-cavitary hyperthermia of carcinoma of the cervix. In: Robinson JE (ed) Biomedical Thermolog. Liss, New York, pp 635–639

Handl-Zeller L (1993) Clinical experience of interstitial thermoradiotherapy using hot water perfusion techniques. In: Seegenschmiedt MH, Sauer R (eds) Interstitial and intracavitary thermoradiotherapy. Springer, Berlin Heidelberg New York, pp 211–222

Hietschold V, Klengel S, Köhler K (1993) Simultaneous dynamic measurement of tissue contrast enhancement and perfusion at 0.5 Tesla: method and postprocessing. In: Proceedings of the Society of Magnetic Resonance in medicine, vol 2, 12th Annual Scientific Meeting, August 14–20, 1993, New York

Herrmann T, Christen N, Alheit HD (1993) Gynäkologische Brachytherapie – von Low-dose-rate zu High-tech. Strahlenther Onkol 169: 141–151

Höckel M, Knoop C, Schlenger K, et al. (1993) Intratumoral pO_2 predicts survival in advanced cancer of the uterine cervix. Radiother Oncol 26: 45–50

Hornback NB, Shupe RE, Shidnia H, Marshall CV, Lauer T (1986) Advanced stage IIIB cancer of the cervix: treatment by hyperthermia and radiation. Gynecol Cncol 23: 160–167

Kolstadt P (1965) The development of the vascular bed in tumours as seen in squamous-cell carcinomas of the cervix uteri. Br J Radiol 38: 216–223

Kottmeier HL (ed) (1988) Annual report on the results of treatments in gynaecological cancer, volume XIX. International Federation of Gynecology and Obstetrics, Stockholm

Lagendijk JJW, Mooibroek J, Crezee (1993) Future developments in respect of thermal modeling, treatment planning, and tretment control for interstitial hyperthermia. In: Seegenschmiedt MH, Sauer R (eds) Interstitial and intracavitary thermoradiotherapy. Spring, Berlin Heidelberg New York, pp 155–159

Li DJ, Chou CK, Luk KH, Wang JH, Xie CF, McDougall JA, Huang GZ (1991) Design of intracavitary mircowave applicators for the treatment of uterine cervix carcinoma. Int J Hyperthermia 7: 693–701

Löffel J, Stahl H, Wust P, Riess H, Felix R (1993) Clinical experience with regional RF-hyperthermia: an overview. In: Proceedings of the 11th Annual Scientific Meeting of the ESHO, June 16–17, 1993, Brussels

Lowrey GC, Mendenhall WM, Million RR (1992) Stage IB or IIA-B carcinoma of the intact uerine cervix treated with irradiation: a multivariate analysis. Int J Radiat Oncol Biol Phys 24: 205–210

Marchal C, Nadi M, Hofstetter S, Bey P, Pernot M, Prieur G (1989) Practical interstitial method of heating operating at 27.12 MHz. Int J Hyperthermia 5: 451–466
Martinez A, Edmundson GK, Cox RS (1985) Combination of external beam irradiation and multiple-side perineal applicator (MUPIT) for treatment of locally advanced or recurrent prostatic, anorectal and gynecological malignancies. Int J Radiat Oncol Biol Phys 11: 391–398
Martinez A, Gersten D, Corry P (1993) Clinical rationale for interstitial thermoradiotherapy of gynecological tumors: review of clinical results and own experiences with continuous mild hyperthermia. In: Seegenschmiedt MH, Sauer R (eds) Interstitial and intracavitary thermoradiotherapy. Springer, Berlin Heidelberg New York, pp 179–186
Meyer JL (1984a) Hyperthermia as an anticancer modality – a historical perspective. Front Radiat Ther Oncol 18: 1–22
Meyer JL (1984b) Ultrasound hyperthermia: the Stanford experience. Front Radiat Ther Oncol 18: 126–135
Müller C (1912) Therapeutische Erfahrungen an 100 mit Kombination von Röntgenstrahlen und Hochfrequenz, resp. Diathermie behandelten bösartigen Neubildungen. Münch Medizin Wschr 28: 1546–1549
Nagano H, Tanohata K, Kusaba T, Kakehi M (1993) Radiohyperthermia for stage III, IV and recurrent uterine carcinioma. 16th Intern. Symposium on Clinical Hyperthermia, June 13–16, 1993, Kyoto
Nagata K, Yamamoto K, Shiga T, Tanaka Y (1993) Clinical results of radiofrequency hyperthermia for malignant pelvic tumors. 16th Intern. Symposium on Clinical Hyperthermia, June 13–16, 1993, Kyoto
Notter M, Schwegler N (1992) Monitoring of deep hyperthermia: what means a complete remission ? Strahlenther Onkol 168: 657–659
Overgaard J (1989) The current and potential role of hyperthermia. Int J Radiat Oncol Biol Phys 16: 535–549
Overgaard J, Horsmann MR (1992) Hyperthermia. In: The ESTRO book of basic clinical radiobiolog, pp 177–188
Parisi S, Raguso A, Portaluri M, Maiorana A, Vittori Antisari P (1990) Intracavitary hyperthermia combined with HDR afterloading irradiation in vaginal recurrences of cervical carcinoma. Adv Exp Med Biol 267: 429–432
Perez CA (1980) Radiation therapy alone in the treatment of the uterine cervix. I. Analysis of tumor recurrence. Cancer 51: 1393–1402
Perez CA, Grigsby PW, Nene SM, Camel HM, Galakatos A, Kao MS, Lockett MA (1992) Effect of tumor size on prognosis of carcinoma of the uterine cervix treated with irradiation alone. Cancer 69: 2796–2806
Probert JC, Saben HS, Gregory JC (1977) Use of the pig for assessing damage in the locally treated pelvis and abdomen. Int J Radiat Oncol Biol Phys 2: 491–503
Petrovich Z, Langholz B, Lam K, et al. (1989) Interstitial microwave hyperthermia combined with iridium-192 radiotherapy for recurrent tumors. Am J Clin Oncol 12: 264–268
Puthawala AA, Syed AMN, Khalid MA, Rafie S, McNamara CS (1985) Interstitial hyperthermia for recurrent malignancies. Endocurietherapy/Hyperthermia Oncol 1: 125–131
Roos D (1993) Review of intracavitary hyperthermia techniques. In: Seegenschmiedt MH, Sauer R (eds) Interstitial and intracavitary thermoradiotherapy. Springer, Berlin Heidelberg New York, pp 75–82
Sapozink MD, Joszef G, Astrahan MA, Gibbs FA Jr, Petrovich Z, Stewart JR (1990) Adjuvant pelvic hyperthermia in advanced cervical carcinoma. I. Feasibility, thermometry and device comparison. Int J Hypertherma 6: 985–996
Schorcht J (1994) Radiothermotherapy of cervical carcinoma. In: Fietkau R, Mould RF (eds) Brachytherapy state of the art in Germany. Proceedings Deutsche Brachytherapie-Konferenz '93, Naumburg/Saale, September 23–25, 1993, Chapter 10 Nucletron, Veenendaal, pp 81–87
Schorcht J, Zimmermann M, Redmann M, Eberhardt HJ (1989) Erste Erfahrungen mit der kombinierten hochdosierten Afterloading-Kurzzeittherapie und Hyperthermie beim nicht-operierten Zervixkarzinom. Radiobiol Radiother 30: 386–390
Seegenschmiedt MH (1993) Clinical experience of interstitial thermoradiotherapy using microwave techniques. In: Seegenschmiedt MH, Sauer R (eds) Interstitial and intracavitary thermo-radiotherapy. Springer, Berlin Heidelberg New York, pp 193–210
Seegenschmiedt MH, Sauer R (1992) The current role of interstitial thermoradiotherapy. Strahlenther Onkol 168: 119–140
Seegenschmiedt MH, Sauer R, Brady LW, Karlsson UL (1990) Interstitial thermoradiotherapy: review on current techniques and clinical experience. Am J Clin Oncol 13: 352–363
Seegenschmiedt MH, Sauer R, Miyamoto C, Brady LW (1993) Interstitial thermoradiotherapy for pelvic tumors: a co-operative phase 1–2 study. In: Seegenschmiedt MH, Sauer R (eds) Interstitial and intracavitary thermoradiotherapy. Springer, Berling Heidelberg New York, pp 271–288
Seegenschmiedt MH, Martus P, Fietkau R, Iro H, Brady LW, Sauer R (1994) Multivariate analysis of prognostic parameters using interstitial thermoradiotherapy (IHT-IRT): tumor and treatment variables predict outcome. Int J Radiat Oncol Biol Phys 29: 1049–1063
Sharma S, Patel FD, Sandhu APS, Gupta BD, Yadav NS (1989) A prospective randomized study of local hyperthermia as a supplement and radiosensitizer in treatment of carcinoma of the cervix with radiotherap Endocurietherapie/Hyperthermia Oncol 5: 151–159
Sharma S, Sandhu APS, Patel FD, Ghoshal S, Gupta BD, Yadav NS (1990) Side-effects of local hyperthermia: results of a prospectively randomized clinical study. Int J Hyperthermia 6: 279–285
Sharma S, Singhal S, Sandhu APS, Ghoshal S, Gupta BD, Yadav NS (1991a) Local thermoradiotherapy in carcinoma cervix: improved local control versus increased incidence of distant meta-stasis. Asia Oceania J Obstet Gynecol 17: 5–12
Sharma S, Patel FD, Gupta PD, Negi PS, Ayyagary S (1991b) Clinical trial of LDR versus HDR brachytherapy in carcinoma of the cervix. Selectron Activity 2: 59–64
Shimm DS, Kittelson JM, Oleson JR, Aristizabal JA, Barlow LC, Cetas TC (1990) Interstitial thermoradiotherapy: thermal dosimetry and clinical results. Int J Radiat Oncol Biol Phys 18: 383–387
Siracky J, Siracka E, Kovac R, Revesz L (1988) Prognostic significance of vascular density and a malignancy grading in radiation treated uterine cervix carcinoma. Neoplasma 35: 289–296
Stea B, Shimm D, Cetas TC (1993) Clinical experience of interstitial thermoradiotherapy using ferromagnetic

implant techniques. In: Seegenschmiedt MH, Sauer R (eds) Interstitial and intracavitary thermoradiotherapy. Springer, Berlin Heidelberg New York, pp 223–232

Sullivan MF, Beamer JL, Cross FT, Lund JE, Mahony TD, Endres GW, Buschbom RL (1980) Pathologic effects of intracavitary irradiation with Californium-252. Int J Radiat Oncol Biol Phys 6: 1613–1627

Surwit EA, Manning MR, Aristizabal SA, Oleson JR, Cetas TC (1983) Interstitial thermoradiotherap in recurrent gynecologic malignancies. Gynecol Oncol 15: 95–102

Touboul E, Lefranc JP, Blondon J, et al. (1992) Preoperative radiation therapy and surgery in the treatment of "bulky' squamous cell carcinoma of the uterine cervix (stages Ib, IIa and IIb) operable tumors. Radiother Oncol 24: 32–40

Turner PF (1993) Recent developments using the BSD-2000 system. In: Issels RD, Wilmanns H (eds) Abstracts of the Conference on Hyperthermia in Clinical Oncology, October 25–27, 1993, Munich, p 40

Vaupel P (1990) Oxygenation of human tumors. Strahlenther Onkol 166: 377–386

Vernon CC (1992) Application of focused ultrasound for local hyperthermia. Strahlenther Onkol 168: 653–656

Vora NL, Luk KH (1993) Interstitial thermoradiotherapy for pelvic tumors: the City of Hope Experience. In: Seegenschmiedt MH, Sauer R (eds) Interstitial and intracavitary thermoradiotherapy. Springer, Berlin Heidelberg New York, pp 257–264

Westermark F (1898) Über die Behandlung des ulcerierenden Cervixcarcinoms mittels konstanter Wärme. Z Gynäkol 49: 1335–1339

Wust P, Nadobny J, Seebass M, Böhm M, Felix R (1992) Concepts for further improvement of RF-hyperthermia. Strahlenther Onkol 168: 657–659

Zee van der J, Rhoon van GC, Koper PC, Treurniet-Donker AD, Wijnmaalen AJ (1991) First clinical experience with deep regional hyperthermia. Strahlenther Onkol 167: 349

Zee van der J, Gonzales-Gonzales D, Putten van WLJ, et al. (1993) Hyperthermia combined with radio-therapy in deep seated tumours: a phase III trial. In: Issels RD, Wilmanns H (eds) Abstracts of the Conference on Hyperthermia in Clinical Oncology, October 25–27, 1993, Munich, p 41

Zimmermann M, Schorcht J, Andree W (1993) Theoretical and experimental investigations of a newly developed intracavitary applicator system for radiothermotherapy of gynaecological tumours. Int J Hyperthermia 9: 463–477

11 Thermoradiotherapy and Thermochemotherapy for Sarcomas

K. LEOPOLD and R.D. ISSELS

CONTENTS

11.1 Introduction

Soft tissue sarcomas are tumors which are derived from mesenchymal tissue and thus may arise in essentially any site in the body. They often infiltrate surrounding normal tissue extensively and aggressively. Local functional loss and pain are frequently quite debilitating when these tumors are uncontrolled. In addition to causing morbidity from local extension, soft tissue sarcomas have a high propensity for distant metastatic spread, usually including the lung (YANG et al. 1993). These connective tissue cancers are unusual (only around 6000 estimated cases for the United States in 1993) but are frequently lethal (3100 deaths from this disease were anticipated in the United States during 1993) (BORING et al. 1993).

K. LEOPOLD, MD, Department of Radiation Oncology, P.O. Box 3085-154, Durham, NC 27710, USA

Priv. -Doz. ROLF D. ISSELS, MD, PhD. GSF-Institut Für Klinische Hâmatologie Institut für Klinische Hâmatologie Marchioninistraße 25, D-81377 München, FRG, and Klinikum Großhadern, Medizinische Klinik III, Marchionistrae 15, D-81377 München, FRG

Soft tissue sarcomas have a propensity for extensive local tissue invasion. The extent of local spread can be fairly well predicted by pathological features and tumor size (LACK et al. 1989; COSTA et al. 1984; TROJANI et al. 1984). More aggressive lesions tend to show large regions of necrosis, high mitotic activity, and morphological atypia. Larger size (5 cm in diameter is generally used as an arbitrary cutoff) independently predicts for increased local recurrence (SUIT et al. 1988; POTTER et al. 1985; BEAHRS et al. 1992). High grade and large size are also associated with a higher propensity for distant metastasis (SUIT et al. 1988; POTTER et al. 1985; BEAHRS et al. 1992).

Conventional treatment of soft tissue sarcomas has, for decades, been based on surgical extirpation. Because of the propensity for moderate- to high-grade lesions to extensively invade adjacent tissues, excision of these tumors without a margin of normal-appearing tissue resulted in a local recurrence rate of about 85% (GERNER et al. 1975; MARKHEDE et al. 1982). When this high recurrence rate was appreciated, tumor excision with a safety margin of several centimeters of normal-appearing soft tissue became the standard surgical resection approach. Although this improved local control compared to "marginal" excisions, local failures still occurred in about 50% of cases (SIMON et al. 1976; GERNER et al. 1975).

As the poor results of conservative excisions became appreciated, and as surgical techniques improved, even more aggressive surgical procedures became the norm. These generally consisted of resection of all of the tissue in the "anatomical compartment" in which the tumor was located, or amputation if this "compartmentectomy" could not be reasonably accomplished. Such radical procedures led to a substantial improvement in local tumor control with several large series reporting local failure rates of around 15% (SIMON et al. 1976; MARKHEDE et al. 1982). These procedures are generally more feasible in

Table 11.1. Univariate logistic regression results of thermal, tumor, and patient variables versus histopathological response of soft tissue sarcomas treated with preoperative radiation and hyperthermia

Covariate	Model chi-square	P
Av. cumulative min $T_{50} \geq 41.5°C$	19.18	<0.001
T_{50}	16.82	<0.001
T_{10}	15.89	<0.001
Av. cumulative min $T_{90} \geq 40.5°C$	15.13	<0.001
T_{90}	11.77	0.001
T_{max}	10.76	0.001
1 vs 2 HT treatments/week	7.54	0.006
T_{min}	6.43	0.01
Tumor volume	3.16	0.08
Number of HT treatments	0.74	0.39
Liposarcoma vs other histology	0.40	0.53
Age	0.05	0.82
Limb vs other tumor site	0.01	0.91
Sex	0.01	0.91

extremity locations. Radical extirpation in these extremity sites, however, is usually associated with significant functional impairment.

In order to improve function without compromising tumor control, oncologists turned to wide excision followed by adjuvant irradiation of the residual compartment (or irradiation of the tumor bed with a 5- to 10-cm margin). Although function was improved with this approach, local failure rates were higher than desired in many instances (Lindberg et al. 1981; Mandard et al. 1989; Potter et al. 1985). During the last 15–20 years, several institutions instituted the practice of preoperative irradiation. Reports indicated an advantage to this approach (Barkley et al. 1988; Suit et al. 1988) and many institutions now regard this as the standard therapy for most resectable soft tissue sarcomas.

Several problems persist in the management of soft tissue sarcomas despite the recent gains noted above. In many circumstances, tumor is located such that wide excision cannot be reasonably performed. These include tumors that are located in the pelvis or abdomen/retroperitoneum, or that involve essential neural or vascular structures. In such instances, local control with radiation alone is unusual unless high doses are used (Lindberg 1980; Tepper and Suit 1985). This would lead to unacceptable morbidity of normal tissues in many instances. Even when wide excision can be performed, local failure after preoperative irradiation of high-grade tumors has been reported to be as high as 17% in one large series (Suit et al. 1988). Also, the appearance of distant metastases after resection remains a problem in the majority of high-grade, large lesions (Suit et al. 1988; Barkley et al. 1988; Mandard et al. 1989). The role of chemotherapy in this regard remains unresolved (Yang et al. 1993).

The combination of anticancer drugs with hyperthermia was only recently introduced as a new clinical strategy. This approach within the field of medical oncology is based on the convincing evidence that hyperthermia enhances the therapeutic effect of several chemotherapeutic agents even in drug-resistant cells. Such a combined modality is of particular interest as a means of overcoming the limited therapeutic efficacy of conventional anticancer agents in the case of many solid human tumors.

In an attempt to improve disease control without unacceptable treatment-induced morbidity, a number of investigators have studied the addition of hyperthermia to the other treatment modalities noted above. The basis for thermoradiotherapy in other settings was well established. The combination of anticancer drugs with hyperthermia was only recently introduced as a new clinical strategy. This approach within the field of medical oncology is based on the convincing evidence that hyperthermia enhances the therapeutic effect of several chemotherapeutic agents even in drug-resistant cells. Such a combined modality approach is of particular interest as a means of overcoming the limited therapeitic efficacy of conventional anticancer agents in the case of many solid human tumors. This chapter summarizes the technical considerations and clinical results of these studies.

11.2 Technical Considerations

The hyperthermia technique employed for the majority of soft tissue sarcomas is dictated by the generally large volume and deep-seated nature of these lesions. Deep-seated tumors, in general, are more difficult to heat than superficial lesions. Soft tissue sarcomas, however, frequently can be heated to relatively high temperatures (Leopold et al. 1992; Egawa et al. 1989). This is likely principally a result of the lower blood flow in soft tissue sarcomas as compared to other cancers (Acker et al. 1990). Such a reduction in blood flow would be expected to yield higher tumor temperatures per specific absorption rate as predicted by bioheat transfer models. Thermal modeling of annular phased-array systems has also stressed the dependence of temperature elevation on blood flow rate (STROHBEHN et al. 1989; ZHOU and FESSENDEN 1993).

We have demonstrated tumor blood flows, using laser-Doppler flow techniques, in the range of 0.1–24.7 ml/min/100 g in soft tissue sarcomas. The average blood flow in the eight sarcomas examined was 0.4 ± 0.37 ml/min/100 g. This compares with an average blood flow rate in carcinomas of 46.4 ml/min/100 g (range of 0.4–0.6 ml/min/100 g) (ACKER et al. 1990). Given these low blood flow values, it would be expected that most soft tissue sarcomas would heat more efficiently than most carcinomas. Furthermore, we have shown, using magnetic resonance imaging (MRI) gradient refocusing and spectral shift techniques, that soft tissue sarcomas have relatively few thermally significant blood vessels (DEWHIRST et al. 1990). Thus, it would be expected not only that high maximum tumor temperatures could be attained, but also that the majority of the tumor would be heated relatively well.

The above theoretical considerations have been borne out in our experience. Whereas the median non-soft tissue sarcoma deep-seated tumor had 50% of measured temperature points (T_{50}) greater than or equal to 40.2°C and $T_{90} \geqslant$ 39.2°C, soft tissue sarcomas had $T_{50} \geqslant$ 41.4°C and $T_{90} \geqslant$ 39.4°C. Others have reported relative success in their ability to heat deep-seated soft tissue sarcomas using microwaves (EGAWA et al. 1989), magnetic induction (JABBOURG et al. 1987; REDDY et al. 1987), and scanned focused ultrasound (BUATTI et al. 1990).

Using electromagnetic (EM) energy for noninvasive heating the field sources are external to the patient and the heating modality and techniques are dictated by the characteristics of the clinical problem (e.g., size, depth, anatomical location). A coherent array of radiating sources can be used for EM energy deposition in deep-seated tissues and there are several reasons for using the phased-array approach for deep heating: The energy sources can be arranged so that the electric field is along the body axis and therefore predominantly tangential to the subcutaneous fat/muscle interface, avoiding the problem of excessive fat heating. It also allows some energy focusing or steering within the exposed tissue region by manipulating the relative phase and amplitude of the external sources.

The array device most widely used is the annular phased array system (BSD Corp., Salt Lack City, Utah) and its technical design and clinical potential have been well documented (TURNER 1984; SAMULSKI et al. 1987). The body region, such as the pelvis, is surrounded by an annular configuration (diameter 60 cm) of the radiating antennas coupled to the patient contour using a water bolus. The frequency used for phased-array devices suitable for heating tissue deep in the pelvis is in the range of 70–100 MHz. Smaller array designs for limb heating (diameter 30 cm) or for the treatment of children (diameter 40 cm) have been developed recently and are also capable of being operated in a phase- and amplitude-controlled mode.

At Duke University the APAS has generally been used for pelvic, abdominal/retroperitoneal, proximal limb, and some trunkal lesions. Tumors involving the lower extremity distal to the mid-thigh or the upper extremity distal to the mid-arm have generally been treated with a miniature annular phased array (BSD Corp., Salt Lake City, Utah). The occasional small, superficial lesion was treated with superficial microwave applicators (433 or 915 MHz) or nonfocused ultrasound (1–3 MHz). Magnetic induction, scanned ultrasound, and perfusion have been used by others, as noted above.

Regional hyperthermia (RHT) using the BSD system for deep-seated tumors has been extensively studied at several institutions in phase I trials (for review) (SAPOZINK et al. 1986). Accurate assessment of the treatment-induced temperature distributions in tumor and surrounding tissues has been essential for the evaluation of RHT treatments. At present, only invasive techniques are possible. These are routinely performed in the clinic by percutaneous or intraoperative insertion of one or more Teflon thermometry catheters across the diameter of the tumor within the field of the planned RHT. Insertion of thermistor probes into the lumen of the catheters immediately before RHT and the use of a semiautomatic thermal mapping system (GIBBS 1983) allow measurements of temperatures mapped along the axis of each thermometry catheter at fixed intervals (0.5 or 1 cm) repeated every 5 min. These enable temperature-time profiles to be obtained in a larger number of spatial points for each probe insertion.

11.3 Treatment Practice (Planning and Performance)

The technique for heating soft tissue sarcomas is similar in most respects to the treatment of other tumors. Prior to positioning the patient in the treatment apparatus, thermometry catheters are placed (fluoroptic probes, thermistors, or, with ultrasound treatments, thermocouples may be used). If hyperthermia is done in the preoperative setting, care must be used to place these catheters through tissue that is to be included in the region of surgical resection in order to avoid tumor seeding. Since the incision site of the biopsy is routinely resected, this is usually the preferred site for thermometry catheter placement. Two to three perpendicularly placed, closed-ended catheters should be placed through the complete tumor volume to its deep edge. Direct on-line computerized tomography (CT) facilitates this placement and allows one to avoid critical structures (Fig. 11.1).

Following interstitial thermometry placement, the patient is positioned within the treatment apparatus. Additional intracavitary and surface temperature sensors should be applied at this time as dictated by normal tissue concerns. For treatment with the Sigma 60 device (which allows electrical field steering), electrical fields should be monitored by dipole sensors placed on the surface of the patient in all four quadrants. For APAS treatments, the water bolus is filled. Cool water (25°C) can be circulated if the tumor does not involve the skin.

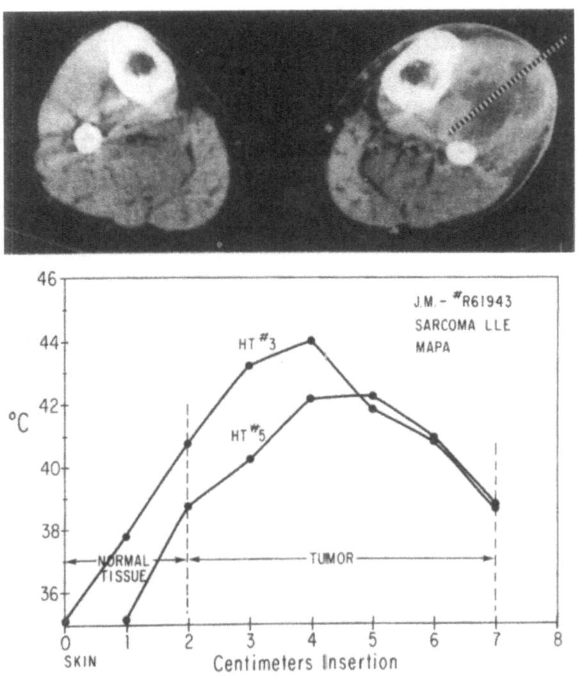

Fig. 11.1. Facilitation and documentation of catheter placement by CT scanning. The catheter tract can be seen entering the leg from a left anterior oblique position and has been enhanced by hatching. The median value temperature map for the third and fifth treatments are shown. The depth of thermometer insertion was measured from the CT scan (from Leopold et al. 1989)

Once the setup is completed, power is turned on. The usual initial power level with the APAS is around 250 W. Power is increased, generally in 50-W increments, until the power-limiting endpoint is reached. These endpoints have been described in detail by the Radiation Therapy Oncology Group (Sapozink et al. 1991). Optimally, all tumor would be raised to ≥43°C with all normal tissue kept below 42°C. In practice, patient discomfort usually limits the achievable power so that monitored temperatures are below these levels. Power can sometimes be increased by phase-amplitude steering of the field, placement of saline-filled bags at regions of discomfort (often the thighs in patients with pelvic lesions or the knees in those with thigh lesions), or use of analgesics. The last-mentioned approach must be used with caution, however, since hot spots can occur at sites which are not being thermally monitored and complications can therefore arise if a patient's pain response is blunted.

Tumor and normal tissue temperatures should be monitored throughout the heat treatment. The detail in which measurements are obtained will dictate the depth and value of thermal analysis that will be possible. We generally obtain temperature measurements along two or three catheters placed through the tumor. Temperature measurements are taken at 0.5-cm intervals through these catheters (temperature mappings) every 5 min during the treatment and the cool-down period. Between mappings, temperatures are constantly monitored at the point of the maximum reading. This monitoring system, including data input into the computer, has largely been automated (Leopold et al. 1992). For those who do not have access to such sophisticated equipment, it is recommended that temperatures be monitored at least every 2 cm (temperature differences of up to 5°C at this distance are not rare in soft tissue sarcomas) every 10 min.

11.4 Results of Clinical Trials

11.4.1 Preoperative Hyperthermia and Radiation Therapy: The Duke University Experience

The goal of preoperative treatment is to improve local control, facilitate conservative resection, and devitalize tumor before surgical manipulation. The latter theoretically could decrease the probability of distant metastases. At Duke University, we initiated thermoradiotherapy in the preoperative setting for moderate- to high-grade soft tissue sarcomas in 1984 and have treated about 70 patients in this fashion. Forty-five of these lesions have been fully evaluated at this time. Lesions were randomized to one versus two hyperthermia treatments per week during radiation therapy with stratification by tumor volume. Details of patients and tumors are given on Table 11.2.

Hyperthermia treatment parameters have been noted in Sect. 11.2 and in prior publications (LEOPOLD et al. 1989, 1992). Radiation fields were based on the location of gross disease as demonstrated by MRI, CT scan, and physical examination. Fields were designed to cover the compartment containing the gross disease for a distance of 10 cm proximal and distal to the gross disease. Alternatively, the origin or insertion of the muscle groups contained within the involved compartment were used as field borders if these occurred within 10 cm of the gross disease. If the tumor was not contained within a well-defined compartment, a wide margin was allowed around neighboring intact tissue planes. A strip of normal tissue was left outside of the radiation fields to facilitate lymphatic drainage. These fields were treated to 44 Gy at 2.0 Gy per fraction or 45 Gy at 1.8 Gy per fraction. The fields were subsequently reduced to give 5-cm proximal and distal margins, and an additional 5.4–6.0 Gy was delivered, yielding a total dose of 50–50.4 Gy.

Table 11.2. Preoperative thermoradiotherapy in soft tissue sarcomas – Duke University Experience

Number of tumors analyzed	45
Age (average)	54
Male/Female	24/21
Tumor Volume[1] (average)	606 cm^3
Site	
Lower Extremity	31
Upper Extremity	2
Trunk	12
Histology	
Liposarcoma	13
MFH	18
Other	14
3–4 + Tumor Necrosis/Response	60%
Local Failure	5 (11%)
3 Year Disease Free Survival	53%

[1] Tumor volume was taken as the product of three perpendicular axes

Surgery was performed approximately 4 weeks after the completion of thermoradiotherapy. This waiting period was found to be optimal in that it allowed for the acute treatment reaction to subside, allowed for some tumor regression, and was short enough for treatment-related fibrosis/vascular problems to be minimized. Preoperative chest x-ray or CT was performed routinely. This continues to be recommended as three patients were found to have developed pulmonary metastases in the interval between their initial workup and time for resection.

The surgical intent was to perform a wide excision of the initially involved region. Great attention was paid to preserving as much function as possible. Vascular flaps were liberally used (BARWICK et al. 1992). It should be stressed that these operative procedures, particularly following thermoradiotherapy, are technically complex and demanding. It is of the utmost importance that they be performed by a team that is skilled and experienced in the treatment of these tumors. Good communication between the surgeons, radiation oncologists, medical oncologists, and other involved medical personnel is also of paramount importance.

The average tumor volume in the studied group was 606 cm^3 (ranging from around 30 cm^3 to 2500 cm^3). About two-thirds of the lesions were of the lower extremities (usually the thigh). No retroperitoneal/intra-abdominal lesions were treated. Histologically, roughly one-third were malignant fibrous histiocytomas, one-third liposarcomas, and the other third various other subtypes. These characteristics are in keeping with the general sarcoma population (YANG et al. 1993).

With an average follow-up of 32 months, there have been five local failures (11%). The estimated 3-year probability of local control was 84%. Two of the local failures were in the deep tumor bed, two were at the proximal resection margins, and one was indeterminate.

There were 12 trunkal lesions, all of which were controlled locally. No difference in local control was noted comparing one versus two hyperthermia treatments per week. The probability of local control was not significantly related to any treatment or tumor variables, although the power to detect such relationships was low given the small number of local failures.

There were ten patients with continuous local control who were noted to develop distant metastases. The 3-year probability of disease-free survival was 53%. These results are better than most series of resection and postoperative radiation therapy (LINDBERG et al. 1981; MANDARD et al. 1989; POTTER et al. 1985) and are similar to preoperative radiation therapy series in which more aggressive radiation therapy was often used (SUIT et al. 1988; BARKLEY et al. 1988).

At Duke University, we learned during the first few years of this treatment that postoperative wound breakdown could be a significant problem. Because of this, vascular flaps were used liberally (LEOPOLD et al. 1989; BARWICK et al. 1992). Serious complications were infrequent after this practice was initiated.

The functional results of the above treatment were good. Nearly all patients, however, did have some level of residual functional impairment. This in general consisted of moderate edema and restriction in the range of motion of affected extremities.

11.4.2 Hyperthermia and Radiation Therapy for Nonresected Tumors

Scant information exists detailing the outcome of soft tissue sarcomas lift in situ after thermoradiotherapy. EGAWA et al. (1989) have described results from the treatment of 26 lesions. Radiation therapy consisted of 2-Gy fractions given five times per week to a dose of 40–60 Gy (depending on tumor location and whether prior radiation therapy had been given). Hyperthermia was given twice a week during radiation therapy. Each hyperthermia treatment was for 30–45 min. The 14 deep-seated lesions were treated with the APAS and/or a radiofrequency system. Six of the ten superficial lesions and four of the 16 deep lesions had responded by 1 month after completion of therapy. In the deep-seated group, however, nine of the 12 nonresponding tumors appeared to be effectively treated as judged by resection or biopsy (four cases) or CT scans (five cases). At Duke University it has also been noted that large tumors might be nearly or totally necrotic histopathologically even though they have not diminished in size by 1 month following treatment. In large sarcomas that we have treated without resection, clinical response was frequently noted to be delayed.

11.4.3 Thermal Dose Considerations

The resection of tumor that had been recently treated with thermoradiotherapy presented an excellent opportunity to perform thermal dose studies with an endpoint that was more sensitive than usually found in clinical practice. This endpoint, the percentage of intact-appearing tumor cells in the studied specimen, had previously been shown by others to have relevance to local tumor control (ROLLO et al. 1981) (Fig. 11.2).

The initial studies at Duke University focused on improving the method of characterizing the inhomogeneous temperature distributions typically created by local and regional heating devices. We found that describing this distribution by noting the temperature that a reference percentile of tumor was heated to or beyond yielded a significant relationship with the percentage of intact tumor cells found in the resected specimen. The T_{min}, T_{max}, best T_{min}, and average of the best two T_{mins} were not as strongly related to this endpoint (LEOPOLD et al. 1989) (Fig. 11.3). Describing measured temperatures via percentile measurements also is more accurate from a theoretical point of view than description using minima and maxima. These latter terms are more dependent on the number of spatial points monitored (CORRY et al. 1988) and the interpretation of the tumor/normal tissue boundary (LEOPOLD et al. 1992).

Subsequent studies in the sarcoma population revealed that thermal descriptors that incorporated both temperature distribution and treatment time were somewhat more strongly related to histopathological outcome than temperature distribution alone (see Table 11.1). This finding was corroborated in studies of superficial tumors and deep-seated tumors (LEOPOLD et al. 1993). The time variable, that was found to be most strongly related to tumor response has been the cumulative minutes that an arbitrary percentile of tumor was raised to or above about 41°C. The model for the soft tissue sarcoma population (assuming 50–50.4 Gy in 1.8- to 2.0- Gy fractions) shows that about 100 cumulative minutes of

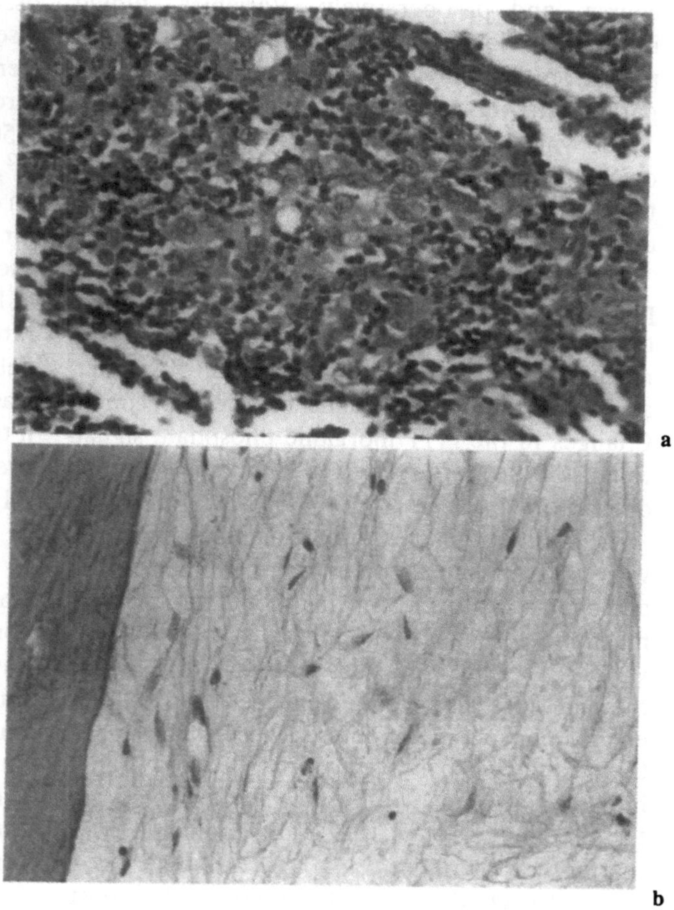

Fig. 11.2a,b. Histopathological response of an undifferentiated sarcoma of the thigh. The patient received ten hyperthermia treatments (2 treatments per week) concurrently with 50 Gy in 5 weeks followed 5 weeks later by wide excision. Pathological examination revealed no intact malignant cells. **a** Pretreatment biopsy. H&E, ×250. **b** Histology at extirpation. H&E. ×250 (from LEOPOLD et al. 1989)

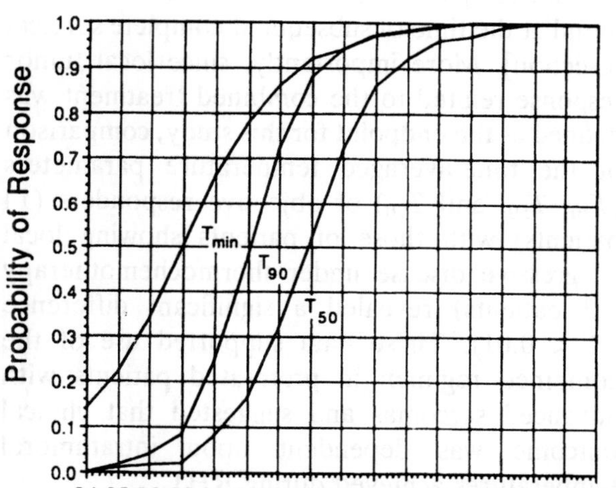

Fig. 11.3. Probability of complete or near-complete histopathological response versus T_{90}, T_{50}, and T_{min}. T_{min} is not as strongly related to response as T_{90} and T_{50} (from LEOPOLD et al. 1993)

hyperthermia (delivered as described above) with a $T_{90} \geqslant 41°C$ is required in order to have a 75% probability of a successful histopathological outcome. It is reasonable to assume that higher radiation and thermal doses would be required for prolonged local tumor control if the lesions are left in situ.

11.4.4 Predictors of Tumor Response

Identifying the probability that a given modality or treatment scheme has of leading to a successful outcome would be critically important in therapeutic decision making. At Duke University we have explored this in our soft tissue sarcoma population with the use of MRI and phosphorus-31 spectroscopy (MRS) (PRESCOTT et al., to be published). Twenty-one soft tissue sarcomas were studied with these tests at the initiation of thermoradiotherapy, after the first hyperthermia treatment, towards the end of the treatment course, and preoperatively. Variables studied included initial T2 relaxation times and various phosphometabolite ratios, and changes in these parameters between the first and second studies. These variables were compared to histopathological (human patients) or clinical (canine patients) response as well as various thermal descriptors.

A decrease in the ratio of adenosine triphosphate (ATP) to phosphomonoester from the initial to the subsequent study was found to be significantly predictive of finding less than 5% intact-appearing tumor cells in the resected specimen. Changes in the ATP/inorganic phosphate signal-to-noise ratio were related to cumulative thermal descriptors.

In addition to the human patients, ten dogs with soft tissue sarcomas were studied in an analogous protocol. In this population, initial magnetic resonance parameters correlated with various thermal dose descriptors. Increases in thermal dose also resulted in decreases in high-energy phosphometabolites. These data suggest that it may be possible to prospectively predict how well a tumor will be able to be heated and the likelihood of a successful outcome with thermoradiotherapy.

EGAWA et al. (1989) have noted that post-thermoradiotherapy CT scans can predict successful outcomes in soft tissue sarcomas that are left in situ. They found that the development of a prominent hypodensity in the tumor predicted long-term tumor control. This information could be useful in determining which tumors can be spared potentially functionally debilitating surgery after treatment.

11.4.5 Thermochemotherapy for Recurrent and Advanced Sarcomas: The Goroßhadern Experience

Because of the potential to target heat delivery to deep-seated tumors, including the adjacent surrounding tissue ("tumor bed"), while simultaneously applying conventional doses of systemic combination chemotherapy, in 1986 the Klinikum Großhadern Medical Center (KGMC) started the first pilot study employing the BSD system for RHT with systemic chemotherapy (ISSELS et al. 1987).

Twelve patients with advanced deep-seated tumors (including seven retroperitoneal soft tissue sarcomas) who had shown progressive disease under conventional treatment protocols were entered in the trial. Patients with soft tissue sarcomas received 4-weekly cycles of ifosfamide (1500 mg/m^2, days 1–5) plus etoposide (100 mg/m^2, days 1, 3, 5) combined with RHT given only on days 1 and 5. In 68% of the RHT treatments for pelvic tumors, the intratumoral temperature exceeded 42.5°C with a minimum temperature of at least 40°C. Subacute toxicity and complication rate were acceptable although pain within the field of the applicator (44% of RHT treatments) was a limiting factor in achieving the prescribed 1-h treatment duration. It is of note that myelosuppression was not increased by the addition of RHT.

Following these encouraging results in regard to feasibility and toxicity, the RHT-86 protocol was activated at the KGMC as a phase II study combining ifosfamide plus etoposide with RHT in patients with locally advanced sarcomas. An interim report on 40 patients (27 pretreated with multiagent chemotherapy, and ten with surgery and/or radiation), including 25 with soft tissue sarcomas, detailed the information on histology, tumor grade, size and localization of the treated tumors, and patient history (ISSELS et al. 1990). In 38 assessable patients, the overall objective response rate was 37% [six complete responses (CRs), four partial responses (PRs), and four pathohistological responses, i.e., >50% necrosis found at the time of subsequent complete surgical resection]. More importantly, since local tumor response related to the combined treatment was defined as the endpoint for this study, comparison of the time-averaged temperature parameters (T_{20}, T_{50}, and T_{90}) of objective responders (14 patients) with those of patients showing local progressive disease under thermochemotherapy (13 patients) revealed a significant difference ($P < 0.01$). These data supported use of the combined regimen in pretreated patients with advanced sarcomas and suggested that clinical outcome was dependent upon intratumoral temperatures achieved during RHT.

An updated report (ISSELS et al. 1991) confirmed the previous results in 65 patients, including 43 with soft tissue sarcomas (mean observation time for all patients: 10.1 months). The results regarding tumor response (overall response 34%) are summarized in Table 11.3. Of the 65 patients, 40 (62%) had received ifosfamide-containing drug regimens before entering the RHT study, 17

Table 11.3. Tumor response in 65 patients entered in a phase II study of thermochemotherapy at the KGMC

Histology	No. of pts.	No. of treatments	NED	PR	NC	PD	n.e.	Alive
Soft tissue sarcoma	43	268	11	2	15	14	1	21/43
Leiomyosarcoma	11	63	1 pCR/1 FHR	1	3	4	1	5/11
Liposarcoma	9	56	1 pCR/2 FHR	1	2	2		5/9
Rhabdomyosarcoma	8	66	2 pCR/2 FHR		3	1		6/8
Malignant fibrous histiocytoma	5	32	1 FHR		3	1		2/5
Others	10	51			4	6		3/10
Ewing's sarcoma	12	82	3 pCR		7	2		6/12
Chondrosarcoma	7	54	1 pCR/1 FHR	2		1	2	3/7
Osteosarcoma	3	22	1 FHR			1	1	1/3
Total	65	426	17 pCR9 FHR8	4	22	18	4	31/65

NED, no evidence of disease; CR, complete response; PR, partial response; FHR, favorable histological response; *P*, pathohistological; n.e., not evaluable

(26%) had been pretreated by surgery and/or radiation, and eight (12%) were undergoing primary treatment. A total of 426 RHT treatments (mean 6.6 RHTs/patient) were applied, predominantly for pelvic tumors (82%). Duration of response was satisfactory; i.e., following CR the patients showed a disease-free survival of 15.6 months at the cutoff date for the analysis. Of the patients with PR and a favorable histological response, three died from metastatic and/or local disease after 4, 17, and 39 months, and one died from other disease (acute myeloid leukemia) after 27 months. The other eight patients remained stable for a mean of 14.1 months. Again, the time-averaged temperature achieved in 20%, 50%, and 90% of all the measured tumor sites differed significantly between responders and nonresponders ($P < 0.01$). The correlation of tumor response with the averaged temperatures in a given fraction of measured tumor points ($T_{\%}$ values) is shown in Fig. 11.4. By taking into account tumor temperature (T_{20}) and temperature difference or gradient as measured within the tumor ($T_{50}-T_{90}$) of each patient, this retrospective analysis allowed the correct classification of responders and nonresponders in most of the cases. An interesting observation is that the descriptors which were most predictive of treatment outcome are not in a temperature range that is known to be particularly cytotoxic (i.e., T_{20} = 41.5°C, T_{50} = 40.9°C, T_{90} = 40.0) but well in the range of thermal chemosensitization.

At the KGMC, the next study (RHT-91) was started in November 1990 for high-risk soft tissue sarcoma using *preoperative* systemic EIA

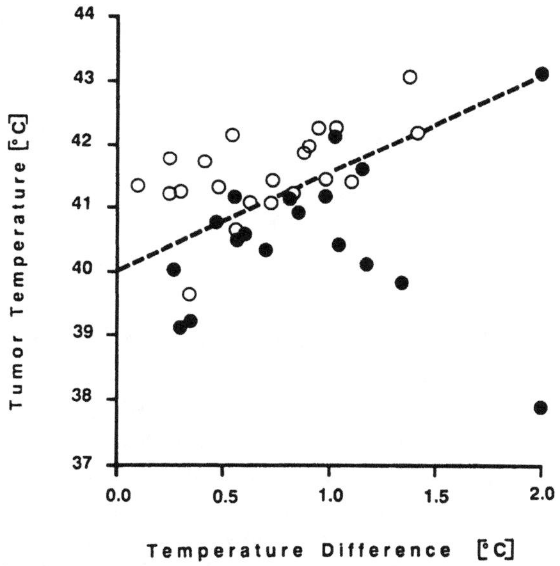

Fig. 11.4. Plot of time-averaged tumor temperature (T_{20}) versus temperature difference ($T_{50}-T_{90}$) calculated for 20%, 50%, and 90% of all measured tumor points within the tumor of each individual patient (n = 39). O, responders (n = 21); ●●, nonresponders (n = 18); *deshed line*, arbitrarily chosen to separate responders (*above*) and nonresponders (*below*)

chemotherapy combined with RHT: etoposide (125 mg/m^2, days 1 and 4), ifosfamide (1.25 g/m^2, days 1–4), Adriamycin (50 mg/m^2, day 1), and mesna (250 mg/m^2 × 3, days 1–4) with RHT given only on days 1 and 4 in repeated EIA/RHT cycles every 3 weeks. The design of the study is shown in Fig. 11.5. By definition, tumor size >8 cm, extracompartmental tumor location (group A), and recurrent disease at presentation

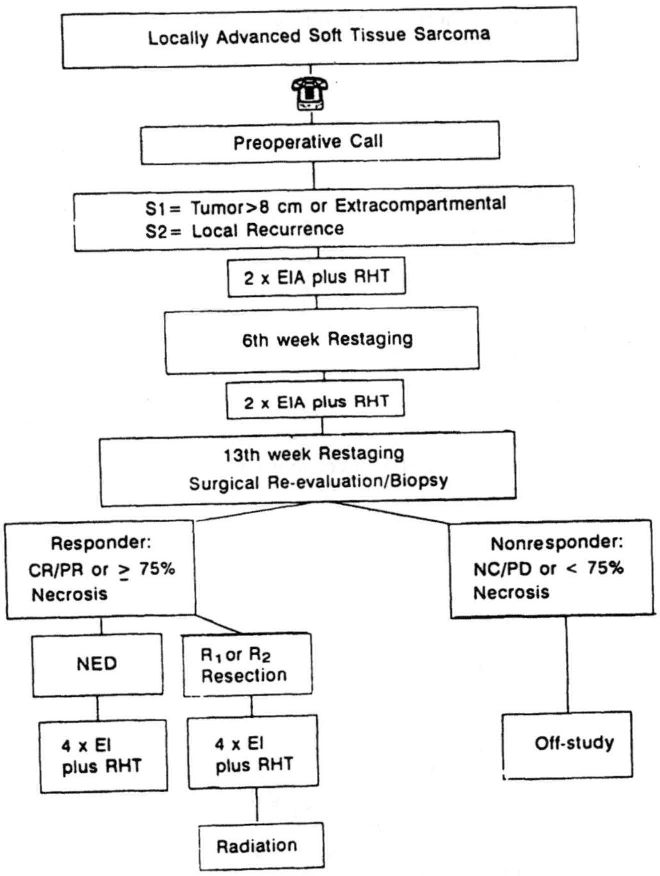

Fig. 11.5. Design of the RHT-91 study at KGMC

(group B) were considered as high-risk factors in addition to tumor grade (II or III).

Evidence that supports the use of systemic, preoperative induction chemotherapy alone to render soft tissue sarcomas resectable or to improve local control has been previously presented (Rouesse et al. 1987; Pezzi et al. 1990).

Our first experience with the RHT-91 study (Issels et al. 1993) has in the meantime been confirmed in 63 evaluable patients. Between November 1990 and November 1993 a total of 63 adults with high-risk, nonmetastatic soft tissue sarcoma were entered in this protocol. Tumor grading (55 patients had grade II or III soft tissue sarcoma), tumor size >8 cm, and extracompartmental tumor extension (28 patients) or local recurrence (35 patients) were the pretreatment high-risk factors. Thirty patients had undergone previous surgery and/or radiation, 17 had received previous multidrug chemotherapy, and 16 had received no previous treatment. A total of 440 RHT treatments were applied within the pelvic region (24 patients), trunk (10 patients), or extremities (29 patients) bearing relatively large tumors (median volume 218 cm^3).

By the cutoff date for this analysis (November 1993), 55 patients had undergone surgery after receiving two to five cycles (mean: 3.6) of EIA chemotherapy combined with RHT; all except seven tumors could be resected without amputation. In 15 patients no surgical procedure had been performed. Among the 63 evaluable patients evaluable for response, the clinical response rate is 41% [one CR, 14 PRb (partial response), 11 PRa (minor response)]. Twenty-seven patients showed stable disease (NC) and ten showed tumor progression. Pathological response to preoperative thermochemotherapy was evaluable in 48 patients, with 19 (=30%) responders having >50% histological necrosis and/or regression. In seven patients (two PRb, one PRa, four NC) a pathological CR was found at the time of surgery. Of the 63 patients, 24 relapsed within 14 months (=median time to progression). At the cutoff date, 39 patients (62%) showed no evidence of disease (median observation time = 20 months). Overall, 51 patients are alive and 12 patients have died.

11.5 Conclusion

Soft tissue sarcomas are unusual cancers that often grow to a large size and have a propensity to cause local problems. Their neovascularization pattern is often such that they are characterized by low tumor perfusion. Given this combination of large size, local invasion, and poor perfusion, they are often good candidates for thermoradiotherapy. Clinical studies have demonstrated the relatively good ability to heat these tumors and the marked tumor necrosis that frequently results from thermoradiotherapy. Soft tissue sarcomas have proved to be a good model for studying thermal dosimetry and predictive variables. The limited data available pertaining to the treatment of these tumors without subsequent resection suggest that the local control rate with thermoradiotherapy is quite good.

The clinical application of hyperthermia combined with chemotherapy also has a strong biological well-documented rationale. Clinical results using thermochemotherapy in far-advanced, either locally (surgery, radiation) or systemically (chemotherapy) pretreated patients with soft tissue sarcomas clearly indicate therapeutic activity of the combined modality in the studies referenced. Currently continuous multipoint thermometry is available, which indicates that it is not justified to speak about the tumor temperature, but rather a distribution of temperatures, which is heterogeneous not only spatially but also temporally. The time/temperature descriptors of hyperthermia treatments showing a strong correlation to treatment outcome (e.g., histopathological and clinical response) can now be tested prospectively along with other prognostic important factors in patients at risk for local or metastatic disease. As the RHT approach allows full-dose systemic standard chemotherapy combined with tumor temperature elevation, this strategy will play an important role in the preoperative treatment of soft tissue sarcomas.

11.6 Summary

- Local control of soft tissue sarcomas with conventional treatment remains problematic in large, high-grade lesions that cannot be resected with a good margin.
- Large sarcomas often have low perfusion rates, making them good candidates for hyperthermia.
- When the spatial and temporal temperature profile demonstrates good heating during a course of thermoradiotherapy, there is a high probability of complete or near complete killing of tumor cells.
- Beside improvement of local control the prevention of distant metastasis in high risk groups of patients with soft tissue sarcomas are the major goals for future multidisciplinary trials using hyperthermia combined with other treatment modalities.

References

Acker, JC, Dewhirst MW, Honore GM, Samulski TV, Tucker JA, Oleson JR (1990) Blood perfusion measurements in human tumours: evaluation of laser Doppler methods. Int J Hyperthermia 6: 287–304

Barkley JT, Martin RG, Romsdahl MM, et al. (1988) Treatment of soft tissue sarcomas by preoperative irradiation and conservative surgical resection. Int J Radiat Oncol Biol Phys 14: 693–699

Barwick WJ, Goldberg JA, Scully SP, Harrelson JM (1992) Vascularized tissue transfer for closure of irradiated wounds after soft tissue sarcoma resection. Ann Surg 216: 591–595

Beahrs HO, Henson DE, Hutter RV, et al. (1992) Staging of soft tissue sarcomas. In: Beahrs OH, Henson DE, Hutter RV, et al. (eds) Manual for the staging of cancer. American Joint Commission on Cancer, 4th edn. Lippincott, Philadelphia

Boring CB, Squires TS, Tong T (1993) Cancer statistics, 1993. CA Cancer J Clin 43: 18–19

Buatti JM, Cassady JR, Cetas TC, et al. (1990) Hyperthermia and radiation for advanced or recurrent sarcomas (abstract). 10th Annual Meeting of the NAHG

Corry PM, Jabboury K, Kong JS, et al. (1988) Evaluation of equipment for hyperthermia treatment of cancer. Int J Hyperthermia 4: 53–74

Costa J, Wesley RA, Glatstein EJ, et al. (1984) The grading of soft tissue sarcomas. Results of a clinicohistopathological correlation in a series of 163 cases. Cancer 53: 530–541

Dewhirst MW, Sostman HD, Leopold KA, et al. (1990) Soft-tissue sarcomas: MR imaging and MR spectroscopy for prognosis and therapy monitoring. Work in progress. Radiology 174: 847–853

Egawa S, Tsukiyama I, Kajiura Y, et al. (1989) Characteristics of the response of soft tissue sarcoma to hyperthermia: the correlation between temperature distribution, radiological examination and histology. Int J Hyperthermia 5: 23–35

Gerner RE, Moore GE, Pickren JW (1975) Soft tissue sarcomas. Ann Surg 181: 803–808

Gibbs FA (1983) "Thermal mapping" in experimental cancer treatment with hyperthermia: description and use of a semiautomatic system. Int J Radiat Oncol Biol Phys 9: 1057–1063

Issels RD, Wadepohl M, Tilling K, et al. (1987) Regional hyperthermia combined with systemic chemotherapy in advanced abdominal and pelvic tumors: first results of a pilot study employing an annular phased array applicator. Recent Results. Cancer Res 107: 236–243

Issels RD, Prenninger SW, Nagele A, et al. (1990) Ifosfamide plus etoposide combined with regional hyperthermia in patients with locally advanced sarcomas: a phase II study. J Clin Oncol 8: 1818–1829

Issels RD, Mittermüller J, Gerl A, et al. (1991) Improvement of local control regional hyperthermia combined with systemic chemotherapy (ifosfamide plus etoposide) in advanced sarcomas: updated report on 65 patients. J Cancer Res Clin Oncol 117 (suppl IV): s141–s147

Issels RD, Bosse D, Abdel-Rahman S, et al. (1993) Preoperative systemic EIA chemotherapy (etoposide + ifosfamide + adriamycin) combined with regional hyperthermia in high-risk sarcoma: a pilot study. Cancer Chemother Pharmacol 31: 233–237

Jabboury K, Corry P, Plager C, Benjamin R (1987) Hyperthermia induction in sarcoma (abstract). Proc Ann Meet Am Assoc Cancer Res 28: 222

Lack EE, Steinberg SM, White DE, Kinsella T, Glatstein E, Chang AE, Rosenberg SA (1989) Extremity soft tissue sarcomas: analysis of prognostic variables in 300 cases and evaluation of tumor necrosis as a factor in stratifying higher-grade sarcomas. J Surg Oncol 41: 263–273

Leopold KA, harrelson J, Prosnitz L, Samulski TV, Dewhirst MW, Oleson JR (1989) Preoperative hyperthermia and radiation for soft tissue sarcomas: advantage of two vs one hyperthermia treatments per week. Int J Radiat Oncol Biol Phys 16: 107–115

Leopold KA, Dewhirst MW, Samulski TV, et al. (1992) Relationships among tumor temperature, treatment time, and histopathological outcome using preoperative hyperthermia with radiation in soft tissue sarcomas. Int J Radiat Oncol Biol Phys 22: 989–998

Leopold KA, Dewhirst MW, Samulski TV, Oleson JR, et al. (1993) Cumulative minutes with T_{90} greater than $TemP_{index}$ is predictive of response of superficial malignancies to hyperthermia and radiation. Int J Radiat Oncol Biol Phys 25: 841–847

Lindberg RD (1980) Soft tissue sarcoma. In: Fletcher GH (ed) Textbook of radiotherapy, 3rd edn. Lea & Febiger, Philadelphia, pp 922–942

Lindberg RD, Martin RG, Romsdahl MM, Barkley HT (1981) Conservative surgery and postoperative radiotherapy in 300 adults with soft tissue sarcomas. Cancer 47: 2391–2397

Mandard AM, Petiot JF, Marnay J, et al. (1989) Prognostic factors in soft tissue sarcomas. A multivariate analysis of 109 cases. Cancer: 63: 1437–1451

Markhede G, Angervall L, Stener B (1982) A multivariate analysis of the prognosis after surgical treatment of malignant soft tissue tumors. Cancer 49: 1721–1733

Meyer JL, Kapp DS, Fessenden P, et al. (1989) Hyperthermic oncology: current biology, physics and clinical results. Pharmacol. Ther 42: 251–288

Pezzi CM, Pollock RE, Evans HL, et al. (1990) preoperative chemotherapy for soft-tissue sarcomas of the extremities. Ann Surg 4: 476–481

Potter DA, Glenn J, Kinsella T (1985) Patterns of recurrence in patients with high grade soft tissue sarcomas. J Clin Oncol 3: 353–366

Prescott DM, Charles HC, Sostman HD, Leopold KA, Dewhirst MW, et al. (1994) Therapy monitoring in human and canine soft tissue sarcomas using magnetic resonance imaging and spectroscopy. Int J Radiat Oncol Biol Phys 15: 28(2): 415–423

Reddy NM, Maithreyan V, Vasanthan A, et al. (1987) Local RF capacitive hyperthermia: thermal profiles and tumour response. Int J Hyperthermia 3: 379–387

Rollo J, Rozenbom CV, Thawley S, et al. (1981) Squamous carcinoma of the base of the tongue: a clinicopathologic study of 81 cases. Cancer 47: 333–342

Rouesse JG, Friedmann S, Sevin DM, et al. (1987) Preoperative chemotherapy in the treatment of locally advanced soft tissue sarcomas. Cancer 60: 296–300

Samulski TV, Kapp DS, Fessenden P, et al. (1987) Heating deep seated eccentrically located tumors with an annular phased array system: a comparative clinical study using two annular phased array operating configurations. Int J Radiat Oncol Biol Phys 13: 83–94

Sapozink MD, Gibbs FA, Egger MJ, et al. (1986) Regional hyperthermia for clinical advanced deep-seated pelvic malignancy. Am J Clin Oncol 9: 162–169

Sapozink MD, Corry PM, Kapp DS, et al. (1991) RTOG quality assurance guidelines for clinical trials using hyperthermia for deep-seated malignancy. Int J Radiat Oncol Biol Phys 20: 1109–1115

Simon M, Enneking WF (1976) The management of soft tissue sarcomas of the extremities. J Bone Joint Surg [AM] 58: 317

Strohbehn JW, Curtis EH, Paulsen KD, Yuan XC, Lynch DR (1989) Optimization of the absorbed power distribution for an annular phased array hyperthermia system. Int J Radiat Oncol Biol Physics 16: 589–599

Suit HD, Mankin HJ, Wood WC (1988) Treatment of the patient with stage M_0 soft tissue sarcoma. J Clin Oncol 6: 854–862

Tepper JE, Suit HD (1985) Radiation therapy of soft tissue sarcomas. Cancer 55: 2273–2277

Trojani M, Contesso G, Coindre JM, et al. (1984) Soft tissue sarcomas of adults. Study of pathological prognostic variables and definition of a histopathological grading system. Int J Cancer 33: 37–42

Turner PF (1984) Regional Hyperthermia with an annular phased array. IEEE Trans Biomed Eng 31: 106–114

Yang JC, Rosenberg SA, Glatstein EJ, Antman KH (1993) Sarcomas of soft tissues. In: Devita VT Jr, Hellamn S, Rosenberg SA (eds) Cancer: principles and practice of oncology, 4th edn. Lippincott, Philadelphia, pp 1436–1488

Zhou L, Fessenden P (1993) Automation of temperature control for large-array microwave surface applicators. Int J Hyperthermia 9: 479–490

12 Thermoradiotherapy for Brain Tumors

P.K. SNEED and B. STEA

CONTENTS

12.1 Introduction

There has been much interest in using thermoradiotherapy in the treatment of primary brain tumors because patients treated conventionally have a poor prognosis despite a wide variety of treatment approaches (DAVIS 1989; NELSON et al. 1986) and because local disease progression is the predominant pattern of failure (BASHIR et al. 1988; GASPAR et al. 1992; HOCHBERG and PRUITT 1980; LIANG et al. 1991; WALLNER et al. 1989), even in patients undergoing aggressive treatment including an interstitial brain implant boost (AGBI et al. 1992).

For at least two decades, it has been hypothesized that adjuvant hyperthermia combined with radiation and/or chemotherapy will result in improved local tumor control and survival of patients with malignant brain tumors. Over the same period, numerous experiments and clinical trials have been performed to test this hypothesis, recently with improved equipment and promising results. This chapter will review pertinent in vitro studies, experiments in animal tumor models, heating techniques, toxicity studies in normal brain, and clinical trials. New directions will be discussed and conclusions will be drawn.

P.K. SNEED, MD, Department of Radiation Oncology, University of California, San Francisco, CA 94143-0226, USA

B. STEA, MD, PhD, Department of Radiation Oncology, University of Arizaona Health Sciences Center, Tucson, AZ 85724, USA

12.2 In Vitro Studies

Many investigators have evaluated the *sensitivity of brain tumor cell lines* to hyperthermia alone and to various combinations of heat, chemotherapy, and radiation. One of the first reports on the thermal sensitivity of human glioma cells in vitro came from GERWECK and RICHARDS (1981).

DASILVA et al. (1987) reported that hyperthermia treatment with 42°C for 60 min increased the cytotoxicity of various chemotherapeutic agents against a human glioblastoma cell line (U-87MG) in tissue culture. Thermal enhancement ratios of 1.1, 1.6, 2.0, and 2.8 were observed for spirohydantoin mustard, 1,3-bis-(2-chloroethyl)-1-nitrosourea (BCNU), cisplatin, and 2,5-diaziridinyl-3, 6-bis[carboxethoxyamino]-1,4-benzoquinone, respectively.

TANAKA et al. (1986) also studied the effects of heat and chemotherapy on a human glioblastoma cell line (SKMG1) and on three rat malignant brain tumor cell lines (T9, EB 679, and TR 481). Treatments given included heat alone (42°C for 1 h), drug alone (1 h), and hyperthermia 42°C for 1 h) before, after, or during 1-h drug exposures to Nimustine (ACNU), Aclarubicin (ACR); or cisplatin. Cytotoxicity was greatest for simultaneous hyperthermia and ACNU, ACR, or cisplatin chemotherapy.

WATANABE et al. (1992) studied the sensitivity of a human malignant glioma cell line (NP-2) to simultaneous hyperthermia and ACNU, Adriamycin, bleomycin, cisplatin, mitomycin C, or vincristine chemotherapy, under both oxygenated and chronically hypoxic conditions. ACNU had similar cytotoxicity under both euoxic and hypoxic conditions. Adrimaycin and mitomycin C were preferentially cytotoxic to hypoxic cells, at 37°C, 42°C for 1 h, and 43°C, and synergism with hyperthermia was observed under both euoxic and hypoxic conditions. Bleomycin, cisplatin, and vincristine were more cytotoxic to oxygenated cells, both at 37°C and at elevated temperatures. Synergism was observed between cisplatin and hyperthermia in oxygenated cells. It was concluded that hyperthermia combined with Adriamycin or mitomycin C may have enhanced efficacy against the hypoxic cell subpopulation within malignant gliomas.

In vitro response to hyperthermia (44°C for 30 min), radiation (5 Gy), BCNU, and cisplatin was studied in a human glioblastoma call line (U-87MG) and in transplantable canine brain tumor (CBT) cells by SALCMAN and EBERT (1991). Hyperthermia was administered immediately before or immediately after radiation and/or chemotherapy, or concurrent with cisplatin exposure. All combinations of radiation, hyperthermia, and BCNU enhanced cell killing, generally with additive effects. Sequencing of cisplatin and hyperthermia had no effect in these experiments. The combination of hyperthermia and cisplatin produced additive effects in the U-87MG cell line and synergistic effects in CBT cells. It was concluded that hyperthermia may be an effective potentiator of radiation and chemotherapy for gliomas.

RAAPHORST et al. (1991) reported on thermal sensitivity and thermal radiosensitization in three human glioma cell lines with a large capacity for recovery from potentially lethal radiation damage (U-87MG, U-138MG, and U-373MG). Cells grown in plastic tissue culture flasks were irradiated with 2, 4, 6, or 8 Gy at 1.3 Gy/min and sealed with paraffin for water-bath heating. Thermal radiosensitizaiton occurred for hyperthermia given either before or after irradiation and the degree of thermal radiosensitization depended on duration of the heat exposure and on temperature. Complete inhibition of repair of potentially lethal damage occurred with 45°C for 60 min.

It has also been reported that hyperthermia (40° or 43°C for 60 min) enhanced the antitumor effect of recombinant murine interferon-β against Rous sarcoma virus-induced mouse malignant glioma cells both in vitro and in vivo after subcutaneous transplantation of the glioma cells into the hind legs of mice (KUROKI et al. 1987).

12.3 In Vivo Studies

As an extension of the in vitro work, tumors were produced in laboratory animals by implanting or inoculating tumor cells for *hyperthermia experiments in vivo*. KOBAYASHI et al. (1986) heated cutaneous tumors in rats produced by inoculation of rat gliosarcoma (T9) cells. Tumors completely disappeared within 4 weeks after treatment with 45°C for 60 min using magnetic-induction heating of a ferromagnetic implant. In subsequent experiments by the same group, T9 glioma cells were inoculated intracerebrally into rats and then heated 10 days later for 30 min with a 45°C ferromagnetic implant. Heated animals had significantly prolonged survival in comparison with untreated control animals (KOBAYASHI et al. 1989).

Combined hyperthermia and chemotherapy were evaluated in the BT_4A rat brain tumor implanted in the hind legs of rats (DAHL and MELLA 1982; MELLA and DAHL 1985). Tumors were treated with water-bath heating at 44°C for 60 min and/or bleomycin or BCNU. Tumors which could not be controlled by any single modality disappeared completely when hyperthermia was combined with either drug (MELLA and DAHL 1985). In later experiments, hind leg tumors were produced in rats by transplantation of BT_4T or BT_4An tumors and treated with locally applied water-bath hyperthermia (44°C for 45 min), BCNU, or both, with or without prior administration of a glucose load to reduce intratumoral pH (SCHEM et al. 1989). Glucose reduced the effect of BCNU alone and failed to enhance the effect of hyperthermia alone, but markedly enhanced the antitumor effect of combined BCNU and hyperthermia. The same group also demonstrated thermal enhancement of both cisplatin and carboplatin against BT_4A or BT_4An tumors in the hind legs of rats (SCHEM et al. 1992).

TANAKA et al. (1989a) implanted VX2 carcinoma cells intracerebrally into 28 Japanese white rabbits. The animals were treated 7 days later with hyperthermia alone for 30 min (by thermal conduction from a 45°C ferromagnetic implant), intravenous ACNU chemotherapy alone, or combined ACNU and hyperthermia. Significant prolongation of survival was noted for both single-treatment groups, but the longest survival was achieved with combination therapy.

SCHEM and DAHL (1991) studied thermochemotherapy with ACNU in a rat model. Subcutaneous hind leg tumors from the BT_4An malignant rat brain glioma cell line underwent water-bath heating to 44°C for 45 min with or without intraperitoneal ACNU. The effect of pretreatment administration of a glucose load to lower tumor pH was also studied. Treatment with ACNU and hyperthermia after glucose was more effective than ACNU and hyperthermia without glucose, which was more effective than hyperthermia alone. Tumor growth was not affected by ACNU alone or by ACNU after glucose administration.

TAMURA et al. (1988, 1989) performed intracerebral inoculation of G-XII glioma tissue into 6-to 8-week-old rats. They studied survival, histopathological changes, and bromodeoxyuridine (BUdR) labelling of tumor after treatment with radiation alone (8 Gy in one fraction to the whole head), hyperthermia alone (44° or 45°C at the surface of a single 2450-MHz antenna for 30 min), or both. Combined hyperthermia and radiation produced longer survival and additive histological changes and tumor cell growth suppression.

12.4 Brain Heating Methods

Ingeneral, brain heating methods may be classified as *external* or *interstitial* (Table 12.1). Three external heating methods include radiofrequency capacitive heating, scanned focused ultrasound, and a small experience with magnetic-loop induction heating using the "Magnetrode." Radiofrequency capacitive heating at 8 to 27 MHz requires bilateral craniectomies for application of large disc-shaped electrodes to both sides of the brain and also has the disadvantage of heating intervening normal brain tissue. Scanned focused ultrasound requires an ipsilateral craniectomy with a margin of at least 1.5 cm around the underlying tumor but makes possible selective tumor heating.

Interstitial hyperthermia involves probes placed directly into the tissue which heat the tissue by radiating an electromagnetic field (as for microwave antennas), by resistive heating as current is passed between pairs of electrodes (as in radiofrequency localized current field technique), or by thermal conduction from hot sources such as heated probes or inductively heated ferromagnetic seeds. Interstitial ultrasound applicators are also under development.

An advantage of microwave antennas is that wider spacing is possible (about 1.5–1.8 cm) and fewer probes are needed to successfully heat tumors. Cooled antennas have been shown to produce more uniform heating than antennas without cooling (MORIYAMA et al. 1988). Though the heating patterns are less predictable than for hot source techniques, the heating patterns of two different microwave antenna designs (helical coil and dipole) have been described in detail and compared for various heating lengths and insertion depths (MECHLING and STROHBEHN 1992; RYAN et al. 1991).

Table 12.1. Brain heating methods: advantages and disadvantages

Heating method	Advantages	Disadvantages
External		
Radiofrequency capacitive heating	–	Requires bilateral craniectomies
Scanned focused ultrasound	Precise localization	Requires ipsilateral craniectomy
Magnetic loop induction	–	Poorly localized heating
Interstitial		
Microwave antennas	Fewer heating sources required	Harder to thermally model
Radiofrequency localized current field electrodes	Good two dimensional control of power deposition	Intermediate number of heating sources required; often no longitudinal control
Radiofrequency capacitively coupled electrodes	Independent power control over each probe and longitudinal control	Intermediate number of heating sources required; undesired current paths possible
Hot sources (ferromagnetic seeds, resistively heated probes, hot water tubes, laser)	Easy to thermally model	More heating sources required
Interstitial ultrasound probes	Excellent control over heating expected	System not commercially available

Hot source techniques generally require closer probe spacing than microwave antennas, on the order of 1.0 cm, but have the advantage of much more predictable and controllable heating (Babbs et al. 1990; DeFord et al. 1990, 1991). With inductively heated ferromagnetic seeds, heating of the implanted tissues is based on the absorption of energy by the ferromagnetic seeds from an externally applied radiofrequency magnetic field. Due to the thermally regulating nature of the seeds, there is no danger of overheating the tissues since the power absorption efficientcy of the seeds drops off rapidly as they approach their Curie point (Hadier et al. 1991). The heated seeds then raise the temperature of the surrounding tissues by thermal conduction. The final temperature achieved in tissues depends on the Curie point of the seeds (a function of alloy composition), the seed spacing, the strength of the applied magnetic field, and, as in the case of other hot source techniques, also on the level of blood flow. A novel hot source technique involves steering of an externally heated metallic sphere or cylinder throughout the target volume by means of magnetic manipulation, with fluoroscopic monitoring (Grady et al. 1989; Molloy et al. 1990, 1991).

In addition, Nd: YAG laser "hyperthermia" has been described by multiple authors. In some cases, the laser was used to induce edge tumor temperatures in the range of 41°–45°C (Nowak et al. 1990; Roux et al. 1992; Sugiyama et al. 1990), whereas very high temperatures were described by other authors (Ascher et al. 1991; Bettag et al. 1991).

12.5 Animal Brain Toxicity Studies

Experiments have been performed in rats, rabbits, cats, and dogs to assess *thermal tolerance of normal brain tissue* (Table 12.2). Electrophysiological studies performed by Harris et al. (1962) with hemispheric heating of dog brain demonstrated significant slowing in the electroencephalogram with a temperature of 43°C for 30 min, disappearance of visual evoked response with temperatures of 43°–46°C for 10 min, and death within 36 h with associated edema and focal hemorrhage and infarction after heating to 44°C for 30 min. Using whole-body heating, other investigators reported increased latency and decreased amplitude of visual, somatosensory, and brainstem auditory evoked response with brain temperatures of 41.0°–42.5°C in cats (Britt et al. 1984a) and deterioration of electroencephalogram and somatosensory evoked potentials with a brain temperature of 44°C in rabbits (Yamada et al. 1985).

Silberman et al. (1982) performed brain hyperthermia in New Zealand white rabbits using an externally applied field from a magnetic-loop applictor ("Magnetrode"). Rabbits survived brain hyperthermia temperatures of 42°–44°C for 1 h but died within minutes of reaching brain temperatures of 45°C.

Moriyama et al. (1991) observed breakdown of the blood-brain barrier in rat brain heated with 2450-MHz microwave antennas to 44.3°C for 30 min or 42.5°C for 60 min.

Using ultrasound to heat normal cat brain for 50 min and interstitial microwave antennas to heat normal dog brain for periods of 50–70 min, Britt and Lyons (Britt et al. 1984b; Lyons et al. 1984) demonstrated a threshold for neuronal damage between 42.2° and 42.5°C, neuronal cell lysis and cerebral edema at 43.0°C, disruption of deep white matter tracts at 43.0°–43.5°C, and complete lysis and disappearance of neurons at 45°C.

Sneed et al. (1986) estimated the threshold for cerebral necrosis to be 44°C for 30 min using interstitial microwave antennas to heat normal dog brain. Fike et al. (1991) also performed interstitial microwave antenna hyperthermia in dogs, heating to 40°, 41°, 42°, 43°, 43.5°, and 44°C for 30 min at a reference points 5 mm from the antenna junction. Maximal changes were observed at 1 week. Computed tomography (CT) scans and histopathological examination revealed a radiolucent area of necrosis with a thin rim of contrast enhancement representing reactive changes including endothelial cell proliferation. The threshold for brain necrosis was 43.9° ± 1.5°C (mean ± standard deviation) and the threshold for contrast enhancement was 40.3° ± 1.0°C (Fike et al. 1991).

Hoopes et al. (1990) used CT, magnetic resonance (MR) imaging, and histopathological examination to assess thermal damage in nomral brains in dogs heated with interstitial microwave antennas for 30, 45, or 60 min. Breakdown of the blood-brain barrier occurred at 42.8° ± 0.27°C (mean ± standard error) for 30 min, 42.4° ± 0.20°C for 45 min, or 42.4° ± 0.04°C for 60 min, and necrosis occurred at 44.3° ± 0.29°C for 30 min, 43.4° ± 0.34°C for 45 min, or 42.8° ± 0.40°C for 60 min.

Table 12.2. Animal brain hyperthermia toxicity experiments

First author	Year	Model: effect	Threshold
HARRIS	1962	Hemispheric heating of dog brain:	
		Slowing in electroencephalogram	43°C × 30 min
		Disappearance of visual evoked response	43°–46°C × 10 min
		Death at ≤36 h with edema and focal hemorrhage and infarction	44°C × 30 min
BRITT	1984a	Whole-body heating in cats:	
		Increased latency and decreased amplitude of visual, somatosensory, and brainstem auditory evoked response	41.0°–42.5°C (brain temperature)
YAMADA	1985	Whole-body heating in rabbits:	
		Deterioration of electroencephalogram and somatosensory evoked potentials	44°C (brain temperature)
SILBERMAN	1982	Magnetic-loop whole-brain heating in rabbits:	
		Death within several minutes	45°C (brain temperature)
MORIYAMA	1991	Interstitial microwave heating in rat brain:	44.3°C × 30 min or
		Breakdown of blood-brain barrier in rat brain	42.5°C × 60 min
BRITT	1984b	Ultrasound heating in cat brain:	
		Neuronal pyknosis	42.5°C × 50 min
		White matter edema and partial loss of gray matter neurons	43°C × 50 min
		Complete lysis and disappearance of neurons	45°C × 50 min
LYONS	1984	Interstitial microwave heating in dog brain:	
		White matter edema	42°C × 50–70 min
		Pyknotic cortical neurons and cerebral edema	43°C × 50–70 min
		Neuronal cell lysis	43°C × 50–70 min
		Disruption of white matter tracts	43.0–43.5°C × 50–70 min
SNEED	1986	Interstitial microwave heating in dog brain:	
		Cerebral necrosis	44°C × 30 min
FIKE	1991	Interstitial microwave heating in dog brain:	
		Contrast enhancement on CT	40.3° ± 10°C × 30 min
		Cerebral necrosis	43.9° ± 1.5°C × 30 min
HOOPES	1990	Interstitial microwave heating in dog brain:	
		Breakdown of the blood-brain barrier on MR imaging	42.8° ± 0.27°C × 30 min, or
			42.4° ± 0.20°C × 45 min, or
			42.4° ± 0.04°C × 60 min
		Cerebral necrosis	44.3° ± 0.29°C × 30 min, or
			43.4° ± 0.34°C × 45 min, or
			42.8° ± 0.40°C × 60 min

12.6 Human Brain Hyperthermia Trials

Numerous human studies of brain hyperthermia have been reported over the last two decades involving a wide variety of heating techniques (BOROK et al. 1988; COUGHLIN 1989; CUMMINS and McINTOSH 1976; GUTHKELCH et al. 1991; HEPPNER 1982, 1986; KOBAYASHI and KIDA 1992; KOBAYASHI et al. 1991; MARCHOSKY et al. 1990a,b; MATSUMOTO et al. 1992; ROBERTS et al. 1986, 1989; SALCMAN and SAMARAS 1983; SILBERMAN et al. 1985, 1986; SNEED et al. 1991, 1992; STEA et al. 1990, 1992; TANAKA et al. 1987, 1989; WEN and DAHELE 1984; WEN et al. 1988; WINTER et al. 1985; YOKOTE et al. 1990) (Table 12.3). Reports of clinical studies of brain hyperthermia date back to at least 1971 when SUTTON heated 7 brain tumors for periods of 7–40 h by thermal conduction from a single probe heated to 42.0°C, with or without intravenous or intratumoral chemotherapy, followed by surgical resection. Necrosis was noted around the heated probe with unaffected tumor tissue peripherally (SUTTON 1971). Like Sutton, most early investigators of brain hyperthermia had relatvely crude heating and thermometry methods available to them.

In 1986, Roberts et al. reported the first clinical brain hyperthermia trial with sophisticated heating and multipoint thermometry. Arrays of four to six 915-MHz or 2450-MHz interstitial microwave

Table 12.3. Clinical brain hyperthermia trials

First author	Year	No. of pts./Dx	Heating method	Thermometry sites	Results
SUTTON	1971, 1984	18 MG	Intraoperative heating with single heated probe	Heating probe only	–
CUMMINS	1976	5 MG	Heating of carotid arterial blood	Carotid arterial blood	2 deaths within 48 h; 1 patient survived 5 months; 2 patients alive at 5–10 months
HEPPNER	1982, 1986	85 GM	Electromagnetic heating of metallic powder lining surgical resection bed	Surface of tumor bed	–
SALCMAN	1983	6 MG	Single interstitial 2450 MHz microwave antenna used for 3 hyperthermia sessions	Antenna	4 of 6 patients survived at least 18 months after treatment
WEN	1984, 1988	6 Gr. I 8 Gr. II 4 Gr. II 4 Gr. IV 2 oligo. 1 epend.	Intraoperative heating of resection cavity with 2450-MHz microwave antenna	Surface of tumor bed	11 patients died at 2 days to 40 months; 14 patients were alive at 21 to 41 months
SILBERMAN	1985, 1986	13 met. or MG	External magnetic-loop induction heating	Single intratumoral point and single brain point	–
WINTER/BOROK	1985/1988	21 MG	One or more interstitial 2450-MHz microwave antennas	Antenna	–
ROBERTS	1986, 1989	18 MG	4–6 interstitial 915- or 2450-MHz microwave antennas + brachytheray ± EBRT	Antenna, tumor, and brain	–
YOKOTE	1990	2 GM 5 AA 8 met.	Radiofrequency localized-current field heating ± MCNU	Heating electrode and several points in tumor	9 patients died at 1–10 months; 6 patients alive at 5–19 months
TANAKA	1987, 1989	17 GM	External 13.56 MHz radiofrequency capactive heating via bilateral craniectomies + EBRT + ACNU	Multiple tumor and brain sites	8 of 15 evaluable tumors showed regression on CT
GUTHKELCH	1991	13 GM 2 AA	Scanned focused ultrasound via craniectomy site + EBRT	Multiple points within 2–4 thermometry catheters	Survival 29–57 weeks for newly diagnosed gliomas and 2–50 weeks for recurrent gliomas; 2 patients alive
MARCHOSKY	1990	33 GM 9 AA 8 met.	Thermal conductive heating from multiple interstitial probes without brachytherapy or EBRT	Heating probes and sites within tumor	Median survival 22 weeks after 1st hyperthermia
KOBAYASHI	1991, 1992	24 MG 8 met. 3 other	Inductively heated ferromagnetic implants + EBRT	One point at ferroseed and one point in tumor	4 complete responses and 7 partial responses
STEA	1990, 1992	19 GM 9 AA	Inductively heated ferromagnetic implants	Multiple points within 3–5 thermometry catheters	Median survival 5.8 months after treatment for recurrent gliomas; 14.9 months after diagnosis for GM
SNEED	1991, 1992	25 GM 16 AA 7 met.	1–6 interstitial 915- or 2450-MHz microwave antennas	Multiple points within 1–3 thermometry catheters	Median survival 49 weeks after treatment for recurrent GM; 140 weeks for recurrent AA

MG, malignant glioma; GM, glioblastoma multiforme; Gr., grade (glioma); oligo., oligodendroglioma; epend., ependymoma; met., metastasis; AA, anaplastic astrocytoma; EBRT, extermal beam radiotherapy; ACNU, Nimustine

antennas were used to heat malignant gliomas for 60 min immediately before and after brachytherapy with iridium-192 delivering 60 Gy (followed by external beam radiotherapy in newly diagnosed tumors). Temperatures were mapped along each antenna catheter and along an additional orthogonal dedicated thermometry catheter. Among 18 patients treated, complications included four cases of permanent worsening of neurological deficit, three transient neurological deficits, one case requiring immediate debulking for swelling, one cerebrospinal fluid leak, one case of meningitis, and one deep venous thrombosis (COUGHLIN 1989; ROBERTS et al. 1986, 1989). A subsequent report from the same institution described temperatures achieved in 23 patients who underwent brain hyperthermia. Minimum tumor temperatures ranged from 37.2° to 44.3°C and maximum tumor temperatures from 46.5° to 60.1°C. Seventy-one percent of all tumor temperatures reached the goal of at least 43°C (RYAN et al. 1992).

Radiofrequency localized-current-field hyperthermia was used to heat 21 metastatic brain tumors and seven deep-seated malignant gliomas less than 30 mm in diameter in 15 patients (YOKOTE et al. 1990). The heating electrode size ranged from 2 to 4 mm and temperature ranged from 60° to 80°C for 2–5 min (short-term high-temperature hyperthermia).

TANAKA et al. (1987, 1989b) treated 17 patients with newly diagnosed or recurrent glioblastoma using 13.56-MHz radiofrequency capacitive heating with cooled radiofrequency applicators 6 or 9 cm in diameter applied directly to the brain intraoperatively or to the scalp over bilateral craniectomies postoperatively. Tumors were heated for 60 min twice weekly for a total of four to ten sessions in combination with external beam radiotherapy (20–50 Gy) and ACNU chemotherapy. Tumor temperatures ranging from 40° to 46°C were attained while limiting normal brain temperatures to 38°–42°C and scalp temperatures to 28°–35°C.

GUTHKELCH et al. (1991) treated ten recurrent glioblastomas, three newly diagnosed glioblastomas, and two newly diagnosed anaplastic astrocytomas with external beam radiotherapy (45–65 Gy for initial tumors and 10–40 Gy for recurrences) and 2- to 4-weekly scanned focused ultrasound treatments for 15, 30, 45, or 60 min through a craniectomy site. Intratumoral temperatures were measured with thermocouples within two to four thermometry catheters. For the best hyperthermia treatment in each patient, minimum tumor temperatures ranged from 37.3° to 42.7°C and maximum tumor temperatures ranged from 41.1° to 45.9°C. Survival ranged from 29 to 57 weeks from diagnosis for initial tumors and 2 to 50 weeks from the end of treatment for recurrences. Two patients were living at last follow-up.

MARCHOSKY et al. (1990a,b) developed a hot-source technique for long-duration hyperthermia using 2.2-mm diameter electrically resistive catheters implanted stereotactically 1.5 cm apart from each other through a template guide in a CT suite under general anesthesia. Computer-control algorithms used catheter power levels and catheter temperature measurements to predict minimum tumor temperature in the region of each catheter in real time and to adjust applied power accordingly (BABBS et al. 1990; DEFORD et al. 1990, 1991). Typically, a complete 96-h treatment cycle consisted of 72 h of heating, given during 3 of every 4 h (i.e., with a 1-h break after every 3 h). Experience was analyzed in 50 patients with recurrent malignant brain tumors treated with hyperthermia alone using this technique (MARCHOSKY et al. 1990a). The average age was 46.5 years (range 16–69 years). Thirty-three of the patients had glioblastoma multiforme (GM), nine had anaplastic astrocytoma (AA), and eight had metastatic tumors. Intratumoral temperatures were not published. For 133 treatments delivered, reported toxicity included generalized seizures in eight patients, focal seizures in 12, mass effect requiring craniotomy for debulking in five, increased intracranial pressure requiring ventriculostomies in two, deep venous thrombosis and/or pulmonary embolism in nine, minimal hemorrhage in 15, major hemorrhage in four, scalp infections in three, and meningitis in one. There was one death from myocardial infarction. The median duration of survival for the whole group measured from the first hyperthermia treatment was 22 weeks.

KOBAYASHI et al. (1991), KOBAYASHI and KIDA (1992) described a series of 42 patients with newly diagnosed or recurrent malignant brain tumors treated with external beam radiotherapy and one to four inductively heated 1.8-mm-diameter, 15-to 20-mm-long ferromagnetic implants placed stereotactically or at craniotomy. Implants were heated two to three times weekly for 60 min using an externally applied magnetic field. Up to 52 hyperthermia treatments were administered, using temperature monitoring at one point within tumor and at one point on a ferromagnetic implant. Tumor temperature 10 mm from the implant ranged from 42° to 46°C. Among 35 evaluable patients, 13 had cortical malignant gliomas, 11 had basal ganglia or thalamic gliomas, eight had a single brain metastasis, and three had other brain tumors. Four complete responses and seven partial responses were observed.

Stea et al. (1990, 1992) performed a phase I study of interstitial irradiation and interstitial hyperthermia by means of inductively heated ferromagnetic implants in adults with newly diagnosed or recurrent supratentorial GM or AA. Patients with preivously untreated tumors underwent external beam radiotherapy (40–54 Gy at 1.8–2.0 Gy per fraction, 5 days per week) prior to brachytherapy. Multiple afterloading plastic catheters spaced at 1.2-cm intervals were implanted stereotactically through a template guide and three to five additional catheters were implanted for thermometry. The target volume for thermoradiotherapy included a margin of up to 1.5 cm beyond the contrast-enhancing tumor edge. Interstitial hyperthermia was given for 60 min immediately before and after brachytherapy (13.9–50 Gy using iridium-192).

A temperature of at least 42°C was attained in 61% of core sensors (>5 mm inside the edge of the implant volume), 35% of peripheral sensors (in the outer 5 mm zone of the implant), and only 3.5% of normal tissue sensors. Among the 29 patients entered on the trial, there was one fatal complication, three major complicaitons (hydrocephalus from edema, pneumoencephalos, and intracranial hemorrhage), six focal seizures, four cases of transient brain edema and neurological deficits, and one case of increased arm weakness. A total of 28 patients underwent hyperthermia, with a median age of 44 years (range 21–79 years) and a median Karnofsky performance score (KPS) of 90 (range 50–90). There were 15 patients with primary (newly diagnosed) GM, four with recurrent GM, seven with primary AA, and two with recurrent AA. The median survival was 14.9 months from diagnosis for all 19 patients with GM (Fig. 12.1) and 5.8 months from thermoradiotherapy for all patients with recurrent tumors. It was concluded that interstitial ferromagnetic brain hyperthermia was feasible and

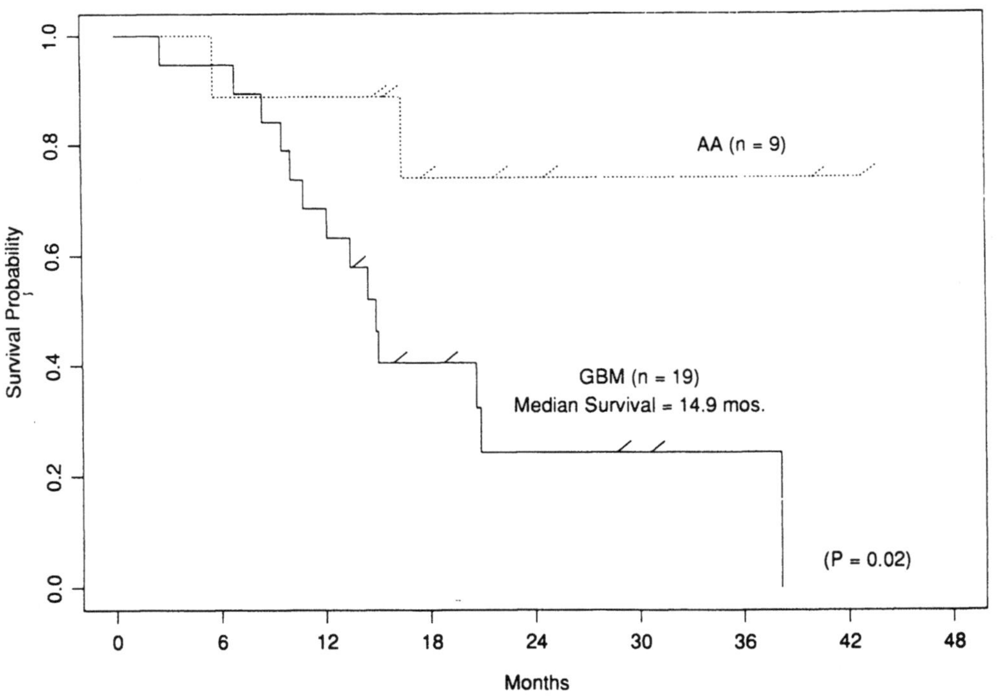

Fig. 12.1. Kaplan-Meier representation of the probability of survival in months, measured from the date of diagnosis, for patients with glioblastoma multiforme (*GBM*) ($n = 19$) and anaplastic astrocytoma (*AA*) ($n = 9$) enrolled in a phase I trial of thermoradiotherapy at the University of Arizona. This analysis includes a group of six patients (four with GBM, two with AA) who were treated at the time of recurrence. (See text for details). *Tick marks* represent censored patients

that toxicity was acceptable when implant volume was limited to 100 cm^3. Further evaluation of brain thermoradiotherapy with ferromagnetic seeds was recommended (Stea et al. 1992).

At the University of California, San Francisco, two brain hyperthermia trials have been undertaken (Sneed et al. 1991, 1992). The initial phase I/II trial of interstitial hyperthermia and brachytherapy alone for recurrent malignant gliomas and recurrent solitary brain metastases laid the groundwork for the later randomized trial for newly diagnosed GM.

Between June 1987 and September 1990, 48 patients with recurrent brain tumors were treated on our first thermoradiotherapy protocol (Sneed et al. 1991, 1992). Brain catheters were implanted stereotactically after CT-based preplanning. Figure 12.2 illustrates the preplan with the stereotactic frame in place for a patient with a GM. Helical coil microwave antennas (Satoh and Stauffer 1988; Satoh et al. 1988) were used to heat as much of the tumor as possible to at least 42.5°C for 30 min immediately before and after brachytherapy, delivering about 10 Gy/day with temporarily implanted high-activity iodine-125 sources. Figure 12.3 shows contrast-enhanced CT scans of a GM immediately before and 2 months after thermoradiotherapy.

The median patient age was 43 years (range 18–71 years) and the median KPS was 90 (range 40–90). There were 25 patients with GM, 16 with AA, and seven with brain metastasis. Brachytherapy dose ranged from 32.6 to 63.3 Gy given at 37–70 cGy/h. A total of 89 hyperthermia treatments were delivered using one to eight antennas and one to three dedicated thermometry catheters. The median steady-state minimum tumor temperature was 40.1°C (range 37.0°–45.7°C) and the median steady-state maximum tumor temperature was 45.7°C (range 39.5°–51.7°C). Of all steady-state tumor temperatures measured, 61% were at least 42.5°C. Acute toxicity included seven cases of transient neurological changes, six reversible neurological changes, six brief focal seizures, one 20-min focal motor seizure, one case of meningitis, one scalp/bone flap infection, and one deep venous thrombosis with pulmonary embolism. There were no deaths or permanent neurological sequelae (Sneed et al. 1992).

The median survival after the date of thermoradiotherapy was 49 weeks for GM and 140 weeks for AA. Multivariate analyses were performed to determine how survival and freedom from local

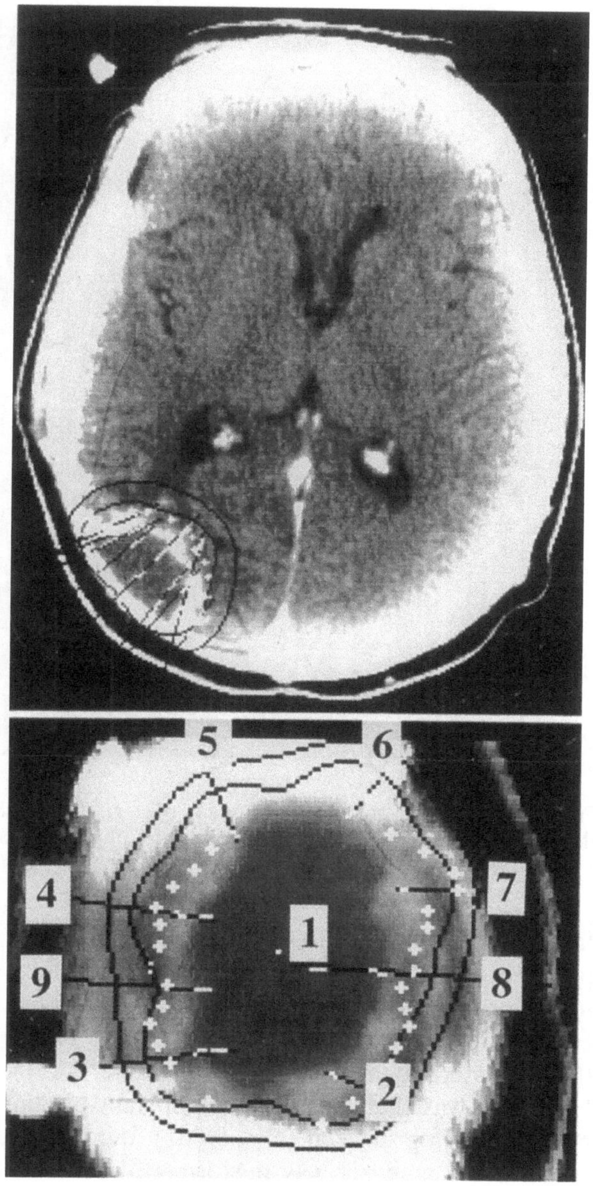

a

b

Fig. 12.2. a Preplanning axial computed tomography (CT) image for a patient with a glioblastoma multiforme. The tumor is demarcated with "+" symbols, the catheter trajectories and seed positions are indicated, and the resulting 0.45 Gy/h and 0.25 Gy/h isodose contours are shown. **b** This end-on view of the same implant preplan shows the arrangement of catheters used to heat the tumor (catheters #2–#8) and two dedicated thermometry catheters (#1 and #9)

tumor progression were influenced by histology, patient age, tumor volume, brachytherapy dose, and various thermal parameters. Minimum tumor temperature and T_{90} (the temperature exceeded by 90% of the monitored tumor points for a given hyperthermia treatment) were the only significant

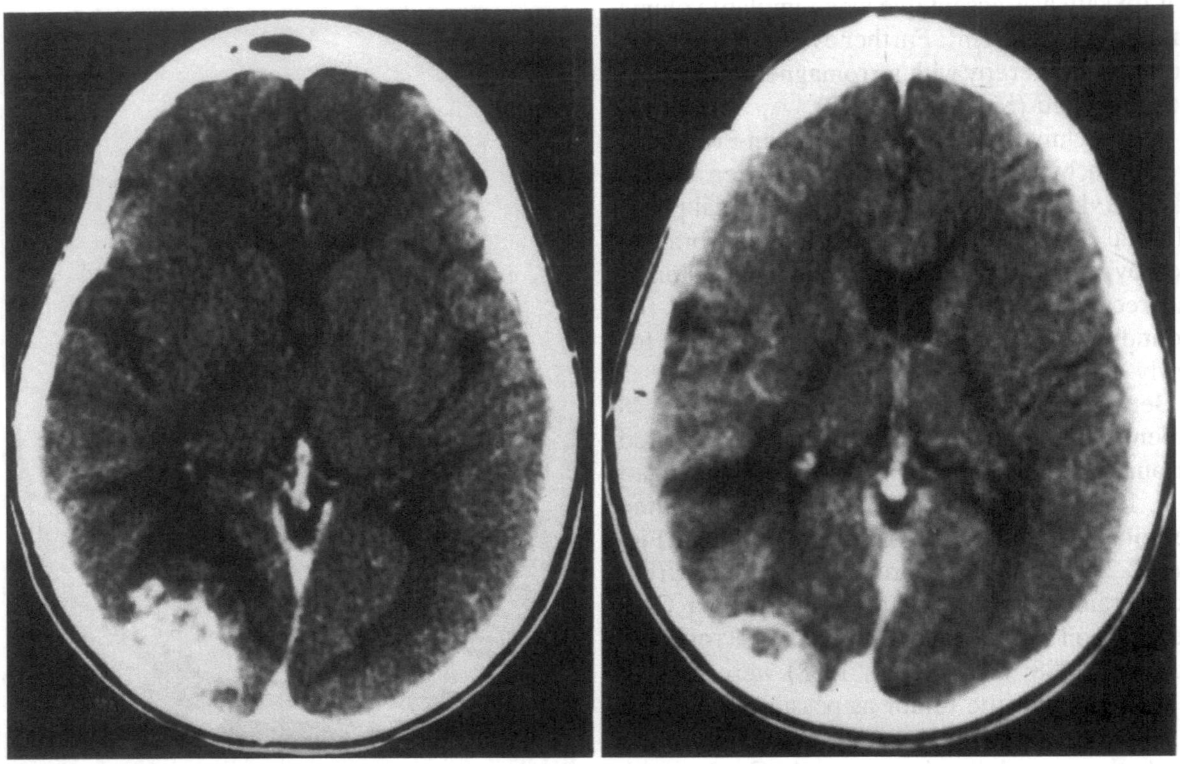

Fig. 12.3. Contrast-enhanced CT scans of a glioblastoma multiforme immediately before (left) and 2 months after thermoradiotherapy (right) showing a partial objective response

factors predicting for freedom from local tumor progression. Kaplan-Meier freedom from local tumor progression curves are shown in Fig. 12.4, comparing gliomas heated to a $T_{90} \geqslant 41.5°C$ and those heated to a $T_{90} < 41.5°C$ ($P < 0.001$). Histology was the single most important parameter influencing survival ($P < 0.001$), but when a multivariate analysis was performed, age ($P = 0.04$) and T_{90} ($P = 0.04$) were identified as other significant factors. Kaplan-Meier survival curves displayed in Fig. 12.5 for patients with GM demonstrate improved survival for patients whose tumors were heated to a T_{90} temperature of at least 41.2°C ($P = 0.008$).

Northern California Oncology Group protocol 6G-90-2 was opened in July 1990 for patients with newly diagnosed glioblastoma. Following surgery, focal external beam radiotherapy (59.4 Gy at 1.8 Gy per daily fraction, 5 days per week) is given in conjunction with oral hydroxyurea, followed by implant boost (60 Gy) with or without interstitial hyperthermia (42.5°C for 30 min immediately before and after brachytherapy). As of July 1993, 75 eligible patients had been entered on the protocol. No results are available to date for this ongoing trial, but when completed, it should help answer whether or not sequential, short-duration brain hyperthermia improves survival in glioblastoma patients undergoing brachytherapy boost.

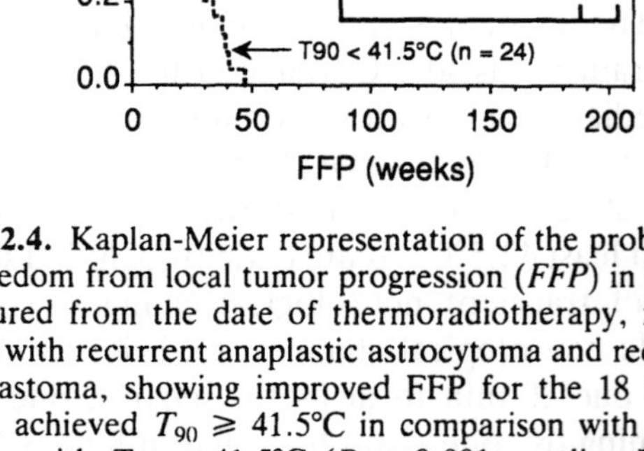

Fig. 12.4. Kaplan-Meier representation of the probability of freedom from local tumor progression (*FFP*) in weeks, measured from the date of thermoradiotherapy, for patients with recurrent anaplastic astrocytoma and recurrent glioblastoma, showing improved FFP for the 18 tumors which achieved $T_{90} \geqslant 41.5°C$ in comparison with the 24 tumors with $T_{90} < 41.5°C$ ($P < 0.001$; median FFP 38 weeks vs 18 weeks). *Tick marks* represent censored patients

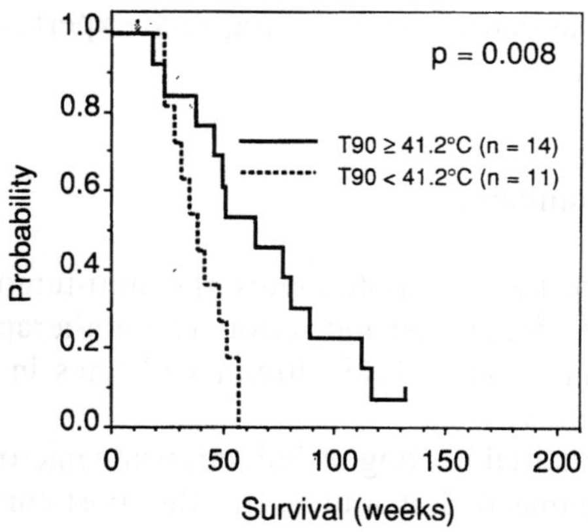

Fig. 12.5. Kaplan-Meier representation of the probability of survival in weeks, measured from the date of thermoradiotherapy, for patients with recurrent glioblastoma comparing patients whose tumors were heated to a T_{90} temperature of at least 41.2°C and those with a T_{90} of less than 41.2°C (P = 0.008). *Tick marks* represent censored patients

12.7 Future Perspectives

Many further technical improvements can be made in existing hyperthermia technologies to allow better localization of heating and uniformity of heating (see Chap. 13 in vol 1 of this book). Computerized three-dimensional hyperthermia treatment planning is also needed, taking into account tissue properties (Lu et al. 1992) and including blood flow as a dynamic parameter (Kato et al. 1992; Moriyama 1990; Patel et al. 1992; Salcman et al. 1989; Satoh et al. 1989; Uda and Tanaka 1990).

Despite much in vitro and in vivo evidence of thermal enhancement when hyperthermia is combined with cisplatin and the nitrosoureas and despite the fact that lower temperatures may be needed for chemosensitization than for radiosensitization, there is little clinical experience with brain thermochemotherapy. At the University of Arizona, a phase I study has been undertaken of scanned focused ultrasound hyperthermia in combination with carboplatin for recurrent glioblastoma multiforme. Patients first undergo a craniectomy with maximal tumor debulking and then receive three courses of thermochemotherapy spaced 4–5 days apart to allow for decay of thermotolerance. This treatment has been well tolerated with no morbidity observed in the first nine patients enrolled. Three patients (all with recurrent glioblastoma multiforme after a full course of fractionated radiotherapy) remain alive at 19–32 months from treatment with hyperthermia and carboplatin. They all continue to have a very high performance status. Further accrual on this protocol and longer follow-up should help to answer the question of whether the thermal chemosensitization observed in vitro for carboplatin (Schem et al. 1992) will translate into a clinical benefit. Finally, it is possible that trimodality therapy would be advantageous, using the higher temperatures attained in the tumor core for radiosensitization and the lower temperatures attained in the margin surrounding the tumor for chemosensitization.

One of the most interesting areas of opportunity lies in the investigation of low-temperature, long-duration, simultaneous heat and radiation. It is well accepted that heat radiosensitization is greatest for simultaneous heat and radiation. Continuous, low-temperature, long-duration hyperthermia (in the range of about 41°–43°C for many hours) concurrent with brachytherapy could result in acceptable toxicity and patient tolerance, substantial radiosensitization, and accumulation of a large thermal dose. Armour et al. (1991) reported radiosensitization of rat 9L gliosarcoma cells to low-dose-rate irradiation by long-duration hyperthermia at 41°C. They also demonstrated that continuous low-dose-rate irradiation at 0.5 Gy/h in the rat 9L gliosarcoma cell line could be replaced by pulsed radiation schemes ranging from 0.25 Gy every 30 min to 3.00 Gy every 6 h (Armour et al. 1992). Furthermore, continuous heating at 41°C resulted in substantial radiosensitization for both continuous low-dose-rate and pulsed radiation (Armour et al. 1992). Finally, although human tumor cell lines (including glioblastoma U-87MG) were more resistant to 43°C hyperthermia than rodent tumor cell lines, they were more sensitive to 41°C hyperthermia than were rodent cells (Armour et al. 1993).

Most brain hyperthermia trials to date have employed sequential, short-duration heat and radiation. Garcia et al. (1992) have undertaken a protocol in newly diagnosed patients with malignant glioma for concurrent conductive interstitial hyperthermia (minimum tumor temperature 41.5°C for 36 h of hyperthermia over a 48-h period) and high-dose-rate iridium-192 interstitial brachytherapy (15 Gy in three fractions administered at equally spaced breaks in the hyperthermia treatment). We await the results of this trial with much interest.

12.8 Conclusions

Experiments in vitro and in vivo have demonstrated that hyperthermia has additive or synergistic effects in combination with radiation and with chemotherapeutic drugs such as cisplatin and the nitrosoureas. Hyperthermia immediately before or after acute exposures to radiation inhibits repair of potentially lethal damage in human glioma cell lines. However, from animal brain toxicity studies we know that the tolerance of normal brain tissue to hyperthermia is quite limited. The best toxicity data probably come from HOOPES et al. (1990), who estimated the threshold for brain necrosis to be 44.3°C for 30 min or 42.8°C for 60 min. Various strategies have been adopted to overcome this seeming lack of a therapeutic window: selective tumor heating with carefully controlled interstitial or scanned focused ultrasound techniques, the combination of hyperthermia with chemotherapy for which lower temperatures may have efficacy, and simultaneous heat and radiation (based on the speculation that thermal enhancement will be greatest for tumor cells with a large capacity to repair potentially lethal damage, and that less thermal enhancement will occur for normal cells with less capacity to repair potentially lethal damage).

One clinical trial in patients with recurrent gliomas provided evidence of a thermal dose-response relationship, with significantly improved freedom from local tumor progression for $T_{90} \geqslant$ 41.5°C (SNEED et al. 1992) and improved survival for patients with GM with $T_{90} \geqslant 41.2$°C. A randomized trial is in progress at the University of California, San Francisco to evaluate the efficacy and toxicity of short-duration, sequential hyperthermia and brachytherapy boost in patients with glioblastoma. Trials in progress at other institutions are investigating thermochemotherapy and long-duration hyperthermia.

Many questions remain, such as the best method of heating, the appropriate thermal dose and sequencing of hyperthermia and radiation and/or chemotherapy, and the appropriate target volume, given the presence of tumor cells beyond the contrast-enhancing volume on CT or MR imaging (BURGER 1983; KELLY et al. 1987). As GASPAR and CAIRNCROSS (1992) editorialized, there is sound rationale for combining heat and radiation, but currently we have more questions than answers and brain thermoradiotherapy needs to be subjected to continued, careful phase I/II testing at centers with the required expertise and interest.

12.9 Summary

- Hyperthermia potentiates the anti-tumor effects of radiation and various chemotherapeutic agents against brain tumor cell lines in vitro and in vivo.
- Interstitial heating techniques using microwave antennas or hot sources are the most common brain heating methods.
- The tolerance of normal brain tissue to hyperthermia is quite limited. Breakdown of the blood-brain barrier occurs with 42.8°C for 30 min or 42.4°C for 60 min and necrosis occurs with 44.3°C for 30 min or 42.8°C for 60 min.
- Recent brain hyperthermia clinical trials have shown that interstitial brain hyperthermia is feasible and that toxicity is acceptable with careful control of the heating and limitation of the implanted volume to less than 100 cm^3. The median survival after thermoradiotherapy was 49 weeks for recurrent glioblastomas and 140 weeks for recurrent anaplastic astrocytomas treated at the University of California, San Francisco. A T_{90} temperature of at least 41.5°C was associated with improved freedom from local tumor progression (SNEED et al. 1992).
- Areas for future research include technical improvements in heat localization and uniformity, combination of hyperthermia with chemotherapy, and investigation of low-temperature, long-duration, simultaneous heat and brachytherapy.
- Further phase I/II clinical trials and eventually phase III trials are needed to evaluate thermoradiotherapy of brain tumors at centers with the required expertise.

References

Agbi CB, Bernstein M, Laperriere N, Leung P, Lumley M (1992) Patterns of recurrence of malignant astrocytoma following stereotactic interstitial brachytherapy with iodine-125 implants. Int J Radiat Oncol Biol Phys 23: 321–326

Armour EP, Wang ZH, Corry PM, Martinez A (1991) Sensitization of rat 9L gliosarcoma cells to low dose rate irradiation by long duration 41 degrees C hyperthermia. Cancer Res 51: 3088–3095

Armour EP, Wang ZH, Corry PM, Martinez A (1992) Equivalence of continuous and pulse simulated low dose

rate irradiation in 9L gliosarcoma cells at 37° and 41°C. Int J Radiat Oncol Biol Phys 22: 109–114
Armour EP, McEachern D, Wang ZH, Corry PM, Martinez A (1993) Sensitivity of human cells to mild hyperthermia. Cancer Res 53: 2740–2744
Ascher PW, Justich E, Schröttner O (1991) A new surgical but less invasive treatment of central brain tumors. Acta Neurochir Suppl (Wien) 52: 78–80
Babbs CF, Fearnot NE, Marchosky JA, Moran CJ, Jones JT, Plantenga TD (1990) Theoretical basis for controlling minimal tumor temperature during interstitial conductive heat therapy. IEEE Trans Biomed Eng 37: 662–672
Bashir R, Hochberg F, Oot R (1988) Regrowth patterns of glioblastoma multiforme related to planning of interstitial brachytherapy radiation fields. Neurosurgery 23: 27–30
Bettag M, Ulrich F, Schober R, Fürst G, Langen KJ, Sabel M, Kiwit JCW (1991) Stereotactic laser therapy in cerebral gliomas. Acta Neurochir Suppl (Wien) 52: 81–83
Borok TL, Winter A, Laing J, Paglione R, Sterzer F, Sinclair I, Plafker J (1988) Microwave hyperthermia radiosensitized iridium-192 for recurrent brain malignancy. Med Dosim 13: 29–36
Britt RH, Lyons BE, Ryan T, Saxer E, Obana W, Rossi G (1984a) Effect of whole-body hyperthermia on auditory brainstem and somatosensory and visual-evoked potentials. In: Hales JRS (ed) Thermal physiology. Raven Press, New York, pp 519–523
Britt RH, Pounds DW, Lyons BE (1984b) Feasibility of treating malignant brain tumors with focused ultrasound. Prog Exp Tumor Res 28: 232–245
Burger PC (1983) Pathologic anatomy and CT correlations in the glioblastoma multiforme. Appl Neurophysiol 46: 180–187
Coughlin TC (1989) Introduction and clinical results of interstitial hyperthermia using microwave for brain tumors. In: Sugahara T, Saito M (eds) Hyperthermic oncology 1988, vol 2. Taylor & Francis, London, p 94
Cummins B, McIntosh I (1976) Experiences with cerebral hemisphere hyperthermia in the treatment of malignant gliomas. Proc Br Inst Radiol 49: 1059–1060
Dahl O, Mella O (1982) Enhanced effect of combined hyperthermia and chemotherapy (bleomycin, BCNU) in a neurogenic rat tumor (BT4A) in vivo. Anticancer Res 2: 395–364
DaSilva VF, Raaphorst GP, Goyal R, Feeley M (1987) Drug cytotoxicity at elevated temperature: in vitro study of the U-87MG glioma cell line. J Neurosurg 67: 885–888
Davis LW (1989) Presidential address: malignant glioma – a nemesis which requires clinical and basic investigation in radiation oncology. Int J Radiat Oncol Biol Phys 16: 1355–1365
DeFord JA, Babbs CF, Patel UH, Fearnot NE, Marchosky JA, Moran CJ (1990) Accuracy and precision of computer-simulated tissue temperatures in individual human intracranial tumours treated with interstitial hyperthermia. Int J Hyperthermia 6: 755–769
DeFord JA, Babbs CF, Patel UH, Bleyer MW, Marchosky JA, Moran CJ (1991) Effective estimation and computer control of minimum tumour temperature during conductive interstitial hyperthermia. Int J Hyperthermia 7: 441–453
Fike JR, Gobbel GT, Satoh T, Stauffer PR (1991) Normal brain response after interstitial microwave hyperthermia. Int J Hyperthermia 7: 795–808
Garcia DM, Marchosky JA, Nussbaum G, Drzymala R (1992) Interstitial HDR brachytherapy and long duration interstitial hyperthermia in the treatment of newly diagnosed malignant glioma. Selectron Brachy J 6: 70–74
Gaspar LE, Cairncross JG (1992) Hyperthermia and brachytherapy for glioma – will cooler heads prevail? Int J Radiat Oncol Biol Phys 24: 803–804
Gaspar LE, Fisher BJ, Macdonald DR, LeBer DV, Halperin EC, Schold SC Jr, Cairncross JG (1992) Supratentorial malignant glioma: patterns of recurrence and implications for external beam local treatment. Int J Radiat Oncol Biol Phys 24: 55–57
Gerweck LE, Richards B (1981) Influence of pH on the thermal sensitivity of cultured human glioblastoma cells. Cancer Res 41: 845–849
Grady MS, Howard MA III, Molloy JA, Ritter RC, Quate EG, Gillies GT (1989) Preliminary experimental investigation of in vivo magnetic manipulation: results and potential application in hyperthermia. Med Phys 16: 263–272
Guthkelch AN, Carter LP, Cassady JR, et al. (1991) Treatment of malignant brain tumors with focused ultrasound hyperthermia and radiation: results of a phase I trial. J Neurooncol 10: 271–284
Haider SA, Cetas TC, Wait JR, Chen JS, Roemer RB (1991) Power absorption in ferromagnetic implants from radiofrequency magnetic fields and the problem of optimization. IEEE Trans Microwave Theory Tech 39: 1817–1827
Harris AB, Erickson L, Kendig JH, Mingrino S, Goldring S (1962) Observations on selective brain heating in dogs. J Neurosurg 19: 514–521
Heppner F (1982) New technologies to combat malignant tumours of the brain. Anticancer Res 2:101–109
Heppner F (1986) The glioblastoma multiforme: a lifelong challenge to the neurosurgeon. Neurochirurgia (Stuttg) 29: 9–14
Hochberg FH, Pruitt A (1980) Assumptions in the radiotherapy of glioblastoma. Neurology 30: 907–911
Hoopes PJ, Ryan TP, DeLeo JA, Roberts DW, Douple EB, Taylor JH (1990) Thermotolerant effects of corticosteroids or preheating on hyperthermia induced lesions in dog brain. Tenth annual meeting of the North American hyperthermia group, New Orleans, Louisiana, Abstract Ac-1, p 7
Kato K, Matsuda J, Yamashita T, Tanaka R (1992) Simultaneous estimation of blood flow rate and tissue temperature. Front Med Biol Eng 4: 135–143
Kelly PJ, Daumas-Duport C, Kispert DB, Wall BA, Scheithauer BW, Illig JJ (1987) Imaging-based stereotaxic serial biopsies in untreated intracranial glial neoplasms. J Neurosurg 66: 865–874
Kobayashi T, Kida Y (1992) Interstitial hyperthermia of malignant brain tumors by an implant heating system using stereotactic techniques. Stereotact Funct Neurosurg 59: 123–127
Kobayashi T, Kida Y, Tanaka T, Kageyama N, Kobayashi H (1986) Magnetic induction hyperthermia for brain tumor using ferromagnetic implant with low Curie temperature. I. Experimental study. J Neurooncol 4: 175–181
Kobayashi T, Tanaka T, Kida Y, Matsui M, Ikeda T (1989) Interstitial hyperthermia of experimental brain tumor using implant heating system. J Neurooncol 7: 201–208

Kobayashi T, Kida Y, Tanaka T, Hattori K, Matsui M, Amemiya Y (1991) Interstitial hyperthermia of malignant brain tumors by implant heating system: clinical experience. J Neurooncol 10: 153–163
Kuroki M, Tanaka R, Hondo H (1987) Antitumor effect of interferon combined with hyperthermia against experimental brain tumour. Int J Hyperthermia 3: 527–534
Liang BC, Thornton AF Jr, Sandler HM, Greenberg HS (1991) Malignant astrocytomas: focal tumor recurrence after focal external beam radiation therapy. J Neurosurg 75: 559–563
Lu Y, Li B, Xu J, Yu J (1992) Dielectric properties of human glioma and surrounding tissue. Int J Hyperthermia 8: 755–760
Lyons BE, Briott RH, Strohbehn JW (1984) Localized hyperthermia in the treatment of malignant brain tumors using an interstitial microwave antenna array. IEEE Trans Biomed Eng 31: 53–62
Marchosky JA, Babbs CF, Moran CJ, et al. (1990a) Conductive, interstitial hyperthermia: a new modality for treatment of intracranial tumors. In: Bicher HI, et al. (eds) Consensus on hyperthermia for the 1990s. Plenum Press, New York, pp 129–143
Marchosky JA, Moran CJ, Fearnot NE. Babbs CF (1990b) Hyperthermia catheter implantation and therapy in the brain. J Neurosurg 72: 975–979
Matsumoto K, Nakagawa M, Higashi H, et al. (1992) Interstitial microwave hyperthermia for malignant glioma: phase I clinical trial. In: Gerner EW (ed) Hyperthermic oncology 1992, vol 1. Arizona Board of Regents, Tucson, Az, p 395
Mechling JA, Strohbehn JW (1992) Three-dimensional theoretical SAR and temperature distributions created in brain tissue by 915 and 2450 MHz dipole antenna arrays with varying insertion depths. Int J Hyperthermia 8: 529–542
Mella O, Dahl O (1985) Timing of combined hyperthermia and 1,3-bis(2-chloroethyl)-1-nitrosourea or *cis*-diaminedichloroplatinum in BD IX rats with BT4A tumours. Anticancer Res 5: 259–264
Molloy JA, Ritter RC, Grady MS, Howard MA III, Quate EG, Gillies GT (1990) Experimental determination of the force required for insertion of thermoseed into deep brain tissue. Ann Biomed Eng 18: 299–313
Molloy JA, Ritter RC, Broaddus WC, Grady MS, Howard MA III, Quate EG, Gillies GT (1991) Thermodynamics of movable inductively heated seeds for the treatment of brain tumors. Med Phys 18: 794–803
Moriyama E (1990) Cerebral blood flow changes during localized hyperthermia. Neurol Med Chir (Tokyo) 30: 923–929
Moriyama E, Matsumi N, Shiraishi T, et al. (1988) Hyperthermia for brain tumors: improved delivery with a new cooling system. Neurosurgery 23: 189–195
Moriyama E, Salcman M, Broadwell RD (1991) Blood-brain barrier alteration after microwave-induced hyperthermia is purely a thermal effect: I. Temperature and power measurements. Surg Neurol 35: 177–182
Nelson DF, Urtasun RC, Saunders WM, Gutin PH, Sheline GE (1986) Recent and current investigations of radiation therapy of malignant gliomas. Semin Oncol 13: 46–55
Nowak G, Rentzsch O, Terzis AJ, Arnold H (1990) Induced hyperthermia in brain tissue: comparison between contact Nd:YAG laser system and automatically controlled high frequency current. Acta Neurochir (Wien) 102: 76–81
Patel UH, Babbs CF, DeFord JA, Bleyer MW, Marchosky JA, Moran CJ (1992) Evidence of changes in regional blood perfusion in human intracranial tumours during conductive interstitial hyperthermia. Med Biol Eng Comput 30: 651–655
Raaphorst GP, Feeley MM, Danjoux CE, DaSilva V, Gerig LH (1991) Hyperthermia enhancement of radiation response and inhibition of recovery from radiation damage in human glioma cells. Int J Hyperthermia 7: 626–641
Roberts DW, Coughlin CT, Wong TZ, Fratkin JD, Douple EB, Strohbehn JW (1986) Interstitial hyperthermia and iridium brachytherapy in treatment of malignant glioma: a phase I clinical trial. J Neurosurg 64: 581–587
Roberts DW, Strohbehn JW, Coughlin C, Ryan T, Lyons B, Douple E, Fratkin J (1989) Hyperthermia of brain tumor: the Dartmouth experience. In: Sugahara T, Saito M (eds) Hyperthermic oncology 1988, vol 2. Taylor & Francis, London, p 88
Roux FX, Merienne L, Fallet-Bianco C, Beuvon F, Devaux B, Leriche B, Cioloca C (1992) Stereotaxic laser interstitial thermotherapy. A new alternative in the therapeutic management of some brain tumors. Neurochirurgie 38: 238–244
Ryan TP, Hoopes PJ, Taylor JH, Strohbehn JW, Roberts DW, Douple EB, Coughlin CT (1991) Experimental brain hyperthermia: techniques for heat delivery and thermometry. Int J Radiat Oncol Biol Phys 20: 739–750
Ryan TP, Roberts D, Trembly BS, Coughlin C (1992) Brain hyperthermia: microwave antenna array techniques and clinical data. In: Gerner EW (ed) Hyperthermic oncology 1992, vol 1. Arizona Board of Regents, Tucson, Az, p 391
Salcman M, Ebert PS (1991) In vitro response of human glioblastoma and canine glioma cells to hyperthermia, radiation, and chemotherapy. Neurosurgery 29: 526–531
Salcman M, Samaras GM (1983) Interstitial microwave hyperthermia for brain tumors: results of a phase I clinical trial. J Neurooncol 1: 225–236
Salcman M, Moriyama E, Elsner HJ, Rossman H, Gettleman RA, Neuberth G, Corradino G (1989) Cerebral blood flow and the thermal properties of the brain: a preliminary analysis. J Neurosurg 70: 592–598
Satoh T, Stauffer PR (1988) Implantable helical coil microwave antenna for interstitial hyperthermia. Int J Hyperthermia 4: 497–512
Satoh T, Staufer PR, Fike JR (1988) Thermal distribution studies of helical coil microwave antennas for interstitial hyperthermia. Int J Radiat Oncol Biol Phys 15: 1209–1218
Satoh T, Nakasone S, Nishimoto A (1989) Cerebral blood flow response to the tissue temperature in tumour and brain tissues. Int J Hyperthermia 5: 683–696
Schem BC, Dahl O (1991) Thermal enhancement of ACNU and potentiation of thermochemotherapy with ACNU by hypertonic glucose in the BT4An rat glioma. J Neurooncol 10: 247–252
Schem BC, Mella O, Dahl O (1989) Potentiation of combined BCNU and hyperthermia by pH reduction in vitro and hypertonic glucose in vivo in the BT4 rat glioma. Int J Hyperthermia 5: 707–715
Schem BC, Mella O, Dahl O (1992) Thermochemotherapy with cisplatin or carboplatin in the BT4 rat glioma in vitro and in vivo. Int J Radiat Oncol Biol Phys 23: 109–114

Silberman AW, Morgan DF, Storm FK, Rand RW, Bubbers JE, Brown WJ, Morton DL (1982) Localized magnetic-loop induction hyperthermia of the rabbit brain. J Surg Oncol 20: 174–178
Silberman AW, Rand RW, Krag DN, Storm FK, Benz M, Drury B, Morton DL (1985) Phase I trial of thermochemotherapy for brain malignancy. Cancer 56: 48–56
Silberman AW, Rand RW, Storm FK, Drury B, Benz ML, Morton DL (1986) Effect of localized magnetic-induction hyperthermia on the brain. Cancer 57: 1401–1404
Sneed PK, Matsumoto K, Stauffer PR, Fike JR, Smith V, Gutin PH (1986) Interstitial microwave hyperthermia in a canine brain model. Int J Radiat Oncol Biol Phys 12: 1887–1897
Sneed PK, Stauffer PR, Gutin PH, et al. (1991) Interstitial irradiation and hyperthermia for the treatment of recurrent malignant brain tumors. Neurosurg 28: 206–215
Sneed PK, Gutin PH, Stauffer PR, et al. (1992) Thermoradiotherapy of recurrent malignant brain tumors. Int J Radiat Oncol Biol Phys 23: 853–861
Stea B, Cetas TC, Cassady JR, et al. (1990) Interstitial thermoradiotherapy of brain tumors: preliminary results of a phase I clinical trial. Int J Radiat Oncol Biol Phys 19: 1463–1471
Stea B, Kittelson J, Cassady JR, et al. (1992) Treatment of malignant gliomas with interstitial irradiation and hyperthermia. Int J Radiat Oncol Biol Phys 24: 657–667
Sugiyama K, Sakai T, Fujishima I, Ryu H, Uemura K, Yokoyama T (1990) Stereotactic interstitial laser-hyperthermia using Nd-YAG laser. Stereotact Funct Neurosurg 54–55: 501–505
Sutton CH (1971) Tumor hyperthermia in the treatment of malignant gliomas of the brain. Trans Am Neurol Assoc 96: 195–199
Tamura M, Zama A, Kunimine H, Tamaki Y, Niibe H (1988) Effect of hyperthermia in combination with radiation therapy in a rat glioma model. No Shinkei Geka 16: 659–663
Tamura M, Tsukahara T, Kunimine H, Zama A, Tamaki Y, Niibe H (1989) Histopathologic changes and tumor cell kinetics after hyperthermia and/or radiation therapy in a rat glioma model: bromodeoxyuridine (BUdR) labelling index. No Shinkei Geka 17: 555–559
Tanaka T, Kobayashi T, Kida Y, Kageyama N (1986) The effect of hyperthermia and antitumor drugs on brain tumor cell lines. Gan To Kagaku Ryoho 13: 2993–2997
Tanaka R, Kim CH, Yamada N, Saito Y (1987) Radiofrequency hyperthermia for malignant brain tumors: preliminary results of clinical trials. Neurosurg 21: 478–483
Tanaka T, Kobayashi T, Takahashi T, Hattori K (1989a) Effect of combined treatment with magnetic induction hyperthermia and chemotherapy in a rabbit brain tumor model. Neurol Med Chir (Tokyo) 29: 377–381
Tanaka R, Hondo H, Yamada N, Kawamata M, Nakajima T, Saito Y (1989b) Radiofrequency capacitive heating for malignant glioma: clinical trials of extracranial heating. In: Sugahara T, Saito M (eds) Hyperthermic oncology 1988, vol 2. Taylor & Francis, London, p 91
Uda M, Tanaka Y (1990) Arterial blood flow changes after hyperthermia on normal liver, normal brain, and normal small intestine. Gan No Rinsho 36: 2362–2366
Wallner KE, Galicich JH, Krol G, Arbit E, Malkin MG (1989) Patterns of failure following treatment for glioblastoma multiforme and anaplastic astrocytoma. Int J Radiat Oncol Biol Phys 16: 1405–1409
Watanabe M, Tanaka R, Hondo H, Kuroki M (1992) Effects of antineoplastic agents and hyperthermia on cytotoxicity toward chronically hypoxic glioma cells. Int J Hyperthermia 8: 131–138
Wen HL, Dahele JS (1984) Invasive microwave hyperthermia for treatment of glioma. Chin Med J (Engl) 97: 813–818
Wen HL, Dahele JS, Mehal ZD (1988) Application of invasive microwave hyperthermia for the treatment of gliomas. J Neurooncol 6: 93–101
Winter A, Laing J, Paglione R, Sterzer F (1985) Microwave hyperthermia for brain tumors. Neurosurg 17: 387–399
Yamada N, Tanaka R, Kanayama T, Takeda N, Suzuki Y, Sekiguchi K, Saito Y (1985) The influence of hyperthermia on cerebral functions – blood flow, metabolism and electroencephalography. In: Overgaard J (ed) Hyperthermic oncology 1984, vol 1. Taylor & Francis, London, pp 743–746
Yokote H, Komai N, Nakai E, Itakura T, Hayashi S (1990) Stereotactic hyperthermia for brain tumors. Stereotact Funct Neurosurg 54–55: 506–513

13 Thermoradiotherapy for Eye Tumors

P.T. Finger

CONTENTS

13.1 Introduction

The most common primary intraocular tumors are retinoblastoma in children and uveal melanoma in adults. Enucleation (removal of the eye) was the standard treatment until radiotherapy techniques were found to offer patients "eye and vision-sparing" alternatives (Stallard 1962, 1966, 1968; Zimmerman et al. 1978).

With up to a mean of 10 years' follow-up, various forms of radiotherapy have been shown to stop the growth of uveal melanomas or achieve tumor shrinkage in more than 85% of cases (Davidorf et al. 1976, 1978; Gragoudas et al. 1987; Karlson et al. 1989; Lindstadt et al. 1990; Lommatzsch 1986; Packer et al. 1992). But, with all forms of radiotherapy, at least 40% of patients have been noted to experience significant radiation associated side-effects (Packer et al. 1992). These complications have been related to the type of radiation used, its method of delivery, the size of the tumor treated (therefore the amount of radiation delivered to the eye), the location of the tumor, and the tumor's response to irradiation (Char et al. 1989).

Radiation-associated adnexal and anterior segment intraocular problems have included eyelash loss, dry eye, keratitis, corneal ulceration, rubeosis iridis, secondary glaucoma, and cataract. Posterior segment intraocular complications have included vitreous hemorrhage, retinal detachment, radiation retinopathy, and radiation optic neuropathy. In addition, tumor destruction sometimes causes an exudative or hemorrhagic retinochoroidopathy which may be limited to an encircling of the tumor, or can diffusely involve the choroid and retina.

The three most commonly used forms of radiotherapy for intraocular tumors have been external beam radiotherapy, plaque radiotherapy, and charged-particle external beam radiotherapy. The use of standard external beam radiotherapy has been largely limited to the treatment of multifocal retinoblastoma and pre-enucleation treatment of uveal melanoma. Solitary or unifocal intraocular tumors have been commonly treated with plaque radiotherapy. This technique has involved affixing a dish-shaped source [e.g., cobalt-60 (^{60}Co), iodine-125(^{125}I), palladium-103 (^{103}Pd), ruthenium-106 (^{106}Ru)] on the sclera over the base of the intraocular tumor (Finger et al. 1991a; Lommatzsch 1974; Packer and Rotman 1980; Shields et al. 1982). With plaque radiotherapy, radiation travels through and is absorbed by the eye wall, the tumor, the vitreous, and finally normal ocular structures as it exits the eye. In vitro dosimetry, preclinical simulations, and phase I clinical data have supported the use of low-energy radionuclides (Chiu-Tsao and

P.T. Finger, MD, Director, The Ocular Tumor Service, The New York Eye and Ear Infirmary, 310 E. 14th Street, New York, NY 10003, USA; and Chief, The Division of Ocular Tumor and Orbital Disease, North Shore University Hospital, 300 Community Drive Manhasset, New York, NY 11036, USA

ANDERSON 1991; EARLE et al. 1987; FINGER et al. 1993, 1994; PACKER et al. 1984). With this type of approach, the only normal structure through which radiation must penetrate (entry site) is the sclera immediately beneath the tumor. Since radioactive plaques deposit most of the radiation around the tumor, radiation retinopathy may be more common with plaque therapies.

Other investigators have advocated charged-particle external beam radiotherapy (e.g., protons or helium ions) (GRAGOUDAS et al. 1982; LINDSTADT et al. 1990). In contrast to plaques, charged particles are derived from a cyclotron, are aimed through a portal, and travel through air towards the patient's eye. Then charged particles must pass through (an entry site) the lids, lashes and lacrimal system, the cornea, the iris, the lens, and finally the vitreous prior to reaching the tumor. An entry dose greater than 70% of the tumor dose has been reported. This may explain why adnexal and anterior segment intraocular complications have been more common with beam therapies (CHAR et al. 1989).

Primarily due to the high incidence of site-threatening complications after radiotherapy of intraocular tumors, investigators have become interested in methods to reduce the amount of radiation delivered to normal ocular structures (FINGER et al. 1990b). Adjuvant hyperthermia offers the possibility of improved local control, and a reduction in the radiation dose required to sterilize intraocular tumors, with a resultant decrease in radiation-associated complications (EMAMIET et al. 1988; KIM et al. 1982; MANNING et al. 1982; MEYER 1984; MOLLS and SCHERER 1987).

In 1980, *Lagendijk* first reported on a microwave stripline applicator designed to treat retinoblastoma. Since that report, as if a microcosm of clinical hyperthermia, conductive (etched element, ferromagnetic) and inductive plaque sources [three microwave, one radiofrequency-localized current field (LCF)], as well as two teletherapy (microwave, ultrasound) hyperthermia systems have been applied to treat intraocular tumors (FINGER et al. 1982, 1984; GODFREY et al. 1986; LIGGETT et al. 1990; MIELER et al. 1989; RIEDEL 1988; SWIFT et al. 1990). They have all been evaluated on normal and tumor-bearing rabbit eyes (FINGER et al. 1991b). In phase I clinical trials, microwave and LCF thermotherapy has been used together with (^{125}I, ^{103}Pd) episcleral plaque radiotherapy (FINGER et al. 1989; LIGGETT et al. 1991). Ultrasound thermotherapy has also been clinically evaluated as an adjuvant to ^{60}Co plaque radiotherapy (COLEMAN et al. 1986).

13.2 Anatomy, Physiology, and Methods

13.2.1 Pertinent Anatomy and Physiology of the Eye and Orbit

The eye is a 3-cm spheroid surrounded by orbital tissues consisting of muscle, fat, skin, and connective and glandular tissue called adnexa (Fig. 13.1.). These orbital tissues are in turn bounded by orbital bones posteriorly. The bony orbit is configured in the shape of a ovoid cone measuring 3.5 cm in height, 4.0 cm in width, and 4.5 cm in depth. Most of the ocular and adnexal arteries enter the orbit posteriorly and course anteriorly. Most venous drainage collects anteriorly and exits through the posterior orbit.

The wall of the eye can be divided into three layers: from the outside into the eye one finds the fibrous sclera, the vascular uvea (e.g. choroid), and the neural retina. Deep to the retina and filling the eye is the vitreous gel (which is almost entirely composed of water). The central retinal artery, a direct branch of the ophthalmic artery, enters the optic nerve 10 mm behind the eyeball, enters the eye, and perfuses the retina. The uvea is supplied by multiple ciliary arteries which also are derived from the ophthalmic artery. They reach the uvea by piercing the sclera both posteriorly and anteriorly. In general, the arteries of the eye are small and have a lower pressure (e.g., 65 to 70 mmHg) than other arteries in the body (e.g., 100 mmHg). Though the rate of blood flow through the retina and choroid is high, these structures carry relatively little blood volume (BILL 1981).

13.2.2 Approaches to the Treatment of Retinoblastoma

The most common intraocular tumor in children is retinoblastoma. These tumors arise from the retina and grow either into the vitreous gel which fills the eye (endophytic), or towards the choroid (exophytic), or both. Since this tumor is relatively friable, clumps of "seeds" have been noted to float into the vitreous gel within the eye and/or to locations beneath tumor-associated retinal detachments. Retinoblastomas are known to exit the eye

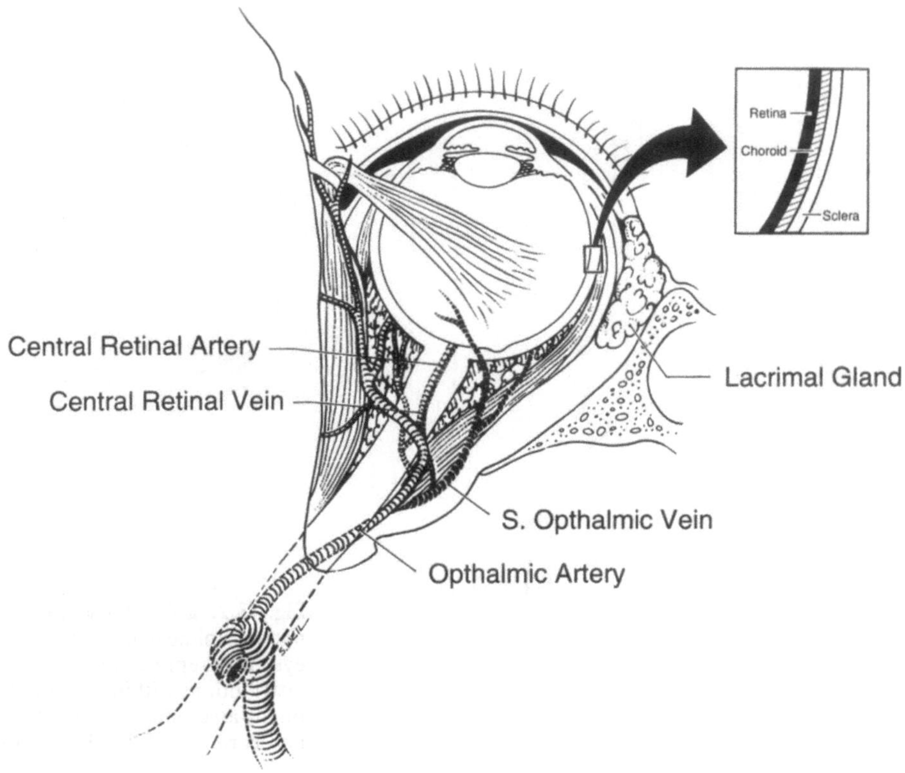

Fig. 13.1. The anatomic relationships of the normal eye and orbit

into the central nervous system by direct extension through the optic nerve. Retinoblastomas are commonly multifocal, and can affect one or both eyes.

Since few retinoblastomas present as small discrete masses suitable for plaque radiotherapy, most have been treated by enucleation or external beam radiotherapy (AMENDOLA et al. 1990). Small unifocal tumors have been treated by plaque radiotherapy (STANNARD et al. 1987).

In an effort to address the problem of heating large and multifocal intraocular retinoblastomas, Lagendijk designed a 2450-MHz microstripline microwave applicator to induce generalized heating of the posterior segment of the eye (BOLLEMEIJER et al. 1989; LAGENDIJK 1982a). With the anterior chamber cooled by water, the microstripline was placed around the ora serrata (Fig. 13.2). In contrast, small unifocal lesions could be treated with plaque-like heat delivery systems.

13.2.3 Approaches to the Treatment of Uveal Melanoma

Malignant melanomas of the eye are usually solitary tumors which arise within the uveal tract (choroid, ciliary body, and iris) of one eye. Therefore uveal melanomas extend from the vascular eye wall and push the retina into the avascular vitreous humor. Since the vitreous is avascular, and the overlying retinal vessels rarely feed the tumor, intraocular melanomas are dependent on basal uveal vessels. Seventy-five percent of these tumors assume a dome shape, and at least 25% mushroom through Bruch's membrane (which separates the choroid and retinal layers) to form a "collar-button" or "mushroom" configuration. It is significant that most uveal melanomas have been found to be located in the posterior half of the eye.

Like radiotherapy, hyperthermic treatment has involved either placing a plaque on the sclera beneath the intraocular tumor or using teletherapy. Six types of episcleral "plaque-like" devices have been devised utilizing conductive and inductive heat delivery systems. Two types of teletherapy heat-deliverys systems have also been developed.

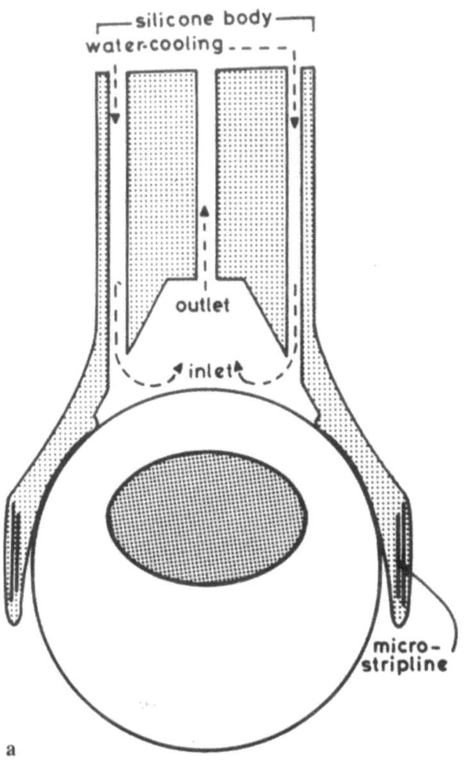

a

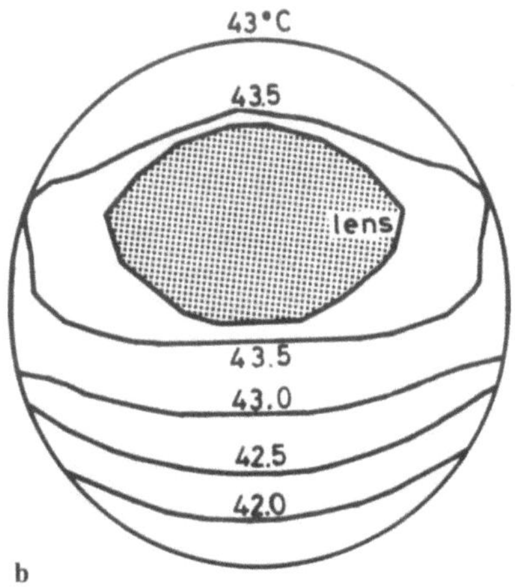

b

Fig. 13.2. a A representation of the Lagendijk 2450-MHz microstripline microwave applicator in place on a schematic eye. **b** A representation of the characteristic temperature distributions within the eye. These calculations were based on the assumption of a constant temperature of the stripline and cornea (43°C). (From BOLLEMEIJER et al. 1989)

13.3 Heat Delivery Systems

13.3.1 Conductive Plaque-Shaped Heat Sources

Both etched-element and ferromagnetic plaques have been evaluated on normal and tumor-bearing rabbit eyes. The etched-element (thermofoil) heater incorporated an etched-foil resistive element (75 ohm) between two layers of electrical insulation. DC power was required to heat the element. A single central thermocouple was used to monitor treatment temperatures. These experiments on normal rabbit eyes demonstrated that 50° to 52°C for 1 h was tolerated by the sclera and cornea (FINGER et al. 1983; GOLDBLATT et al. 1989). Slightly lower temperatures were found to stimulate scleral fibroblasts to produce new scleral collagen (FINGER et al. 1986).

Ferromagnetic seeds have been used alone and together with ^{125}I seeds in episcleral plaques on an animal model of uveal melanoma (Fig. 13.3). Within an oscillating magnetic field, the ferromagnetic seeds generated heat within the plaque (MEILER et al. 1989; STEEVES et al. 1992). Like the etched-element heater, this technique deposited heat onto the sclera, and intraocular heating resulted from thermal conduction.

13.3.2 Inductive Plaque-Shaped Heat Sources

Three microwave plaques and one LCF 500-kHz radiofrequency-emitting episcleral plaque have been designed. All microwave and LCF plaques were tested on normal and tumor-bearing rabbit eyes prior to clinical trials. Ophthalmic hyperthermia plaques have deposited most of their heat at the base of the tumor and therefore have targeted its vascular supply (REINHOLD and ENDRICH 1986). Of the four microwave techniques investigated, a noncooled microwave applicator design has been demonstrated to offer the steepest thermal gradient outside the targeted zone (Fig. 13.4) (FINGER et al. 1989, 1993a). Therefore its energy deposition pattern may have provided less heating of normal ocular structures. Measurements of intraocular heating as proved by noncooled microwave plaque applicators have consistently demonstrated a decrease of approximately 1°C per central axial (intraocular) millimeter (FINGER et al. 1985; RIEDEL et al. 1991).

One group has constructed a microwave coil antenna-plaque (KINDY-DEGNAN et al. 1986). This design offered scleral surface cooling capability and potentially greater intraocular penetration as evaluated in preclinical studies (Fig. 13.5).

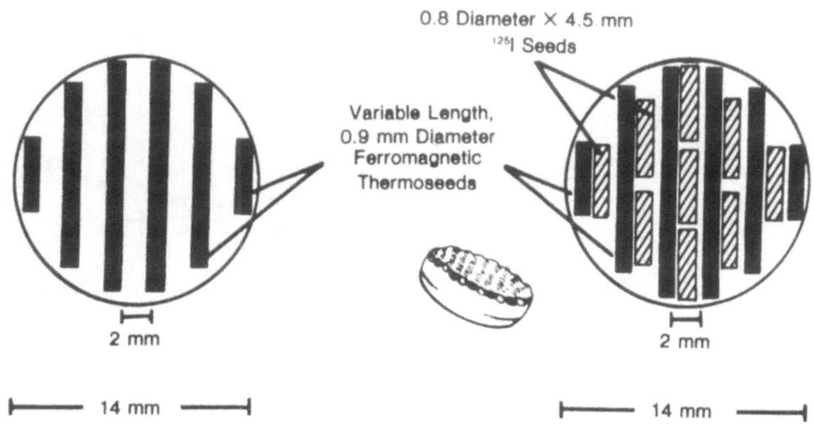

Fig. 13.3. Left: The ferromagnetic thermoseed plaque design. Right: A combined ferromagnetic thermoseed and ^{125}I seed plaque design. (From MIELER et al. 1989)

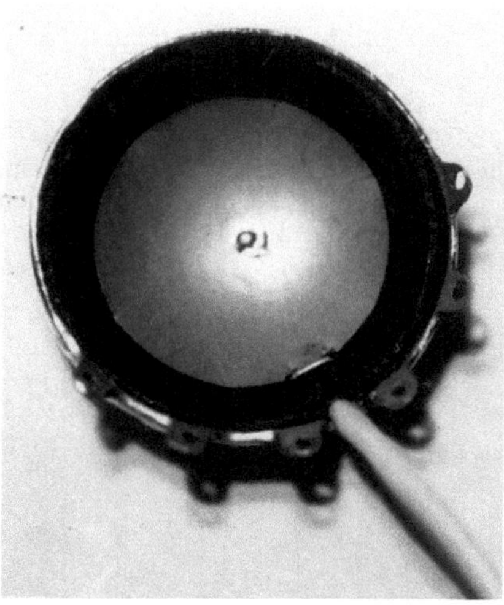

Fig. 13.4. A plaque-shaped microwave antenna affixed within a gold episcleral plaque. A white miniature coaxial cable is noted leaving the plaque. The plaque is shown prior to thermocouple assembly and silicone insulation for better visualization. (From FINGER 1992)

The LCF (radiofrequency) plaques have been used alone or together with radioactive seeds. Intraocular heating has been characterized by deep intraocular penetration with a slower (−0.3°C per axial mm) thermal drop-off (Fig. 13.6). This group evolved a heating technique on a rabbit model, and then began a phase I clinical trial (ASTRAHAN et al. 1987; LIGGEETT et al. 1991; PETROVICH et al. 1992).

13.3.3 Hyperthermic Teletherapy

Much like charged-particle therapy, hyperthermic teletherapy for intraocular tumors has involved the production of a beam which enters the front of the eye in order to treat tumors which are most commonly located in the posterior segment of the eye. Though low-power external beam microwave exposures were tolerated by monkey eyes, the literature is replete with articles describing the production of "microwave" cataracts (GUY et al. 1975; LIPMAN et al. 1988; MCAFEE et al. 1979). Whether these cataracts were truly due to microwaves or to microwave-induced heating has not been established. One group has reported success treating experimental choroidal melanomas in rabbits using an external beam microwave generator (GODFREY et al. 1986).

An ultrasound teletherapy heat delivery system has also been investigated alone or in combination with charged-particle irradiation in preclinical studies (RIEDEL et al. 1985). For treatment, the beam entered anterior to the equator of the eye and traveled through the vitreous gel prior to reaching the tumor (Fig. 13.7). Since ultrasound preferentially heats interfaces where there are changes in acoustic impedance, selective heating occurred at the tumor's surface, the sclera, and lastly the orbital bones (RIEDEL et al. 1985). In contrast to plaque techniques which exactly place and surgically attach the heat source over the base of the tumor (fixed target volume), therapeutic ultrasound relies on a focusing mechanism (A-scan) to locate the tumor. Teletherapies could also be affected by eye movements (mobile target volume).

13.4 Thermometry

Clinical thermometry has been hampered by ophthalmologists' reluctance to penetrate an eye

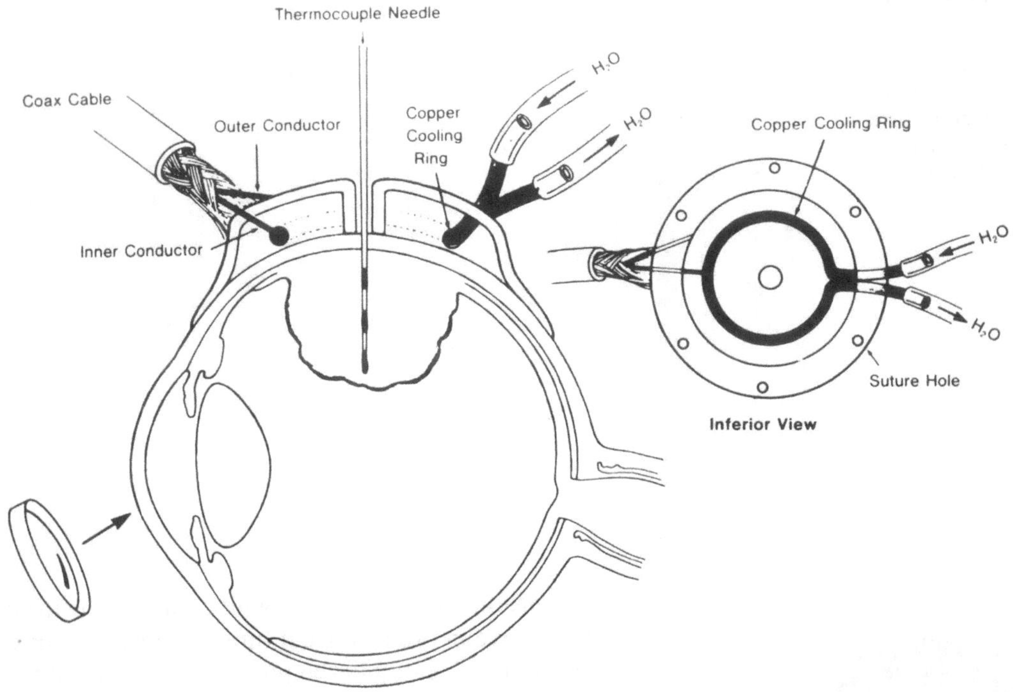

Fig. 13.5. A schematic drawing of a water-cooled 2450-MHz microwave plaque applicator (coil-type antenna) with integral surface cooling. Temperature monitoring was accomplished with an intraocular 25-gauge thermal probe with three separate sensors 3 mm apart on a rabbit model. (From KINDY-DEGNAN et al. 1989)

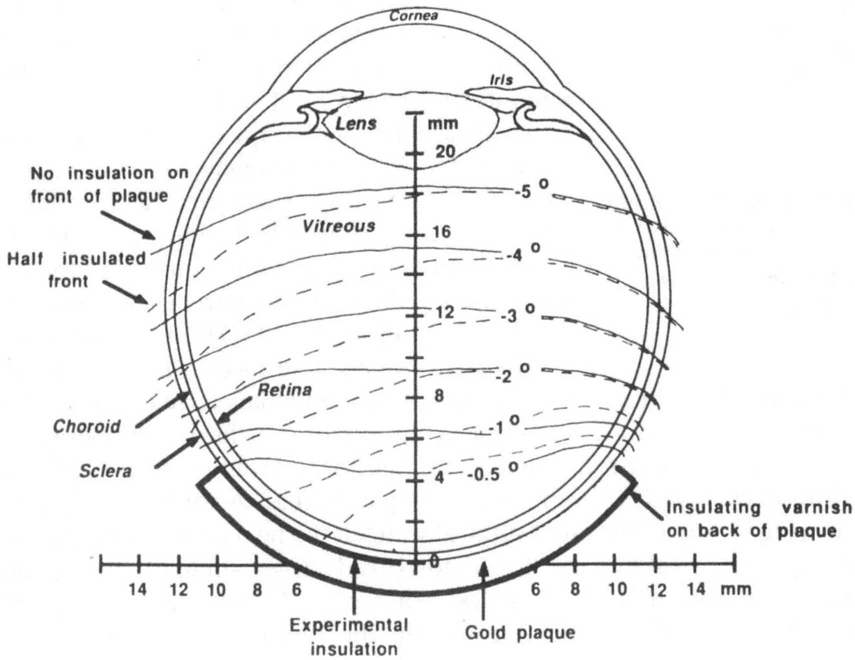

Fig. 13.6. Temperature isotherms of a 500-kHz LCF plaque on phantom material and in a steady-state condition. Measurements were taken in a plane containing the central and the long axis of the plaque surface. isotherms were referenced to the average temperature at the plaque surface. The *solid lines* are for the conventional plaque. The *dashed lines* are for the same plaque in which half of the concave (front) surface has been electrically insulated. ^{125}I seeds could be glued into slots on the inner surface of the plaque. The second electrode was placed approximately 30 mm directly above the plaque. As illustrated, the isotherms were super-imposed on a cross-section of a human eye to illustrate the scale. (From ASTRAHAN et al. 1987)

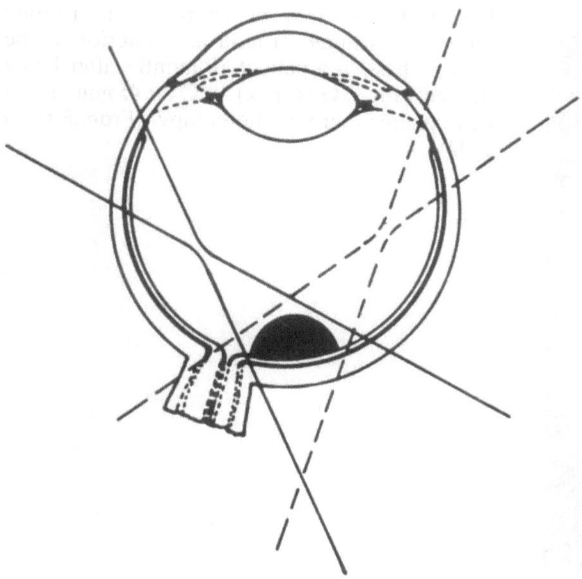

Fig. 13.7. Positions of the ultrasound beam in relation to normal ocular structures and a tumor. (From COLEMAN et al. 1986)

with intraocular thermometers. This has related to concerns about dissemination of tumor cells into the periocular orbit, with subsequent metastasis. Most centers have performed laboratory evaluations of intraocular thermometry on rabbit eyes and phantom materials (ASTRAHAN et al. 1987; FINGER et al. 1985, 1993a; RIEDEL et al. 1991; SWIFT et al. 1990). Based on these experiments, clinical applications have largely inferred intraocular temperature distributions from boundary (scleral) measurements (HAND 1987). Two techniques have relied on mathematical modeling of intraocular and intratumor temperature during clinical applications (COLEMAN et al. 1986; LAGENDIJK 1982b).

13.5 Results

Investigators have consistently demonstrated that heat used alone and in combination with radiation causes destruction of intraocular tumors in a rabbit model. Most have added hyperthermia to plaque brachytherapy, and one group investigated combinations of ultrasonic heating and charged-particle therapy. Though heat-related complications have included scleral damage, orbital vascular occlusions, retinal detachment, and vitreous hemorrhage, most centers have been encouraged by evidence of tumor damage and regression. Such preclinical investigations have allowed for modifications in applicator and systems design with resultant improvements in safety for patients.

Several centers have undertaken phase I clinical trials to investigate intraocular thermoradiotherapy. Microwave, LCF (radiofrequency) applicator, and ultrasonic heat delivery systems have been employed. As in the preclinical investigations, most have used hyperthermia as an adjuvant to ophthalmic plaque brachytherapy. Evidence of early tumor regression and excellent local control rates has led one group to lower the minimum tumor dose (apex dose) to 50 Gy (FINGER 1992, 1994). Though the clinical data have not yet shown that these dose reductions have decreased radiation-associated complications, comparative clinical dosimetry has suggested this may occur (FINGER et al. 1990a). At relatively short mean follow up intervals, all groups have reported that thermoradiotherapy has demonstrated at least equivalent local control rates as compared to brachytherapy alone.

Certain complications have been attributed to the addition of heat to radiotherapy. As with radiotherapy, heat-related intraocular complications have been related to the energy deposition characteristics of each heat delivery system, the size and location of the tumors and their response to treatment. Specifically the groups using ultrasonic transocular hyperthermia reported cataract formation, ectopic heating, and orbital vascular occlusions (BRAAKMAN et al. 1989; COLEMAN et al. 1986; RIEDEL et al. 1985). Plaque-like microwave applicators were reported to induce chorioretinal scar formation around and anterior to the tumor's base, and to decrease intraocular pressure (without hypotony) after treatment of anterior tumors (Fig. 13.8) (FINGER 1992). This may be helpful if the tumor is associated with increased intraocular pressure. In the treatment of very large tumors, LCF hyperthermia was reported to induce cataracts, vitreous hemorrhages, and retinal detachments (LIGGETT et al. 1991). A decrease in mean scleral (boundary) temperature to less than or equal to 44°C and the inclusion of medium-sized tumors in the series has reduced the incidence of these complications (PETROVICH et al. 1992). Microwave plaque applicators have thus far been associated with the fewest significant heat-related complications.

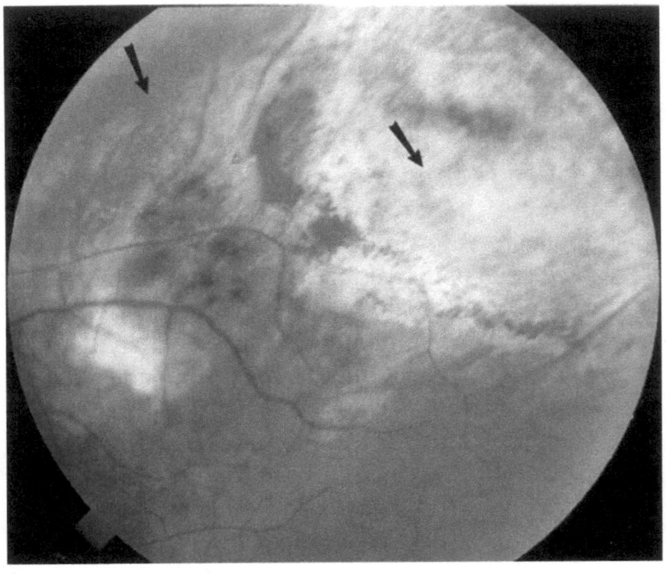

Fig. 13.8. An area of chorioretinal atrophy (arrow) was noted around and anterior to the tumor's base in a patient 10 months after being treated with 55 Gy (apex) 48°C for 45 min microwave plaque thermoradiotherapy. (From FINGER 1992)

13.6 Discussion

It has been generally believed that therapeutic enhancement of radiotherapy by adjuvant hyperthermia could lead to a reduction in the amount of ionizing radiation required to sterilize intraocular tumors. Thereby, the incidence of ionizing radiation-associated complications could be reduced for currently employed plaque radiotherapy (e.g. ^{125}I, ^{106}Ru, and ^{103}Pd), as well as beam therapies (proton, helium ion). In the treatment of retinoblastoma, lowered radiation doses would diminish the exposure of the bony orbit. This may (if dose dependent) decrease the incidence of secondary cancers (e.g., osteogenic sarcomas) within the radiation field (ROARTY et al. 1988; SAGERMAN et al. 1969).

In one series, 36 patients with uveal melanoma have already been treated with reduced apical doses of plaque brachytherapy (^{125}I, ^{103}Pd) together with adjuvant microwave thermotherapy (FINGER 1992). By reducing the amount of radiation delivered to the tumor apex to a target dose of 50 Gy, the amount of radiation delivered to normal ocular structures was decreased by 50% or more compared with most centers using radiotherapy alone (EARLE et al. 1987).

As it relates to the effectiveness of apex dose reductions, it is important to consider that the tumor's apex has been the historical standard prescription point for plaque brachytherapy. That was because it was the farthest point of intraocular tumor extension, the farthest point to which the radiation must travel, and therefore the point of the minimum tumor dose. Though apical dose reductions will allow for comparisons of thermoradiotherapy-induced complications with historical standards of data, this form of radiation prescription carries forward the legacy ot variable average tumor doses. For example, a large tumor (or eye) treated to an apex prescription dose of 50 Gy apex receives much more radiation than a small tumor (or eye) treated to the same apex prescription dose. Though this gradient phenomenon would be less significant with charged-particle treatment, one must consider the relatively large entry dose and high dose rates associated with beam radiotherapy. With any form of radiation therapy, reductions of radiation dose to normal ocular structures should result in fewer radiation-associated complications.

Though there has been tremendous academic interest in hyperthermic treatment of intraocular tumors, we must remember that the most common primary intraocular malignancies (uveal melanoma and retinoblastoma) are rare tumors. There are too few patients to interest most medical technology companies. The hope for the production of commercially available hyperthermia units for treatment of intraocular tumors may lie in other applications for low-level, thermometry-controlled heating (FINGER et al. 1991c,d, 1993b). Heat delivery systems manufactured for more common ophthalmic diseases may allow for the production of accessory applicators for the treatment of intraocular tumors.

13.7 Conclusion

Intraocular hyperthermia has undergone an evolution from conceptualization, laboratory evaluations, and most recently phase I clinical trials. So far no long-term or comparative studies have been reported. The world's experience with adjuvant hyperthermia reflects an optimism that multimodality therapy may play a role in the treatment of intraocular tumors, and that future randomized comparative studies are warranted.

13.8 Summary

- Several heat delivery systems have been developed to treat intraocular tumors.
- Invasive thermometry techniques have been avoided in order to keep tumor-cells from exiting the eye.
- Phase I clinical trials have been started for microwave, LCF, and ultrasound thermoradiotherapy.
- The frequency and type of complications attributed to intraocular heating have largely been acceptable.
- Future comparative trials designed to compare radiotherapy alone versus thermoradiotherapy are warranted.

References

Amendola BE, Lamm FR, Markoe AM, Karlsson UL, Shields J, Shields CL, et al. (1990) Radiotherapy of retinoblastoma. A review of 63 children treated with different irradiation techniques. Cancer 66: 21–26

Astrahan M, Liggett P, Petrovich Z, Luxton G (1987) A 500 KHz localized current field hyperthermia system for use with ophthalmic plaque therapy. Int J Hyperthermia 3: 423–432

Bill A (1981) Ocular Circulation. In Moses RA, (ed), Adler's Physiology of the Eye, Mosby, St. Louis, pp 184–203

Bollemeijer, JG, Lagendijk JJW, van Best JA, de Leeuw AA, van Delft JL, de Wolff-Rouendaal D, Oosterhuis JA, Schipper J (1989) Effects of microwave induced hyperthermia on the anterior segment of healthy rabbit eyes. Graefe's Arch Clin Exp Ophthalmol 227: 271–276

Braakman R, van der Valk P, van Delft JL, de Wolff-Rouendaal D, Oossterhuis JA (1989) The effects of ultrasonically induced hyperthermia on exaperimental tumors in the rabbit eye. Invest Ophthalmol Vis Sci 30: 835–844

Char DH, Castro JR, Quivey JM, Phillips TL, Irvine AR, Stone RD, Kroll S (1989) Uveal melanoma radiation. I-125 brachytherapy versus helium-ion irradiation. Ophthalmology 96: 1708–1715

Chiu-Tsao ST, Anderson LL (1991) Thermoluminescent dosimetry for Pd-103 seeds (Model 200) in a solid water phantom. Med Phys 18: 449–452

Coleman DJ, Lizzi FL, Burgess SE, Silverman RH, Smith ME, Driller J, Rosado A (1986) Ultrasonic hyperthermia and radiation in the management of intraocular malignant melanoma. Am J Ophthalmol 101: 635–642

Davidorf FH, Makley TA, Lang JR (1976) Radiotherapy of malignant melanoma of the choroid. Trans Am Acad Ophthalmol Otolaryngol 81: 849–861

Davidorf FH, Pajka JT, Makley TA, Kartha MK (1978) Radiotherapy of choroidal melanoma, an 18-year experience with radon. Arch Ophthalmol 105: 352–355

Earle J, Kline RW, Robertson DM (1987) Selection of iodine-125 for the Collaborative Ocular Melanoma Study. Arch Ophthalmol 105: 763–764

Emami B, Perez CA, Konefal J, Pilepich MV, Leybovich L, Straube W, Von Gerichten D, Hederman MA (1988) Thermoradiotherapy of malignant melanoma. Int J Hyperthermia 4: 373–381

Finger PT, Packer S, Albert DM (1982) The effect of hyperthermia on the normal rabbit eye. Invest Ophthalmol Vis Sci (suppl) 22: 8

Finger PT, Packer S, Svitra PP, Paglione RW, Albert DM, Chess J (1983) A 5.8 GHz ophthalmic microwave applicator for treatment of choroidal melanoma. IEEE Trans Microwave Theory Tech MTT-S International Microwave Symposium Digest F-1: 177–179 (83CH 1871–1873)

Finger PT, Packer S, Svitra PP, Paglione RW, Chess J, Albert DM (1984) Hyperthermic treatment of intraocular tumors. Arch Ophthalmol 102: 1477–1481

Finger PT, Packer S, Svitra PP, Paglione RW, Anderson LL, Kim JH, Jakobiec FA (1985) Thermoradiotherapy for intraocular tumors. Arch Ophthalmol 103: 1574–1578

Finger PT, Curtin BJ, Packer S, Svitra PP, Iwamoto T, Whitmore WG, Jakobiec FA (1986) Scleral hyperplasia induced by heat. Am I Ophthalmol 102: 25–32

Finger PT, Packer S, Paglione RW, Gatz JF, Ho TK, Bosworth JL (1989) Thermoradiotherapy of choroidal melanoma. Clinical experience. Ophthalmology 96: 1384–1388

Finger PT, Packer S, Ho TK, De Blasio, D.S., Bosworth, JL (1990a) 50 Gray (Apex) I-125/Microwave plaque thermoradiotherapy for treatment of choroidal melanoma. Invest Ophthalmol Vis Sci (suppl) 31: 500

Finger PT, Ho TK, Fastenberg DM, Hyman RA Stroh EM, Packer S, Perry HD (1990b) Intraocular Radiation Blocking. Invest Ophthalmol Vis Sci 31: 1724–1730

Finger PT, Moshfeghi DM, Ho TK (1991a) Palladium-103 ophthalmic plaque radiation therapy. Arch Ophthalmol 109: 1610–1613

Finger PT, Svitra PP, Packer S, Riedel KG, Albert DM (1991b) Models of uveal melanoma. In Bornfeld N, Gragoudas ES, Hopping W, Lommatzsch PK, Wessing A, Zografos L (eds) International symposium on tumors of the eye, Essen, FRG, Sept. 21–23, 1989. Kugler, Amsterdam, pp 207–213

Finger PT, Paglione RW, Packer S (1991c) Microwave thermotherapy for choroidal hemangioma. Am J Ophthalmol 111: 240–241

Finger PT, Moshfeghi DM, Smith PD, Perry HD (1991d) Microwave thermotherapy for glaucoma in a rabbit model. Arch Ophthalmol 109: 1001–1004

Finger PT (1992) Microwave plaque thermoradiotherapy for choroidal melanoma. Brit J Ophthalmol 76: 358–364

Finger PT, Selkin R, Grabczyk J, Fetter RW (1993a) A phantom system for microwave treatment of intraocular tumors. Retina 13: 63–68
Finger PT, Svitra PP, McCormick SA, Pressor A (1993b) Microwave diathermy of the retina and choroid. Arch Ophthalmol 111: 254–258
Finger PT, Lu DF, Buffa A, DeBlasio, DM, Bosworth, JL (1993) Palladium-103 versus iodine-125 for ophthalmic plaque radiotherapy. Int J Radiat Oncol Biol Phys 27: 849–854
Finger PT, Buffa A, Mishra S, Berson A, Bosworth JL, Vikram B (1994) Palladium-103 plaque radiotherapy of uveal melanoma: clinical experience. Ophthalmology 101: 256–263
Godfrey R, Gordon R, Schlosser JV, Yamanouchi K, Salpeter J (1986) Hyperthermia and radiation treamtent of intraocular melanoma. Invest Ophthalmol Vis Sci (suppl) 27: 86
Goldblatt WS, Finger PT, Perry HD, Stroh EM, Weiser DS, Donnenfeld ED (1989) Hyperthermic treatment of rabbit corneas. Invest Ophthalmol Vis Sci 30: 1778–1783
Gragoudas ES, Goitein M, Verhey L, Munzenreider J, Urie M, Suit M, Koehler A (1982) Proton beam irradiation of uveal melanoma. Results of a 5½-year study. Arch Ophthalmol 100: 928–934
Gragoudas ES, Seddon JM, Egan K, Glynn R, Munzenrider J, Austin-Seymour M, Goiten M, Verhey L, Koehler (1987) Long-term results of proton beam irradiated uveal melanomas. Ophthalmology 94: 349–353
Guy AW, Lin JC, Kramar PO, Emery AF (1975) Effect of 2450-MHz Radiation on the rabbit eye. IEEE Trans Microwave Theory Tech 23: 492–498
Hand JW (1987) Heat delivery and thermometry in clinical hyperthermia. Recent Results Cancer Res 104: 1–23
Karlsson UL, Augsburger JJ, Shields JA, Markoe AM, Brady LW, Woodleigh R (1989) Recurrence of posterior uveal melanoma after cobalt-60 episcleral plaque therapy. Ophthalmol 96: 382–388
Kim JH, Hahn EW, Ahmed SA (1982) Combination hyperthermia and radiation therapy for malignant melanoma. Cancer 50: 478–482
Kindy-Degnan N, Char DH, Swift P, Kaleta S, Ljung BM (1989) Bromodeoxyuridine uptake in the assessment of hyperthermic therapy for intraocular tumors. Arch Ophthalmol 107: 746–750
Lagendijk JJW (1980) Microwave applicator for hyperthermic treatment of retinoblastoma. Natl. Cancer Inst. Monograph 61: 469–471
Lagendijk JJW (1982a) A microwave heating technique for the hyperthermic treatment of tumours in the eye, especially retinoblastoma. Phys Med Biol 27: 1313–1324
Lagendijk JJW (1982b) A mathematical model to calculate temperature distributions in human and rabbit eyes during hyperthermic treatment. Phys Med Biol 27: 1301–1311
Liggett PE, Pince KJ, Astrahan M, Rao N, Petrovich Z (1990) Localized current field hyperthermia: effect on normal ocular tissue. Int J Hyperthermia 6: 517–527
Liggett PE, Ma C, Astrahan M, Pince KJ, Green R, McDonnell J, Petrovich Z (1991) Combined localized current field hyperthermia and irradiation for intraocular tumors. Ophthalmology 98: 1830–1836
Lindstadt D, Castro J, Char D, Decker M, Ahn D, Petti P, Nowakowski V, Quivey J, Phillips TL (1990) Long-term results of helium-ion irradiation of uveal melanoma. Int J Radiat Oncol Biol Phys 19: 613–618
Lipman RM, Tripathi BJ, Tripathi RC (1988) Cataracts induced by microwave and ionizing radiation. Surv Ophthalmol 33: 200–210
Lommatzsch PK (1974) Treatment of choroidal melanomas with 106Ru/106Rh beta-ray applicators. Surv Ophthalmol 19: 85–100
Lommatzsch PK (1986) Results after Beta-irradiation (Ru-106/Rh-106) of choroidal melanomas: 20 years experience. Br J Ophthalmol 70: 844–851
Manning MR, Cetas TC, Miller RC, Oleson JR, Conner WG, Gerner EW (1982) Clinical hyperthermia: Results of a phase I trial employing hyperthermia alone or in combination with external beam or interstitial radiotherapy. Cancer 49: 205–216
McAfee RD, Longacre A, Bishop RR, Elder ST, May JG, Holland MG, Gordon R (1979) Absence of ocular pathology after repeated exposure of unanesthetized monkeys to 9.3-GHz microwaves. J Microwave Power 14: 42–44
Mieler WF, Jaffe GJ, Steeves RA (1989) Ferromagnetic hyperthermia and Iodine-125 brachytherapy in the treatment of choroidal melanoma in a rabbit model. Arch Ophthalmol 107: 1524–1528
Molls M, Scherer E (1987) The combination of hyperthermia and radiation: Clinical investigations. Recent Results in Cancer Res 104: 110–135
Meyer JL (1984) The clinical efficacy of localized hyperthermia. Cancer Res 44(suppl 10): 4745s–4751s
Packer S, Rotman M (1980) Radiotherapy of choroidal melanoma with Iodine-125. Ophthalmology 87: 582–590
Packer S, Rotman M, Salanitro P (1984) Iodine-125 irradiation of choroidal melanoma. Clinical experience. Ophthalmol 91: 1700–1708
Packer S, Stoller S, Lessor ML, Mandel FS, Finger PT (1992) Long-term results of iodine-125 irradiation of uveal melanoma. Ophthalmology 99: 767–774
Petrovich Z, Astrahan MA, Luxton G, Green R, Langholz B, Liggett P (1992) Episcleral plaque thermoradiotherapy in patients with choroidal melanoma. Int J Radiat Oncol Biol Phys 23: 599–603
Riedel KG, Svitra PP, Seddon JM, et al. (1985) Proton beam irradiation and hyperthermia: Effects on experimental choroidal melanoma. Arch Ophthalmol 103: 1862–1869
Riedel KG (1988) Hypertherme Therapieverfahren Erganzung zur Strahlenbehandlung maligner intraokularer Tumoren. Klin Mbl Augenheilkd 2(193): 131–137
Riedel KG, Plischke H, Turkner KH, Russer P (1991) Thermoradiotherapy of choroidal melanoma: New compact 2.45 GHz microstrip applicators. Invest Ophthalmol Vis Sci (suppl) 32(4): 1196
Reinhold HS, Endrich B (1986) Invited review: Tumor microcirculation as a target for hyperthermia. Int J Hyperthermia 2: 111–137
Roarty JD, McLean IW, Zimmerman LE (1988) Incidence of second neoplasms in patients with bilateral retinoblastoma. Ophthalmol 85: 1583–1587
Sagerman RH, Cassady JR, Tretter P, Ellsworth RM (1969) Radiation induced neoplasia following external beam therapy for children with retinoblastoma. Am J Roentgenol Radium Ther Nucl Med 105: 529–535
Stannard C, Sealy R, Shackleton D, Hill J, Korrubel J (1987) The use of iodine-125 plaques in the treatment of retinoblastoma. Ophthalmic Paediatr Genet 8: 89–93

Shields JA, Augsburger JJ, Brady LW, Day JL (1982) Cobalt plaque therapy of posterior uveal melanomas. Ophthalmol 89: 1201–1207
Stallard HB (1962) Doyne Memorial Lecture, 1962. The conservative treatment of retinoblastoma. Trans Ophthalmol Soc UK 82: 473–535
Stallard HB (1966) Radiotherapy for malignant melanoma of the choroid. Br J Ophthalmol 50: 147–155
Stallard HB (1968) Malignant melanoblastoma of the choroid. Bibl Ophthalmol 75: 16–38
Steeves RA, Murray TG, Moros EG, Boldt HC, Mieler WF, Paliwal BR (1992) Concurrent ferromagnetic hyperthermia and I-125 brachytherapy in a rabbit choroidal melanoma model. Int J Hyperthermia 8: 443–449
Swift PS, Stauffer PR, Fries PD, Kaleta-Michaels S, Murray T, Sneed PK, Phillips TL, Char DH (1990) Microwave hyperthermia of choroidal melanoma in rabbits. Invest Ophthalmol Vis Sci 31: 1754–1760
Zimmerman LE, McLean IW, Foster WD (1978) Does enucleation of the eye containing a malignant melanoma prevent or accelerate the dissemination of tumour cells. Br J Ophthalmol 62: 420–425

14 Thermoradiotherapy and Thermochemotherapy for Pediatric Tumors

R. VAN HEEK-ROMANOWSKI, F. D'OLEIRE, and W. HAVERS

CONTENTS

14.1 Introduction: The Special Challenge in Introducing Thermotherapy to Pediatric Oncology

The spectrum of malignant diseases of children and adolescents is different from that in adults. The neoplasms associated with childhood show a relative abundance of leukemia, lymphoma, brain tumors, sarcomas, and embryonal tumors (Table 14.1). Most of these entities are of high malignancy.

R. VAN HEEK-ROMANOWSKI, MD, Universitätskinderklinik Essen, Hufelandstraße 55, D-45147 Essen, FRG
F. D'OLEIRE, MD, Department of Human Oncology, The University of Wisconsin, Madison, WI 53792, USA
W. HAVERS, MD, Universitätskinderklinik Essen, Hufelandstraße 55, D-45147 Essen, FRG

High-grade malignancies with low differentiation are often correlated with a high sensitivity to chemotherapy and ionizing radiation. This could contribute to the relatively high response rates achieved in childhood cancer. Table 14.1 summarizes the frequencies, therapeutic modalities, and cure rates of malignant diseases in childhood in a very simplified manner: it does take into consideration the different subgroups of the diseases and highly sophisticated treatment stratifications. Cure rates are given as percentage of the first continuous complete remission as expressed by the stable plateau of a life table according to Kaplan and Meyer.

The annual incidence of cancer in children under 15 years of age is approximately 14 cases in a population of 100000. In the United States this rate has increased by 4.1% from 1972 to 1988 (BLEYER 1993). However, during this same period the overall mortality in this age group has decreased by 38%, mainly due to a striking drop on mortality from leukemia, lymphoma, and soft tissue sarcoma of more than 50% (BLEYER 1993). The rarity of certain neoplasms compromises the enrollment of a sufficient number of patients into a clinical trial within a reasonable period. Consequently testing a new treatment modality, such as hyperthermia, for a given malignancy in childhood can present an extremely challenging task. This is especially true as the necessary technology for hyperthermia is only available at a few oncological centers. In addition, another impediment for new trials can be concluded from Table 14.1: cure can be achieved in more than half of the patients. Accordingly, the introduction of a new treatment modality should not jeopardize "standard" good results. Hence the new approach to therapy should have a rationale of improving efficacy and/or reducing toxicity.

Currently pediatricians are facing severe problems with regard to prevailing treatment regimens. These include late side-effects of chemotherapy and radiotherapy, e.g., growth inhibition, inferti-

Table 14.1. Frequency[a], treatment and outcome of cancer in children

Type of disease	Relative frequency (%)	Established treatment modalities	Level of 1st CCR (%)	References
Leukemias	**34.7**			
Acute lymphoblastic leukemia	28.0	ChT	70	Riehm et al. (1990); Reiter et al. (1992)
Acute nonlymphoblastic leukemia	4.7	ChT	45	Creutzig et al. (1993)
Lymphomas	**14.6**			
Non-Hodgkin's lymphoma	5.5	ChT	80	Riehm et al. (1990)
Hodgkin's disease	4.6	RT, ChT	80–90	Brämswig et al. (1990)
CNS tumors	**15.9**			
Medulloblastoma	3.9	S, RT, ChT	70	Packer et al. (1991)
Embryonal tumors	**16.7**			
Neuroblastoma	7.2	S, ChT, (RT)	20–80[b]	Berthold et al. (1992)
nephroblastoma	6.1	S, ChT, RT	80	D'Angio et al. (1989)
Retinoblastoma	2.6	S, RT, (ChT)	90	Havers et al. (1986)
Hepatoblastoma	0.8	S, ChT	60–80	von Schweinitz et al. (1992)
Bone tumors	**5.2**			
Osteosarcoma	2.8	S, ChT	60	Winkler et al. (1991)
Ewing's sarcoma	1.9	S, ChT, RT	50–60	Burgert et al. (1990)
Soft tissue sarcomas	**6.9**			
Rhabdomyosarcoma	3.9	S, ChT, RT	50–70	Rodary et al. (1991)
Germ cell neoplasms	**3.1**	S, ChT, (RT)	80–90	Haas et al. (1989); Göbel et al. (1993)
Epithelial neoplasms	**0.9**			

S, surgery; ChT, chemotherapy; RT, radiotherapy; CCR, continuous complete response
[a] Relative frequency from data from the German Registry for Childhood Cancer (Haaf et al. 1993), which are rather similar to data from other western European countries and the United States
[b] According to stage and age of the child

lity, impairment of renal, cardiac, and endocrine function, cerebral dysfunction, and secondary malignancies (Blatt and Bleyer 1989). Mutilating surgical procedures are still unavoidable and cause severe physical and especially psychosocial problems during adolescence. Furthermore there are still diseases with a poor prognosis, e.g., stage IV neuroblastoma, stage IV soft tissue sarcomas, or brain tumors of moderate- or high-grade malignancy. Therefore, the introduction of new treatment modalities to improve cure rates, to diminish toxicity or even to decrease the costs of therapy is compelling.

In contrast to adults, the majority of children with cancer need chemotherapy or ionizing radiation to be cured (Table 14.1). Hyperthermia could be integrated into a broad spectrum of multimodal treatments, if it is shown in clinical trials to enhance the efficacy of cytotoxic drugs or of irradiation, without boosting normal tissue toxicity. Clearly the potential utility of hyperthermia can only be demonstrated in the context of randomized trials.

Prior to phase III studies (addressing hyperthermia as an independent variable), phase I and II studies are necessary, since there are still many unanswered questions in the field of clinical hyperthermia. An important problem is the *localization of heat application*, e.g., should heat be directed at only the tumor, the whole tumor-bearing region (even after resection of the tumor), a whole limb, the clearing lymph nodes or the whole body? Other critical questions relate to hyperthermia as an adjunctive therapy: Should heat be used together with ionizing radiation or with specific chemotherapeutic agents? Which drugs should be selected?

The *sequencing of hyperthermia and other antineoplastic therapies* is still an open issue. Preclinical studies should answer these questions. In vitro and in vivo research should precede any clinical trial to ascertain optimal temperatures, doses, fractionation, and sequencing of drugs/irradiation. Dose (or thermal) enhancement ratios have to be determined for any agent used in combination with hyperthermia. In addition clinical results obtained in adults should be most helpful for the pediatrician, but, clearly, not all results obtained in adults can be extrapolated to children or vice versa.

Nowadays, preclinical research has provided us with numerous facts about the effects of heat, and there are also results from studies in adults. Nevertheless, our experience in children is still limited. Thus, we are at the very beginning of the evaluation of thermotherapy in pediatric oncology. In the following section we will outline the preclinical basis for introducing hyperthermia into clinical investigations centered on pediatric malignancies.

14.2 Biological and Clinical Studies Relevant for Pediatric Thermotherapy

It has been proven in numerous studies in vitro as well as in vivo that hyperthermia enhances the cytotoxicity of ionizing radiation (STREFFER and VAN BEUNINGEN 1987; see Chap. 4 in volume 1) as well as of several antineoplastic drugs (ENGELHARDT 1987; see Chap. 5 in volume 1). In general, higher temperatures produce more enhancement but drug efficacy can be significantly increased in a temperature range as low as 40°–42°C (FISHER and HAHN 1982; COHEN and ROBINS 1987; NEUMANN et al. 1985; WIEDEMANN et al. 1993).

Toxic thermal effects on *normal tissues* are also well known (FAJARDO 1984). Acute toxicity of thermoradio- or thermochemotherapy is extensively reported in clinical trials. In contrast, there is little if any information about late or chronic toxicity of thermotherapy, which is especially important in pediatric oncology in view of growth and development. Cellular and physiological reactions to hyperthermia are of critical importance for clinical studies. Thermotolerance, drug resistance, tumor immunogenicity, perfusion, and microenvironment are changed by hyperthermia. These interesting topics are broadly covered in other chapters of the previous volume. Such effects must be regarded for the design of treatment protocols especially under the aspect of sequencing the different treatment modalities.

Preclinical hyperthermia studies on tumor models representing childhood cancer are rare. For a human neuroblastoma cell line (LAN 1) it could be shown in vitro that the cytotoxicity of doxorubicin as well as of cisplatin and carboplatin is enhanced by a temperature elevation to 40°C or 42°C for 1 h (Fig. 14.1; ROMANOWSKI et al. 1992a; KREMENS et al. 1993). The effect of etoposide on the same cell line was enhanced neither at 40°C nor at 42°C for 1 h (own unpublished data). This observation is consistent with results in other in vitro or in vivo models (Wiedemann, personal communication). WILLNOW (1981) studied the incorporation of ^{3}H-thymidine in primary tissue cultures of 44 solid tumors of children treated by doxorubicin or hyperthermia alone and with simultaneous administration. Hyperthermia of 42.5°C for 120 min resulted in a decrease in ^{3}H-thymidine uptake by 47.5% for heat alone, 62% for drug alone, and 81.4% for the combined treatment. KOOLE and SCHIPPER (1990) implanted human Y-79 retinoblastoma cells into eyes of athymic mice. The eyes were treated with x-rays in six fractions of 3 Gy with or without two hyperthermia treatments of 43°–45°C for 30 min after irradiation. Tumor regrowth occurred in 10 out of 15 eyes treated by irradiation alone and in 3 out of 15 eyes after combined treatment. This result was statistically significant ($P = 0.035$).

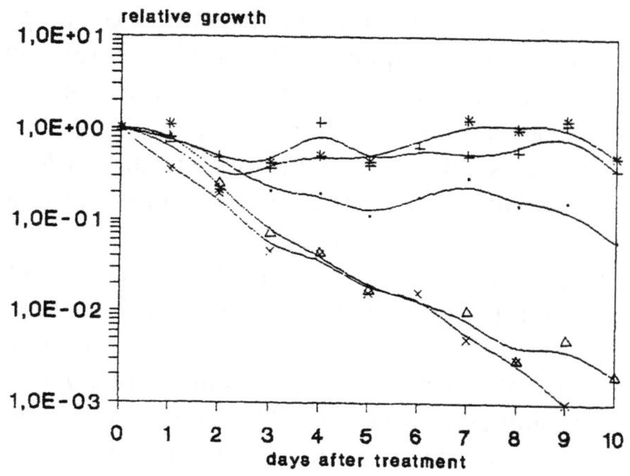

Fig. 14.1. Growth of human neuroblastoma cells (LAN 1) in vitro related to untreated control. Heating to 40°C (+) or 42°C (*) for 1 h does not change the proliferation of LAN 1 cells. Incubation with cisplatin (8 μg/ml) (●) clearly decreases subsequent cell counts (logarithmic scale). The toxicity of the same drug dose is significantly enhanced if the incubation temperature is elevated to 40°C (△) or 42°C (×). (From KREMENS et al. 1992)

Clinical experiences in adults concerning feasibility and therapeutic efficacy of thermotherapy are of major relevance for pediatric oncology adopting this new treatment modality. These topics are covered in other chapters of this volume. Most important in pediatrics is the feasibility of different heating techniques relevant for malignancies of childhood as well as the efficacy of chemotherapy with heat. Late sequelae of combined treatment are much more important in pediatrics than they are in general oncology. Regarding these aspects a short review of relevant clinical experience with thermotherapy outside pediatrics is presented here.

It is possible to heat tumors of various locations locally above 40°C by different methods. This can be accomplished in superficial (see Chaps. 3 and 5 in this volume) and deep-seated tumors of the pelvis (ISSELS et al. 1991; FELDMANN et al. 1993). Experience with local thermotherapy of central nervous system malignancies is increasing (IACONO et al. 1992; SNEED et al. 1992; Chap. 12 in this volume). Tumors of the upper abdomen are difficult to heat (see Chap. 7 in this volume). Limited experience and many unresolved problems are associated with local thermotherapy for tumors of the skull base and the bony face as well as for pulmonary or mediastinal tumors.

The acute toxicity of regional hyperthermia combined with radiotherapy or chemotherapy was acceptable (KAPP et al. 1990; ISSELS et al. 1991). The simultaneous application of thermochemo- and thermoradiotherapy is also feasible (HERMAN et al. 1989; own unpublished experience). It should be noted, however, that severe toxicity has been described in previously irradiated treatment fields (BORNSTEIN et al. 1993), but was probably dependent on the heating technique as well as dose and fractionation of reirradiation.

In prospective randomized clinical trials it has been proven that local hyperthermia enhances radiotherapy, resulting in better local tumor control as well as in improved survival in patients with malignant melanoma (OVERGAARD et al. 1993) or head and neck cancer (VALDAGNI et al. 1988; DATTA et al. 1990). In a randomized phase II study on 64 dogs with spontaneous soft tissue sarcomas local tumor control was significantly better in the group treated by thermoradiotherapy than after radiotherapy alone (MCCHESNEY GILLETTE et al. 1992).

No clinical study has yet been published that proves the efficacy of deep regional hyperthermia with ionizing radiation. A prospective randomized trial on recurrent rectal cancer is in progress (VAN DER ZEE et al. 1993). In nonrandomized clinical trials statistically significant dose-response relationships indicate thermal enhancement (OLESON et al. 1993; FELDMANN et al. 1993). However, it is evident that high temperatures induced by electromagnetic heating arise in necrotic areas with decreased perfusion (FELDMANN et al. 1992). Thus it is also possible that high temperatures indicate good response rather than producing it. Furthermore it has not directly been shown that the proven thermal enhancement of ionizing irradiation is superior to an increase in irradiation dose applied with modern techniques.

As regards *regional hyperthermia with systemic chemotherapy*, statistically significant correlations have been shown between tumor temperatures and tumor response in soft tissue sarcomas (ISSELS et al. 1990). Furthermore, a special pattern of tumor response has been observed in this study, i.e., complete necrosis of some tumors of unchanged volume (ISSELS et al. 1990). The clinical courses of these patients were generally good.

Whole-body hyperthermia up to 41.8°C can be induced in adults without severe toxicity (BULL et al. 1979; ROBINS et al. 1984) in combination with drugs (ROBINS et al. 1993; see also Chap. 17 in this volume) as well as with total-body irradiation (ROBINS et al. 1990). If thermal drug enhancement involves not only the tumor but the whole organism, the therapeutic gain will probably be lost due to increased toxicity (ROBINS et al. 1992). Hence only drugs for which the toxicity is not equally enhanced in all organ systems are useful. In this context, a recent report is of great relevance: systemic hyperthermia induces high plasma levels of IL-1β and G-CSF (D'OLEIRE et al. 1993). This observation can explain in part why the bone marrow toxicity of carboplatin and ifosfamide is not increased by systemic hyperthermia while clinical efficacy is improved (ROBINS et al. 1993; Wiedemann, personal communication).

Concerning the combination of *chemotherapy with systemic hyperthermia*, one randomized phase III trial was performed on 55 patients suffering from small cell lung cancer. Patients were treated in six cycles with doxorubicin, vincristine and cyclophosphamide, and randomized to undergo systemic hyperthermia (41° ± 0.5°C, 1 h) within the first three cycles. In the evaluable group of 22 patients treated at normothermia there were eight complete or partial responses (mean duration 105 days), while in the hyperthermia group the response rate was 15/22 (mean duration 130 days). Despite the small number of patients in this study, this result is encouraging.

Another randomized clinical study was performed on dogs, but nevertheless it is of some interest. In a study on 46 dogs with high-grade lymphoma, animals which were in complete remission after doxorubicin treatment alone were randomized to receive five treatments of doxorubicin either with or without systemic hyperthermia. The median duration of disease-free survival was 189 days after chemotherapy alone and 239 days after combined treatment. Again, this difference was not statistically significant (PAGE et al. 1992), but the study group was small, too.

It was shown in a randomized clinical trial for melanoma of the extremities that *regional hyperthermic perfusion* with melphalan after surgery produced significantly better results than surgery alone (GHUSSEN et al. 1988). Such a study – of course – does not prove the enhancement of chemotherapy by hyperthermia.

14.3 Clinical Thermotherapy in Children

14.3.1 Clinical Experience

Clinical studies on thermotherapy in children and adolescents are rare. Sometimes such experience is reported within larger studies with adults without giving special attention to pediatric items (EGAWA et al. 1989; SEEGENSCHMIEDT et al. 1993a). Many clinical studies are published without information about the age of the patients; hence it cannot be excluded that there is experience with the treatment of children. BAAS et al. (1989) reported on six children and eight adolescents with melanoma who were treated by hyperthermic isolated limb perfusion with melphalan. Nine patients were in stage IA, five in stage IIIB. The 5-year survival rate was 93%, and the 10-year survival rate, 81%. Issels and co-workers were the first to treat children with solid tumors by regional hyperthermia combined with systemic chemotherapy. These patients were part of a larger phase I/II study mainly recruiting adult patients (ISSELS et al. 1990). A multicenter phase I study of the German Society for Pediatric Oncology and Hematology (GPOH) recruited 34 patients (mean age of 11.6 years, range 0.6–18) and showed that deep regional hyperthermia is feasible in children of all ages by external radiofrequency electromagnetic induction. Hyperthermia was combined with systemic high-dose chemotherapy mainly consisting of etoposide (4 × 150 mg/m^2 per course) simultaneously with carboplatin at the same dose or ifosfamide (4 × 2 g/m^2 per course) repeated every 3–4 weeks after hematological recovery. Tumors of the pelvis, abdomen, spine, and limbs were heated. Temperatures were taken every 5 min every 5–10 mm along the track of implanted catheters. Temperature distribution was expressed by T_{index} values, i.e., those values which were exceeded by x% of the measured values (T_x) (according to ISSELS et al. 1990). T_{90} was 39.8°C, T_{20}, 41.7°C. In 221 hyperthermia treatments there occurred two superficial burns and two complex events associated with accidental overheating in general anesthesia during the early phase of the study. All hyperthermia-related damage was restituted completely, though in two patients a treatment delay was necessary due to the complications. Twenty-five patients did not have distant metastases before thermochemotherapy, but still had many unfavorable prognostic factors. Twelve patients of this group achieved complete remission by subsequent surgery and irradiation. Seven of these remained in complete remission for more than 6 months, some of them promising to result in long-term success (ROMANOWSKI et al. 1993a). These cases are listed in Table 14.2. We conclude from this study that: (a) the toxicity of the combined treatment is tolerable; (b) temperatures are in a range where significant drug enhancement can be expected on the basis of preclinical studies; (c) the outcome is at least not worse than what could be expected without thermotherapy; (d) this work should be continued as a phase II study.

A special pattern of response, as mentioned above, is noteworthy in this group. Four tumors resected after clinical nonresponse, and one after partial response, proved to be completely necrotic when examined histopathologically. Another tumor showed almost complete necrosis with subtotal liquefaction and only minimal viable tumor in the outer areas (Fig. 14.2). EGAWA et al. (1989) also published such cases and stated this phenomenon to be typical for regional hyperthermia treament. It is associated with high intratumoral temperatures.

KRUCK et al. (1991) reported the thermochemotherapy of three children with huge pelvic *osteosarcomas*, which were heated by a similar method without complications. However, temperature was only measured in a single point at the tumor edge; hence the information about temperature elevation is not sufficient. TSEITLIN

Table 14.2. Patients in complete remission after combined therapy including regional hyperthermia with systemic chemotherapy (modified from ROMANOWSKI et al. 1993a)

Age at start of thermochemotherapy (years)	Sex	Diagnosis	Pretreatment status	Duration of remission (months)
16	f	Ewing's sarcoma	No response	7
14	m	Ewing's sarcoma	1st local relapse	11
16	m	Liposarcoma	1st manifestation	14
15	f	Rhabdomyosarcoma[a]	1st local relapse	29
3	f	Fibrosarcoma	7th local relapse	35
15	m	Ewing's sarcoma	No response	54
14	f	Rhabdomyosarcoma[a]	2nd local relapse	64

All tumors localized in the pelvis
[a] Embryonal

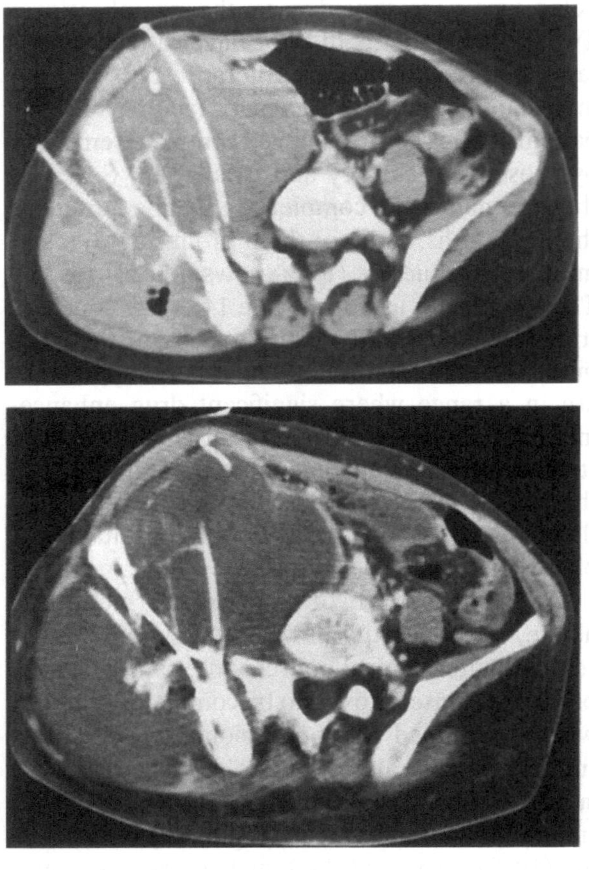

Fig. 14.2a,b. Remarkable pattern of response to regional hyperthermia with systemic chemotherapy in a 12-year-old boy with primitive neuroectodermal tumor of the pelvis. **a** Solid tumor before thermotherapy. **b** Liquefied and mainly necrotic tumor 10 weeks later, following three cycles of thermochemotherapy

and ZAITSEV (1993) treated six children by regional hyperthermia combined with radiotherapy for *soft tissue sarcomas*. Intratumoral temperatures reached 42°C. Complications were stated to be tolerable. However, the quality of heating is difficult to estimate since temperatures were only measured at three points. Using the same method the authors treated five children with *aggressive fibromatosis*. Three cases resulted in a partial remission, and complete resection became possible in one of them (Tseitlin, personal communication).

Experience with thermoradiotherapy of *retinoblastoma* is described in Sect. 14.4.3.

There is only a small amount of experience with whole-body hyperthermia in children. CRILE (1962) reported complete regression of *cutaneous metastases of a neuroblastoma* in a "baby" after "immersion of the affected areas" in a water bath of 46°–47°C. The patient died 2 months later from other metastases without cutaneous tumor recurrence. It cannot be excluded that the infant had a stage IVs neuroblastoma, where spontaneous tumor regression is common.

PETTIGREW et al. (1974) treated two children with *neuroblastoma* and one with *nephroblastoma*. The effects were described as good initial response in one case and as "initial improvement" in two of the patients who died a short time after treatment from "respiratory difficulties." Treatment temperatures were not reported, nor was it stated whether the patients received additional chemotherapy.

LAMPERT (1975) reported on an 11-year-old boy with *acute leukemia* who was cured in 1967. Mild induction chemotherapy with vincristine and steroid was followed by maintenance therapy consisting of 6-mercaptopurine for 1 year and more than 100 systemic hyperthermia treatments up to 40°C for 20 min in 2 years. In his pioneer study the same author treated four other patients by the same hot water bath hyperthermia. Systemic temperatures above 39°C were well tolerated without any toxicity (LAMPERT 1968, unpublished work).

WILLNOW et al. (1989) combined systemic hyperthermia with vincristine (1.5 mg/m^2), cyclophosphamide (600–800 mg/m^2), and actinomycin D (0.4 mg/m^2). Hyperthermia was induced by a modified hemodialysis machine by which the blood was heated extracorporeally in conjunction with general anesthesia. By this method 16 children with *metastatic tumors* and one with an unresectable *brain stem tumor* were treated by elevation of body temperature up to or above 42.0°C in 58 sessions. Beside myelosuppression, neurological and hepatic toxicity were observed, especially after three or more treatments or particularly high temperatures. The investigators observed one complete and eight partial remissions (WILLNOW et al. 1989). The remissions achieved were of short duration. In view of the poor prognosis and sometimes poor general condition of this group of patients, these results are very promising (Table 14.3). Probably a more frequent treatment schedule would result in a better outcome.

There are limited data about the pharmacokinetics of the cytotoxic drugs during dialysis and hyperthermia. The same method used by WILLNOW et al. was recently utilized by Wiedemann and Wagner (personal communication) to treat two children with *metastatic osteosarcoma* and one with metastatic primitive *neuroectodermal tumor* (within a study involving a larger group of adult patients). They gave ifosfamide (10 g/m^2) and actinomycin D (2 mg/m^2) at 41.8°C core temperature. All three patients had progressive disease under chemotherapy alone. After either two or three combined treatment sessions, the two patients suffering from osteosarcoma showed partial remission in all tumor sites. The disease of the third patient remained unchanged during therapy. Remarkably the myelodepression was unexpectedly low. Pharmacokinetic studies indicated that dialysis decreases drug levels by approximately one-third compared to nondialysed patients (Wagner, personal communication). Of note, the method is very consuming in terms of time and manpower.

An easier heating method, e.g., using a radiant heating device, would allow a higher frequency of systemic thermochemotherapy as well as reliable drug doses. ROBINS et al. (1986) treated two adolescents, one with *refractory leukemia and one with Burkitt's lymphoma*, with a preconditioning regimen before allogenic bone marrow transplant. Whole-body hyperthermia at 41.8°C (induced by a radiant heat device) was combined with total-body irradiation and chemotherapy. The method was extensively used and found to be safe in adult patients (ROBINS et al. 1990). The most important observation in these two cases was an early engraftment of the transplant which could be noted at the eighth and the ninth day respectively. In adult patients treated by this method the same group observed significant cytokine induction after heat treatment, by which the early engraftment could be explained (D'OLEIRE et al. 1993).

Table 14.3. Results of systemic thermochemotherapy in children with advanced solid tumors (modified from WILLNOW et al. 1989)

Diagnosis	CR	PR	NR	NE	Total
Neuroblastoma		2		3	5
Nephroblastoma	1	2			3
Hepatoblastoma		1		1	2
Ewing's sarcoma		2	1[a]		3
Osteosarcoma			1	1	2
Liver cell carcinoma		1			1
Brain stem tumor			1[a]		1
Total	1	8	3	5	17

CR, complete response; PR, partial response; NR, no response; NE, not evaluable
[a] Good palliative effect

14.3.2 Special Oncological Problems and Risks

Most of the childhood malignancies grow faster and metastasize earlier than carcinomas and sarcomas of adulthood. More often than adults, pediatric patients can be cured by intensive and aggressive therapy consisting of high-dose multidrug therapy, surgery, and irradiation. Therefore any treatment delay that could become necessary, e.g., due to traumatic lesions caused by heat or by the insertion of thermometry catheters, might give rise to tumor relapse or drug resistance. Furthermore there is strong evidence that traumatizing especially a highly malignant tumor may cause distant or local metastases: VAN DER ZEE et al. (1992) observed tumor growth along a thermometry catheter track in a case of rectal cancer. Nevertheless, most authors agree that thermometry channels must finally be resected or irradiated completely in a curative approach to avoid recurrences in this area.

There is also some evidence that thermoradiotherapy itself may increase the risk of distant metastases. An increased rate of distant metastases of Yoshida sarcoma in rats (DICKSON and ELLIS 1976) and of C3H mouse mammary carcinoma (WALKER et al. 1978) was found after local hyperthermia alone. In contrast to this observation, ANDO et al. (1987) observed a prevention of distant metastases by localized hyperthermia of a xenotransplanted mouse fibrosarcoma alone, and HAHN et al. (1979) reported a similar result in mouse osteosarcomas. In a clinical study on spontaneous soft tissue sarcomas in dogs, distant metastases were insignificantly more frequent after thermoradiotherapy than after radiotherapy alone. One year after completion of the treatment 7.4% of the animals treated by radiation alone had developed distant metastases, compared with 20% of animals after the combined treatment (11.5% vs 25% after 2 years). Invasive thermometry was utilized in this study (MCCHESNEY GILLETTE et al. 1992). LORD et al. (1981) treated spontaneous osteosarcoma in dogs by local irradiation with systemic hyperthermia. At the time of relapse they showed widespread skeletal metastases in six out of seven cases. In reviewing this report, however, ROBINS et al. (1992) pointed out that the natural history of disease may have changed (i.e., osteosarcoma in dogs usually metastasizes to lungs) due to an increase in survival.

Hyperthermia can induce not only thermotolerance but also drug resistance. Stress-induced proteins might function in reducing the desired cytotoxic effects of drugs or ionizing radiation (see Sect. 14.2). Other considerations related to thermotherapy include a functional and anatomical decrease in blood flow (REINHOLD and ENDRICH 1986; Sect. 14.2) which could affect drug delivery or irradiation effects. Thus there is a hypothetical risk that hyperthermia could lead to "treatment failure" in patients who would otherwise have a good prognosis. It is therefore critical that hyperthermia should only be utilized in the context of well-defined clinical trials and well-defined clinical endpoints.

14.3.3 Side-effects of Oncological Treatment

Clearly, the potential short- and long-term toxicity of thermotherapy must be considered. In current multimodal, highly aggressive treatment regimens the growing organism of children is stressed to a maximum. The introduction of hyperthermia into the therapeutic strategies adds new stress, which could cause complications. Multidrug regimens including specific drugs could cause fatal side-effects if combined with systemic hyperthermia. This is, for example, assumed for the *cardiotoxic effect of doxorubicin*. WILLNOW et al. (1989) saw reduced cardiac function in children following systemic hyperthermia with doxorubicin. In a study on dogs receiving doxorubicin with or without systemic hyperthermia, the clinical incidence of cardiac dysfunction was not increased in the group with hyperthermia. However, the animals on the thermochemotherapy arm showed significantly more myocyte degeneration and cardiac fibrosis (PAGE et al. 1992).

It is interesting that there is evidence that addition of whole-body hyperthermia to a drug regimen did not increase or could even decrease *myelosuppression* (ROBINS et al. 1993; Wiedemann, personal communication). This interesting effect is probably due to cytokine induction by systemic hyperthermia (D'OLEIRE et al. 1993) and could allow an intensification of therapy.

There is little knowledge about late complications caused by thermotherapy, especially if combined with chemotherapy. It is possible that effects of drugs and radiation on growth plates, gonads, heart, kidneys, and other organs could be enhanced by local or systemic hyperthermia if vulnerable organs are included in the treatment field. Thermochemotherapy could enhance side-effects already caused at normothermia, such as restricted myocardial function (doxorubicin), pulmonary fibrosis (bleomycin), nephrotoxicity (ifosfamide, cisplatin), or deafness (cisplatin). In combination with ionizing radiation, local hyperthermia may increase the risk of severe fibrosis and ulceration inside the treatment area. VALDAGNI et al. (1986) and HOWARD et al. (1987) observed these complications only in patients treated by thermoradiotherapy and not in those treated by irradiation alone. However, this finding was not confirmed by other groups (BEN-YOSEF and KAPP 1992). A nonsignificant correlation was found between maximal tumor temperature and the risk of late complications (BEN-YOSEF and KAPP 1992).

Hyperthermia's potential to effect cellular transformation and possibly carcinogenesis is another area of consideration. An increase in the transforming potential of bleomycin and cisplatin due to hyperthermia was observed by an in vitro assay (HEI et al. 1986). In contrast KOMATSU et al. (1988) demonstrated that the transforming potential of actinomycin D, BCNU, and mitomycin was reduced by hyperthermia. It has also been shown that after heating the transforming potential of x-rays was decreased compared to unheated cells (MILLER et al. 1989). In an animal model it was found that hyperthermia given 90 days following irradiation increased the risk of cancerogenesis due to x-rays (SMINIA et al. 1990). Clinical reports on this topic are rate. In 64 adult patients observed for 24 months or more after radiotherapy with hyperthermia there was one second malignant tumor inside the treatment field (BEN-YOSEF and KAPP 1992).

14.3.4 Anesthesia for Clinical Hyperthermia

Regional hyperthermia can cause discomfort or pain due to the fixed position of the patient, the equipment-induced pressure, or the heat itself. In whole-body hyperthermia this problem can be solved by general anesthesia (CRONAU et al. 1984; WILLNOW et al. 1989) or by sedation (ROBINS et al. 1985). However, this is more complicated in regional induced hyperthermia, as hot spots may be noticed only by the patient himself. Thus, general anesthesia can result in unrecognized, undesired localized thermal lesions. In older patients who are able to give precise information, hot spots can often be avoided. Sedatives and analgesics can be used judiciously to ease the treatment and discomfort. Children below the age of 10 (–12) years tend to panic and will often not give precise information about the localization of pain. Frequently, regional hyperthermia is not possible without strong sedation. Our best experience has been with continuous infusion of propofol. Propofol has a very short half-life and it can be titrated such that the patient is in a hypnotic stage but still reacting to localized pain, comparable to the first stage of tolerance in classical general anesthesia. It should be noted that such drugs can affect thermoregulation and may accidentally promote whole-body hyperthermia above 39.5°C during regional hyperthermia (ROMANOWSKI et al. 1993b).

14.3.5 Associated Medical Matters, Nursing, and Psychosocial Support

Typical pediatric clinical concerns include imbalances of water and electrolytes due to sweating. Seizures in febrile children below 5 years of age are common and may be triggered by elevated body temperatures. Ifosfamide can cause central nervous system toxicity (PRATT et al. 1986). This rare phenomenon will probably be seen more often under systemic hyperthermia (ROMANOWSKI et al. 1993b).

Due to body size, the eyes of a child are more likely to be inside the stray field of a microwave applicator, causing an increased risk of cataract formation. This, however, has not been a problem in our experience.

During chemotherapy invasive thermometry catheters for regional hyperthermia often remain in local body sites for several months. They must be fixed in such a way that they will not be dislocated and do not disturb the normal activity of the child. The exact catheter location has to be confirmed by CT scans before each treament cycle; this often requires general anesthesia.

As long as thermotherapy is still an experimental treatment, clinical studies will preferentially recruit patients with a poor prognosis. Thus, patients and families are under maximal emotional stress. Frequently families must travel to distant centers. We believe that much of the anxiety and discomfort due to the treatment can be overcome by a careful preparation process. The children should become familiar with the heating equipment prior to the treatment; possibly they should experience the strange feeling of the induced heat and find a convenient position in the device in advance. These preparations are often more useful than sedation. A nurse must always be present during the treatment. If the children are awake, a comforting person, most often the mother or father, should be present. During the treatment some diversion such as reading or listening to music may be helpful. If a little pain is unavoidable, sometimes "visualization" (SIMONTON 1984) can be a useful coping mechanism.

14.3.6 *Special Techniques of Regional Hyperthermia for Children*

With the exception of the small annular phased array of the BSD system (Sigma 40, BSD-Medical Corp., Utah, USA) the hyperthermia devices are rarely designed to treat children. Lower energy levels or perfusion rates are required to heat the target volume, and the distance between skin surface and tumor is smaller in young patients. A single radiofrequency antenna designed for superficial hyperthermia may be sufficient for deep pelvic heating in a 3-year-old child. Disadvantages include problems relating to the positioning and fixation of applicators; hence special constructions may be necessary. The people present during treatment must be protected against the electromagnetic stray field (in accordance with the different national laws). Measurement of the field power, proper placement, or protecting clothes are demanded.

14.3.7 *Quality Assurance in Clinical Trials*

With regard to the small number of patients it is absolutely necessary to perform cooperative multiinstitutional trials. This requires detailed treatment protocols and documentation standards. It is mandatory to guarantee minimal technical and treatment standards and to develop special terms to describe treatment quality and thermal profile. Quality assurance guidelines as developed by the Radiation Therapy Oncology Group (Shrivastava et al. 1989; Sapozink et al. 1991) or by the European Society for Hyperthermic Oncology (Hand et al. 1989) should be followed. Temperature data should be given in precise raw data rather than in transformed biological equivalence doses, so that different thermal dose models can be utilized later. This is difficult in the case of electromagnetically induced heating; with such methods temperatures are heterogeneous due to inhomogeneous energy absorption and tissue perfusion. Temperature percentiles seem to be the best way to report these temperatures.

It is also important to know the spatial representation of the tumors by invasive thermometry. The quality of thermometry could be expressed by the ratio of measured points to tumor size. In interstitial heating systems a high ratio is inherent (Seegenschmiedt et al. 1993b). This is not the case for externally induced hyperthermia; the more extensive a tumor, the lower will be the ratio of measured points to the tumor volume. It is necessary to have at least a minimum quantification of this ratio for quality assurance in multicenter trials. The S-quotient is a simple but practical description of the *spatial quality of thermometry*: the intratumoral length of the thermometry catheters is divided by the sum of the tumor diameters (Romanowski et al. 1991). For example, one catheter passing a complete diameter of a round tumor will produce an S of 0.3. The same could be achieved by two catheters each passing a half of the diameter. Some clinical examples are given in Figs. 14.3 and 14.4.

14.4 Thermotherapy for Specific Pediatric Tumors: Special Considerations

High-quality regional hyperthermia still demands some technical improvements, especially for deep-seated tumors. The development of non-invasive thermometry techniques is still the major task in this field. For disease limited to limbs, hyperthermic perfusion is a promising method in combination with chemotherapy (Ghussen et al. 1988; Lienard et al. 1992; see Chap. 18 in this volume). Indwelling catheters and repeated perfusion may be beneficial (Krause et al. 1991). Several other heating techniques are available for various tumor locations: focused ultrasound (see Chap. 12 in volume 1), interstitial heating (especially for combination with brachyradiotherapy; see Chap. 13 in volume 1 and Chap. 15 in this volume), special heating devices for eye tumors (see Chap. 13 in this volume). From the data reviewed above we can conclude that whole-body hyperthermia can be performed reliably and safely, especially by radiant heating in adolescents (Robins et al. 1992). For children this still has to be shown.

The utilization of various heating techniques may be necessary to encompass all clinical situations in which hyperthermia is shown to be useful. The most difficult task currently is to define hyperthermia's place among other treatment modalities within highly sophisticated treatment protocols that promise cure for the majority of patients. Clearly new studies should address patients in high-risk situations, such as are listed in Table 14.4. There is no alternative to phase I and II studies of hyperthermia until various clini-

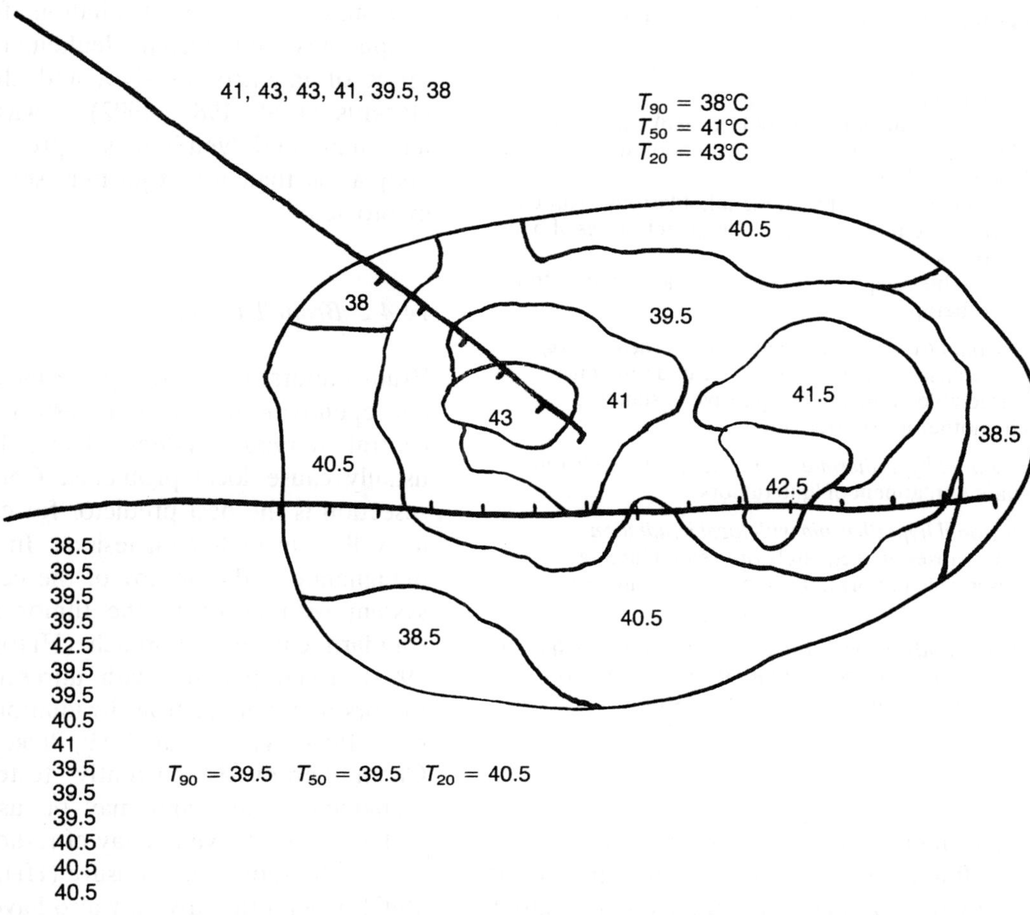

Fig. 14.3. Heterogeneity of intratumoral temperature distribution and reliability of temperature percentiles. The thermal parameters in this illustrative tumor are different for each of the thermometry catheters. The second catheter, which has a longer intratumoral part, seems to be more valid

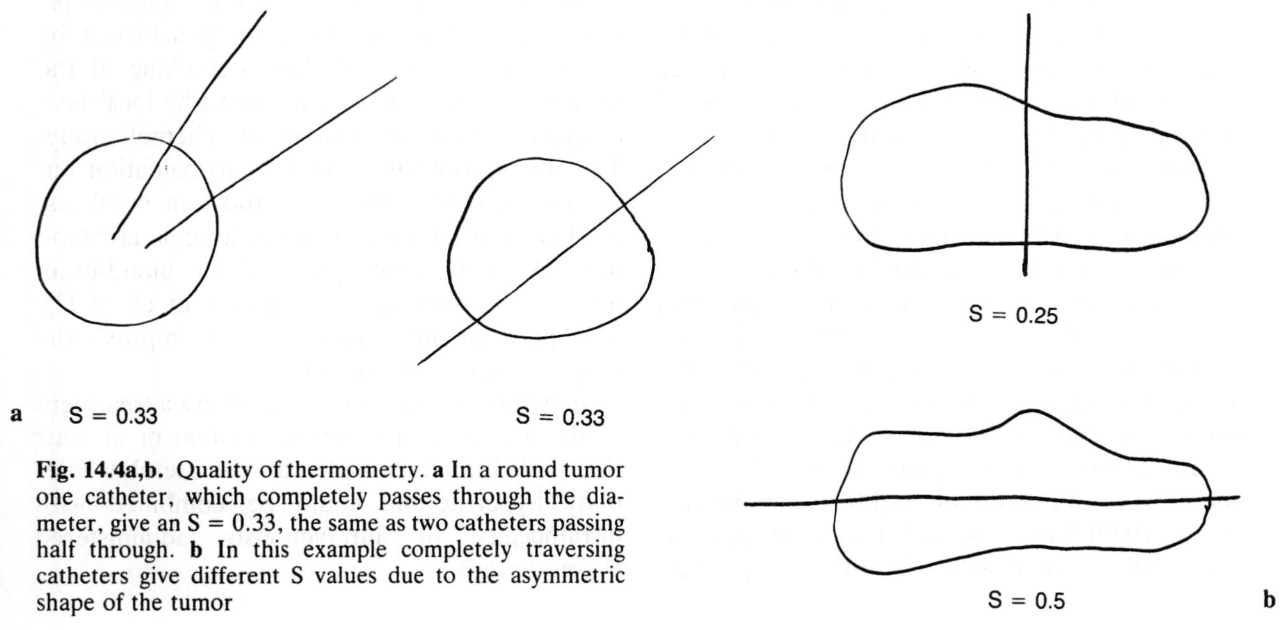

Fig. 14.4a,b. Quality of thermometry. **a** In a round tumor one catheter, which completely passes through the diameter, give an S = 0.33, the same as two catheters passing half through. **b** In this example completely traversing catheters give different S values due to the asymmetric shape of the tumor

Table 14.4. Objects for clinical trials with thermochemotherapy

– *Systemic thermochemotherapy*
Relapse of: acute nonlymphoblastic leukemia, non-Hodgkin's lymphoma, acute lymphoblastic leukemia, Hodgkin's disease
Metastatic: neuroblastoma, medulloblastoma, soft tissue sarcoma, retinoblastoma, skeletal metastases of bone sarcomas
Unresectable relapses of malignant brain tumors after radiotherapy
– *Regional hyperthermia with systemic chemotherapy*
Local relapses of adequately pretreated sarcomas
Unresectable tumors not responsive to standard chemotherapy or irradiation
– *Regional hyperthermia with regional chemotherapy*
Palliative treatment of limb tumors
– *Regional hyperthermia with local irradiation*
Local relapses of adequately pretreated sarcomas
Unresectable tumors not responsive to standard chemotherapy or irradiation
– *Whole-body hyperthermia with total-body irradiation*
For systemic thermochemotherapy if bone marrow transplantation is intended and possible

cal parameters, including response and toxicity, are defined. Preclinical studies and thermoradiotherapy of superficial carcinomas do not supply a stable basis and rationale for phase III studies on children.

14.4.1 Leukemia and Lymphoma

Leukemia and lymphoma must always be considered to be systemic in nature. Local manifestations rarely cause complications; hence conventional treatment is sufficient, and regional or local hyperthermia is not indicated in these malignancies. Thus, thermotherapy for leukemia and lymphoma, if indicated, should be *systemic hyperthermia*. Current indications for thermochemotherapy could be induction of remission in refractory cases. Whole-body hyperthermia with either chemotherapy or total-body irradiation, or even both modalities, could be integrated into a conditioning regimen for bone marrow transplantation. This was successfully tested by Robins et al. (1986) in some patients, including two adolescents (see Sect. 14.2). Moreover, Robins et al. (1990) have reported a series of patients successfully treated with whole-body hyperthermia and total-body irradiation for favorable lymphomas and chronic leukemia. In a large series of in vitro, in vivo, and clinical studies (Robins et al. 1984, 1992) it was shown that leukemias and lymphomas represent a class of neoplasms that are exquisitely sensitive to heat cytotoxicity.

14.4.2 Brain Tumors

Brain tumors, even high grade medulloblastoma and ependymoma rarely metastasize outside the central nervous system. Thus, brain tumors usually cause local problems. Complete tumor resection is the best predictor for cure in benign as well as in malignant lesions. In cases of high malignancy, radiotherapy of the central nervous system with boost to the tumor region is the standard curative approach (Heidemann et al. 1993). Even patients with unresectable benign tumors may benefit from irradiation (Flickinger et al. 1988; Weiss et al. 1989; Pierce et al. 1990). Chemotherapy is currently tested in highly malignant tumors and may be useful in small children, to achieve a delay of radiotherapy or to reduce the radiation exposure (Heidemann et al. 1993). Chemotherapy may also have a role in the treatment of low-grade gliomas (Packer et al. 1988).

Local hyperthermia of well-circumsribed brain tumors is possible with interstitial or ultrasound heating techniques (see Chap. 12 in this volume). The toxicity of these techniques is rather low. However, heating of peripheric microscopic tumor infiltrations is insufficiently achieved by these methods. Nevertheless, debulking of the main tumor mass may be achieved by local heat combined with irradiation or chemotherapy. This might contribute not only to palliation but possibly also to cure. In a study on monkeys, local heating caused an increase in regional blood flow. At 43°C a disruption of the blood-brain barrier was observed (Nakagawa et al. 1992). This phenomenon could probably improve the drug delivery to the tumor.

In highly malignant tumors, where a treatment of the whole central nervous system or at least the whole brain is considered to be useful, whole-body hyperthermia could be combined with intrathecally or intravenously administered chemotherapy.

14.4.3 Embryonic Tumors

Embryonic neoplasms, with the exception of retinoblastoma, have to be considered as systemic diseases. Usually they are extremely sensitive to chemotherapy but surgery and – dependent on the extension – radiotherapy are required for cure (see Table 14.1). Despite relatively high cure rates, however, many patients do not survive. More than 50% of *neuroblastomas* are metastatic at diagnosis (stage IV according to Evans). The survival probability is only about 20% (Brodeur and Castleberry 1993). Even very aggressive myeloablative treatment has not improved outcome (Garavent et al. 1993). This represents a major challenge for pediatric oncology. Experimental therapies, including systemic hyperthermia combined with chemotherapy or total-body irradiation, are therefore indicated. Willnow et al. (1989) reported two remissions after systemic thermochemotherapy in five refractory end-stage cases (see Table 14.3). However, more experience with this group of patients, usually below an age of 6 years, is required before a larger trial can be started.

Local problems of neuroblastoma are rarely the cause of treatment failure (Brodeur and Castleberry 1993; Prokop et al. 1993). Compression of the spinal cord can be relieved by conventional means (Hayes et al. 1989). Thus there are only very rare conditions in which local hyperthermia treatment of a neuroblastoma could be indicated. Hyperthermia and radiation for spinal cord disease may even be contraindicated in view of the increased risk of transverse myelitis (Neville et al. 1984; Sminia et al. 1987).

Nephroblastoma (Wilms' tumor) of a higher tumor stage of unfavorable histology requires local irradiation (Green et al. 1993). Theoretically, a reduction of radiation dose might be possible by the addition of hyperthermia to avoid radiation-induced late sequelae. Currently there is no indication for regional thermotherapy in nephroblastoma. Nevertheless, considering the relapse-free survival rates in metastatic nephroblastoma of above 50% (Green et al. 1993), systemic thermochemotherapy should be discussed in case of drug-resistant metastasized tumors. In a prognostically poor case of metastatic rhabdoid tumor, Willnow et al. (1989) achieved a complete remission after systemic thermochemotherapy.

Retinoblastoma – if discovered early enough – rarely metastasizes to the central nervous system or to other organs. However, in those exceptional cases the disease is comparable to other metastatic embryonal neuroectodermal tumors such as neuroblastoma and peripheral neuroectodermal tumor. Therefore systemic thermochemotherapy could have a place in its treatment. The therapy of localized retinoblastoma depends on the extent of the tumor. Coagulation of the tumor with laser or freezing is as well established as radioplaque irradiation. The success of such localized treatments is limited by tumor size. These measures and also external beam irradiation are useful to save the vision of an eye, especially in bilateral cases (Havers et al. 1986). Most tumors will be cured; however, the success carries a new threat: 25% of the patients with bilateral retinoblastoma develop secondary malignancies within 25 years. These may be related to external ionizing irradiation (Romanowski et al. 1992b; Eng et al. 1993). Local hyperthermia might be indicated in bilateral retinoblastoma for the conservative treatment of the less involved eye. With the addition of local hyperthermia it would probably be possible to reduce the radiation dose and this might decrease the risk of secondary cancers within the radiation field. Lagendijk (1982) developed a microwave applicator which is designed to heat the entire eye. Twenty-seven children with advanced primary or recurrent tumors were treated by this method in combination with different radiation regimens. The authors observed dramatic responses and continuous complete remissions; however, many eyes had to be enucleated later. The need for enucleation was due to either tumor residues (which proved to be necrotic in most cases) or severe damage of the eyes caused by the tumors (Schipper and Lagendijk 1986; Schipper et al. 1987). Unfortunately no further clinical study on patients with a better prognosis has been performed with this method.

It has been shown that local remission of retinoblastoma can also be achieved by systemic chemotherapy with carboplatin combined with local hyperthermia (Murphree, personal communication). In the study of Murphree and coworkers, hyperhthermia was induced by a laser technique. Temperature parameters can be estimated from preclinical data and will be rather high in the center of the beam and the apex of the tumor, and moderate to low at the base, especially at the edge. Clinical cases are very promising and further studies seem to be indicated in this field. Although different heating systems for the eye have been developed (see Chap. 13 in this volume), they are usually not designed for homogeneous heating of the entire eye. This should be a desired goal in technology development for the treatment of retinoblastoma.

Hepatoblastoma can be cured in the majority of the cases by resection of the tumor either primarily or after chemotherapy (VON SCHWEINITZ et al. 1992). In case of resistance or metastatic disease, systemic chemothermotherapy may be beneficial. Even chemotherapy alone is often able to control disseminated hepatoblastoma (GREENBERG and FILLER 1993). Hepatocellular carcinoma is generally less sensitive to drugs and thermal enhancement might be useful to achieve resectability.

Malignant germ cell tumors are most often sensitive to chemotherapy. Localized tumor residues that cannot be controlled by surgery, and radiotherapy may represent a rare indication for regional hyperthermia. Metastatic cases with primary drug resistance or after relapse may be another indication for systemic thermochemotherapy.

14.4.4 Sarcomas

Therapy of sarcomas often results in severe mutilation. *Osteosarcoma* is not curable without radical excision, but even with local control of the tumor as many as 80% of the patients will develop metastatic disease without chemotherapy (EILBER et al. 1987). Since radiotherapy has not proven to be useful, regional hyperthermia may be indicated in future to avoid mutilation. Due to the risk of promoting local or distant metastases (LORD et al. 1981) in a situation where cure seems probable, we do not see an indication for *local* hyperthermia. Hence, indications for *regional* hyperthermia for osteosarcoma are restricted to unresectable cases, especially those involving the spine. In two such cases treated with a palliative intent by means of regional hyperthermia and systemic chemotherapy, we saw stagnation of the primary tumor while pulmonary metastases progressed (ROMANOWSKI et al. 1993a). Another osteosarcoma involving the spine was treated by the same method. The tumor was incompletely resected but was found to be necrotic in the remaining areas. The patient has been free of disease for 2 years (LAUX et al. 1993). Patients with pulmonary metastases can be saved by radical metastasectomy and chemotherapy (WINKLER et al. 1989). However, patients with systemic relapse during chemotherapy and those with skeletal metastases have a very poor prognosis (WINKLER et al. 1989; LINK and EILBER 1993). Systemic thermochemotherapy could be experimentally implemented in this group of patients.

Ewing's tumor can be locally controlled either by irradiation or by radical surgery or – best – by a combination of both (DUNST et al. 1991). Local relapse justifies a trial with local hyperthermia with chemotherapy as well as combined with irradiation. In a phase I/II study four patients with Ewing's sarcoma (two who had not responded to the initial chemotherapy, and two with first local relapse) achieved complete remissions for more than a year after regional hyperthermia with systemic chemotherapy, followed by resection and/or irradiation. One patient relapsed after 36 months; one is in complete remission for more than 4 years (ROMANOWSKI et al. 1993a; see Table 14.2).

Relapse of Ewing's sarcoma after primary therapy will be systemic in the majority of patients. The prognosis is poor after systemic relapse as well as with initial skeletal metastases. Disease-free survival after initial pulmonary metastasis is better, but did not exceed 30% in a multicenter trial (PAULUSSEN et al. 1993). Since myeloablative chemotherapy and total-body irradiation have been tried with some success (BURDACH et al. 1993), systemic hyperthermia could be added to these therapies. WILLNOW et al. (1989) observed a partial response in two of three patients after systemic thermochemotherapy (see Table 14.3).

Soft tissue sarcoma is regarded as a subject of study for regional hyperthermia after local relapse, or if an unresectable tumor does not respond to chemo- and radiotherapy. In case of local relapse of a rhabdomyosarcoma the probability of survival is less than 30% (KLINGEBIEL et al. 1993). Some cases of amazing long-term remissions have been observed in prognostically very poor cases after regional hyperthermia with systemic chemotherapy followed by tumor resection and often radiotherapy. A special pattern in five patients treated with regional hyperthermia and systemic chemotherapy was complete necrosis of tumors with unchanged volume. These high-risk patients should probably be treated by combined thermoradiochemotherapy. Aggressive fibromatosis – a semimalignant tumor – can be successfully treated by regional hyperthermia with either systemic chemotherapy or irradiation if other therapies fail (see 14.3.1). Systemic thermochemotherapy could also be tried in metastatic soft tissue sarcoma, e.g., integrated into a myeloablative treatment with autologous stem cell rescue.

14.4.5 Carcinomas

The most frequent carcinomas in childhood occur in the liver, the thyroid, the nasopharnynx, and the adrenal cortex. The prognosis is only good if complete resection is possible (Chrousos 1993). Nasopharyngeal carcinoma can be cured by radiotherapy and chemotherapy (Pao et al. 1989). Thus, patients with such disease refractory to conventional therapy might be candidates for combined hyperthermia approaches, using protocols adopted from adults. In this regard, isolated hyperthermic perfusion also proved a useful therapeutic approach in a group of children with malignant melanoma (Baas et al. 1989).

14.5 Conclusions and Future Perspectives

Hyperthermia combined with chemo- or radiotherapy is an experimental therapy still in its infancy in pediatric oncology. It bears several risks which are not well defined. Thus, it is only indicated in situations where the established therapy protocols cannot offer a good chance of long-term survival, i.e., disease refractory to a first- (or second-)line treatment or cases that relapse. There are only rare indications where such experimental treatment can be introduced into the primary treatment (e.g., metastatic neuroblastoma, Ewing's sarcoma, soft tissue sarcoma, some brain tumors, and unresectable osteosarcoma). For these diseases phase II studies are desirable (see Table 14.4). However, special techniques such as radiative induced systemic hyperthermia or local hyperthermia of the brain or eye still demand phase I studies in children since these methods are only used in adults. Pediatric oncologists are looking forward to positive results from prospective randomized studies on thermochemotherapy and deep regional hyperthermia in adults which are currently in progress or about to be started. Nevertheless, thermotherapy should be initiated in children with cancer without awaiting the results of trials in adults, since it is known from the past that treatment modalities which fail in adults may still be successful in treating neoplasms of children and adolescents!

Inherent to progress in this field is the accessibility of efficient technology for a sufficient number of patients to be treated. Technical improvements, especially in local hyperthermia (in particular noninvasive thermometry) are urgently required. Among many other experimental approaches and beneath the ongoing refinement of chemotherapy, surgery, and radiotherapy, thermotherapy may meet the two major challenges faced by pediatric oncology over the next 20 years: to further increase cure rates and to decrease late sequelae.

14.6 Summary

- Hyperthermia enhances the efficacy of many antineoplastic drugs and of ionizing radiation as been shown in different experimental models and clinical studies. There are only few experimental data about specific cancer of children.
- Regional hyperthermia is feasible in children of all ages in different tumor locations. There is little experience with whole body hyperthermia but those also indicate feasibility.
- More informations are needed about interactions of heat and drugs and cellular tolerance mechanims for designing optimal treatment schemes.
- Data about late sequelae in children following combined thermotherapy compared to conventional oncological treatments are completely missing.
- Clinical efficacy of combined thermotherapy in specific neoplastic diseases of children must be proven in respective studies.
- Since combined thermotherapy is still experimental in children clinical studies may only recrute patients with poor prognosis.

Acknowledgments. This work was supported by the Deutsche Krebshilfe and the Cancer Research Institute, New York City, USA. F. d'Oleire is supported by the Midwest Athletes Against Childhood Cancer, USA.

References

Ando K, Urano M, Kenton L, Kahn J (1987) Effect of thermochemotherapy on the development of spontaneous lung metastases. Int J Hyperthermia 3: 453–458

Baas PC, Hoekstra HJ, Schraffordt Koops H, Oosterhuis WJ, van der Weele LT (1989) Hyperthermic isolated regional perfusion in the treatment of extremity melanoma in children and adolescents. Cancer 63: 199–203

Ben-Yosef R, Kapp DS (1992) Persistent and/or late complications of combined radiation therapy and hyperthermia. Int J Hyperthermia 8: 733–745

Berthold F, Trechow R, Utsch S, Zieschang J (1992) Prognostic factors in metastatic neuroblastoma. A multivariate analysis of 182 cases. Am J Pediatr Hematol Oncol 14: 207–215

Blatt J, Bleyer WA (1989) Late effects of childhood cancer and its treatment. In: Pizzo PA, Poplack DG (eds) Principles and practice of pediatric oncology. Lippincott, Philadelphia, pp 1003–1025

Bleyer WA (1993) What can be learned about childhood cancer from cancer statistics review 1973–1988. Cancer 71: 3229–3236

Bornstein BA, Zouranjian PS, Hansen HL, Flaser SM, Gelwan LA, Teicher BA, Svensson GA (1993) Local hyperthermia, radiation therapy and chemotherapy in patients with local-regional recurrences of breast carcinoma. Int J Radiat Oncol Biol Phys 25: 79–85

Brämswig JH, Hörnig-Franz I, Riepenhausen M, Schellong G (1990) The challenge of pediatric Hodgkin's disease – where is the balance between cure and long-term toxicity? A report of the West German multicenter studies dal-hd 78, dal-hd 82 and dal-hd-85. Leukemia and Lymphoma 3: 183–193

Brodeur GM, Castleberry RP (1993) Neuroblastoma. In: Pizzo PA, Poplack DG (eds) Principles and practice of pediatric oncology, 2nd edn. Lippincott, Philadelphia, pp 739–767

Bull JM, Lees D, Schuette W, et al. (1979) Whole body hyperthermia: a phase I trial of potential adjuvant chemotherapy. Ann Intern Med 90: 317–323

Burdach S, Jürgens H, Peters C, et al. (1993) Myeloablative radiochemotherapy and hematopoietic stem-cell rescue in poor prognosis Ewing's sarcoma. J Clin Oncol 11: 1482–1488

Burgert EO, Nesbit ME, Garnsey LA (1990) Multimodal therapy for the management of nonpelvic localized Ewing's sarcoma of bone: intergroup study. IESS-II. J Clin Oncol 8: 1514–1524

Chrousos GP (1993) Endocrine tumors. In: Pizzo PA, Poplack DG (eds) Principles and practice of pediatric oncology, 2nd edn. Lippincott, Philadelphia, pp 889–912

Cohen JD, Robins HI (1987) Hyperthermic enhancement of *cis*-diamine-1,1-cyclobutate dicarboxylate platinum (II) cytotoxicity in human leukemia cells in vitro. Cancer Res 47: 4335–4337

Cohen JD, Robins HI, Schmitt CL (1989) Tumoricidal interactions of hyperthermia with carboplatin, cisplatin and etoposide in human leukemia cells in vitro. Cancer Lett 44: 205–210

Creutzig U, Ritter J, Zimmermann M, Schellong G (1993) Does cranial irradition reduce the risk for bone marrow relapse in acute myelogenous leukemia? Unexpected results of the childhood acute myelogenous leukemia study BFM-87. J Clin Oncol 11: 279–186

Crile G (1962) Selective destruction of cancer after exposure to heat. Ann Surg 156: 404–407

Cronau LH, Bourke DL, Bull JM (1984) General anesthesia for whole body hyperthermia. Cancer Res 44(Suppl): 4873–4877

D'Angio GJ, Breslow N, Beckwith JB (1989) Treatment of Wilm's tumor. Results of the third national Wilm's tumor study. Cancer 64: 349–360

Datta NR, Bose AK, Kapoor HK, Gupta S (1990) Head and neck cancers: results of thermoradiotherapy versus radiotherapy. Int J Hyperthermia 6: 479–486

Dickson JA, Ellis HA (1976) The influence of tumor volume and the degree of heating on the response of the solid Yoshida sarcoma to hyperthermia (40–42°C). Cancer Res 36: 1188–1195

D'Oleire F, Schmitt CL, Robins HI (1993) Cytokine induction in humans by 41.8°C whole body hyperthermia. J Natl Cancer Inst 85: 833–834

Dunst J, Sauer R, Burgers JMV, et al. (1991) Radiation therapy as local treatment in Ewing's sarcoma studies CESS 81 and CESS 86. Cancer 67: 2818–2825

Egawa S, Tsukiyama I, Kajiura Y, et al. (1989) Characteristics of the response of soft tissue sarcoma to hyperthermia: the correlation between temperature distribution, radiological examination and histology. Int J Hyperthermia 5: 23–25

Eilber F, Guiliano A, Eckhardt J, Patterson K, Moseley S, Goodnight J (1987) Adjuvant chemotherapy for osteosarcoma: a randomized prospective trial. J Clin Oncol 5: 21–26

Eng C, Li FP, Abramson DH, et al. (1993) Mortality from second tumors among long-term survivors of retinoblastoma. J Natl Cancer Inst 85:1121–1128

Engelhardt R (1987) Hyperthermia and drugs. Recent Results Cancer Res 104: 136–203

Engelhardt R (1988) Summary of recent clinical experience in whole body hyperthermia combined with chemotherapy. Recent Results Cancer Res 107: 200–204

Fajardo LF (1984) Pathological effects of hyperthermia in normal tissue. Cancer Res 44: 4826s–4835s

Feldmann HJ, Molls M, Hoederath H, Krümpelmann S, Sack H (1992) Blood flow and steady state temperatures in deep seated tumors and normal tissues. Int J Radiat Oncol Biol Phys 23: 1003–1008

Feldmann HJ, Romanowski R, Strehl K, Baumhoer W, Sack H (1993) Long-term analysis of thermoradiotherapy of pelvic recurrences: influence of total radiation dose. ESHO 93, Brussels, June 16th–19th, p 11

Fisher GA, Hahn GM (1982) Enhancement of cis-platinum (II) diamine dichloride cytoxicity by hyperthermia. Natl Cancer Inst Monogr 61: 255–257

Flickinger JC, Torres C, Deutsch M (1988) Management of low grade gliomas of the optic nerve and chiasma. Cancer 61: 635–642

Garavent A, Ladenstein R, Chauvin F, et al. (1993) High dose chemotherapy with autologous bone marrow rescue in advanced stage IV neuroblastoma. Eur J Cancer 29A: 487–491

Ghussen F, Krueger I, Groth W, Stuetzer H (1988) The role of regional hyperthermic cytostatic perfusion in the treatment of extremity melanoma. Cancer 61: 654–659

Göbel U, Calaminus G, Teske C, et al. (1993) BEP/VIP bei Kindern und Jugendlichen mit malignen nichttestikulären Keimzelltumoren. Ein Vergleich der Behandlungsergebnisse der Therapiestudien MAKEI 83/86 und 89P/89. Klin Pädiatr 205: 231–240

Green DM, Finkelstein JZ, D'Angio GJ, Kelalis P, Beckwith JB, Thomas PRM, Breslow NE (1993) Wilm's tumor (nephroblastoma, renal embryonal). In: Pizzo PA, Poplack DG (eds) Principles and practice of pediatric oncology, 2nd edn. Lippincott, Philadelphia, pp 713–737

Greenberg M, Filler RM (1993) Hepatic tumors. In: Pizzo PA, Poplack DG (eds) Principles and practice of pediatric oncology, 2nd edn. Lippincott, Philadelphia, pp 697–711

Haaf HG, Kaatsch P, Michaelis J (1993) Jahresbericht 1991 des Deutschen Kinderkrebsregisters. IMSD, Mainz

Haas RJ, Göbel U, Harms D, Schmidt P, Weißbach L (1989) Maligne Hodentumoren im Kindesalter. Konzept der kooperativen Therapiestudie MAHO 88 auf der Basis von MAHO 82. Klin Pädiatr 201: 269–274

Hahn EW, Alfieri AA, Kim JH (1979) The significance of local tumor hyperthermia/radiation on the production of disseminated disease. Int J Radiat Oncol Biol Phys 5: 819–823

Hand JW, Lagendijk JJW, Bach-Andersen J, Bolomey JC (1989) Quality assurance guidelines for ESHO protocols. Int J Hyperthermia 5: 421–428

Havers W, Alberti W, Messmer EP, Rath B, Höpping W (1986) Retinoblastoma. Monogr Paediatr 18: 342–358

Hayes FA, Green AA, O'Connor DM (1989) Chemotherapeutic management of epidural neuroblastoma. Med Pediatr Oncol 17: 6–8

Hei TK, Hall EJ, Kushner S, Osmak RS (1986) Hyperthermia, chemotherapeutic agents and oncogenic transformation. Int J Hyperthermia 2: 311–320

Heidemann RL, Freeman CR, Packer RJ, Borke LB, Albright LA (1993) Tumors of the central nervous system. In: Pizzo PA, Poplack DG (eds) Principles and practice of pediatric oncology, 2nd edn. Lippincott, Philadelphia, pp 633–681

Hermann TS, Jochelson MS, Teicher BA, et al. (1989) A phase I-II trial of cisplatin, hypothermia and radiation in patients with locally advanced malignancies. Int J Radiat Oncol Biol Phys 17: 1273–1279

Honess DJ, Hu DE, Bleehen NM (1991) A study of the mechanism of hydralazine enhancement of thermal damage in KHT tumour. Int J Hyperthermia 7: 667–679

Howard GCW, Sathiaseelan V, Freedman L, Bleehen NM (1987) Hyperthermia and radiation in the treatment of superficial malignancies: an analysis of treatment parameters, response and toxicity. Int J Hyperthermia 3: 1–8

Iacono RP, Stea B, Lulu BA, Citas T, Cassady JR (1992) Template-guided stereotactic implantation of malignant brain tumors for interstitial thermoradiotherapy. Stereotact Funct Neurosurg 59: 199–204

Issels RD, Prenninger SW, Nagele A, et al. (1990) Ifosfamide plus etoposide combined with regional hyperthermia in patients with locally advanced sarcomas: a phase II study. J Clin Oncol 8: 1118–1129

Issels RD, Mittermüller J, Gerl A, et al. (1991) Improvement of local control by regional hyperthermia combined with systemic chemotherpay (ifosfamide plus etoposide) in advanced sarcomas: updated report of 65 patients. J Cancer Res Clin Oncol 117:s141–s147

Kampinga HH, Kruk GVD, Konings AWT (1989) Reduced DNA break formation and cytotoxicity of the topoisomerase II drug 4′-(9′acridinylamino) methansulfon-m-anisidide when combined with hyperthermia in human and rodent cell lines. Cancer Res 49: 1712–1717

Kapp DS, Petersen IA, Cox RS, Hahn GM, Fessenden P, Prionas SD, Lee ER, Meyer JL, Samulski TV, Bagshaw MA (1990) Two or six hyperthermia treatments as an adjunct to radiation therapy yield similar tumor responses: results of a randomised trial. Int J Radiat Oncol Biol Phys 19: 1481–1495

Klingebiel T, Bode U, Hess C, et al. (1993) Treatment of relapse in soft-tissue and Ewing's sarcoma patients – a phase II trial (CESS/CWS Rez 91). Med Pediatr Oncol 21: 573

Komatsu K, Miller RC, Hall EJ (1988) The oncogenic potential of a combination of hyperthermia and chemotherapy agents. Br J Cancer 57: 59–63

Koole P, Schipper J (1990) Treatment of human retinoblastoma cell line Y-79 growing in the athymic mouse eye with fractionated Hyperthermia and/or radiation. Int J Hyperthermia 6: 203–211

Krause U, Beyer M, Hartwig T, Galati G (1991) Isolierte Mehrfachperfusion der Extremitäten am Hund – eine experimentelle Studie. In: Waclawiczek HW, Gebhardt W, Manfreda D, Schlag P (eds) Das maligne Melanom. Springer, Berlin Heidelberg New York, pp 199–202

Kremens B, Romanowski R, Zölzer F, et al. (1992) Adriamycin (ADR) and Cis-Platinum (CDDP) with moderate hyperthermia for in-vitro treatment of human neuroblastoma (NBL) cells. Klin Pädiatr 204: 315

Kremens B, Romanowski R, Zölzer F, et al. (1993) Cytostatic drugs and moderate hyperthermia: in-vitro data on neuroblastoma cells. In: Evans AE, Biedler JL, Brodeur GM, D'Angio GJ, Nahagawora A (eds) Advances in neuroblastoma research 4, Wiley-Liss, New York, p 437

Kruck H, Wolff F, Gutjahr G (1991) Regionale Tumor-Hyperthermie und Zytostatika bei Kindern mit osteogenen Sarkomen – Erfahrungen nach 20 Behandlungen. Monatsschr Kinderheilkd 139: 506

Lagendijk JJW (1982) A microwave heating technique for the hyperthermic treatment of tumours in the eye, especially retinoblastoma. Phys Med Biol 27: 1313–1324

Lampert F (1975) Hämatologische Befunde im Kindesalter (10). Pädiatr Prax 15: 585–588

Laux C, Feldmann H, Basu O, et al. (1993) Systemic chemotherapy combined with regional hyperthermia in the treatment of advanced sarcoma: quality and toxicity of treatment. ESHO 93, June 16th–19th, Brussels, p 30

Lienard D, Ewalenko P, Delmotte JJ, Renard N, Lejeune FJ (1992) High dose recombinant tumor necrosis factor alpha in combination with interferon gamma and melphalan in isolation perfusion of the limbs for melanoma and sarcoma. J Clin Oncol 10: 52–60

Link MP, Eilber F (1993) Osteosarcoma. In: Pizzo PA, Poplack DG (eds) Principles and practice of pediatric oncology, 2nd edn. Lippincott, Philadelphia, pp 841–866

Lord PF, Kapp DS, Morrow D (1981) Increased skeletal metastases of spontaneous canine osteosarcoma after fractionated systemic hyperthermia and local x-irradiation. Cancer Res 41: 4331–4334

McChesney Gillette S, Dewhirst MW, et al. (1992) Response of canine soft tissue sarcomas to radiation or radiation plus hyperthermia: a randomized phase II study. Int J Hyperthermia 8: 309–320

McWilliams NB (1986) Stage IV-s neuroblastoma: treatment controversy revisited. Med Pediatr Oncol 14: 41–44

Miller RC, Roizin-Towle L, Komatsu K, Richards M, Hall EJ (1989) Interaction of heat with X-rays and cis-platinum; cell lethality and oncogenic transformation. Int J Hyperthermia 5: 697–705

Nakagawa M, Higashi H, Ono Y, et al. (1992) Effects of hyperthermia on the blood brain barrier of normal monkey brain. In: Gerner EW (ed) Hyperthermic oncology 1992, vol 1. Summary papers. Arizona Board of Regents, Tucson, Az, p 176
Neumann HA, Fiebig HH, Loehr GW, Engelhardt R (1985) Effects of cytostatic drugs and 40.5°C hyperthermia on human clonogenic tumor cells. Eur J Cancer Clin Oncol 21: 515–523
Neville AJ, Robins HI, Martin P, Gilchrist KW, Dennis WH. Steeves RA (1984) Effect of whole body hyperthermia and BCNU on the development of radiation myelitis in the rat. International Journal of Radiation Biology 46: 417–420
Österreich S, Schunck H, Benndorf R, Bielka H (1991) Cisplatin induces the small heat shock protein hsp25 and thermotolerance in Ehrlich ascites tumor cells. Biochem Biophys Res Commun 180: 243–248
Oleson JR, Samulski TV, Leopold KA, Clegg ST, Dewkirst MW, Dodge RK, George SL (1993) Sensitivity of hyperthermia trial outcomes to temperature and time: implications for thermal goals of treatment. Int J Radiat Oncol Biol Phys 25: 29–297
Overgaard J, Bichel P (1977) The influence of hypoxia and acidity on the hyperthermic response of malignant cells in vitro. Radiology 123: 511–514
Overgaard J, Gonzales-Gonzales D, Arcangeli G, Dahl O, Bentzen SM (1993) ESHO protocol 3–85: as multicenter trial randomized trial evaluating hyperthermia as an adjuvant to radiation therapy of recurrent or metastatic malignant melanoma. ESHO 93, Brussels, June 16th–19th, p 41
Packer RJ, Sutton LN, Bilaniuk LT, et al. (1988) Treatment of chiasmatic / hypothalamic gliomas of childhood with chemotherapy: an update. Ann Neurol 23: 79–85
Packer RJ, Sutton LN, Goldwein JW (1991) Improved survival with the use of adjuvant chemotherapy in the treatment of medulloblastoma. Neurosurgery 74: 433–440
Page RL, Macy DW, Ogilvie GK, et al. (1992) Phase III evaluation of doxorubicin and whole body hyperthermia in dogs with lymphoma. Int J Hyperthermia 8: 187–198
Pao WJ, Hustu HO, Douglass EC, Beckford NS, Kun LE (1989) Pediatric nasopharyugeal carcinoma in long-term follow up of 29 patients. Int J Radiat Oncol Biol Phys 17: 299–305
Paulussen M, Braun-Munziger G, Burdach S, et al. (1993) Behandlungsergebnisse beim primär ausschließlich pulmonal metastasierten Ewingsarkom: eine retrospektive Analyse von 41 Patienten. Klin Pädiatr 205: 210–216
Pettigrew RT, Galt JM, Ludgate CM, Smith AN (1974) Clinical effects of whole body hyperthermia in advanced malignancy. Brit Med J 4: 679–682
Pierce SM, Barnes P, Loeffler JS (1990) Definitive radiation therapy in the management of symptomatic patients with optic glioma. Cancer 65: 45–52
Pratt CB, Green AA, Horowitz ME, et al. (1986) Central nervous system toxicity following the treatment of pediatric patients with ifosfamide / mesna. J Clin Oncol 4: 1253–1261
Prokop A, Pichlmaier H, Berthold F (1993) Periphere neurogene Tumoren – Chirurgische Therapie des Neuroblastoms. Zentralbl Chir 118: 315–321
Reinhold HS, Endrich B (1986) Tumour microcirculation as a target for hyperthermia. Int J Hyperthermia 2: 111–137
Reiter A, Schrappe M, Ludwig WD, et al. (1992) Favorable outcome of B-cell acute lymphoblastic leukemia in childhood: a report of three consecutive studies of the BFM group. Blood 80: 2471–2478
Riehm H, Gadner H, Hanze G, et al. (1990) Results and significance of six randomized trials in four consecutive ALL-BFM studies. In: Büchner T, Schellong G, Hiddemann W, Ritter J (eds) Haematology and blood transfusion, acute leukemias II, vol 33. Springer, Berlin Heidelberg New York, pp 439–449
Robins HI, Dennis WH, Steeves RA, Sondel PM (1984) A proposal for the addition of hyperthermia to treatment regimens for acute and chronic leukemia. J Clin Oncol 2: 1050–1056
Robins HI, Dennis WH, Neville AJ, et al. (1985) A nontoxic system for 41.8°C whole body hyperthermia: results of phase I study using a radiant heat device. Cancer Res 45: 3937–3944
Robins IH, Longo WL, Hugander A, Steeves A, Flynn B, Schwartz B, Sondel PM (1986) Whole body hyperthermia combined with total body irradiation and chemotherapy as a preparative regimen for allogeneic bone marrow transplantation in a patient with Burkitt's lymphoma. Cancer J 1: 180–183
Robins HI, Longo WL, Steeves RA, et al. (1990) Adjunctive therapy (whole body hyperthermia versus lonidamine) to total body irradiation for the treatment of favourable B-cell neoplasm: a report of two pilot clinical trials and laboratory investigations. Int J Radiat Oncol Biol Phys 18: 909–920
Robins HI, Neville AJ, Cohen JD (1992) Whole body hyperthermia: biological, physical, and clinical aspects. Springer, Berlin Heidelberg New York
Robins HI, Cohen JD, Schmitt CL, et al. (1993) Phase I clinical trial of carboplatin and 41.8°C whole body hyperthermia in cancer patients. J Clin Oncol 11: 1787–1794
Rodary C, Gehan EA, Flamant F, Treuner J, Carli M, Auquier A, Maurer H (1991) Prognostic factors in 951 nonmetastatic rhabdomyosarcoma in children: a report from the international rhabdomyosarcoma workshop. Med Pediatr Oncol 19: 89–95
Romanowski R, Schött C, Feldmann J, Molls M (1991) Numeric description of thermometry quality in regional microwave hyperthermia: the S-quotient. Strahlenther Onkol 167: 33
Romanowski R, Kremens B, Zölzer F, Günther K, Klecker G, Havers W, Streffer C (1992a) Proliferation, DNA-content and DNA-synthesis of human neuroblastoma cells treated by adriamycin (ADM), cis-platinum (CDDP) and moderate hyperthermia in vitro. In: Gerner EW (ed) Hyperthermic oncology 1992, vol I, Arizona Board of Regents, Tucson, Az, p 148
Romanowski R, Timmermann M, Höpping W, Sauerwein W, Bornfeld N, Havers W (1992b) Second tumors in retinoblastoma patients. Med Pediatr Oncol 20: 465
Romanowski R, Schött C, Issels R, et al. (1993a) Regionale Hyperthermie mit systemischer Chemotherapie bei Kindern und Jugendlichen. Durchführbarkeit und klinische Verläufe bei 34 intensiv vorbehandelten Patienten mit prognostisch ungünstigen Tumorerkrankungen. Klin Pädiatr 205: 249–256
Romanowski R, Havers W, Schött C, et al. (1993b) Regional hyperthermia combined with systemic chemotherapy in 30 patients under 18 years: a phase I study. In: Gerner EW, Cetas TC (eds) Hyperthermic oncology 1992, vol II. Arizona Board of Regents, Tucson, Az, pp 289–291

Sapozink MD, Corry PM, Kapp DS, et al. (1991) RTOG quality assurance guidelines for clinical trials using hyperthermia for deep seated tumors. Int J Radiat Oncol Biol Phys 20: 1109–1115

Schipper J, Lagendijk JJW (1986) The treatment of retinoblastoma by fractionated radiotherapy combined with hyperthermia. In: Anghileri LJ, Robert J (eds) Hyperthermia in cancer treatment, vol III. CRC Press, Boca Raton, FI, pp 79–87

Schipper J, Lagendijk JJW, Hofman P, Tan Ke WP (1987) Treatment of retinoblastoma by radiotherapy combined with hyperthermia. Int J Hyperthermia 3: 588–589

Seegenschmiedt MH, Sauer R, Miyamoto C, Chalal JA, Brady LW (1993a) Clinical experience with interstitial thermoradiotherapy for localized implantable pelvic tumors. Am J Clin Oncol 16: 210–222

Seegenschmiedt MH, Sauer R, Fiethau R Jro H, Chalal JA, Brady LW (1992): Interstitial thermal radiation therapy: five-year experience with head and neck fumors. Radiology 184: 795–804

Shrivastava P, Luk K, Oleson J, et al. (1989) Hyperthermia quality assurance guidelines. Int J Radiat Oncol Biol Phys 16: 571–587

Simonton SM (1984) The healing family: the Simonton approach for familiar facing illness. Bantam Books, Toronto

Sminia P, Haveman J, Wondergem J, Van Dijk JDP, Lebesque JV (1987) Effects on 434 MHz microwave hyperthermia applied to the rat in the region of the cervical spinal cord. Int J Hyperthermia 3: 441–452

Sminia P, Jansen W, Haveman J, Van Dijk JDP (1990) Incidence of tumours in the cervical region of the rat after treatment with radiation and hyperthermia. Int J Radiat Biol 57: 425–436

Sneed PK, Gutin PH, Stauffer PR, et al. (1992) Thermoradiotherapy of recurrent malignant brain tumors. Int J Radiat Oncol Biol Phys 23: 853–861

Streffer C, Van Beuningen (1987) The biological basis for tumor therapy by hyperthermia and radiation. Recent Results Cancer Res 104: 24–70

Tseitlin GY, Zaitsev AV (1993) Hyperthermia modifying effect on superfractionation. Med Pediatr Oncol 21: 597

Valdagni R, Kapp DS, Valdagni C (1986) N3 (TNM-UICC) metastatic neck nodes managed by combined radiation therapy and hyperthermia: clinical results and analysis of treatment parameters. Int J Hyperthermia 2: 189–200

Valdagni R, Amichetti M, Pani G (1988) Radical radiation alone versus radiation plus microwave hyperthermia for N3 (TNM-UICC) neck nodes: a prospective randomized trial. Int J Radiat Oncol Biol Phys 15: 33–24

Van der Zee J, Veeze-Kuijpers B, Wiggers T, Van de Merve SA, Treuniet-Donker AD (1992) Risk of tumor growth along thermometry catheter track: a case report. Int J Hyperthermia 8: 621–624

Van der Zee J, Gonzales-Gonzales D, Van Putten LJ, et al. (1993) Hyperthermia combined with radiotherapy in deep seated tumour – a phase III trial. Hyperthermia in clinical oncology, München, Nov 25th–27th, abstracts, p 41

von Schweinitz D, Bürger D, Weinel P, Mildenberger H (1992) Die Therapie maligner Lebertumoren des Kindesalters. Ein Zwischenbericht der multizentrischen Studie HB-89 der GPOH. Klin Pädiatr 204: 214–220

Walker A, McCallum HM, Wheldon TE, Nias AH, Abdlaac AS (1978) Promotion of metastasis of C3H mouse mammary carcinoma by local hyperthermia. Br J Cancer 35: 561–563

Weiss M, Sutton L, Marcial V, et al. (1989) The role of radiation therapy in the management of childhood craniopharyngioma. Int J Radiat Oncol Biol Phys 17: 1313–1321

Wiedemann G, Siemens HJ, Mentzel M, Biersack A, Wössmann W, Weiss C, Wagner T (1993) Effects of temperature on the therapeutic efficacy and pharmacokinetics of ifosfamide. Cancer Res 53: 4268–4272

Willnow U (1981) The effect of hyperthermia alone or in combination with actinomycin D on the RNA metabolism of solid tumors in children. Neoplasm 28: 721–727

Willnow U, Lindner H, Brock D, Wild L, Diestelhorst C, Greiner C, Eichstädt H (1989) Behandlung konventionell inkurabler Tumorerkrankungen im Kindesalter mit Ganzkörperhypertherie und Chemotherapie. Dtsch Med Wochenschr 114: 208–213

Winkler K, Torggler S, Beron G, et al. (1989) Behandlungsergebnisse bei primär disseminiertem Osteosarkom. Onkologie 12: 92–96

Winkler K, Bieling P, Bielack S, et al. (1991) Local control and survival from the co-operative osteosarcoma study group studies of the German Society of Pediatric Oncology and the Vienna Bone Tumor Registry. Clin Orthop 270: 79–86

15 Clinical Practice of Interstitial Thermoradiotherapy

M.H. SEEGENSCHMIEDT, G. KLAUTKE, R. SEIDEL, and P. R. STAUFFER

CONTENTS

M. HEINRICH SEEGENSCHMIEDT, MD, GUNTHER KLAUTKE, MD, RALPH SEIDEL, MD, Department of Radiation Oncology, University of Erlangen-Nürnberg, Universitätsstrabe 27, D-91054 Erlangen, FRG
PAUL R. STAUFFER, MD, Department of Radiation Oncology, University of California, San Francisco, CA 94143-0226, USA.

15.1 Introduction

Since the beginning of this century radioactive isotopes have been successfully applied in oncology. Initially, radiotherapists used radium implants, but later various refinements of brachytherapy techniques were developed; recently, in response to the need for radiation protection, the "afterloading technique" has been advocated. This technique requires placement of needles or plastic tubes into the target tissue in various geometrical configurations depending on the individual tumor extension. Iridium-192 or iodine-125 isotopes are loaded into these tubes in the form of ribbons, seeds, or malleable wires. When, in the 1970s, it became known that hyperthermia (HT) acts as a cytotoxic agent by itself or synergistically with ionizing radiation, an attempt was made to combine *internal heating devices* with radioactive implants. *External heating devices* were shown to be inadequate for the production of uniform temperatures in many body sites, as they lacked sufficient depth penetration, resulting in critical tumor portions not reaching the desired therapeutic temperatures. In order to overcome these problems, interstitial hyperthermia (IHT) was tested as an alternative in certain clinical situations. IHT was expected to allow more homogeneous and more selective heating.

The development of the presently available IHT techniques dates back to 1975, when Doss and McCABE presented their concept of radiofrequency IHT at the 1st International Symposium on Cancer Therapy by Hyperthermia and Radiation: "I want to talk ... about a modality for the use of electromagnetic energy which is really quite different from (external) microwaves. It has a disadvantage – that is, the technique ... is usually very invasive." (Doss 1975; see also Doss and McCABE 1976).

At that time, crude "external" HT methods were available, but the idea of placing a hot source directly "inside" a tumor dates back to the beginning of this century (Gottschalk 1899; Persy 1916; Westermark 1898). It stimulated researchers worldwide to invent "internal" HT methods. Interstitial HT is just one of these internal HT methods by which energy is supplied directly to the tumor in situ; other internal HT methods are: (a) endocavitary HT with devices being introduced into natural body cavities (vol. 1, Chap. 14: Roos et al.; vol. 2, Chap. 16: Petrovich et al. 1995), (b) *perfusional HT* with extracorporeal blood perfusion (vol. 2, Chap. 19: Cavaliere et al.) and (c) *intraoperative HT* (vol. 2, Chap. 17: Colacchio and Ryan 1995) using different HT devices during surgery. In this chapter we review studies in extracranial tumors which were performed with various *interstitial HT techniques* including microwave (MW), radiofrequency (RF), ferromagnetic (FM) implants, and hot source (HS) devices. The technical background of these IHT techniques has been addressed in Chap. 13 in volume 1 of this book, by Stauffer et al. In writing this chapter we also complement the in-depth coverage of technology and clinical studies in previous reviews (Cosset 1990; Cosset et al. 1986; Coughlin 1990, 1992; Coughlin and Strohbehn 1989; Emami 1992; Emami and Perez 1985; Gautherie 1989; Hand 1987, 1990, 1992; Handl-Zeller 1992; Luk 1992; Manning and Gerner 1983; Neyzari and Cheung 1985; Perez et al. 1992; Seegenschmiedt and Sauer 1989, 1992; Seegenschmiedt et al. 1990a; Stauffer 1990, 1991, 1992).

15.2 Basic Considerations and Concepts

15.2.1 Biological Rationale

Excellent radiobiological reviews (Hahn 1992; Hall 1985,1988; Jones 1993; Jones and Douple 1992) and several studies have outlined the potential radiosensitization when combining heat and low-dose-rate (LDR) irradiation (Ben-Hur et al. 1974; Jones et al. 1986, 1989a,b; van Geel 1994; Gerner et al. 1983; Harisiadis et al. 1978; Miller et al. 1978; Moorthy et al. 1980,1984; Peschke et al. 1993; Sapozink et al. 1983). The studies on thermal enhancement of brachytherapy (IRT) by additional heat revealed thermal enhancement ratio (TER) values ranging from 1.1 to 6.5 and hyperthermic potentiation of LDR irradiation both in vitro and in vivo. It is also evident that the TER depends on other parameters, too, including the dose rate of the radioisotope, the chosen biological endpoint, the individual tumor system, the specific treatment schedule and many others.

In vivo studies revealed a decreased D_0 of the survival curve due to hyperthermic radiosensitization (Ben-Hur et al. 1974; Harisiadis et al. 1978; Gerner et al. 1983), while in vivo studies showed an increased radiation-induced growth delay and in situ cell killing (Jones et al. 1989a; Miller et al. 1978; Moorthy et al. 1984; Papadopoulos et al. 1989; Peschke et al. 1993; Sapozink et al. 1983) (Fig. 15.1). When comparing effects of acute and continuous LDR RT plus heat, it was found that with decreasing dose rate the TER of the RT response was either maintained or increased, but never decreased (Ben-Hur 1974; Gerner et al. 1983; Jones et al. 1986). Recent studies indicate that even a moderate HT exposure of 39°–41°C can enhance tumor cell killing when combined with simultaneous LDR RT (Armour et al. 1991, 1992; Mackey 1993; Raaphorst et al. 1994; Spiro et al. 1991). This is encouraging, as in the clinical situation often only relatively low temperatures are feasible given the constraints on heating deep-seated tumors.

Further research – especially on combined LDR RT and HT – is required to uncover all the involved cellular mechanisms and possible applications of this combined treatment. The complex molecular and cellular interactions of HT-RT and the impact of environmental conditions on thermal sensitivity of tumors and normal tissues have been reviewed (Hall 1988; Leeper 1985; Reinhold and Endrich 1986; Song 1984; Streffer 1988; Streffer and van Beuningen 1987; Vaupel et al. 1988), but are not addressed in this context.

15.2.2 Clinical Rationale

The clinical rationale for IHT has been widely discussed (Arcangeli et al. 1988; Overgaard 1989; Seegenschmiedt and Sauer 1992; Seegenschmiedt and Vernon 1993), including special considerations in respect of different tumor sites (Fietkau et al. 1993; Kapp 1986; Martinez et al. 1993). All IHT applications can be combined with present brachytherapy (IRT) techniques for head and neck, brain, pelvic, and other tumors (Hilaris and Henschke 1985; Müller 1991) (Fig. 15.2) and

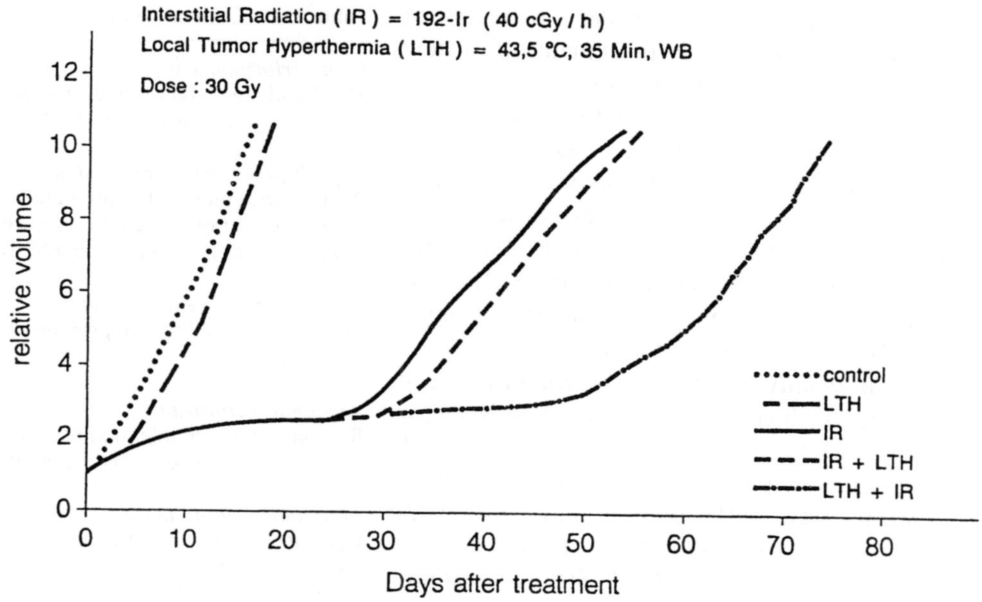

Fig. 15.1. Regrowth curves for the Dunning prostate tumor receiving 30 Gy interstitial radiotherapy (*IR*) delivered with one iridium-192 seed (dose rate: 40 cGy/h) over a period of 3 days and local hyperthermia (*LTH*). (From PESCHKE et al. 1993)

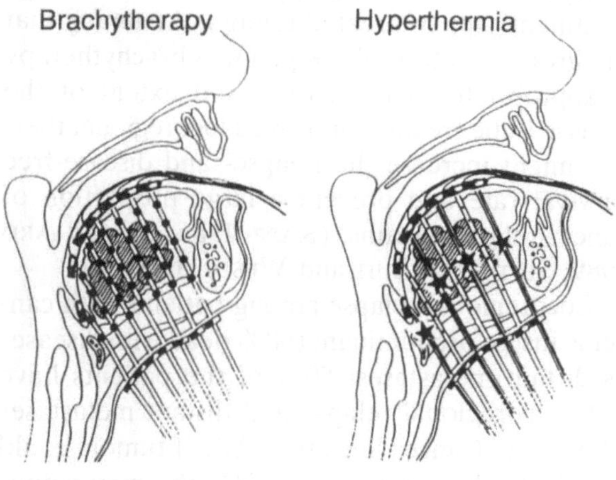

Fig. 15.2. Principles of thermoradiotherapy illustrated on a base of tongue lesion. The implanted plastic tubes are sequentially loaded with low-dose-rate iridium-192 seed strands for brachytherapy (*left*) and interstitial 915-MHz microwave antennas for hyperthermia (*right*)

can be delivered sequentially to or simultaneously with IRT. IHT may provide the following advantages:

1. *Adequate tumor coverage* is possible at any body site with established implant guidelines. Sophisticated diagnostic tools (CT, MRI) assist the physician and physicist in appropriately selecting candidates, planning the implant procedures in advance, and controlling the implant quality.
2. *Sparing of normal tissues* can be achieved by individually loading or unloading radioisotopes and HT applicators from the catheters or by designing HT applicators with better "steering" capabilities (PRIONAS et al. 1989; PRIONAS and KAPP 1992). In contrast, external HT devices provide less discrimination in terms of energy deposition in intervening normal tissues.
3. *Extensive thermometry* is available for treatment control within the implant volume due to the indwelling brachytherapy catheters. Some or all of the latter can be utilized for multipoint thermometry or thermal mapping. Correlation of thermometry and imaging studies (CT, MRI) may identify "biological" and "physiological" prognostic parameters (FELDMANN et al. 1993).
4. *Automatic feedback control* can be incorporated, allowing steering of the power deposition through input of either power level or relative duration of power activation time (duty cycle). Thereby inhomogeneous heat distribution may be avoided.
5. *No additional invasive procedures* are necessary other than those required for brachytherapy. All IRT techniques can be modified to allow additional IHT treatments, and conversely all IHT techniques are able to cope with different

IRT techniques. Certain physical or technical conditions require the placement of a few additional temperature probes.
6. Some *IHT systems* are already commercially available, and a large body of experience has been collected which provides many practical guidelines. Excellent clinical results have been achieved in single-institution trials, but there is still a lack of randomized phase III trials demonstrating the advantage of the combined IHT-IRT treatment modality.
7. Several *quality assurance criteria* have been developed which provide a very good basis for the consistent application of all available IHT techniques in prospective multicenter studies (EMAMI et al. 1991; PRIONAS and KAPP 1992; SEEGENSCHMIEDT and VISSER 1991; SEEGENSCHMIEDT and VERNON 1993; SEEGENSCHMIEDT et al. 1989a; VISSER and KAATEE 1993; vol. 1, Chap. 21: VISSER and VAN RHOON).

Selection of tumors for HT-RT depends on whether the patient may benefit from additional HT and on how safely and "effectively" and with which technique the specific site may be best heated. Clinical indications for IHT-IRT are listed in Table 15.1. However, one should not implement an investigational method like IHT if there are obvious contraindications (Table 15.2). The use of IHT-IRT offers intrinsic advantages which allow it to be applied for localized lesions not only as adjunctive "boost therapy" but also as "salvage treatment" for pretreated tumors. Assuming that the invasive nature of the planned brachytherapy is appropriate to the nature and extent of the disease to be treated, improved locoregional therapy might increase the relapse- and disease-free survival rate and prevent a large proportion of cancer-related deaths (KAPP 1986; OVERGAARD 1989; SUIT 1982; SUIT and WESTGATE 1986).

Table 15.1. Clinical indications for IHT-IRT

Primary advanced tumors
When initial or long-term tumor control is poor using conventional therapy (relapse rate > 20%–25%), IHT-IRT may be used as dditional "boost" therapy.

Persistent primary tumors
When a tumor mass persists and is prone to regrowth after completion of conventional therapy, IHT-IRT may be used as additional "boost" therapy.

Local recurrent tumors
When a radical pretreatment has been delivered and a local relapse needs to be aggressively approached, IHT-IRT may be used to enhance a limited RT dose.

Local metastatic tumors
When surgery cannot completely remove a local metastasis and the patient's general condition and tumor stage offer good evidence for improved quality of life, IHT-IRT may be used to enhance a limited RT dose.

Reduction of treatment toxicity
If standard radiotherapy produces excessive toxicity (>20%–25%), combined IHT-IRT may offer a differential response of normal and tumor tissue.

Table 15.2. Clinical contraindications to IHT-IRT

Poor performance status
Moribund, age >80 years; Karnofsky score <70%; severe pulmonary, cardiovascular or other medical risks.

Rapidly progressive or metastatic disease
Patients with metastatic spread to vital organs (lung, liver, brain) should not be treated, as the expected survival is usually too short to permit benefit from the treatment.

Previous extensive treatments
Prior RT dose >70 Gy to provide enough margin for reirradiation.

Anatomical constraints
Regions not accessible to implantation or in the vicinity of critical structures (e.g., base of skull, spinal cord).

Poor patient compliance
Lack of cooperation with and consent to IHT-IRT is an absolute contraindication.

Locoregional relapse among patients with cancer is just as predominant (68% dead with disease) as distant metastases: 50% of the patients have both locoregional relapse and distant metastases (American Cancer Society 1993). If tumors could be effectively approached by HT, this may reduce locoregional failures and result in a remarkable increase in the survival rate in patients with cancer (KAPP 1986). Improved disease-free survival after salvage or primary therapy could be regarded as proof of the better management of the primary lesions. In some tumors a correlation has been established between the incidence of local failure and the rate of metastases (MILLION et al. 1985; PEREZ et al. 1986a, 1988; SUIT and WESTGATE 1986).

15.2.3 Treatment Planning

Each IHT technique has specific advantages and disadvantages which should be taken into account in the planning of IHT-IRT. Generally, no compromise in the quality of the radioisotope dose distribution should be accepted. Conventional implantation techniques should be used in accordance with established brachytherapy guidelines. This includes the use of templates with rigid needles, free-hand implants with closed-end flexible plastic tubes, or looping techniques. The most appropriate IHT technique should be chosen and adapted to the specific tumor site and individual implant. Sometimes additional probes for invasive thermometry have to be placed.

A flow chart of procedures (adapted to microwave IHT) includes the following steps: diagnostic workup, preimplant planning, tube implantation, postimplant planning, performance of IHT-IRT possibly supplemented by external RT, and posttreatment evaluation (Table 15.3). Details of a typical implant and setup together with a block diagram of an IHT system are shown in Fig. 15.3.

Careful physical examination and imaging studies (CT, MRI) are necessary to assess the exact tumor volume and its relation to surrounding normal tissues. During the implant procedure in the operating room the target volume is determined by the operating physician in close consultation with the attending radiation oncologist and physicists. Established IRT guidelines are applied to achieve optimal implant geometry. Sufficient coverage of the tumor periphery should be provided, i.e., with a margin of ≥0.5 cm beyond the tumor volume. Most IHT techniques rely on a parallel implant geometry and equidistant separation between neighboring heating applicators (Emami et al. 1991; Seegenschmiedt and Visser 1991; Visser and Kaatee 1993; vol. 1, Chap. 21: Visser and van Rhoon).

After completion of the implant, orthogonal radiographs are taken with tumor margins and important anatomical structures outlined, based upon previous CT or MR scans. For treatment planning it is advisable to place "dummy seeds" firstly inside all implanted catheters (IRT planning) and secondly in those assigned to house thermometry probes (IHT planning). On both radiographs the intratumoral and normal tissue sections of all probes are marked properly. A postimplant CT scan provides the most realistic overview of the implant quality and allows possible consequences. This is the required standard of multi-institutional protocols (Emami et al. 1991). All implantation and thermometry requirements

Table 15.3. Flow chart of procedures for IHT-IRT treatment

Diagnostic workup
Clinical examination, histological workup, and imaging studies: definition of tumor location and extension, tumor type and histology; check of inclusion/exclusion criteria; start of preimplant planning
Surgical procedure: tube placement
Placement of tubes with both the surgeon and the radiation oncologist present
Planning procedures
Interstitial brachytherapy (IRT):
Orthogonal radiographs, CT scan, isodose distribution; planning of differential loading and unloading
Interstitial hyperthermia (IHT):
Setup of generators, antennas, and thermometry probe (sensor) distribution; test run (10 min) for setup optimization
Interstitial hyperthermia
60 min at 41°C (minimum) to 44°C (maximum temperature)
One IHT session during IRT or two IHT sessions before and after IRT
Interstitial brachytherapy
20–30 Gy at 50 cGy/h isodose line (48–72 h); tube explantation
1- to 2-week break between interstitial and external beam radiotherapy
External beam radiotherapy
Untreated lesions: up to 50 Gy with photons/electrons to 70–80 Gy
Preirradiated lesions: up to 110 Gy cumulative total RT dose
Follow-up evaluation
First evaluation at 6–12 weeks after completion of therapy; further follow-up every 3 months for 2 years and thereafter every 6 months
Critical comparison of clinical, histological, and imaging studies (CT/MRI)

for the different IHT techniques are summarized in Table 15.4.

15.2.4 Invasive Thermometry

Specific aspects of thermometry have to be considered with regard to IHT technology and implant configuration. Although precise energy deposition is possible with all IHT techniques, steep thermal gradients of 1°–2°C/mm can be expected within the heated target volume. To obtain a realistic but still incomplete thermometry chart of the target volume, invasive measurements are

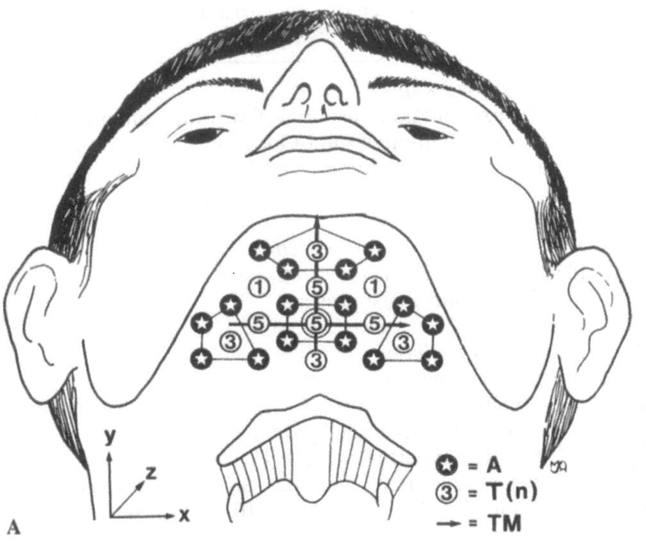

A

Implanted Target Volume

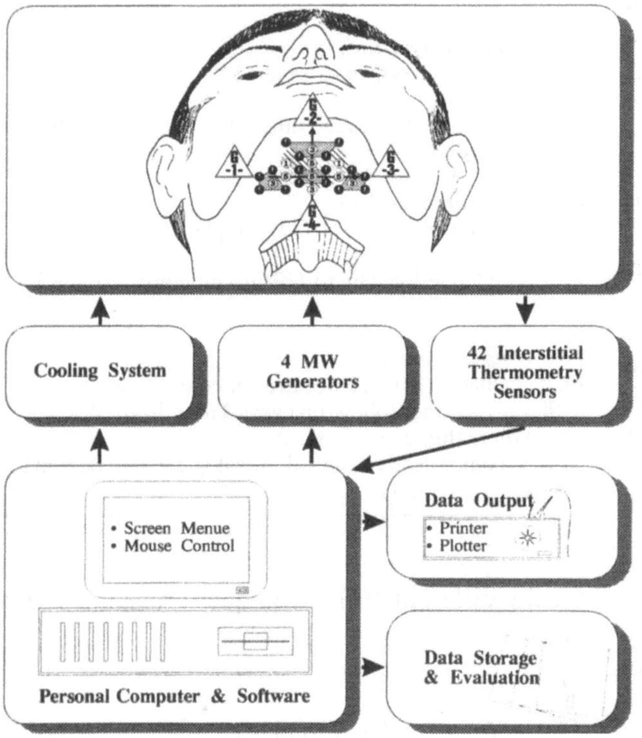

B

Fig. 15.3. A Schematic representation of a head and neck implant and setup for interstitial hyperthermia. The heating applicators (*A*; *black circles*) and thermometry probes (*T*; *white circles with figures indicating the number of thermometry sensors per track*) are equally distributed within the target volume. The *thin lines* connect the heating applicators which are controlled by one of four power generators. The *arrows* indicate the orientation of two of the thermal mapping (*TM*) axes. **B** Block diagram of an interstitial hyperthermia system illustrated for a 915-MHz microwave system with four power generators (*G*), 16 microwave antennas (*black circles*), and 18 temperature probes (*white circles*). IHT treatments are controlled by a PC-based software menu

Table 15.4. Implanatation requirements and thermometry setup

	RF technique	MW technique	FM technique	HS technique
Coverage of target volume	← Routine brachytherapy implantation →			
Distance of heat sources	10–15 mm	12–20 mm	8–12 mm	8–12 mm
Geometry of heat sources	Equidistant, strictly parallel orientation	More or less parallel orientation	Equidistant, ±30° of magnetic field axis	Equidistant, strictly parallel orientation
Brachytherapy techniques	Plastic catheters[a], template technique	Plastic catheters, template technique	Plastic catheters, template technique	Plastic catheters, template technique
	Rigid needle implant	Free hand and/or looping techniques	Permanent or preliminary implant	Rigid needle implant
Distribution of thermal probes	← 2–6 temperature probes depending upon the target volume →			
Thermometry 1st choice	← Fiberoptic thermometry →			
2nd choice	← High-resistance lead thermistors →			
3rd choice	RF-shielded thermocouples	–	RF-shielded thermocouples	RF-shielded thermocouples

RF, radiofrequency; MW, microwaves; FM, ferromagnetic; HS, hot source
[a] Only possible for capacitively coupled 27-MHz RF technology

mandatory. Noninvasive thermometry methods are still not fully developed and routinely available (Fabre et al. 1993; Prevost et al. 1993). Each IHT technique requires a slightly different approach to thermometry. These invasive thermometry guidelines have been previously reviewed (Emami et al. 1991; Seegenschmiedt and Visser 1991; Seegenschmiedt and Sauer 1992; vol. 1, Chap. 15: Waterman) and are compiled in Table 15.4.

Usually many thermometry probes are required. The minimum number depends on the implant configuration and the vicinity of critical structures. The following locations are recommended: (a) center of implant; (b) center of each subarray of three or four heat probes; (c) periphery of implant; and (d) surrounding normal tissue, or near critical organs. At least two to six thermometry probes have to be employed (Emami et al. 1991). A perpendicular probe at the central plane of the tumor is also advisable. In order to record as many thermometry points as possible, stationary multiple-sensor probes and computer-controlled automatically mapped single-sensor probes are used (Engler et al. 1987; Tarczy-Hornoch et al. 1992). Unfortunately, most commercial HT systems are poorly equipped and require manual mapping procedures, i.e., repeated incremental movements of one or multiple sensors along their implanted tracks.

It is important to differentiate thermometry conducted *within catheters containing heating applicators* and thermometry *within nonheated catheters*. Examples of the first approach are measurements directly at the surface of MW antennas or RF needles. This has the advantage of individual control of maximum temperatures and avoidance of thermal toxicity, but the disadvantage of overestimation of minimum temperatures. Artifacts, e.g., self-heating and thermal conduction, have to be carefully taken into account (Astrahan et al. 1988). Even with reliable thermometry close to HT applicators only regions with significantly higher temperatures than in regions between HT applicators are observed. Thus, the measured temperatures may not correlate with treatment outcome. Some IHT methods allow only thermometry outside of the tubes containing HT applicators. This leads to an underestimation of the thermal maximum. Within nonheated catheters one may truly measure *interstitial temperatures* with minimal artifacts, but may also underestimate the high temperatures which occur close to the heat sources. This can be quite hazardous, especially if the patient is being treated under general anesthesia. As a consequence, the measured maximum temperatures outside the heating probes may not correlate with the actually observed thermal toxicity.

15.2.5 Heating Device Selection

The choice of the IHT method for a particular tumor site depends on availability, tumor location, tissue and perfusion characteristics, and implant accessibility (spacing, template or pull-through implant, flexible vs rigid implants, etc.). Our recommendations for clinical practice are as follows (see also vol. 1, Chap. 13: STAUFFER et al.):

1. *RF techniques* are useful for sites which are implanted with an array of equidistant and equal length needles (template technique). Applications in the pelvis for gynecological and colorectal tumors are appropriate. There are also options for chest wall, neck, and extremity tumors and intraoperatively for abdominal and pelvic tumors. When bare metallic needles are used, good insulation at entry and exit points on the skin or mucosa is important to prevent toxicity. Software-controlled multiplexing systems are suited for LDR IRT and simultaneous long-duration HT (CORRY et al. 1993; MARTINEZ et al. 1993), while capacitive-coupled RF systems allow independent source control for nonparallel implants (DEURLOO et al. 1989, 1991; VISSER et al. 1989, 1991).
2. *MW techniques* are best suited for non-parallel implants (free-hand implants, looping techniques), near critical structures where individual control of each heat source is required, and in highly vascularized tissues, e.g., tumors of the head and neck, pelvis, and brain and some extremity lesions. Implantation close to bony structures should be avoided to prevent "hot spots" at the bone-soft tissue interface. For optimization of the heat distribution the use of muscle-equivalent bolus is recommended (SUNDARARAMAN 1990). Body sites which demand precise heat localization at depth call for special MW antennas which provide surface sparing (e.g., choke design). Improved antenna designs have been proposed to cope with complex implant configurations and anatomical sites (ROOS and HUGANDER 1988; RYAN et al. 1990; RYAN 1991, 1993; SATOH and STAUFFER 1988; SATHIASEELAN et al. 1991; TREMBLY et al. 1986, 1988, 1991). Small-diameter ultrasound transducers may assume some of the mentioned MW IHT applications, especially in situations where precise longitudinal specific absorption rate (SAR) control is required.
3. *FM techniques* allow heating without invasive thermometry. They are recommended for lesions which require a high degree of localization and few externalized connections. FM implants are useful where high-precision implants can be achieved, including for thoracic, abdominal, and brain tumors. Clinical applications include intra- (STEA et al. 1989, 1992a,b, 1993) and extracranial sites (AU et al. 1989; MACK et al. 1992, 1993a,b; SHIMM et al. 1989a,b; STEA et al. 1993). As heating relies only on thermal conduction, close spacing and parallel orientation of the inserted FM seeds or wires are essential.
4. *HS techniques* like hot water perfusion (HWP) or resistively heated wires have very similar characteristics to the previously described FM techniques, but they are more restricted due to the external connection requirements; thus, as with MW and RF techniques, localized deep heating may not be possible in all body sites. Nevertheless, clinical applications in a variety of body sites have been reported (HANDL-ZELLER 1993). So far no exclusive application for these thermal conduction techniques has been shown. As these techniques are relatively simple to handle, they may be especially useful in large implants to overcome the rapidly increasing complexity of heat application and control. Due to the well-evolved feedback control capability, the DC resistance wire technique may have a distinct advantage over other HS techniques.
5. *Laser and ultrasound techniques* have only recently been introduced as options for the treatment of liver metastasis and focal tumor sites (STEGER 1993; DIEDERICH and HYNYNEN 1993) but so far have not been used routinely. No other clinical applications have been found to be advantageous for these IHT techniques.

In summary, some groups prefer MW IHT due to the excellent radial power deposition characteristics (DENMAN et al. 1988a,b; MECHLING and STROHBEHN 1986; MECHLING et al. 1992; PAULSEN 1990; RYAN 1991, 1993; STROHBEHN 1987), while others prefer RF IHT due to the small variability in heating along the applicators and when dealing with complex implants (PRIONAS and KAPP 1992; PRIONAS et al. 1989; STAUFFER 1990; STAUFFER et al. 1989). Tumor and treatment parameters and treatment prescription also influence which IHT technique may be preferred in a given situation.

Advantages and disadvantages of each IHT technique have been previously summarized (COSSET 1990; COUGHLIN and Strohbehn 1989; EMAMI and PEREZ 1995; GAUTHERIE 1989; HAND 1992; MANNING and GERNER 1983; NEYZARI and CHEUNG 1985; PEREZ et al. 1992; SEEGENSCHMIEDT and SAUER 1989, 1992; SEEGENSCHMIEDT et al. 1990a; STAUFFER et al. 1989; STAUFFER 1990, 1991, 1992; STROHBEHN 1987; vol. 1, Chap. 13: STAUFFER et al.).

IHT is an ideal test site for *treatment planning*. The challenge for engineers and physicists is to predict thermal distributions inside the tumor and surrounding tissues. This requires different algorithms to compute SAR distributions within "ideal" arrays of IHT applicators. To obtain a realistic prediction, input of anatomical details, electrical tissue properties, and perfusion characteristics is necessary. Details of anatomical, vascular, and physiological data (vessel size, blood flow velocity, and direction within discrete large vessels) are expected to change our treatment planning and treatment performance considerably (LAGENDIJK et al. 1993, 1995). The present methods of thermal modeling and their impact on IHT planning have been reviewed by RYAN (1993).

15.2.6 Treatment Prescription

Clinical IHT-IRT trials demonstrate a wide variation of treatment prescription with regard to: (a) interstitial and external RT dose, (b) number of IHT sessions, (c) sequence of IHT and IRT treatments, (d) fractionation between IHT sessions, (e) "thermal dose" prescription, i.e., temperature level to be considered effective, and (f) overall treatment time. Despite these obvious variations, most clinical series have demonstrated encouraging results.

IHT-IRT treatment schedules can be divided into two groups: (a) IRT combined with *only one* IHT session, which is applied before, after, or parallel to IRT; (b) IRT combined with *two* IHT sessions, which are delivered *before* and *after* IRT. Rarely other schedules have been implemented: (c) multiple IHT sessions combined with external RT, (d) multiple IHT sessions combined with both interstitial and external RT, and (e) multiple interstitial plus external HT sessions combined with external and/or interstitial RT (ENGIN 1993; MITTAL et al. 1990; TUPCHONG et al. 1988). Some groups use two implants separated by 2–4 weeks, the IRT being combined with two IHT sessions on each occasion (PUTHAWALA et al. 1985, 1990). The different treatment schedules are shown in Fig. 15.4.

The HT prescription also varies with respect to the "thermal dose", i.e., total treatment time, steady state time at prescribed "therapeutic" temperature, and temperature level to be considered "therapeutic". The HT can be characterized according to whether the "therapeutic temperature" is based on *one* sensor (registering the minimum or maximum temperature) or on *all* sensors within the target volume (the mean temperature being used as reference). In the literature, the prescription ranges from 41°C for 30 min (VORA et al. 1982) to 43.5°C for 60 min (GAUTHERIE et al. 1989) or 44°C for 45 min (COSSET et al. 1985). Another way of defining HT treatments has been to apply the "thermal dose" concept (SAPARETO and DEWEY 1984), prescribing a HT session of 20 min equivalent to 43°C (DUNLOP et al. 1986). Recent series have used the "index temperature concept," taking all sensors within the target volume into account (SEEGENSCHMIEDT et al. 1994c; SHIMM et al. 1990). In contrast, trials using moderate continuous HT maintain a lower temperature of 41°C for up to 72 h and apply simultaneous LDR brachytherapy (CORRY et al. 1992, 1993; GARCIA et al. 1992a,b; MARCHOSKY 1990a,b; MARTINEZ et al. 1993) or chemotherapy (MARCHOSKY et al. 1992). In some experimental in vitro studies, new concepts have been tested, e.g., HT together with continuous LDR or pulsed HDR radiotherapy (ARMOUR et al. 1991, 1992).

Treatment designs of larger IHT-IRT series are compiled in Table 15.5, including all important treatment parameters, i.e., sequence of HT-RT, number of implants, and RT prescription. In contrast to groups using RF IHT, patients receiving MW IHT have been treated without general anesthesia, but with mild sedation and analgesic medication during the HT session. As plastic afterloading tubes are available, most groups perform two HT sessions, i.e., before *and* after IRT. This contrasts with the practice in RF IHT studies, where patients often receive one IHT session under general anesthesia. In order to apply IHT-IRT in preirradiated sites, several treatment modifications are necessary. Sometimes the radiation oncologist is forced to reduce the concurrent RT dose to avoid an excessive cumulative dose of the

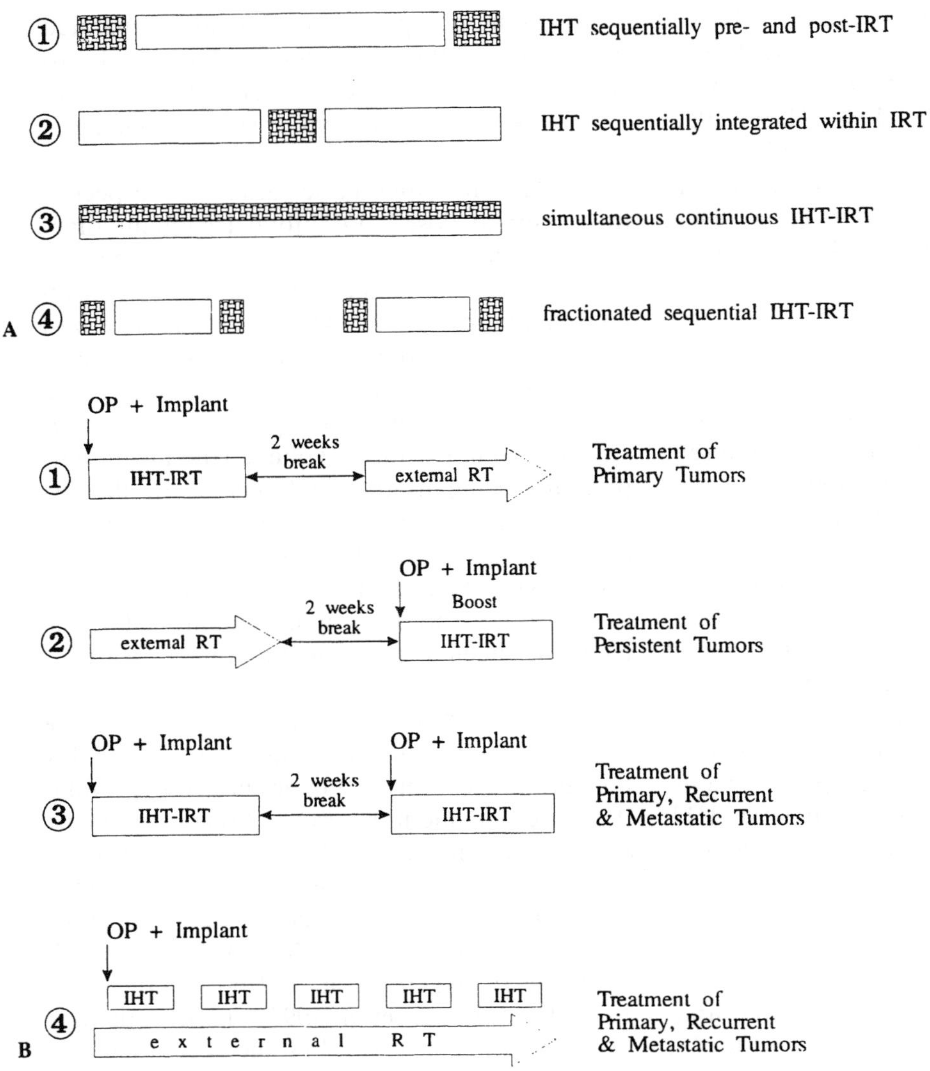

Fig. 15.4. A Different prescription options of combined interstitial HT (*grey*) and interstitial RT (*white*). **B** Different combinations and treatment schedules of interstitial HT-RT and external RT

previously applied and concurrent interstitial or external RT dose. A dose of 100–110 Gy was the limit in the RTOG 84-19 protocol (RTOG 1986).

15.3 Clinical Experience Related to IHT Techniques

Clinical studies with almost 1300 patients have been published in the literature: the primary study goals have been the characterization of IHT equipment and the analysis of the feasibility, efficacy, and treatment toxicity. The clinical rationale of these IHT-IRT studies has been addressed in Table 15.1. Treatments were considered justified if conventional treatments were found to promise insufficient local tumor control, if improved local tumor control could have resulted in a higher cure rate or better prevention of treatment morbidity, if improved tumor effects were expected with less toxicity and patient discomfort, if organ preservation was offered instead of mutilating surgery, and if other effective treatment options were not available. Therefore patients with locally advanced or recurrent tumors of the head and neck, breast, pelvis (gynecological, urogenital and colorectal tumors), extremities, and brain were thought to be the best candidates for such experimental studies (KAPP 1986; OVERGAARD 1989).

Most studies have been performed in specialized hospitals and institutions as intra-institutional nonrandomized phase I–II trials. These trials have concerned the feasibility of original or im-

Table 15.5. Design and treatment prescription of large IHT-IRT studies

Study	Implant (n)	Treatment sequence of IHT/IRT	Temperature (°C)	Time (min)	RT parameters (Gy)
Borrego et al. (1990)	1	IHT/IRT/IHT	41.5–43.0	60	1 × 20–35 Gy (LDR)
Cossett et al. (1985)	1	IHT/IRT/IHT	44.0	45	1 × 30 Gy (LDR)
Coughlin et al. (1991)	1	IHT/IRT/IHT	42.5–43.0	60	1 × 20–60 Gy (LDR)
Emami et al. (1987)	1	IHT/IRT/IHT	42.0	60	1 × 20–60 Gy (LDR)
Gautherie et al. (1989)	1	IHT/IRT/IHT	42.0–43.5	45–60	1 × 15–60 Gy (LDR)
Goffinet et al. (1990)	1	IHT/IRT/IHT	43.0–44.0	45	1 × 20–45 Gy (LDR)
Levendag et al. (1992; 1993)	1	IHT/IRT + ERT	43.0	45–60	1 × 20–34 Gy (LDR) up to 50 Gy ERT
Linares et al. (1986)	1–2	IHT/IRT	43.5	45	1 × 20–40 Gy (LDR)
Martinez et al. (1993)	1	IHT/IRT	41.0	48–72 h	1 × 25–35 Gy (LDR)
Oleson et al. (1984a,b)	1	IHT/IRT/IHT	42.0	30	1 × 30 Gy (LDR)
Petrovich et al. (1989)	1	IHT/IRT/IHT[a]	42.5	45–60	1 × 25–50 Gy (LDR)
Prevost et al. (1993)	1	IHT/IRT/ ± IHT + ERT	41.0–43.0	60	1 × 30–50 Gy (LDR) up to 45 Gy ERT
Puthawala et al. (1985, 1990)	1–2	IHT/IRT + IHT/IRT	41.5–43.0	45–60	2 × 20–25 Gy (LDR)
Rafla et al. (1989)	1	IHT/IRT/IHT	42.5	60	1 × 30–60 Gy (LDR)
Schreiber et al. (1992)	1	IHT/IRT/ ± IHT + ERT	41.5–43.0	45	1 × 20–50 Gy (LDR) up to 50 Gy ERT
Seegenschmiedt et al. (1994a–c)	1	IHT/IRT/ ± IHT ± ERT	41.0–44.0	60	1 × 20–30 Gy (LDR) up to 50 Gy ERT
Tupchong et al. (1988)	1	IHT/IRT + EHT/ERT; EHT after ERT	42.0–45.0	60	15 × 3 Gy ERT (LDR) fractionated ERT
Vora et al. (1989)	1–2	IHT/IRT	42.0–43.0	30	2 × 20–30 Gy (LDR)

IHT, interstitial hyperthermia; IRT, interstitial radiotherapy; EHT, external HT; ERT, external RT; LDR, low dose rate

[a] 20% received no 2nd IHT

proved IHT methods or evaluation of new commercial HT systems or equipment components. So far only one clinical study, the RTOG 84-19 study (Rtog 1986), has been designed and conducted as a prospectively controlled randomized multicenter study to compare treatment outcome with interstitial RT alone and with combined IHT-IRT treatment.

The following sections of this chapter address clinical IHT-IRT studies with respect to: (a) the applied interstitial HT techniques (Sect. 15.3), (b) the treated tumor sites (Sect. 15.4); (c) the addressed clinical endpoints (Sect. 15.5), (d) the observed treatment toxicity (Sect. 15.6), and (e) the prognostic tumor and treatment parameters (Sect. 15.7). In a further section important aspects of quality assurance and future perspectives of clinical IHT applications are addressed.

15.3.1 Radiofrequency Techniques

Resistive RF techniques using rigid needle pairs or single needles together with an external electrode were the first means of inducing IHT (Joseph et al. 1981; Vora et al. 1982). To date, 16 groups have published clinical results on about 500 lesions in various body sites (Table 15.6). Most clinical trials have been performed in the United States (City of Hope Medical Center, University of Arizona, Washington University, M.D. Anderson Hospital, and the Memorial Sloan-Kettering

Table 15.6. Institutions using radiofrequency (RF) IHT techniques

Institution(s)	Studies	No. of cases[a]	Technique	Special features
Stanford University, Stanford, Calif. (USA)	Bagshaw et al. (1993), Goffinet et al. (1990), Kapp and Prionas (1992), Prionas et al. (1989, 1994)	10 31	0.5-MHz LCF	Flexible catheters, Multisegmented or insulated needles
City of Hope Medical Ctr., Duarte, Calif. (USA)	Vora et al. (1982, 1986, 1988, 1989), Vora and Luk (1993)	78	0.5-MHz LCF	Paired needles
University of Arizona, Tucson, Ariz. (USA)	Surwit et al. (1983), Aristizabal and Oleson (1984), Manning et al. (1982b), Oleson and Cetas (1982), Oleson et al. (1984a,b), Shimm et al. (1990, 1992)	(52) 72	0.5-MHz RF-R	Paired needles
Washington University, St. Louis, Mich. (USA)	Emami (1992), Emami et al. (1984, 1987, 1992a), Perez and Emami (1989)	9	0.5-MHz LCF	Paired needles
William Beaumont Hosp., Royal Oak, Ill. (USA)	Borrego et al. (1990), Corry et al. (1992, 1993), Martinez et al. (1993)	16 9	0.5-MHz LCF	HUPIT automatic multiplexed system
M.D. Anderson University, Houston, Tex. (USA)	Frazier and Corry (1984)	12	0.5-MHz RF-R	Needles, wires
Memorial Sloan-Kettering, New York, N.Y. (USA)	Linares et al. (1986)	10	0.5-MHz LCF	Paired needles
French Multistudy Group: Paris, Lyon, Dijon (France)	Gautherie et al. (1989), Gerard et al. (1992), Marchal et al. (1993)	(96) 168	0.5-MHz RF-R	Paired needles
Institute Gustave-Roussy, Villejuif (France)	Cosset (1990), Cosset et al. (1982, 1984a,b, 1985, 1986)	29	0.5-MHz RF-R	Paired needles, insulated electrodes
Curie Institute, Paris (France)	Fourquet et al. (1990) (cited in: Marchal 1993)	11	0.5-MHz RF-R	Paired Needles
Centre Alexis Vautrin, Nancy (France)	Marchal (1992, 1993), Marchal et al. (1985, 1989, 1992, 1993)	5	27-MHz RF-C	Paired and independent capacitive needles, insulated electrodes
Daniel den Hoed Cancer Center, Rotterdam (NL) and University of Utrecht (NL)	Deurloo et al. (1989, 1991), Visser et al. (1989, 1991), Levendag et al. (1992, 1993), Lagendijk et al. (1995)	11	27-MHz RF-C	Paired and independent capacitive needles, insulated electrodes
MRC Hammersmith Hospital, London (UK)	Dunlop et al. (1986)	9	0.5-MHz RF-R	Paired needles
Tokyo University (Japan)	Nakagawa et al. (1989)	7	0.5-MHz RF-R	Paired needles
Shiga University (Japan)	Yabumoto and Suyama (1985) Yabumoto et al. (1989)	14	0.5-MHz RF-R	Paired needles
16 clinical institutions	52 clinical reports	501	4 techniques	Different features

RF-R, resistively coupled radiofrequency; RF-C, capacitively coupled radiofrequency; LCF, local current field; HUPIT, hyperthermia universal perineal interstitial template.

[a] Case numbers in parentheses are included in the larger number of the same group

Table 15.7. Clinical results with radiofrequency (RF) IHT techniques

Institution	No. of cases[a]	Tumor sites	CR (%)	PR (%)	Toxicity (%)	Follow-up
Stanford University						
GOFFINET et al. (1990)	10	Head and neck	80	0	10	Long-term
BAGSHAW et al. (1993)	31	Prostate	NA[b]	NA	42	NA[b]
City of Hope Medical Ctr.						
VORA et al. (1982)	(16)	Cervical tumours	69	6	6	1–3 mos
VORA et al. (1989)	78	Various sites	53	19	18	1–13 mos
University of Arizona						
OLESON et al. (1984a,b)	(52)	Various sites	38	42	21	3–18 mos
SHIMM et al. (1990)	72	Various sites	36	–	24	Long-term
Washington University						
EMAMI et al. (1984, 1987)	9	Pelvic sites	56	33	25	6–48 mos
William Beaumont Hosp.						
BORREGO et al. (1990)	13	Pelvic sites	31	37	50	2–20 mos
MARTINEZ et al. (1993)	9	Pelvic and other sites	66	33	NA	NA
M.D. Anderson University						
FRAZIER and CORRY (1984)	12	Thoracic and other sites	–	50	9	2–12 mos
Memorial Sloan-Kettering						
LINARES et al. (1986)	10	Various sites	30	70	40	Short-term
French Multistudy Group						
GAUTHERIE et al. (1989)	(96)	Various sites	61	15	26	Long-term
MARCHAL et al. (1993)	168	Various sites	69	–	23	Long-term
Institute Gustave-Roussy						
COSSET et al. (1984a,b, 1985)	29	Various sites	66	14	35	2 mos
Curie Institute						
FOURQUET et al. (1990)	11	Head and neck	82	–	27	NA
Centre Alexis Vautrin						
MARCHAL et al. (1993)	5	Head and neck	60	40	20	2–36 mos
DDHCC Rotterdam LEVENDAG et al. (1993)	11	Head and neck	54	9	10	4–36 mos
MRC Hammersmith DUNLOP et al. (1986)	9	Various sites	–	44	NA	1–6 mos
Tokyo University						
NAKAGAWA et al. (1989)	7	Various sites	71	29	–	Short-term
Shiga University						
YABUMOTO and SUYAMA (1985)						
YABUMOTO et al. (1989)	14	Various sites	57	14	31	3–13 mos
15 clinical institutions	~500	Various sites	~55	~25	~25	variable

CR, complete response; PR, partial response; NA, no information available
[a] Case numbers in parentheses are included in the larger number of the same group
[b] No short- and long-term analysis published

Cancer Center), with only very few in Europe and Japan. The largest trial was a French multicenter trial (GAUTHERIE et al. 1989) which accumulated 168 patients and was recently updated (GERARD et al. 1992; MARCHAL et al. 1993). Updated reports on other phase I–II studies are not available. The clinical results with RF IHT techniques are encouraging (Table 15.7): the mean complete response (CR) rate reached 55%, ranging form 30% (LINARES et al. 1986) to 82% (FOURQUET et al. 1990); the mean partial response (PR) rate was 25%; thus, the mean response was 80%. Treatment-related acute toxicity was low: superficial burns or tissue necrosis occurred in 25%

(6%–50%). The follow-up periods ranged from 1 to 48 months, but often were not specified.

The following RF IHT techniques were applied: (a) resistively coupled FR needle pairs and resistively coupled local current field (LCF) techniques, each powered by 0.5-MHz generators; (b) capacitively coupled RF techniques powered by 8- or 27-MHz generators; and (c) resistively coupled automatic multiplexing RF IHT systems (CORRY et al. 1992; 1993; MARTINEZ et al. 1993). A drawback of early RF IHT systems was the inconvenience of using rigid steel needles, which precluded multiple HT sessions with one implant. As a consequence, RF IHT was performed under general anesthesia to avoid patient discomfort and pain during the IHT treatment, but also to facilitate patient handling. When using stainless steel needles as guides for brachytherapy, IHT sessions were delivered just once, mostly before IRT.

The stainless steel trocars caused considerable tolerance problems and complications. This stimulated development of partially insulated electrodes with improved longitudinal power deposition characteristics (GOFFINET et al. 1990; PRIONAS and KAPP 1992). These applicators have a thin layer of electrically insulating paint or are surrounded by plastic tubes in areas where heating is not desired. Further need to improve control of longitudinal heating has triggered the development of multisegmented electrodes that provide individual control of power deposition along the longitudinal axis of each needle (PRIONAS et al. 1989; PRIONAS and KAPP 1992). Recently, flexible RF electrodes have been designed to enable the implantation of sites that are anatomically difficult to access, e.g., in the head and neck and presacral region (GOFFINET 1990).

On the basis of a working principle that underlies LCF methods, MARCHAL et al. (1985) suggested capacitive RF IHT with 27 MHz; thereby direct contact of needles with tissue is replaced by capacitive coupling. The length of the active electrode can be adapted to each anatomical and clinical situation. Recently, this RF IHT technique was improved by using separate 27-MHz generators and a matching network (DEURLOO et al. 1989, 1991; VISSER et al. 1991; LAGENDIJK 1995). Good control of power deposition in various clinical situations has been reported by clinical users (LEVENDAG et al. 1992, 1993).

RF IHT equipment is often complicated to set up and cumbersome, and it is time consuming to connect the RF electrodes to the needle pairs. Moreover, once all of them are connected, it is difficult to make any changes during the HT treatment, as it is difficult visually to separate the individual electrode connectors, be they color coded or not, and physically to manipulate the connectors in a complex implant. Usual RF IHT systems lack appropriate numbers of electrical connections to accommodate the number of needle pairs required to perform adequate HT in very large tumors.

In order to overcome these technical problems and to reduce treatment toxicity, CORRY et al. (1993) developed a new RF IHT system that applies a special "hyperthermia universal perineal template" (HUPIT) which attaches to the MUPIT template (MARTINEZ et al. 1985). It can be coupled both to the microselectron LDR system and to the RF generator (Fig. 15.5). From preliminary clinical experience (BORREGO et al. 1990) it was concluded that the electronic template permits unlimited 2D power deposition control within the

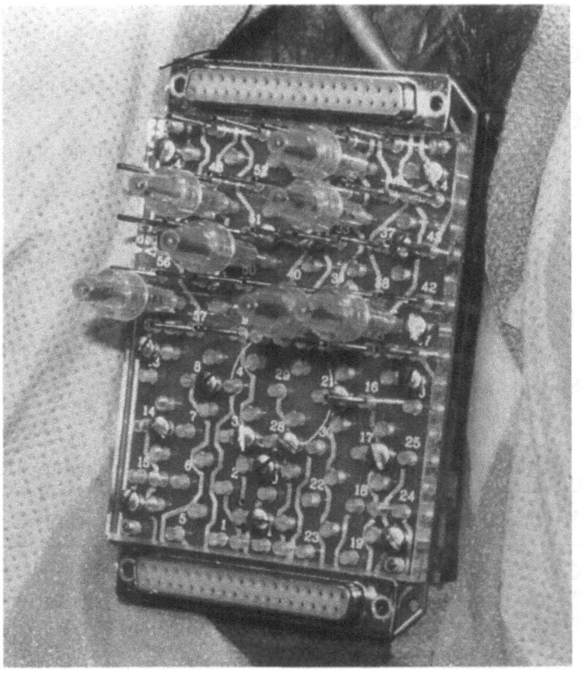

Fig. 15.5. The HUPIT template, which is placed intraoperatively during the implant procedure. The electronic portion of the template is incorporated into the cover section and is attached at the end of the procedure. The connectors at the top and bottom are for power introduction. The plastic hubs represent the removable obturators for the thermometry catheters. Afterloading connections are made to the end of each needle in a conventional manner. (From MARTINEZ et al. 1993)

tumor by effectively generating and controlling power to a total of 1670 electrode pairs. The applicator had a significant beneficial impact on patient comfort, and reduced staff setup and treatment interrupt time; it also seemed to improve the response of very large tumors (Martinez et al. 1993; Corry et al. 1993).

A specific problem related to RF IHT is the performance of invasive thermometry. Often the commercial RF IHT systems provide only the option of thermal measurements within heated needle probes. High-impedance thermistors (Bowmann probes) are recommended which should be placed parallel and if possible perpendicular to the IHT applicators. Unsurprisingly, large discrepancies between temperatures measured inside heated versus nonheated probes have been reported (Levendag et al. 1993). Therefore careful quality control and quality assurance (QA) are necessary (Emami et al. 1991; Prionas and Kapp 1992; Seegenschmiedt and Visser 1991; vol. 1, Chap. 21: Visser and van Rhoon).

In summary, the RF IHT techniques and especially the LCF and the sophisticated multiplexing RF IHT systems have been shown to be efficient in inducing therapeutic temperatures and attaining good clinical results with acceptable though significant toxicity of about 25%. However, toxicity is only partly due to technical factors, e.g., the risk of creating "hot spots" near the tip of converging planes of RF needles. The most recently developed capacitive RF IHT techniques appear very promising in that standard afterloading catheters, conventional implantation techniques, and even irregular implants can be applied.

15.3.2 Microwave Techniques

Interest in the use of interstitial MW antennas as a means to heat tumors arose in the late 1970s (Mendecki et al. 1977, 1978; Taylor 1978, 1980), but clinical work started in the mid 1980s. So far 16 groups have published clinical results (Table 15.8). While the first clinical series involved few patients and discussed technical aspects, more recently, since MW techniques have become better known and accepted, clinical series have included a broader spectrum of diseases and more patients.

Most groups working with MW IHT are located in the United States (Memorial Medical Center, Long Beach; University of Southern California, Los Angeles; Washington University; Dartmouth Medical College, Hanover; Porter Memorial Hospital, Denver; Methodist Hospital, Brooklyn; St. Josephs Cancer Center, Albuquerque; and Hahnemann University, Philadelphia); a few others are located in Europe (Centre Oscart Lambret, Lille; University of Erlangen-Nürnberg) or Japan (Osaka, Tokyo). So far more than 520 lesions in various body sites have been treated. The largest reported trials have been conducted at Long Beach Memorial Medical Center (Puthawala et al. 1990) and at the University of Erlangen-Nürnberg (Seegenschmiedt et al. 1994a–c), and the emphasis has been on the treatment of head and neck tumors.

The clinical results using MW IHT are compiled in Table 15.9. Overall, the mean CR rate was 65% ranging from 10% (Inoue et al. 1989) to 84% (Prevost et al. 1993). The mean PR rate was 25%; thus the mean overall response reached 90%, which is slightly higher than with RF IHT. Treatment toxicity (superficial burns or deep tissue necrosis) was about 20% (range 10%–44%). Follow-up periods ranged from 1 to 68 months, but often were not specified. MW IHT was rarely performed with patients under general anesthesia; instead, mild sedation and analgesics were applied. In most trials the IHT sessions were delivered twice, before and after IRT. Only in one trial were two implants used; they were separated by several weeks and each was accompanied by two IHT sessions, before and after IRT (Puthawala et al. 1985).

MW power sources can be operated at 300–2450 MHz, but often 915 MHz has been used in commercial IHT systems (BSD Medical, Salt Lake City, USA; Clini-Therm, Dallas, USA; Lund/Buchler, Lund, Sweden). Most systems include up to 16 MW antennas and one to eight generators. Through switchboxes power is controlled for single antennas or groups of two to four antennas depending upon the number of power channels (Fig. 15.3). Power deposition along the longitudinal axis of MW antennas is about one-half wavelength in tissue, i.e., different frequencies provide shorter or longer heating patterns. Typical and clinically useful half wavelength patterns are 2.5 cm (at 2450 MHz), 7 cm (915 MHz), and 12 cm (at 433 MHz). MW antennas can be directly inserted into conventional plastic brachytherapy catheters. Thus, MW IHT is fully compatible with standard IRT approaches, but is especially suitable for all free-hand implants

Table 15.8. Institutions using microwave (MW) IHT techniques

Institution	Studies	No. of cases	Technique(s)	Special features
Freeman Memorial, Inglewood, Calif. (USA)	BICHER et al. (1985a,b)	8	300, 915 MHz	Flexible antennas (PdM), air cooling
Memorial Medical Center, Long Beach, Calif. (USA)	PUTHAWALA et al. (1985, 1990)	108	915 MHz	Flexible antennas (PdM; Clini-Therm)
Univ. Southern California, Los Angeles, Calif. (USA)	LAM et al. (1988), PETROVICH et al. (1989)	44	300, 630, 915 MHz	Semirigid antennas (BSD Medical)
Washington University, St. Louis, Miss. (USA)	EMAMI (1992), EMAMI et al. (1984, 1987, 1992a), PEREZ and EMAMI (1989)	63	915 MHz	Flexible or semirigid antennas (BSD Medical; Clini-Therm)
Dartmouth Medical College, Hanover, N.H. (USA)	COUGHLIN et al. (1983, 1985, 1991, 1992), COUGHLIN and STROHBEHN (1989)	35	433, 915, 2450 MHz multi-channel system	IMAAH system with home-built antennas and various generators
Porter Memorial Hospital, Denver, Colo. (USA)	SCHREIBER et al. (1992)	40	915 MHz	Flexible antennas (Clini-Therm)
Jefferson University Hosp., Philadelphia, Pa. (USA)	TUPCHONG et al. (1988), ENGIN et al. (1993)	14	915 MHz	Flexible antennas (Clini-Therm)
Methodist Hospital, Brooklyn, N.Y. (USA)	RAFLA et al. (1988, 1989)	35	915 MHz	Semirigid antennas (BSD Medical)
City of Hope Medical Ctr., Duarte, Calif. (USA)	WONG et al. (1988)	1	915 MHz	Flexible antenna (Cheung System-100)
Northwestern Memorial, Chicago, Ill. (USA)	MITTAL et al. (1990)	1	915 MHz	Semirigid antennas (BSD Medical)
St. Josephs Cancer Center, Albuquerque, N.M. (USA)	KHAN et al. (1992)	35	915 MHz	Semirigid antennas (BSD Medical)
Hahnemann University, Philadelphia, Pa. (USA)	PHROMRATANAPONGSE et al. (1990)	45	915 MHz	Flexible antennas (Clini-Therm)
Centre Oscart Lambret, Lille (France)	PREVOST et al. (1993)	25	915 MHz with 3 GHz radiometry	Flexible antennas (HIMCAR System)
University Erlangen-Nbg., Erlangen (Germany)	SEEGENSCHMIEDT et al. (1989a, 1990b, 1992, 1993a,b, 1994a–c)	90	915 MHz	Semirigid antennas (Lund/Buchler 4010)
Osaka University, Osaka (Japan)	INOUE et al. (1989)	10	915 MHz	Semirigid antennas (BSD Medical)
Yikei University, Tokyo (Japan)	AOYAGI et al. (1989)	10	915 MHz	Flexible antennas (Clini-Therm)
16 clinical institutions	35 publications	564	4 techniques	Different features

BSD Medical, Salt Lake City (USA); PdM System, van Nuys, Calif. (USA); Clini-Therm System, Dallas, Tex. (USA); Lund/Buchler System 4010, Lund/Buchler HT System (Sweden/Germany)

with flexible or curved catheters. The MW IHT technique is also the technique least sensitive to geometrical irregularities.

Many antenna refinements have been proposed (GOTTLIEB et al. 1990; ISKANDER and TUMEH 1989; JAMES et al. 1989; LEE et al. 1986; LIN and WANG 1987; ROOS and HUGANDER 1988; RYAN 1991; SATHIASEELAN et al. 1991; SATOH and STAUFFER 1988; TREMBLY et al. 1986, 1988, 1991a,b; WONG et al. 1989). Recently the following MW designs have been introduced: (a) multisegmented antennas for improved longitudinal heating; (b) helical coil antennas for homogeneous longitudinal heating; (c) hot tip antennas for improved tip heating; (d) choked antennas for tissue shielding to avoid unnecessary heating of the proximal

Table 15.9. Clinical results with microwave (MW) IHT techniques

Institution	No. of cases[a]	Tumor sites	CR (%)	PR (%)	Toxicity (%)	Follow-up
Freeman Memorial, Inglewood,						
BICHER et al. (1985a,b)	8	Various sites	63	25	13	Short-term
Long Beach Memorial Center	(43)	Various sites	74	26	21	Long-term
PUTHAWALA et al. (1985, 1990)	108	Head and neck	75	–	NA	Long-term
University of Southern California						
PETROVICH et al. (1989)	44	Various sites	64	34	20	3–36 mos
Washington University						
PEREZ and EMAMI (1989),	(39)	Various sites	54	23	25	6–48 mos
EMAMI et al. (1987, 1992a)	63	Various sites	51	–	22	Long-term
Dartmouth Medical College						
COUGHLIN et al. (1985, 1992)	35	Various sites	66	23	NA	1–62 mos
Porter Memorial Hospital						
SCHREIBER et al. (1992)	40	Various sites	53	45	15	1–30 mos
Jefferson University Hospital						
TUPCHONG et al. (1988)	14	Head and neck	64	14	NA	NA
ENGIN et al. (1993)	(9)	Head and neck	67	33	44	Long-term
Methodist Hospital Brooklyn,						
RAFLA et al. (1988, 1989)	35	Various sites	54	37	23	Short-term
City of Hope Medical Center						
WONG et al. (1988)	1	Bile duct	NA[b]	NA	NA[b]	Short-term
Northwest Memorial Chicago						
MITTAL et al. (1990)	1	Head and neck	NA[b]	NA	NA[b]	Short-term
Hahnemann Univ. Philadelphia						
PHROMRATANAPONGSE et al. (1990)	(45)	Various sites	69	22	27	6–39 mos
St. Josephs Hospital, Albuquerque						
KHAN et al. (1992)	35	Prostate	NA[b]	NA	NA[b]	1–29 mos
Centre Oscart Lambret, Lille						
PREVOST et al. (1993)	25	Tongue	84	–	<10	3–27 mos
University of Erlangen-Nürnberg						
SEEGENSCHMIEDT et al. (1994a–c)	90	Various sites	66	28	24	4–68 mos
Osaka University						
INOUE et al. (1989)	10	Various sites	10	70	10	1–6 mos
Yikei University, Tokyo						
AOYAGI et al. (1989)	10	Various sites	20	40	20	NA
16 clinical institutions	~520	Various sites	~65	~25	~20	variable

CR, complete response; PR, partial response; NA, no information available
[a] Case numbers in parentheses are included in the larger number of the same group
[b] No short- and long-term analysis published

antenna leads; and (e) surface-cooled antennas to overcome "hot stops" and to increase the radial power deposition pattern (EPPERT et al. 1991). Despite some improvements in the design and performance of MW antennas, further improvements are necessary, namely reduction of the impact of implantation and geometrical parameters, e.g., insertion depth, and improvement of the axial and longitudinal heating and the power deposition at the antenna tip.

At Dartmouth Medical College a sophisticated MW IHT system [interstitial microwave antenna array hyperthermia (IMAAH)] was developed. It provides unique features including independent power control, coherent and incoherent power steering, and phase shifting (COUGHLIN 1990, 1992; COUGHLIN et al. 1985, 1991; STROHBEHN 1987). An integrated automated thermometry system provides instant feedback control to each of the MW antennas such that temperatures can be maintained uniformly throughout the target volume.

MW IHT has distinct advantages over other IHT methods. It allows a wider applicator spacing as compared to other IHT techniques and can better compensate "thermal washout". This is very important, as blood flow is the most critical factor in the uniformity of temperatures. Thermal dosimetry is usually governed by the geometry and separation of the implanted afterloading catheters necessary to deliver uniform IRT dose and to provide uniform heating. Thus, variability of spacing has less impact on MW IHT than on other IHT techniques. Further improvements of MW IHT depend on the development of MW antennas with insertion depth-independent power deposition and improved longitudinal control of power deposition.

In summary, compared to RF IHT, the MW IHT techniques are slightly more effective in inducing therapeutic temperatures and attaining good clinical results (65% CR, 90% overall response), and have a slightly lower toxicity rate of about 20%. Toxicity is partially due to "hot spots" at tissue interfaces or tissue entry and exit points. Several improved MW antenna designs have become available. Depending on the complexity of a tumor volume, it may be desirable to use a "family of different heating-length antennas" in order to cover the entire volume adequately. In the future, complete 3D treatment planning and thermal modeling need to be integrated into clinical implementations of MW IHT systems (Ryan 1993).

15.3.3 Ferromagnetic Techniques

Ferromagnetic (FM) seed HT is based on energy absorption from an external magnetic field of a large RF coil which is placed around the body segment of interest. Thereby eddy currents are induced within the implanted seeds, which in turn heat the seeds resistively. Heat is distributed by thermal conduction. Physical studies appeared in the early 1970s (Burton et al. 1971; Merry et al. 1973; Moidal et al. 1976). Later technical feasibility and in vivo toxicity were analyzed (Atkinson et al. 1984; Brezovich et al. 1984; Forsyth et al. 1985; Stauffer et al. 1984). Nowadays seeds with Curie points near the therapeutic temperature are available. Since FM seeds are thermally self-regulating, invasive thermometry is not necessary. Clinical trials were initiated in several institutions which are listed in Table 15.10. Most of them are in the United States (University of Alabama, Birmingham; University of Arizona, Tucson; University of California, San Francisco; University of Wisconsin, Madison; City of Hope Medical Center), and only a few in Europe (University of Amsterdam) and Japan (Nagoya University). So far about 100 lesions have been treated in various sites in humans.

The largest trial was a multicenter phase I–II study under the auspices of the NCI which involved 44 patients with extracranial tumors (Mack et al. 1992, 1993a,b). Another study involving 35 intracranial tumors was conducted at Nagoya University (Kida et al. 1989; Kobayashi and Kida 1992; Kobayashi et al. 1986, 1991, 1992). The clinical results using FM IHT techniques are summarized in Table 15.11. Overall, the mean CR rate in extracranial sites was 60%, ranging from 31% (Kobayashi and Kida 1992) to 100% (Tohnai et al. 1992). The mean PR rate was 30% and thus the overall response rate reached 90%, which is slightly higher than with RF IHT. Treatment-related toxicity (superficial burns or deep tissue necrosis) was 20% (range 7%–66%), which is comparable to that with other IHT techniques. Follow-up periods ranged from 1 to 53 months, but often were not reported. For intracranial sites the mean CR rate reached 40% (range 31%–50%), while the toxicity data were not fully available or were difficult to interpret.

The advantage of FM IHT is its independence from the composition of the implanted tissues. Heating relies on seed composition, implant geometry (Atkinson et al. 1984), and perfusion (Hand 1992). FM IHT is compatible with all IRT techniques and can be applied simultaneously. By using one surgical procedure, FM seeds can be placed temporarily (Meridith et al. 1989) in afterlogading probes or permanently, which allows the delivery of interstitial or external RT and multiple IHT sessions. Another positive feature is the ease of operation: patients can be treated without general anesthesia, which allows close operator-patient interaction. There are also no restrictions on the number of HT sessions; thus, patient tolerance can be optimized over time. Another advantage is that no internal connections to the heating sources are required. Therefore clinical applications included malignancies of the brain, head and neck, and prostate. Unfortunately, so far no commercially available FM IHT system has been developed.

FM implants also have disadvantages: One relates to poor biocompatibility, which needs to be solved when permanent implants are envisaged. When temporary implants are used, this problem is circumvented, as the seeds are inserted into afterloading tubes and do not come into direct contact with the tissue. Another disadvantage is that no effective power is deposited between implants, which can leave "cold spots" in the target volume. In order to improve the heating performance, seed spacing has to be optimized. Generally, a spacing of about 10 mm is required

Table 15.10. Institutions using ferromagnetic (FM) IHT techniques (including animal and brain lesions)

Institution(s)	Studies	No. of cases	Technique	Special features
University of Arizona, Tucson (USA)	Atkinson et al. (1984), Stauffer et al. (1984), Forsyth et al. (1985)	9	1.8 MHz Induction coil	Animal study: Ni-Si seeds (Curie point 45°–50°C)
	Au et al. (1989), Shimm et al. (1989a,b), Mack et al. (1992, 1993a,b)	14[a]	86–96 kHz Induction coil (1500–2400 A/m)	Head and neck and pelvic tumors: Ni-Si seeds (Curie point 55°–80°C)
	Stea et al. (1989, 1992a,b, 1993)	28	80–100 kHz Induction coil (1500–2400 A/m)	Brain tumors: Ni-Si seeds (Curie point 50°–65°C)
University of Alabama, Birmingham (USA)	Brezovich et al. (1984, 1990), Brezovich and Meridith (1989), Meridith et al. (1989)	15	89 kHz Induction coil (4000 A/m)	Animal study: Ni-Cu seeds and wires (Curie point 45°C): seed migration
University of Wisconsin, Madison (USA)	Partington et al. (1989), Steeves et al. (1992), Tompkins et al. (1992)	8	120 kHz Induction coil	Animal study: Ni-Cu seeds (Curie point 42°–48°C)
Multicenter study (USA): University of Arizona, University of California, City of Hope Medical Ctr., University of Wisconsin	Mack et al. (1992, 1993a,b)	44[a]	80–100 kHz Induction coil (1500–2000 A/m)	Advanced primary and recurrent tumors: Ni-Si seeds (Curie point 50°–80°C)
Amsterdam University, Amsterdam (NL)	van Dijk et al. (1993)	–	80–100 kHz	Preliminary study: home-built seeds: Pd-Ni 26.0/27.0 (Curie point 45°–60°C)
Nagoya University, Nagoya (Japan)	Tohnai et al. (1990), Tohnai et al. (1992)	6 7	240 kHz Induction coil	Head and neck tumors: Fe-Pt seeds (Curie point: 68°C)
	Kobayashi et al. (1986, 1991, 1992), Kida et al. (1989), Kobayashi and Kida (1992)	35	240 kHz Induction coil	Brain tumors: Fe-Pt seeds (Curie point: 68°C)
7 clinical institutions	25 publications	166[a]	5 techniques	Different features

Ni-Cu, nickel-copper seeds; Ni-Si, nickel-silicon seeds; Fe-Pt, iron-platinum seeds; Pd-Ni, palladium-nickel seeds
[a] Number includes some cases twice

(Stauffer et al. 1984). Pretreatment planning is also very critical, as it is impossible to redistribute the FM seeds once they are in place. Power control of individual seeds is only possible through Curie point regulation. A problem relates to seed migration in permanent implants, as many tissues in the human body move relative to each other, especially when tumors continue to grow or shrink and disintegrate in response to effective HT treatments. More in vivo research is needed in this respect.

Important research objectives for FM IHT include the following topics: (a) development and clinical implementation of multitemperature seeds within an array of seeds; (b) optimization of seed location and spacing; (c) development of a preplanning program and special routines to optimize the implant procedures. Optimization of the thermal distribution will also require methods for predetermining relative tumor blood flow although the treatment plan will still be static, as the typical dynamics of perfusion over time and with treatment cannot be accommodated. Only by using special afterloading techniques, which will offset an advantage of FM IHT, may it be possible to exchange seeds and vary thermal dis-

Table 15.11. Clinical results with ferromagnetic (FM) IHT techniques (including animal and brain lesions)

Institution	Tumor sites	No. of cases[a]	CR (%)	PR (%)	Toxicity (%)	Follow-up
University of Arizona						
FORSYTH et al. (1985)	Animal tumors	9	66	33	66	1–8 mos
AU et al. (1989)	Head and neck	4	50	25	50	Short-term
STEA et al. (1990)	Brain	(14)	50	–	43	1–19 mos
STEA et al. (1992b)	Brain	28	43	–	NA	Long-term
Multicenter study (USA)						
MACK et al. (1992, 1993a,b) STEA et al. (1993)	Various sites	44	61	32	7	1–53 mos
Nagoya University						
TOHNAI et al. (1990)	Tongue	6	66	33	NA	NA
TOHNAI et al. (1992)	Oral cavity	7	100	–	NA	NA
KOBAYASHI and KIDA (1992) KOBAYASHI et al. (1992)	Brain	35	31	–	NA	NA
6 clinical institutions	Various sites	~130	~60	~30	~50	variable

CR, complete response; PR, partial response; NA, no information available
[a] Case numbers in parentheses are included in the larger number of the same group
[b] No short- and long-term analysis published

tributions manually over time. Adverse effects of high tissue perfusion may be solved by higher temperature Curie point seeds or a closer spacing.

In summary, compared to RF IHT and MW IHT techniques, clinical results with FM IHT are still preliminary. However, they seem to demonstrate good efficacy in inducing therapeutic temperatures and attaining good clinical results (60% complete, 90% overall response) in extracranial lesions. The observed toxicity rate of 20% is acceptable and comparable with other IHT methods. This toxicity is mostly due to uncontrolled migration of seeds, relatively poor biocompatibility, or uncontrolled "hot spots" in the vicinity of FM seeds. Although a high implant density is required, the FM IHT technique is less demanding of a perfect implant geometry due to the individual thermal regulation within each FM seed. In the future, careful planning of FM IHT treatments will be required. The access to a "family of different seeds" with a wide range of Curie point temperatures is likely to be necessary to overcome at least some of the perfusion variability within the implanted volume.

15.3.4 Hot Source Techniques

Heating with hot source (HS) devices is based on thermal conduction. The technique can be applied in various clinical situations. HANDL-ZELLER (1992, 1993) and co-workers (HANDL-ZELLER et al. 1987a,b, 1992) designed a hot water perfusion (HWP) system by passing hot water with high flow through an array of implanted tubes. Another approach using metallic probes which are resistively heated by electrical elements was designed to treat brain tumors (MARCHOSKY et al. 1990a,b, 1992) Generally, HS IHT systems are simple and very cost-effective methods. Two commercial systems are presently available: the Hydrotherm hyperthermia system (Ottmar Handl, Vienna, Austria), which has been used for extracranial tumors, and the Cook interstitial hyperthermia system VH 8500 (Cook Inc., Bloomington, USA), which has been applied in treating intracranial tumors.

First technical reports date back to the late 1980s (HANDL-ZELLER et al. 1987a,b, 1992; HANDL-ZELLER 1992, 1993). When HS IHT techniques became better known and more widely accepted, clinical trials in humans started in many hospitals. The ten institutions where HS IHT has been applied are listed in Table 15.12. Most of them are in Europe (Universities of Graz and Vienna, Austria; University of Düsseldorf; Oncological Institute of Ljubljana, Slowenia; Curie Institute, Paris; Centre Leon Bertrand, Lyon; Centre Alexis Vautrin, Nancy) and only two of them in the United States (Washington

Table 15.12. Institutions using other HS IHT techniques

Institution(s)	Studies	No. of cases	Technique	Special features
Washington University, St. Louis (USA)	GARCIA et al. (1992a,b)	7	Hot wires 45°C	Prostate carcinoma: resistive heating (Cook VH 8500)
Missouri Baptist Medical Center, St. Louis (USA)	MARCHOSKY et al. (1990a, 1990b, 1992)	50	Hot wires 50°C	Brain tumors: resistive heating (Cook VH 8500)
Multicenter evaluation:	HANDL-ZELLER (1993):	154[a]	Hot water 45°–50°C	Various human tumors
University Clinic, Graz (Austria)	Arian-Schad, Stückl-schweiger	(10)	with water flow: 2.5–4.0 ml/s	Hydrotherm system KHS 9 W 18
University Clinic, Vienna (Austria)	Handl-Zeller, Seitz, Stanek	(72)		Perfusion with either unidirectional or counterflow mode, flexible catheters or
Institute of Oncology, Ljubljana (Slovenia)	Budihna, Lesnicar, Burger	(16)		
University Hospital, Düsseldorf (Germany)	Zamboglou, Kolotas	(34)		
Curie Institute, Paris (France)	Campana, Fourquet, Gaboriaud	(8)		rigid steel needles, simultaneous or sequential LDR/HDR brachtherapy
Centre Leon Berard, Lyon (France)	Ardiet	(2)		
Centre Alexis Vautrin, Nancy (France)	Marchal, Pernot, Hofstetter	(7)		
University of Alabama, Birmingham (USA)	Meredith, Brezovich	(5)		
Institute of Oncology, Ljubljana (Slovenia)	BUDIHNA et al. (1992)	NA	Hot water 45.5°–48°C with water flow: 1.5–2.5 ml/s	Animal experiments (rabbits, pigs): hydrotherm system KHS 9-W 18
Universities of Vienna and Graz (Austria)	STUECKLSCHWEIGER et al. (1991, 1993)	23[a]	Hot water 48°–50°C with water flow: 1.5–2.0 ml/s	Pelvic and other human tumors: hydrotherm system KHS 9-W 18
University of Graz (Austria)	KAPP et al. (1994)	14[a]	Hot water 46°–50°C with water flow: 1.5 ml/s	Anal carcinoma: hydrotherm system KHS 9-W 18
University of Düsseldorf (Germany)	KOLOTAS et al. (1994)	68[a]	Hot water 48°–50°C with water flow: 1.5–2.0 ml/s	Advanced breast ca: hydrotherm system KHS 9-W 18
10 clinical institutions	10 publications	316[a]	2 techniques	Different features

KHS 9-W 18 Hyperthermia System (Ottmar Handl GmbH, Vienna, Austria); Cook VH 8500 Interstitial Hyperthermia system (Bloomington, Ind., USA)
[a] Numbers include some cases twice; numbers in parentheses are already included

University, St. Louis; Missouri Baptist Medical Center). Presently about 300 human lesions have been treated with this method.

A large series was reported from the University of Vienna; this intrainstitutional phase I–II study involved 72 patients with various extracranial tumors (HANDL-ZELLER 1993). In a multicenter study 154 patients have been retrospectively analyzed (HANDL-ZELLER 1993). The clinical results using HS IHT techniques are encouraging (Table 15.13). The mean CR rate in extracranial sites was about 60% (range: 40%–90%) and the mean PR rate, 25%; thus, the overall response rate was 85%, which is comparable to all other IHT techniques. However, the observed treatment toxicity (superficial burns or deep tissue necrosis) was the lowest of all IHT techniques, at only 10% (range: 0%–40%). Follow-up periods ranged from 3 to 56 months, but most studies reported no follow-up data. The analysis of tumor response and treatment toxicity for intracranial sites (MARCHOSKY et al. 1990a,b, 1992) and in the prostate (GARCIA et al. 1992a,b) is still preliminary.

Table 15.13. Clinical results with HS IHT techniques (including animal and brain lesions)

Institution(s)	No. of cases	Tumor sites	CR (%)	PR (%)	Toxicity (%)	Follow-up
Hot wire technique						
Washington University GARCIA et al. (1992a,b)	7	Prostate	86	–	14	2–12 mos
Missouri Baptist Medical Ctr. MARCHOSKY et al. (1990a,b, 1992)	50	Brain tumors	NA	NA	40	Median survival 22 weeks
Hot water perfusion technique						
Multicenter evaluation: HANDL-ZELLER (1993)	154[a]	Various tumors	60	31	3	
University Clinic, Graz ARIAN-SCHAD, STÜCKLSCHWEIGER	(10)	Pelvic tumors	40	50	10	4–16
University Clinic, Vienna HANDL-ZELLER, SEITZ, STANEK	(72)	Various tumors	55	42	4	3–56
Inst. of Oncology, Ljubljana BUDIHNA, LESNICAR, BURGER	(16)	Head and neck	43	36	7	3–56
University Hosp., Düsseldorf ZAMBOGLOU, KOLOTAS	(34)	Breast ca.	90	10	–	Short-term
Curie Institute, Paris CAMPANA, FOURQUET, GABORIAUD	(8)	Breast ca.	75	25	–	3–24 mos
Centre Leon Bernard, Lyon ARDIET	(2)	Head and neck	NA	NA	NA	NA
Centre Alexis Vautrin, Nancy MARCHAL, PERNOT, HOFSTETTER	(7)	Head and neck	NA	NA	NA	NA
Univ. of Alabama, Birmingham MEREDITH, BREZOVICH	(5)	Head and neck	80	20	–	NA
Universities of Vienna and Graz STUECKLSCHWEIGER et al. (1991, 1993)	23[a]	Various tumors	NA	NA	NA	Short-term
University of Graz KAPP et al. (1994)	14[a]	Anorectal ca.	71	21	14	Long-term
University of Düsseldorf KOLOTAS et al. (1994)	68[a]	Breast ca.	56	44	–	NA
10 clinical institutions	~300	Various sites	~60	~25	~10	variable

CR, complete response; PR, partial response; NA, no information available
[a] Case numbers in parentheses are included in the larger number of the same group
[b] No short- and long-term analysis published

Various combinations of HS IHT with LDR IRT or HDR IRT have been implemented in the past. An attractive treatment approach using *simultaneous IHT-IRT* has been applied for prostate tumors (GARCIA et al. 1992) and is also applicable in other sites (HANDL-ZELLER 1993). MARCHOSKY et al. (1990a,b, 1992) applied continuous IHT at 41°C for more than 48–72 h with resistive wire HT. An advantage of the HWP technique is its variability of clinical applications: the implanted HS applicators may be stainless steel tubes or plastic catheters which comply with all standard IRT techniques. In addition, depending upon the specific implant configuration, different flow patterns either through open-ended tubes or within closed-end tubes can be easily implemented (SCHREIER et al. 1990; HANDL-ZELLER 1992, 1993).

A principal advantage of HWP IHT is the fact that maximum temperatures cannot exceed the temperature of the circulating water. Thus, the thermal toxicity of HWP HT can be well controlled. Another problem of many other HT techniques, namely the fact that tissues with different thermal conductivity or thermal flow patterns may induce great variability of the thermal distribution, occurs to a lesser extent with HWP IHT, as the water flow is automatically adjusted in the high and low-temperature regions of the tissue. With the HWP IHT approach patient tolerance has been excellent. Sensations of pain and/or pressure, which often occur with electromagnetic IHT techniques, have rarely been observed (HANDL-ZELLER 1992, 1993).

The required spacing of HS applicators is, however, narrow (8–12 mm). Thermal modeling predicts that HWP with *laminar flow* of 1.5 ml s^{-1} through 1.6-mm-diameter applicators can achieve therapeutic temperatures (42°C) within the target volume when the water temperature is 46°C, tube spacing is 10 mm, and the local perfusion is similar to that of resting muscle. A larger spacing (10–14 mm) and increased perfusion (5 times that of resting muscle) require a *turbulent flow* of >2.5 ml s^{-1} through 1.6-mm tubes and a water temperature of 48°–49°C in order to obtain sufficient tissue temperatures. When the perfusion reaches 10 times that of resting muscle, the tube spacing should not exceed 10 mm and the water temperature should be about 54°C. Thus, performance of all HS IHT systems is very susceptible to blood perfusion changes. To reduce this susceptibility, tubes should have the largest possible diameter and be implanted with minimum spacing.

The advantage of HS IHT is that heating depends only on implant geometry and perfusion patterns, not on tissue composition. It is compatible with any thermometry technique, as there is no electromagnetic interference. HS IHT can be easily handled and patients can be treated awake, allowing good operator-patient interaction. Clinical implementations include all accessible human body sites. Future research objectives are optimization of tube location and spacing, development of preplanning programs, and special routines to optimize the implant procedures. This will require specific methods to predetermine the relative tumor blood flow.

In summary, clinical results with HS IHT are encouraging, as they demonstrate good efficacy in inducing therapeutic temperatures and attaining good clinical results (60% CR) with a low toxicity rate of about 10%. However, a high implant density is required and the technique demands a nearly perfect implant geometry although thermal regulation in the tubes is possible. Careful treatment preplanning is required. Access to a "family of individual tubes" with a range of different cooling zones is likely to improve the selectivity of the tumor heating within the implanted volume.

15.4 Clinical Experience Related to Different Tumor Sites

IHT has been applied in various tumor sites (Fig. 15.6), but many series lack details about the distribution of the treated tumor sites. Thus, a complete survey in this respect is not available. Nevertheless, some conclusive data exist: (a) there are differences in the distribution of tumor sites and applied IHT techniques; (b) most treated lesions are located superficially or at medium depth, while only a few lesions are located at deep-seated sites; (c) tumors of the head and neck (43%), tumors of the breast and chest wall (17%), gynecological tmumors (17%), and colorectal tumors (11%) in the pelvis have been most commonly treated in the past; (d) MW IHT (46%) and RF IHT (33%) are the most often applied IHT techniques. Details on the correlation of IHT techniques and treatment sites are shown in Fig. 15.7. The limited use of IHT in deep-seated tumors is obvious: (a) these sites require the same

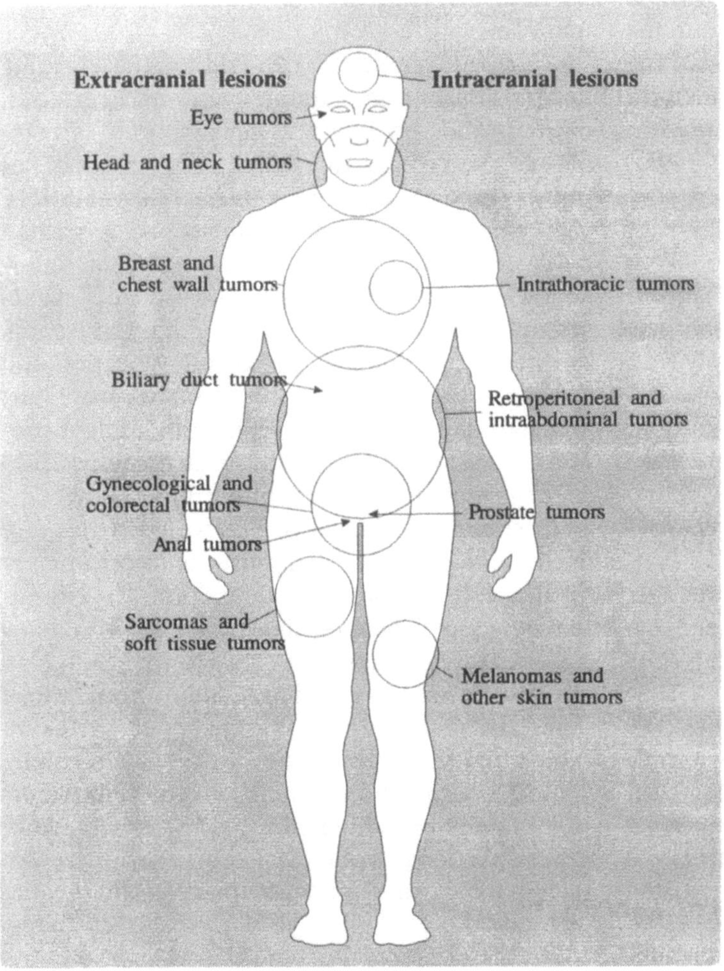

Fig. 15.6. Survey of possible human treatment sites for interstitial thermoradiotherapy

high degree of localization as superficial lesions, which is difficult to achieve from the outside; (b) the necessity of externalizing heating source connections limits the range of clinical applications.

The following section reviews large and more recent clinical series with more details on the tumor distribution and the short- and long-term treatment outcome. If some clinical data were found to be missing, the site-specific results (CR and toxicity rates for a specific treatment site) were assumed to be equal to the reported values for the entire patient group of the clinical series in question.

15.4.1 Head and Neck Tumors

In the literature 559 head and neck lesions have been reported to have received IHT, including tumors of the body, edge and base of tongue, floor of mouth, tonsillar fossa, and other accessible oropharyngeal sites. These tumors can be easily implanted, and IRT has been traditionally applied in these locations. While any of the available IHT techniques can be configured to operate in head and neck tumors, MW IHT has been preferred by many groups due to the types of implants performed in this region (free-hand implants, looping techniques, etc.), the use of flexible afterloading tubes, and the high perfusion in this region. The cumulative CR rate for head and neck lesions was excellent (65%), and the toxicity rate acceptable (20%) (Table 15.14).

The largest series was reported from Long Beach Memorial Medical Center (Puthawala et al. 1990): 98 patients and 108 lesions were treated with two IHT sessions (45–60 min, 42.5°–44°C) immediately before and after LDR brachtherapy (40–60 Gy). The initial CR rate was 82%. At 1 year of follow-up, 75% of the lesions were locally controlled, and at the last follow-up, 54% of the patients were alive and had been free of relapse at

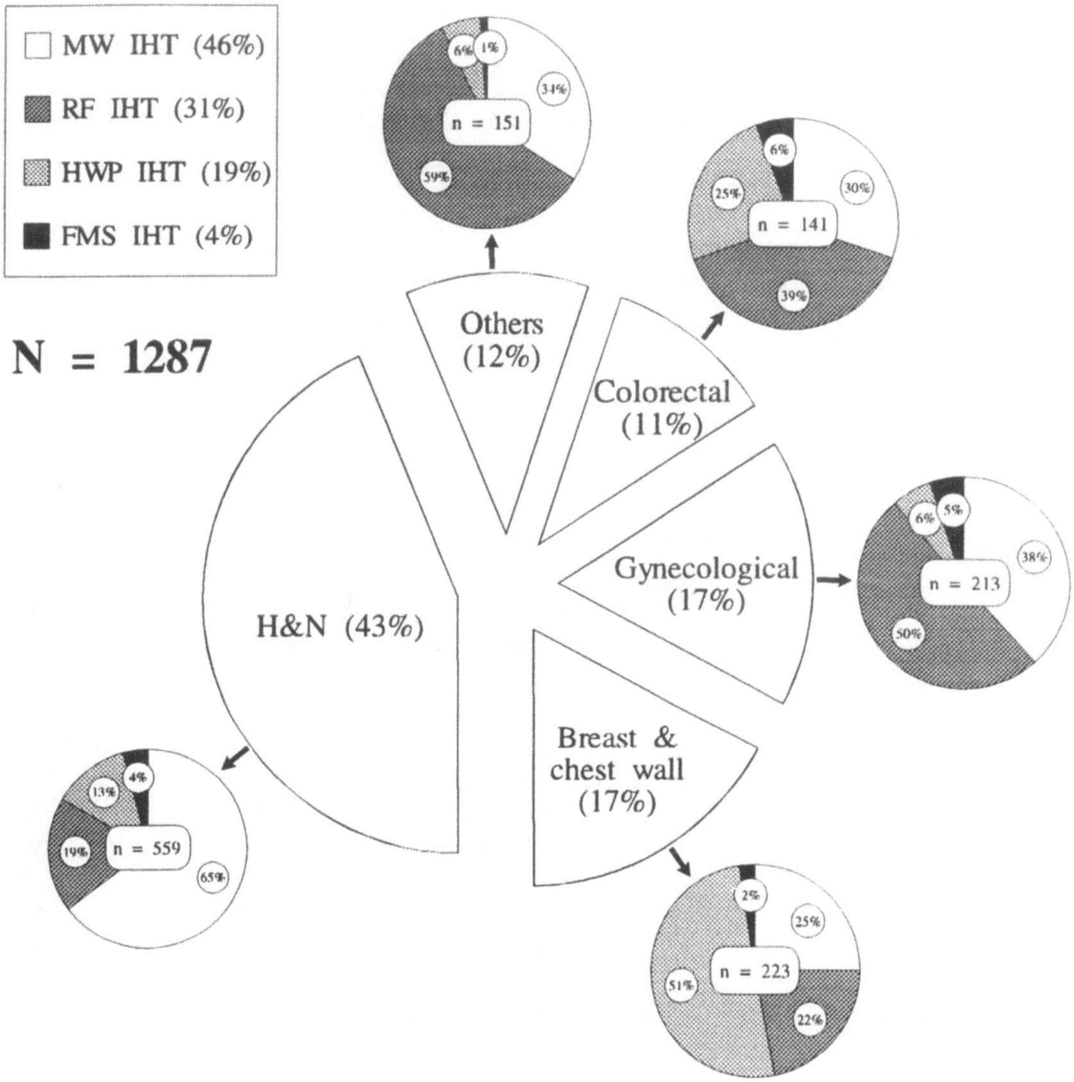

Fig. 15.7. Correlation of applied IHT techniques and treated tumor sites in published IHT-IRT series

the treated site for up to 30 months (median follow-up). Treatment-related complications occurred only in 12% of the patients and were mostly observed in the early phase of the clinical series.

In another large phase I–II trial at the University of Erlangen-Nürnberg (SEEGENSCHMIEDT et al. 1994a–c), 74 patients with localized head and neck tumors were treated with a commercial MW IHT system (Lund, Sweden). The mean tumor volume was $63\,cm^3$ (range: $8–361\,cm^3$). The treatment protocol prescribed two IHT sessions at 41°–44°C before and after LDR IRT and additional external RT if applicable. The initial CR rate was 64% for the whole group, i.e., 85% for 33 primary or persistent and 46% for 41 recurrent or metastatic lesions. At 12 months' follow-up, 62% were still locally controlled, and at last follow-up, 38% of the patients were still alive and free of relapse. Treatment-related severe late complications occurred in 11% of patients.

15.4.2 Breast and Chest Wall Tumors

According to reports in the literature 223 malignant lesions of the breast and chest wall have been treated with combined IHT-IRT. They had advanced primary breast carcinomas, uncontrolled local-regional lymph node metastases, or chest wall recurrences. The malignant disease manifestations in this site can produce significant morbi-

Table 15.14. Clinical results with IHT-IRT for head and neck tumors

Study	Tumors (n)[a]	IHT technique (frequency)	CR rate [n (%)]	Toxicity [n (%)]	Follow-up (months)
Aoyagi et al. (1989)	6 (10)	915-MHz MW	2 (33%)	NA (20%)	NA
Au et al. (1989)	3 (4)	90-kHz FMS	2 (66%)	NA (50%)	Short-term
Cosset et al. (1984a,b, 1985)	9 (29)	0.5-MHz RF	NA (66%)	NA (35%)	2
Coughlin et al. (1991)	9 (35)	915/2450-MHz MW	NA (66%)	NA	1–62
Emami et al. (1987)	29 (48)	915-MHz MW	NA (54%)	NA (25%)	6–48
Emami et al. (1992a)	26 (63)	915-MHz MW	NA (53%)	10 (38%)	Long-term
Engin et al. (1993)	9 (9)	915-MHz MW	6 (67%)	4 (44%)	Long-term
Fourquet et al. (1990)	11 (11)	0.5-MHz RF	9 (82%)	3 (27%)	NA
Gautherie et al. (1989)	35 (96)	0.5-MHz RF	24 (69%)	NA (16%)	Long-term
Goffinet et al. (1990)	5 (10)	0.5-MHz RF	5 (100%)	1 (10%)	Long-term
Handl-Zeller (1993)	70 (154)	HWP System	NA (60%)	NA (3%)	3–56
Inoue et al. (1989)	8 (10)	915-MHz MW	1 (13%)	NA (10%)	1–6
Levendag et al. (1992, 1993)	11 (11)	27-MHz RF	6 (55%)	1 (9%)	4–36
Mack et al. (1992, 1993a,b)	19 (44)	80-120-kHz FMS	NA (61%)	NA (43%)	1–53
Marchal et al. (1993)	5 (5)	27-MHz RF	3 (60%)	1 (20%)	2–36
Oleson et al. (1984a,b)	9 (64)	0.5-MHz RF	NA (38%)	NA (13%)	3–18
Petrovich et al. (1989)	23 (44)	915-MHz MW	16 (70%)	NA (20%)	3–36
Prevost et al. (1993)	25 (25)	915/2450-MHz MW	21 (84%)	2 (8%)	3–27
Puthawala et al. (1985)	20 (43)	915-MHz MW	15 (75%)	NA (21%)	Long-term
Puthawala et al. (1990)	106 (108)	915-MHz MW	90 (85%)	13 (12%)	Long-term
Rafla et al. (1988, 1989)	15 (35)	915-MHz MW	6 (40%)	NA (29%)	Short-term
Schreiber et al. (1992)	11 (40)	915-MHz MW	6 (55%)	NA (15%)	1–30
Seegenschmiedt et al. (1994c)	62 (90)	915-MHz MW	39 (63%)	15 (24%)	4–68
Tupchong et al. (1988)	14 (14)	915-MHz MW	9 (64%)	NA	NA
Vora et al. (1989)	9 (81)	0.5-MHz RF	NA (56%)	NA (17%)	1–13
Yabumoto and Suyama (1985), Yabumoto et al. (1989)	5 (14)	8-MHz RF	NA (60%)	NA (29%)	3–13
Total experience	554	MW: 363; RF: 99; HWP: 70; FMS: 22	~65%	~20%	variable

NA, no data available; MW, microwaves; RF, radiofrequency; HWP, hot water perfusion; FMS, ferromagnetic seeds
[a] Numbers in parentheses represent the total number of tumors in each series

dity including bleeding, ulceration, pain, arm edema, and brachial plexus neuropathy. Usually there is a clear indication to treat the entire chest wall and not just a small circumscribed area. It is known that recurrent lesions of even less than 3 cm diameter may require RT doses of at least 60 Gy to achieve a sufficient local tumor control rate, while for larger tumors about 65–70 Gy is necessary (BEDWINEK et al. 1981; DEUTSCH et al. 1986). Although several other RT options are available to effectively irradiate malignant breast and chest wall lesions, brachytherapy techniques have often been used to boost the primary tumor site as an alternative to the application of an external electron boost.

Adding HT to conventional RT is a reasonable approach in a dismal therapeutic situation, where permanent local-regional control with RT alone or together with chemotherapy is as low as 40%–50%. In the past, external HT has been combined with external RT. Recently, several clinical groups have summarized their experience using combined external HT-RT (GONZALES GONZALES et al. 1988; KAPP et al. 1991; LINDHOLM et al. 1987; PEREZ et al. 1986b; SEEGENSCHMIEDT et al. 19889b; VAN DER ZEE et al. 1988). In contrast, clinical experience with interstitial HT-RT techniques is limited. When breast and chest wall lesions are treated by an interstitial implant, they often require the use of a template technique, and under these conditions the RF IHT technique has been the method of choice (VORA et al. 1988,1989). Using this approach requires that the tissue entry and exit points of the IHT applicators need to be protected from excessive heating. To avoid such complications when using the MW IHT technique, an additional bolus application is recommended (SUNDARARAMAN et al. 1990). The compiled clinical data for breast and chest wall tumors are good and reveal an estimated cumulative CR rate of 60% and a treatment toxicity rate of about 10% (Table 15.15).

The largest clinical series has been reported from the University of Düsseldorf (KOLOTAS et al. 1994). In this trial HWP IHT was applied in 68 females suffering from locally advanced primary breast carcinomas (mean tumor diameter: 7.6 cm). IHT was applied as "boost therapy" which was part of a neoadjuvant radiochemotherapy treatment protocol followed by tumor biopsy and axilla clearing surgery. The first chemotherapy cycle (mitoxantrone 12.5 mg/m^2) was delivered at the time of IHT, while subsequent cycles were delivered simultaneously with external RT (50 Gy). The irradiated volume included the whole breast and the regional lymph nodes. After completion of the fourth chemotherapy cycle, breast-conserving surgery or mastectomy was performed. Histological evaluation revealed 56% of the specimens without any tumor (pathological CR) and 44% with only microscopic residual tumor. The clinical result was significantly better than for a historical control group in which radiochemotherapy without HT was applied. Despite being promising, these results need further validation in randomized controlled trials.

15.4.3 Pelvic Tumors (Gynecological)

According to the literature reports, 354 pelvic lesions have been treated with IHT. Among these were 213 gynecological and 141 colorectal tumors, but in some series no differentiation was made between the two tumor types. Many patients had advanced or recurrent cancers of the uterus, cervix, or ovaries that were considered unresectable. Sometimes small tumors which had failed within the pelvis following radical surgery and/or full-dose external or intracavitary RT were considered for retreatment with IHT-IRT. Without an effective retreatment option, the survival and quality of life for these patients with pelvic recurrences would have been rather dismal. Thus, besides the aim of palliation, the major rationale for the use of IHT-IRT for pelvic tumors was to support therapeutic strategies which aimed to achieve tumor downstaging and eventually complete tumor resectability.

The preferred IRT methods in the pelvis are endocavitary afterloading and interstitial template techniques with rigid needle implants. Sometimes the rigid needles are replaced by flexible plastic tubes. In large series, IHT-IRT has been performed with RF IHT (ARISTIZABAL and OLESON 1984; GAUTHERIE et al. 1989; OLESON et al. 1984a,b; SURWIT et al. 1983; VORA et al. 1988, 1989). The major advantage of rigid RF needles as compared to flexible MW antennas is a fairly homogeneous longitudinal heating pattern. With good insulation of entry and exit points, RF IHT appears to be an optimal approach for deep-seated pelvic tumors. Another subset of patients has been treated with MW IHT (COUGHLIN et al. 1991; GRIGSBY and EMAMI 1993; RAFIA et al. 1989; SEEGENSCHMIEDT et al. 1994c; SCHREIBER et al. 1992), FMS IHT (MACK et al. 1993a,b) or HWP

Table 15.15. Clinical results with IHT-IRT for breast and chest wall tumors

Study	Tumors (n)[a]	IHT technique (frequency)	CR rate [n (%)]	Toxicity [n (%)]	Follow-up (months)
Cosset et al. (1984a,b, 1985)	11 (29)	0.5-MHz RF	NA (66%)	NA (35%)	2
Dunlop et al. (1986)	6 (9)	0.5-MHz RF	NA (0%)	NA	1–6
Emami et al. (1987)	6 (48)	915-MHz MW	NA (54%)	NA (25%)	6–48
Emami et al. (1992)	16 (63)	915-MHz MW	NA (53%)	6 (38%)	Long-term
Handl-Zeller (1993)[b]	45 (154)	HWP System	NA (60%)	NA (3%)	3–56
Gautherie et al. (1989)	14 (96)	0.5-MHz RF	11 (79%)	NA (16%)	Long-term
Kolotas et al. (1994)[b]	68 (68)	HWP System	38 (56%)[c]	0 (0%)	3–36
Mack et al. (1992, 1993a,b)	5 (44)	80-120-kHz FMS	NA (61%)	NA (7%)	1–53
Petrovich et al. (1989)	9 (44)	915-MHz MW	7 (78%)	NA (20%)	3–36
Puthawala et al. (1985)	8 (43)	915-MHz MW	5 (63%)	NA (21%)	Long-term
Rafla et al. (1988, 1989)	6 (35)	915-MHz MW	3 (50%)	NA (29%)	Short-term
Schreiber et al. (1992)	9 (40)	915-MHz MW	NA (53%)	NA (15%)	1–30
Seegenschmiedt (1994c)	2 (90)	915-MHz MW	1 (50%)	0 (0%)	4–68
Vora et al. (1989)	24 (81)	0.5-MHz RF	18 (75%)	NA (17%)	1–13
Total experience	229	HWP: 113; MW: 56; RF: 55; FMS: 5	~60%	~10%	variable

NA, no data available; IHT, interstitial hyperthermia; MW, microwaves; RF, radiofrequency; HWP, hot water perfusion; FMS, ferromagnetic seeds
[a] Numbers in parentheses represent the total number in each series
[b] Some patients may have been counted twice
[c] Pathologically confirmed complete response

IHT (Handl-Zeller 1993; Stuecklschweiger et al. 1991, 1993). Clinical results in gynecological tumors are compiled in Table 15.16. The cumulative CR rate was about 50% and the toxicity rate 20%. Especially confined lesions of less than 6 cm in diameter, which are accessible to a precise IRT implant, were suitable sites for additional IHT.

A large series on gynecological tumors was reported and recently updated from the University of Arizona in Tucson (Aristizabal and Oleson 1984; Manning et al. 1982b; Oleson et al. 1984a,b; Shimm et al. 1990; Surwit et al. 1983). Initially 21 females with preirradiated recurrent gynecological tumors of 40–1000 cm^3 size were reviewed (Surwit et al. 1983). Intraoperative resistive RF IHT (one IHT session at 43°–44°C for 30 min) and LDR IRT (mean: 22 Gy for about 30 h) were applied. Seven (33%) achieved a CR and ten (48%) a PR, which resulted in an overall response rate of 81%; in addition, good palliation was achieved in 13 of 17 (76%) patients who were symptomatic with moderate to severe pain before therapy. Acute complications were minimal and severe late complications were encountered in four patients who developed gastrointestinal and urinary tract fistulas. CR correlated significantly with survival prolongation. An update (Aristizabal and Oleson 1984) stated that 36 of the 47 treated pelvic tumors derived from gynecological organs, but no site-specific results were given; instead the CR (38%) and complication rate (15%) of the whole group of 64 lesions were reported. The latest update (Shimm et al. 1990) on 49 pelvic tumors also lacked data about the site-specific results.

15.4.4 Pelvic Tumors (Colorectal)

Of the 354 pelvic lesions reported in the literature, 141 were colorectal or anal tumors, but in some series differentiation between colorectal and gynecological lesions is difficult. Most of these advanced or recurrent colorectal tumors were considered to be unresectable or were preirradiated. Usually this group of tumors accounts for about 10%–25% of all colorectal cancers (Pahlman et al. 1985). Overall, patients with advanced or recurrent colorectal tumors have a

Table 15.16. Clinical results with IHT-IRT for pelvic (gynecological) tumors

Study	Tumors (n)[a]	IHT technique (frequency)	CR rate [n (%)]	Toxicity [n (%)]	Follow-up (months)
ARISTIZABAL and OLESON (1984)[b]	36 (64)	0.5-MHz RF	14 (39%)	NA (13%)	3–18
BORREGO et al. (1990)	8 (13)	0.5-MHz RF/HUPIT	NA (46%)	NA (50%)	2–20
COUGHLIN et al. (1991)	12 (35)	915-MHz MW	8 (67%)	NA	1–62
EMAMI et al. (1984, 1987)[b]	4 (48)	915-MHz MW	NA (54%)	NA (25%)	6–48
GAUTHERIE et al. (1989)	23 (96)	0.5-MHz RF	11 (48%)	NA (16%)	Long-term
GRIGSBY and EMAMI (1993)[b]	9 (63)	915-MHz MW	NA (64%)	NA (43%)	Long-term
HANDL-ZELLER (1993)[b]	7 (154)	HWP system	NA (60%)	NA (3%)	3–56
MACK et al. (1992, 1993a,b)	11 (44)	80-120-KHz FMS	6 (55%)	NA (43%)	1–53
PETROVICH et al. (1989)	4 (44)	915-MHz MW	3 (75%)	NA (20%)	3–36
PUTHAWALA et al. (1985)	9 (43)	915-MHz MW	7 (78%)	3 (43%)	Long-term
RAFLA et al. (1988, 1989)	4 (35)	915-MHz MW	2 (50%)	NA (20%)	3–36
SEEGENSCHMIEDT et al. (1994c)	15 (90)	915-MHz MW	9 (60%)	4 (27%)	4–68
SCHREIBER et al. (1992)[c]	15 (40)	915-MHz MW	NA (53%)	NA (15%)	1–30
STÜCKLSCHWEIGER et al. (1991, 1993)[b]	6 (23)	HWP system	NA (50%)	0 (0%)	4–16
SURWIT et al. (1983)[b]	21 (21)	0.5-MHz RF	7 (33%)	4 (19%)	2–18
VORA et al. (1989)	20 (81)	0.5-MHz RF	10 (50%)	1 (5%)	1–13
Total experience	204	RF: 108; MW: 72 HWP: 13; FMS: 11	~50%	~20%	variable

NA, no data available; IHT, interstitial hyperthermia; MW, microwaves; RF, radiofrequency; HWP, hot water perfusion; FMS, ferromagnetic seeds
[a] Numbers of parentheses represent the total number in each series
[b] Some patients may have been counted twice
[c] No differentiation between gynecological and colorectal lesions of the pelvis

poor prognosis unless resection is possible. Therefore among other treatment modalities, adjuvant HT-RT was tested to ascertain whether it might improve resectability and prolong survival. Even if a tumor becomes unresectable, the patient could benefit from adjuvant RT-HT as a dose-response relationship has been shown for control of recurrent colorectal cancers (OVERGAARD et al. 1984) and radiation tolerance of adjacent normal tissues is limited. Thus, addition of HT may increase the options for obtaining short- or long-term local control (FELDMANN et al. 1993).

Brachytherapy has rarely been applied for colorectal and anal tumors. Therefore the options for delivering additional HT in conjunction with interstitial or conventional RT are restricted. For large colorectal lesions regional HT techniques may be better suited (FELDMANN et al. 1993; this volume, Chap. 8: GONZALES GONZALES et al.; HIRAOKA et al. 1984; NISHIMURA et al. 1992), and for accessible tumors endocavitary HT has been recommended (BERDOV and MENTESHASHVILI 1990; MORI et al. 1991). Nevertheless, small accessible tumors could also be approached by template techniques and rigid needle implants. For curved implants along the presacral space flexible plastic tubes can be applied, but most IHT series have used rigid needle resistive 0.5-MHz RF IHT techniques (ARISTIZABAL and OLESON 1984; GAUTHERIE et al. 1989; OLESON et al. 1984; SURWIT et al. 1983; VORA et al. 1988, 1989).

The advantages of RF needles versus MW antennas have been pointed out previously. With an unlimited longitudinal heating pattern, RF IHT techniques appear to be the best approach for deep-seated colorectal and anal tumors, but careful attention has to be paid to the insulation of the needle entry points to avoid complications. A small subset of patients has been treated with MW IHT (COUGHLIN et al. 1991; GRIGSBY and EMAMI 1993; RAFIA et al. 1989; SEEGENSCHMIEDT et al. 1994c; SCHREIBER et al. 1992), FMS-IHT (MACK et al. 1993a,b) and HWP-IHT (HANDL-

Zeller 1993; Stücklschweiger et al. 1991, 1993). Clinical results for colorectal and anal lesions are shown in Table 15.17. The CR rate was about 50% and the toxicity about 20%. In summary, confined accessible lesions of less than 6 cm in diameter can be treated with IHT-IRT.

15.4.5 Other Extracranial Tumors

Other lesions in various body sites have been treated with IHT-IRT (Fig. 15.6). Within larger series 151 lesions have been reported to have received combined IHT-IRT. It was used for intrathoracic, retroperitoneal, intra-abdominal, and extremity tumors including sarcomas in both children and adults, melanomas, lymph node metastases, and tumors in deep body sites, e.g., confined prostatic and genitourinary and biliary duct tumors. Indications for IHT-IRT have also been reported for eye tumors (Astrahan et al. 1987; this volume, Chap. 13: Finger; Finger et al. 1984, 1989; Handl-Zeller and Menapace 1992; Steeves et al. 1992). Adjuvant intraoperative HT by means of various techniques combined with intra- and/or postoperative RT has been applied for thoracic, pancreatic, and colorectal tumors (this volume, Chap. 17: Colacchio and Ryan; Colacchio et al. 1990, 1993; Coughlin et al. 1985; Frazier and Corry 1984; Merrick et al. 1987, 1988). As the clinical experience in these locations is rather preliminary and scattered among the various clinical series, so far no conclusive answers can be given with regard to the observed site-specific efficacy and induced treatment toxicity. Some of the published studies will be specifically addressed in the following sections.

15.4.5.1 Prostate Carcinoma

Tumor relapses about the prostatic gland remain a great problem in the management of locally advanced prostatic cancer. In a recent study, 36 patients were treated with transperineal thermobrachytherapy utilizing a specially designed template (Bagshaw et al. 1993; Prionas et al. 1992, 1994). Resistive RF IHT and iridium-192 brachy-

Table 15.17. Clinical results with IHT-IRT for pelvic (colorectal) tumors

Study	Tumors (*n*)[a]	IHT technique (frequency)	CR rate [*n* (%)]	Toxicity [*n* (%)]	Follow-up (months)
Aristizabal and Oleson (1984)	11 (64)	0.5-MHz RF	4 (39%)	NA (15%)	3–18
Borrego et al. (1990)	5 (13)	0.5-MHz RF/HUPIT	NA (46%)	NA (50%)	2–20
Emami et al. (1984, 1987)[b]	3 (48)	915-MHz MW	NA (54%)	NA (25%)	6–48
Gautherie et al. (1989)	16 (96)	0.5-MHz RF	12 (75%)	NA (16%)	Long-term
Goffinet et al. (1990)	5 (10)	0.5-MHz RF	3 (60%)	NA (10%)	Long-term
Grigsby and Emami (1993)[b]	2 (63)	915-MHz MW	NA (64%)	NA (43%)	Long-term
Handl-Zeller (1993)[b]	23 (154)	HWP System	NA (60%)	NA (3%)	3–56
Mack et al. (1992, 1993a,b)	8 (44)	80-120-kHz FMS	7 (87%)	NA (43%)	1–53
Puthawala et al. (1985)	4 (43)	915-MHz MW	3 (75%)	NA (21%)	Long-term
Rafla et al. (1988, 1989)	10 (35)	915-MHz MW	6 (60%)	NA (20%)	3–36
Seegenschmiedt et al. (1994c)	9 (90)	915-MHz MW	5 (56%)	2 (22%)	4–68
Schreiber et al. (1992)[c]	15 (40)	915-MHz MW	NA (53%)	NA (15%)	1–30
Stücklschweiger et al. (1991, 1993)[b]	12 (23)	HWP system	NA (50%)	0 (0%)	4–16
Vora et al. (1989)	18 (81)	0.5-MHz RF	NA (56%)	NA (17%)	1–13
Total experience	141	RF: 55; MW: 43 HWP: 35; FMS: 8	~60%	~20%	variable

NA, no data available; IHT, interstitial hyperthermia; MW, microwaves; RF, radiofrequency; HWP, hot water perfusion; FMS, ferromagnetic seeds
[a] Numbers in parentheses represent the total number in each series
[b] Some patients may have been counted twice
[c] No differentiation between gynecological and colorectal lesions of the pelvis

therapy were applied. Initially placement of rigid needles was performed under general anesthesia during laparatomy, but recently trocars have been placed percutaneously under transrectal ultrasonic guidance. Surgery and HT treatment were well tolerated. Each needle was electrically insulated along the length which traversed surrounding normal tissues. Extensive invasive thermometry and thermal mapping were performed within the tumor volume. Considerably higher temperatures were achieved within tumor than within surrounding normal tissues. So far the follow-up is too short to show an increased therapeutic efficacy, but no patients have succumbed to the cancer, though four have already experienced local relapses. A total of 13 (36%) patients encountered complications.

At Washington University a phase I study was conducted with HS IHT for recurrent prostate carcinoma (GARCIA et al. 1992a,b). IHT was administered concomitantly with LDR iridium-192 brachytherapy for up to 45 h. Catheters were separated by 1.5 cm and placed through a lucite silicone rubber template under transrectal ultrasonic guidance and fluoroscopy. IHT was induced with the Cook VH 8500 System, which is computer-programmed to maintain a minimum temperature of 41°C within the target volume. During the application of moderate-temperature (41°C) long-duration HT, tumor temperatures were monitored at 16 points. The study recruited seven patients, who tolerated the treatment well. Tumor response was dramatic and far more rapid than that produced by interstitial or external RT alone. Good experiences were also reported from the St. Josephs Cancer Center, Albuquerque (KHAN et al. 1992). In summary, IHT-IRT for prostate cancer is feasible, well tolerated, and effective, but optimization is still being sought. Future studies must assess optimal sequencing, extent of acute and long-term morbidity, and the possible impact of this additional therapy on long-term tumor control and overall survival.

15.4.5.2 Thoracic and Intra-abdominal Tumors

Results of extensive surgery and external beam and intraoperative RT for control of local recurrences of thoracic and abdominal cancers demonstrate that lack of local control continues to be the major cause of failure in these tumor sites. Thus, it appears reasonable to investigate other avenues like intraoperative and/or interstitial HT. Today noninvasive deep-heating devices are available, including ultrasound arrays, focused ultrasound, RF capacitive devices, and annular phased array HT systems. All of these HT systems present a variety of physical and logistical problems – both at the time of surgery and postoperatively – that need to be surmounted in order to achieve selective heating of the tumor and sparing of surrounding normal tissues (COLACCHIO et al. 1993).

At the M.D. Anderson Hospital 12 unresectable thoracic, retroperitoneal, and abdominal tumors were treated with resistive RF IHT (FRAZIER and CORRY 1984). Needle electrodes were fashioned at the time of surgical exploration and implanted parallel to each other. Connecting cables were externalized through the skin at a convenient location. An alternating current was set up between pairs of electrodes. IHT was performed at the time of operation with extensive thermometry controlling heat delivery to avoid thermal toxicity. Additional chemo- or radiotherapy was given postoperatively along with further IHT sessions. All tumors were successfully heated to an average temperature >43°C. Side-effects were minimal; the only significant complication was a small bowel perforation in a patient with metastatic adenocarcinoma. Six thoracic cavity tumors responded and were controlled and two patients were still alive at last follow-up. In contrast, the experience with six retroperitoneal (three sarcomas) and intra-abdominal tumors (bladder and colon cancers) was not successful because of the difficulty in encompassing the tumor and isolating the small bowel from heat injury; only two patients achieved a long-term tumor response and the rest died of metastatic disease.

A similar clinical experience was reported from Dartmouth Medical College (COUGHLIN and STROHBEHN 1989; COUGHLIN et al. 1983, 1985, 1991). In this series 915-MHz MW antennas were utilized to induce HT of various thoracic, abdominal, and intracranial tumors intraoperatively. Due to inherent problems including localization of tumor margins along multiple catheters and lack of appropriate treatment planning, the HT was later changed to external ultrasound HT under direct observation at the time of the surgical exploration (COLACCHIO et al. 1990, 1993).

15.4.5.3 Anal Canal Cancer

Function preservation therapy of anal canal cancers with external or interstitial RT alone or combined with chemotherapy has been shown to improve survival to the level which is achieved by surgery while retaining a normal sphincter function in 60%–85% (CUMMINGS 1992; PAPILLON 1990). Due to the low incidence of metastatic disease at the time of initial tumor presentation, the prognosis of the disease can be significantly improved by successful local-regional treatment. Although a CR rate of 60%–90% has been attained in most series, local-regional failure remains a major problem in patients presenting with advanced tumors. Only 30%–50% of these patients with relapse can be salvaged by radical surgery; the remainder die of disease even in the absence of distant metastases (SCHLIENGER et al. 1989). IHT-IRT is considered a reasonable therapeutic approach to improve the local-regional treatment for patients at high risk for local failures.

In a phase I–II study at the University Medical School Graz combined iridium-192 HDR IRT and external beam RT with or without additional chemotherapy and HWP IHT was applied in 14 patients with advanced T_{2-3} N_{0-1} carcinomas of the anal canal (KAPP et al. 1994). Five patients with large tumors (>3 cm diameter) were scheduled to receive chemotherapy (two courses of 5-fluorouracil and mitomycin C) given concomitantly with external beam RT. IHT-IRT was well tolerated. A clinical CR was obtained in 11 and a pathological CR (PCR) in ten patients. One patient with pCR relapsed and succumbed to the disease, but eight were still alive and disease-free at last follow-up. Treatment toxicity was limited to two patients who developed persistent ulcers. The sphincter function was maintained in seven patients. The study showed that HWP IHT was feasible and caused no further complications compared to external beam RT and IRT alone.

15.4.5.4 Biliary Duct Tumors

A series of ten patients with obstructive biliary duct tumors was published by COUGHLIN et al. (1992). MW IHT and iridium-192 LDR IRT were applied through a standard biliary drainage catheter together with thermometry probes for thermal control. During the IHT session the tumor was heated to 45°–55°C while keeping the proximal and distal margins at 43°C. Immediately after IHT, antenna and thermometry probes were removed and a single strand of iridium-192 seeds was placed for irradiation. A dose of 55–79 Gy calculated at 0.5 cm radially from the catheter was delivered over 5–7 days. Upon removal of the seeds a second IHT session was performed. The procedure was tolerated well and no acute toxicity was observed. Complete symptomatic relief or removal of draining tubes was achieved in eight patients, while in two others the laboratory findings improved. The survival ranged from 3 to 57 weeks. A positive experience was also reported from the City of Hope Medical Center (WONG et al. 1988). In summary, IHT treatment of bile duct tumors is feasible and well tolerated and provides palliation of disease.

15.5 Clinical Endpoints and Treatment Outcome

Many IHT-IRT series report CR rates but lack additional information on long-term tumor control, relapse, and survival rates. Only a few large series have addressed these details adequately. Often data regarding the specific method of assessment of initial and long-term tumor response are missing or incomplete. Clinical judgment based on physical examination, imaging studies (x-ray, US, CT or MRI), and histological specimens taken from the tumor site may produce different results in respect of treatment outcome. Effective palliation of relevant clinical symptoms is also rarely addressed. A better standard of reporting of clinical endpoints is required for future IHT-IRT studies. Large IHT-IRT series which have addressed at least some of the treatment endpoints are listed in Table 15.18. The collective CR rates of RF IHT (55%), MW IHT (65%), FM IHT (60%), and HS IHT (60%) were quite similar. Likewise, only small differences were observed between the collective CR rates for different tumor sites (Fig. 15.8).

15.5.1 Initial Tumor Response

Except for technical studies, the initial tumor response has been reported in most published trials, but there has been considerable variation with regard to the time at which the initial tumor response was assessed and to the methods used to establish the certainty of the tumor response. The time for CR evaluation has varied from "directly after therapy" or "1, 2, 3 months after completion of therapy" to "time of best tumor response" and "time without tumor progression or recurrence."

Table 15.18. Local control and relapse in large IHT-IRT clinical studies

Study	Tumors (*n*)	Specific definition of "local control"	Local relapse after CR (%)	Local control [*n* (%)]
Cosset et al. (1985)	29	Sustained complete tumor regression	6/19 (32%)	4/23 (17%) NED at last FU
Coughlin et al. (1991)	35	Complete response	NA	NA
Emami et al. (1987)	48	Sustained complete tumor response	NA	23/48 (48%) LC at last FU
Emami et al. (1992a)	63	Sustained complete tumor response	NA	20/61 (33%); at 3 years FU: 24%
Gautherie et al. (1989)	96	Complete response	NA	NA
Oleson et al. (1984a,b)	52	Complete response	NA	Duration of response was not evaluable
Mack et al. (1992, 1993a,b)	44	Freedom from tumor progression	NA	Median duration of freedom from progression not yet reached
Petrovich et al. (1989)	44	Complete response for >1 month FU	0%	Median survival: 39 weeks 2-year survival: 22%
Phromratanapongse et al. (1990)	45	Sustained complete response at 1 year	3/31 (10%)	27/45 (68%) LC at 1 year FU
Prevost et al. (1993)	25	Long-term control	4/21 (19%)	17/25 (68%) LC at last FU
Puthawala et al. (1985)	43	Total regression of tumor at 12 months' FU	5/37 (14%)	32/43 (74%) LC after 1 year FU
Puthawala et al. (1990)	108	Local tumor control	9/90 (10%)	53/98 (54%) NED at median FU 2-year survival: 40%
Rafla et al. (1988, 1989)	35	No progression or relapse during 6 months' FU	NA	19/35 (54%) LC at last FU
Schreiber et al. (1992)	40	Freedom from tumor progression at last FU	1/21 (5%)	16/40 (40%) LC at last FU
Seegenschmiedt et al. (1994c)	90	Sustained complete tumor response	10/59 (17%)	54/84 (64%) LC at 1 year FU 2-year survival: 47%; at last FU 34% alive, Relapse-free survival 31%
Shimm et al. (1990)	72	Duration of complete response	10/25 (40%)	Median duration of CR: 18 months
Tupchong et al. (1988)	14	Stabilization of locoregional disease	3/9 (33%)	6/14 (43%) LC at last FU
Vora et al. (1989)	78	Complete response	NA	NA

FU, follow-up (observation period in weeks or months); NA, no data available; LC, local control; NED, no evidence of malignant disease

Only in a few studies was the pathological tumor response established. One study from the University of Düsseldorf reports carefully on histopathological data after combined IHT-IRT treatment of advanced breast carcinomas (Kolotas et al. 1994). In this study, patients received HDR IRT, HWP IHT, and neoadjuvant mitoxantrone chemotherapy. All patients underwent surgery 12 weeks after completion of the IHT and radiochemotherapy course. Histopathological results were available to assess the tumor response. This approach was possible because IHT-IRT was part of a neoadjuvant therapy which was followed by surgery. It is more difficult to implement this approach for pretreated and recurrent tumors.

15.5.2 Long-term Tumor Control

Data on long-term tumor control and local relapse following IHT-IRT are difficult to obtain and are not standardized. The reported time points and methods of assessment vary between the different studies and many groups provide no data on long-term tumor control, which can be influenced by patient and tumor selection. Moreover, few groups apply a stringent definition of "local control" (Parsons et al. 1990) or report "survival rates" according to the actuarial method. Thus, not surprisingly data reported in the literature reveal large variations among the different groups (Table 15.18): Petrovich et al. (1989) reported an overall median survival of only 39 weeks and a 2-year

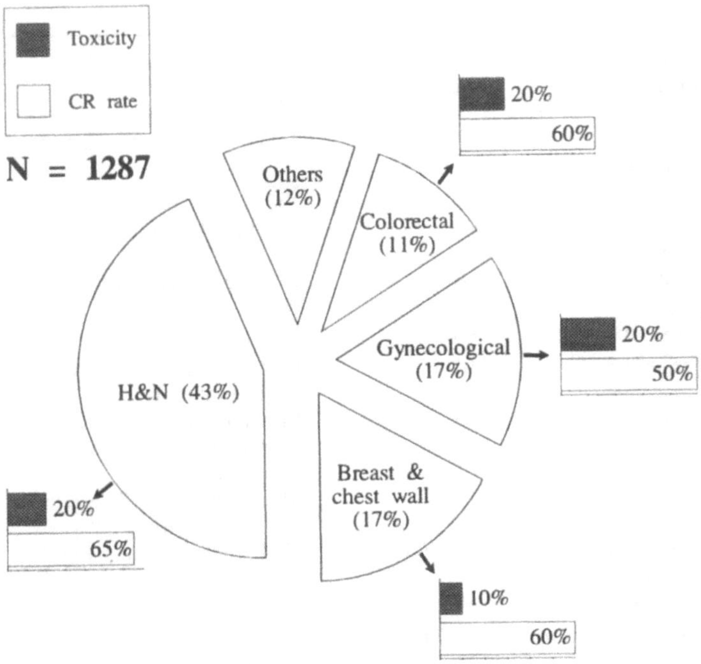

Fig. 15.8. Correlation of applied IHT techniques and treatment outcome (complete tumor response and toxicity rate) in published IHT-IRT series

survival of 22% in a group of 44 patients with recurrent tumors despite a high initial CR of 64%. In contrast, PUTHAWALA et al. (1985) observed a high local control rate of 74% after a minimum follow-up of 12 months for primary advanced and recurrent tumors. Due to the lack of follow-up information even less meaningful data are available for the assessment of local relapses and distant metastases.

15.6 Treatment Toxicity

Generally, combined IHT-IRT is well tolerated with side-effects similar to those observed with IRT alone. When IHT is conducted without general anesthesia (MW IHT and HS IHT), about 20%–25% patients experience pain, general discomfort, and/or systemic stress (e.g., hypertension, tachycardia) during the application of IHT; sometimes this leads to a poor and ineffective heating performance. Surprisingly, when patients were treated under general anesthesia (e.g., as in most trials using RF IHT), the reported complication rate was not increased; however, general anesthesia should be avoided if clinically possible to allow optimal operator-patient interaction during the treatment.

The overall complication rates in the published IHT-IRT series have ranged from 3% (HANDL-ZELLER 1993) to 43% (MACK et al. 1993a,b). While the overall complication rate varied little between RF IHT (about 25%) (Table 15.7) and MW IHT (20%) (Table 15.9), it appeared high for FM IHT (50%) (Table 15.11) and low for HS IHT (10%) series (Table 15.13). Smaller differences in the overall complication rates were observed between different tumor sites (Fig. 15.8), i.e., between head and neck (about 20%) (Table 15.14), breast and chest wall (10%) (Table 15.15), and pelvic tumors (20%) (Tables 15.16, 15.17). These complication rates are acceptable considering the large tumor burden and extensive pretreatment in most treated patients. When analyzing the toxicity data more carefully, the reported details vary between different studies. Some series report an overall complication rate, but lack details on acute toxicity (during IHT treatment) and early (≤90 days after treatment start) and/or late treatment sequelae (>90 days after treatment start). Only in some series can the reported details be retrospectively translated into these established toxicity categories (Table 15.19).

15.6.1 *Acute Treatment Toxicity*

Acute treatment toxicity develops during the IHT-IRT session. It can be associated with pain, general

Table 15.19. Treatment toxicity in large IHT-IRT clinical studies

Study	Tumors (*n*)	Specific toxicity distribution [*n* (%)]	Overall toxicity [*n* (%)]
Cosset et al. (1985)	29	8 (28%) Superficial necrosis 4 (14%) Deep necrosis	Early: 8 (28%) Overall: 10 (25%)
Emami et al. (1987)	48	8 (17%) Delayed wound healing 2 (4%) Cutaneous sinus 2 (4%) Various fistulas	Early: 8 (17%) Late: 4 (8%) Overall: 12 (35%)
Handl-Zeller (1993)	154	5 (3%) Grade 1–3 toxicity	Overall: 5 (3%)
Gautherie et al. (1989)	96	17 (18%) Superficial burns and blistering 8 (8%) Hemorrhage and skin necrosis 15 (16%) Deep necrosis and fistula	Early: 25 (26%) Late: 15 (8%) Overall: NA
Mack et al. (1993a,b)	44	22 (50%) Grade 1 + 2 toxicity 3 (7%) Grade 3 toxicity	Early/late: NA Overall: 19 (43%)
Oleson et al. (1984a,b)	52	6 (12%) Grade 1 + 2 toxicity 7 (13%) Grade 3 toxicity	Early/late: NA Overall: 13 (25%)
Petrovich et al. (1989)[a]	44	6 (14%) Acute erythema 9 (20%) Moist desquamation and blistering 2 (4%) Soft tissue necrosis/ulcer 1 (2%) Aspiration pneumonitis	Acute: 6 (14%) Early: 9 (20%) Late: 2 (4%) Overall: 11 (25%)
Prevost et al. (1993)	25	2 (8%) Superficial and deep necrosis	Early: 2 (8%) Overall: 2 (8%)
Puthawala et al. (1985)	43	2 (5%) Superficial burns 5 (12%) Soft tissue necrosis 3 (7%) Fistula formation 1 (2%) Brachioplexopathy	Early: 4 (9%) Late: 5 (12%) Overall: 9 (21%)
Puthawala et al. (1990)[b]	98	8 (8%) Skin burns and soft tissue necrosis 2 (2%) Severe fibrosis 2 (2%) Osteoradionecrosis 2 (2%) Fistula (1) and carotid blowout (1)	Early: 8 (8%) Late: 6 (6%) Overall: 12 (12%)
Rafla et al. (1988, 1989)	35	2 (6%) Immediate pain and discomfort 1 (3%) Blistering Several ulcers after tumor necrosis	Acute: 2 (6%) Early: 1 (3%) Overall: NA
Schreiber et al. (1992)	40	2 (5%) Blistering 2 (5%) Soft tissue necrosis 2 (5%) Fistula formation	Early: 4 (10%) Late: 2 (5%) Overall: 6 (15%)
Seegenschmiedt et al. (1994c)	90	23 (26%) Acute side-effects 12 (13%) Mucositis, blister 8 (9%) Ulceration and fistula formation 2 (2%) Massive soft tissue breakdown	Acute: 23 (26%) Early: 24 (27%) Late: 14 (16%) Overall: 24 (27%)
Shimm et al. (1990)	70	9 (12%) Recto-/vesicovaginal fistual 3 (4%) Tissue necrosis/ulcer 5 (7%) Skin reactions	Early: 5 (7%) Late: 12 (17%) Overall: 17 (24%)
Vora et al. (1989)	78	7 (9%) Superficial burns 2 (3%) Local inflammation 4 (5%) Fistula formation 1 (1%) Rib fracture	Early: 9 (12%) Late: 5 (6%) Overall: 14 (18%)

NA, no data available
[a] IHT performed under general anesthesia
[b] 2nd IHT not performed due to patient intolerance in >50% of cases

symptoms, and distress (tachycardia, dizziness, and a feeling of unease). Only a few series have actually addressed the question of how many patients have a poor heating session owing to poor subjective tolerance and its possible impact on treatment outcome (Cosset et al. 1985; Emami et al. 1987). Our clinical data using MW IHT revealed that about one-quarter of patients (26%) had suffered from acute treatment toxicity (Seegenschmiedt et al. 1990b, 1992, 1993a,b,

1994a–c). Only in some situations we could find a plausible reason for the problems encountered, such as: (a) interstitial MW antennas located too close to bony structures, thereby inducing "hot spots" close to the bone; (b) irregularly implanted and converging IHT applicators; or (c) short implantation lengths of the MW antennas with an exposed junction region. In about half of these cases we were able to overcome the specific problems by readjusting the heating sources or by applying bolus material at appropriate sites. In our series about one-third of patients had a poor heating performance, while the remainder achieved good thermal parameters. Interestingly, a correlation was observed between patients with good thermal performance and good tumor response.

15.6.2 Early and Late Treatment Sequelae

According to the RTOG/EORTC, early treatment sequelae appear shortly or up to 90 days after the treatment, while late treatment sequelae appear several months or even years later or comprise persistence of early complications beyond 90 days after treatment. Usually, minor early complications including blisters and thermal burns heal within days or weeks and do not provoke development of late sequelae. In contrast, most severe early complications, such as massive and rapid tumor necrosis and soft tissue breakdown, which have occasionally been observed after application of IHT-IRT, are prone to persist for long time. Often these complications are characterized by a deep necrotic crater or delayed wound healing despite a concomitant CR at the tumor site. However, the question of whether toxicity is related to RT or HT damage or both is often difficult to answer.

For example, soft tissue and osteoradionecrosis may occur after IRT or combined IHT-IRT of floor of mouth and base of tongue tumors. Orocutaneous fistulas can arise from initially large mucosal ulcers and soft tissue defects in the oral cavity. Patients with bulky gynecological, urogenital, and colorectal tumors are prone to develop fistulas in the small pelvis. Depending on the tumor type and the site of necrosis, the fistulas occur as vesicovaginal or rectovaginal fistulas. They rarely heal spontaneously and often require complicated plastic surgery. Management of these complications starts with careful nursing care, administration of local or systemic antibiotics, and pain medication if required. Debridement, skin grafts, and plastic surgery may become necessary for long-term and/or nonhealing defects of the mucosa or the skin.

The incidence of complications related to thermal exposure can be reduced by following precautions: (a) increasing power deposition during treatment initiation in small increments either up to the desired thermal level or to the subjective tolerance of the patient; (b) use of extensive multipoint thermometry and (manual or computerized) thermal mapping within the implanted volume to better identify and avoid "hot spots"; (c) manual control of power deposition during the treatment; (d) acknowledgment of the patient's subjective tolerance no matter what temperature is achieved or recorded; (e) not allowing temperatures to exceed 45°C in tumor and 44°C in normal tissues.

15.6.3 Prognostic Factors for Treatment Toxicity

In the literature, thermal toxicity is not correlated with the number of applied IHT sessions nor with the tumor type and site nor with the extent of pretreatment. However, thermal parameters have been associated with "thermal" complications, e.g., high maximum temperatures above 44°–45°C in normal or tumor tissue (Oleson et al. 1984a,b; Puthawala et al. 1985; Seegenschmiedt et al. 1994c) or "thermal doses" of T_{max} Eq 43°C $\geq$160 min (Dewhirst et al. 1984; Dewhirst and Sim 1986). It is important to realize that in all patients with malignant lesions, besides specific thermal treatment components additional radiation treatment components and intrinsic patient and tumor factors may contribute to the development of treatment complications. So far no conclusions can be drawn with regard to prognostic parameters for treatment complications. As long as no uniform criteria are applied to report the type and the severity of toxicity, comparisons between studies, tumor sites, and IHT techniques are not possible.

15.7 Prognostic Factors

Improved knowledge of prognostic factors will elucidate whether or not individual patients will benefit from treatment with combined IHT-IRT.

A careful analysis of previous clinical series can provide knowledge about parameters which might predict poor treatment performance and outcome and clarify the conditions under which IHT-IRT will contribute to a favorable outcome. Treatment outcome can be evaluated in various ways by analyzing initial and long-term tumor control, local recurrence, overall and/or relapse-free survival, or toxicity. For IHT-IRT studies it is useful to differentiate between two types of prognostic factors, i.e., those depending on *tumor biology* (patient's condition, tumor characteristics) and those describing *treatment conditions* (observed IHT and IRT treatment performance).

Unfortunately, only a few series provide sufficient details to permit careful interpretation of prognostic factors correlating with specific treatment endpoints. Moreover, the scientific value of many series is compromised by a low rate of patient accrual, a lack of detailed reporting of relevant IRT and IHT treatment parameters, insufficient analysis of confounding tumor and treatment factors, and lack of sufficient follow-up. Historical series are compromised by less developed thermal and heating technology. Most series also vary considerably with regard to the type of statistical analysis: some apply only a simple comparative analysis and others use uni- and bivariate testing, while only a few groups have applied multivariate logistic regression analysis.

The first report to address important prognostic parameters concerned a large series of patients treated with RF IHT at the University of Arizona, Tucson (Aristizabal and Oleson 1984; Oleson et al. 1984a,b). In a careful evaluation of 64 out of 161 patients receiving RF IHT, CR was significantly ($P < 0.05$) correlated with increasing RT dose, increasing time-averaged tumor temperature, and decreasing tumor volume. Using multivariate logistic regression analysis, the most significant parameters in predicting tumor response were identified as tumor volume, RT dose, and high minimum intratumoral temperature. Among the applied HT technologies, the RF IHT technique achieved the best thermal performance and yielded the highest CR rate.

Lately similar prognostic parameters have been identified by several other groups: small tumor volume, high (total) RT dose, and thermal parameters which are associated with a high time-averaged intratumoral minimum temperature or good "quality of heating" were all correlated with higher CR and lower recurrence rate. CR was also closely associated with increased local tumor control and decreased locoregional relapse rate (Table 15.20).

15.7.1 Patient Parameters

General conditions, such as Karnofsky index, age, metastatic status, and pain control, play a decisive role in how well the IHT-IRT treatment can be conducted in an individual patient. Only those patients with good cooperation, close operator-interaction during the HT treatment, and optimal compliance during follow-up may benefit from the treatment. Thus, the specific selection criteria of each study reflect some of the intrinsic prognostic parameters, which may contribute to the different outcome in the different studies.

Some groups have experienced a "learning process" when using IHT-IRT, reporting that as more patients have been treated, so the IHT-IRT treatment has been better applied and controlled. This has also been reflected in a reduction in the observed toxicity rate (Puthawala et al. 1985, 1990). The changing therapeutic alternatives in a given tumor site, e.g., the introduction of combined radiochemotherapy for advanced head and neck tumors, may also leave the therapist with a changing group of patients with different general conditions as compared with former years. Thus, various aspects can confound the analysis with regard to patient parameters.

In our own series (Seegenschmiedt et al. 1994a–c) and a recent series of City of Hope (Vora and Luk 1993), *younger* patients had a significantly better treatment outcome. In addition, the latter study also reported on the impact of *race* on treatment outcome (Vora and Luk 1993), but this was probably only a very specific and not a systematic finding. Otherwise, no other patient-related prognostic parameters have been reported in the literature.

15.7.2 Tumor Parameters

A careful review of the published literature reveals no conclusive correlation between tumor response and *tumor site*. An exception is the recent study by the University of Arizona, Tucson (Shimm et al. 1990), which reported a better CR rate for head and neck than for pelvic tumors, while in

Table 15.20. Prognostic parameters in large IHT-IRT clinical studies

Study	Statistical analysis	Tumor site or type	Tumor volume	Radiation dose	Thermal parameter
ARISTIZABAL and OLESON (1984)	Uni- and multivariate	–	Small volume → p(CR) ↑	High RT dose → p(CR) ↑	High *T* min(av) → p(CR) ↑
COSSET et al. (1985)	Univariate	NA	Large volume → p(REC) ↑	High RT dose → p(CR) ↑	High *T* min(av) → p(REC) ↓
COUGHLIN et al. (1991)	Comparative	–	Small volume → p(CR) ↑	High RT dose → p(CR) ↑	–
EMAMI et al. (1987)	Comparative	–	Small volume → p(CR) ↑	NA	High temperature → p(CR) ↑
GAUTHERIE et al. (1989)	Comparative	Head and neck > thoracic	NA	NA	NA
GRIGSBY and EMAMI (1993)	Uni- and multivariate	NA	Small volume → p(CR) ↑	High RT dose → p(CR) ↑	High thermal dose → p(CR) ↑
PETROVICH et al. (1989)	Univariate	–	Small volume → p(CR) ↑	High RT dose → p(CR) ↑	High thermal dose → p(CR) ↑
PATHAWALA et al. (1985, 1990)	Comparative	–	NA	NA	High *T* min(av) → p(REC) ↓
RAFLA et al. (1988, 1989)	Univariate	–	Small volume → p(CR) ↑	High RT dose → p(CR) ↑	NA
SCHREIBER et al. (1992)	Univariate	Primary tumors >persistent tumors	Small volume → p(CR) ↑	High RT dose → p(CR) ↑	High *T* min(av) → p(CR) ↑
SEEGENSCHMIEDT et al. (1994c)	Uni- and multivariate	Tumor site –; primary tumors >recurrences	Small volume → p(CR) ↑	High RT dose → p(CR) ↑; implant quality	High *T* min(av), TQ41, *T*10, TEM; *T*(init) → p(CR) ↑
SHIMM et al. (1990)	Uni- and multivariate	Head and neck >pelvic sites	Small volume → p(CR) ↑	High RT dose → p(CR) ↑	High *T* min(av) → p(CR) ↑
VORA et al. (1989)	Comparative	Primary tumors >recurrences	NA	–	–
VORA and LUK (1993)	Uni- and multivariate	Primary tumors >recurrences	NA	High RT dose → p(CR) ↑	–

NA, not analysed; >, first variable better than second; p(CR) ↑, probability of CR increasing; p(REC) ↓, probability of recurrences decreasing; –, parameter not found to be significant

contrast a longer response duration was found for pelvic than for head and neck tumors. An advantage for head and neck patients was detected in the French multicenter study (GAUTHERIE 1989), while PUTHAWALA et al. (1985) reported a higher toxicity rate for pelvic tumors as compared to other tumor sites. In contrast, most other authors (COUGHLIN et al. 1985; EMAMI et al. 1987; PETROVICH et al. 1989; RAFLA et al. 1989), including ourselves, have not found a site-specific difference for the analyzed study endpoints, i.e., complete response, local tumor control, tumor relapse, and survival (SEEGENSCHMIEDT et al. 1994c). Different findings among the clinical series are probably related more to treatment technique, tumor volume, and accessibility of the tumors for implants rather than to truly intrinsic differences. The tumor accessibility also has an obvious impact on the quality of the implant and the quality of the heating performance.

In several series significant outcome differences have been observed for different *tumor types*. Primary tumors and tumors without previous RT fared better than recurrent or metastatic lesions or preirradiated lesions. Clearly the latter lesions represent a worse selection of tumors to begin with, which cannot be aggressively irradiated. Even if a cumulative RT dose of 110 Gy may be accepted, the retreatment provides only a margin of 40–50 Gy. Moreover, these lesions are more radioresistant and have larger volumes than primary tumors. Thus, the findings in the literature are well explained (SCHREIBER et al. 1992; SEEGENSCHMIEDT et al. 1994a–c; VORA and LUK 1993; VORA et al. 1989).

The parameter *tumor volume* has been reported to have had a significant impact on treatment outcome in many series (ARISTIZABAL and OLESON 19484; COSSET et al. 1985; COUGHLIN et al. 1991; EMAMI et al. 1987; GRIGSBY and EMAMI 1993; PETROVICH et al. 1989; RAFLA et al. 1989; SCHREIBER et al. 1992; SEEGENSCHMIEDT et al. 1994a–c; SHIMM et al. 1990). However, different cut-off values have been reported, e.g., a 4 cm average tumor diameter (EMAMI et al. 1987) or volumes ranging from 22 cm^3 (SHIMM et al. 1990) and 80 cm^3 (SEEGENSCHMIEDT et al. 1994a–c) to as high as 150 cm^3 (PETROVICH et al. 1989). In these series tumor volume was negatively correlated with tumor response, but positively with relapse (COSSET et al. 1985) or treatment toxicity (PUTHAWALA et al. 1985; SHIMM et al. 1990). It is important to note that the parameter "tumor volume" cannot be separated from other parameters such as tumor site, accessibility for implantation, and the resulting thermal distribution within the tumor, as small tumors are much easier and more homogeneous to implant, thereby enabling a higher and more uniform thermal pattern to be achieved.

15.7.3 Radiation Treatment Parameters

Although it is difficult to account for different biological effects of interstitial and fractionated external RT, several groups have corroborated the prognostic impact of the total radiation dose (COSSET et al. 1985; COUGHLIN et al. 1991; GRIGSBY and EMAMI 1993; OLESON et al. 1984a,b; PETROVICH et al. 1989; RAFLA et al. 1989; SCHREIBER et al. 1992; SEEGENSCHMIEDT et al. 1994a–c); SHIMM et al. 1990; VORA and LUK 1993). Only in one trial did neither the interstitial nor the external or total RT dose correlate with treatment outcome (VORA et al. 1989). Different prognostic cut-off values have been reported, starting from as low as 29 Gy (ARISTIZABAL and OLESON 1984; COSSET et al. 1985; OLESON et al. 1984; SHIMM et al. 1990) when additional parameters like tumor volume and minimum tumor temperature were taken into account in the analysis. In contrast, our series (SEEGENSCHMIEDT et al. 1994a–c) and the Methodist Hospital, Brooklyn series (RAFLA et al. 1989) suggest a much higher minimum RT dose of 50 Gy or 60 Gy, respectively, but tumor type and site also influence the RT dose that can be applied in a given patient.

15.7.4 Thermal Treatment Parameters

The definition of an effective "thermal dose" and how it should be recorded and reported is a very controversial issue in thermoradiotherapy. Even with available HT techniques, homogeneous heating over the entire tumor volume is not achievable. Moreover, different concepts exist with regard to where thermometry has to be performed and which temperature should be recorded. It is important that all thermal sensors should be taken into account, while the clinically most significant recordings are the *minimum* and *maximum* temperatures, which are often associated with tumor response and treatment toxicity, respectively.

Assuming that all HT sessions yield satisfactory heating, it has also not been established how many sessions are necessary to achieve the best tumor response and long-term control. In the literature from one to eight and sometimes even more HT sessions have been applied, but no significant differences in response rate have been observed. It should also be borne in mind that only one or two treatment sessions can be applied with IHT due to obvious technical and clinical limitations. Thus it appears that *one satisfactory HT session* (i.e., with good thermal coverage of the target volume) is as effective as a large number of HT sessions. In addition, the biological superiority of LDR RT over HDR RT in combination with HT is an unsettled issue. Even simultaneous HT-RT using concomitant long-term HT at moderate temperatures (41°C) plus IRT appears to be an interesting treatment approach (GARCIA et al. 1992a,b).

In several of the series subjected to uni- and multivariate analysis, a better CR was observed when *high minimum* and *mean tumor temperatures* and *good thermal performance* were achieved. Thus, different cut-off values and endpoints have been correlated: CR or local tumor control was associated with "satisfactory heating" and $T_{min(av)} \geqslant 42.5°C$ (SHIMM et al. 1990), with $T_{(tumor)} > 42°C$ (EMAMI et al. 1987), with $T_{min(av)} \geqslant 41.0°C$, $T_{mean} \geqslant 42.0°C$, or thermal quality TQ41°C >

75% (Seegenschmiedt et al. 1994a–c), with $T_{90} \geqq 40°C$ (Leopold et al. 1992), and with the thermal quality calculated as hyperthermia equipment performance rate (Coughlin et al. 1991). In contrast, poor thermal tumor parameters were correlated with increased relapse rate (Cosset et al. 1985; Puthawala et al. 1985). Often several thermal parameters were closely associated with each other and yielded similar prognostic information in different predictive multivariate models; so far this aspect has not been fully considered in clinical reports, but it was demonstrated in our study.

Some series suggest that a high maximum temperature is correlated with treatment toxicity, thus greater toxicity has been found at $T_{max(av)} \geqslant$ 44°–45°C (Aristizabal and Oleson 1984; Oleson et al. 1984a,b; Puthawala et al. 1985; Shimm et al. 1990) and following a thermal dose of $TEM_{max} \geqslant$ 160 min (Dewhirst et al. 1984, 1986) in an animal study. Our own series revealed only a statistical trend towards a correlation of complications and maximum temperatures (Seegenschmiedt et al. 1994a–c), but in this instance invasive thermometry was not performed within catheters containing the IHT applicators. The correct maximum temperatures in the vicinity of the interstitial MW antennas may have been missed. This points to a general problem, which is related to invasive thermometry, as only a random selection of thermometry points represents the actual "heating performance." Even a uniform power deposition throughout the target volume may not prevent large thermal gradients between poorly perfused necrotic areas of large tumors and well-perfused areas or areas close to vessels.

15.8 Quality Assurance for Interstitial Thermoradiotherapy

Regardless of the choice of IHT technique, heating quality has been shown to be one of the most important factors in achieving tumor control. It is important that the physical characteristics of the IHT system and its relationship to the clinical situation at hand are fully recognized. To obtain both a reasonable *radiation* and *thermal distribution*, quality assurance measures have to be applied (Emami et al. 1991; Hand et al. 1989; Seegenschmiedt and Visser 1991; vol. 1, Chap. 21: Visser and van Rhoon), but the most important step is for the entire target volume (gross tumor volume with 1-cm margin) to be homogeneously implanted.

15.8.1 Implant Quality

Two proposals have been made to define the implant quality and quantify the specific "implant density." The proposal from the Daniel den Hoed Cancer Center (Levendag et al. 1993) assumes that the central implant plane (S), which is perpendicular to the main direction of the implant and contains all implanted catheters, represents the distribution of the heating and thermometry probes most adequately. The proposed algorithm defines the "mean spacing" (X) as the square root of S divided by the number of implanted HT applicators (n). In this respect, not all HT applicators are equally weighted, but each is given a specific weight, depending on its position within the implant. While all applicators within the boundary of S have a weight 1, applicators in catheters at the boundary of S are less weighted depending upon the specific angle under which the neighboring intersections are viewed. A clinical example is illustrated in Fig. 15.9.

Another proposal was made by our group (Seegenschmiedt et al. 1994c). Herein the implant quality is simply calculated as the ratio of the tumor volume and the number of activated heating probes. In our hands and for our applied MW IHT technique a volume of 5–10 cm^3 per MW antenna was a reasonable cut-off value to indicate an adequate volume coverage when assuming that each MW antenna could reach an effective heating volume at the 50% isospecific absorption rate which has about the same volume. In univariate analysis this "implant density" proved to differentiate well between responders and nonresponders, but it was also closely associated with the parameter "tumor volume," and in multivariate analaysis the implant density was completely outweighted by the tumor volume. Thus, it is recognized that with increasing implant volume the IRT and IHT techniques reach a definitive limit of technical applicability and clinical handling. In our experience, this volume limit is about 100–125 cm^3 (5 cm diameter or 5 cm × 5 cm × 5 cm) for the employed MW IHT technique, but this may vary considerably for other IHT techniques.

$$\text{'Mean Spacing'}\ X = \sqrt{\frac{S}{n}} \quad [\text{cm}]$$

S = the smallest area which contains all catheters (= plane that is perpendicular to the main direction of the implant

n = number of applicators

Example of the calculation of the mean spacing:

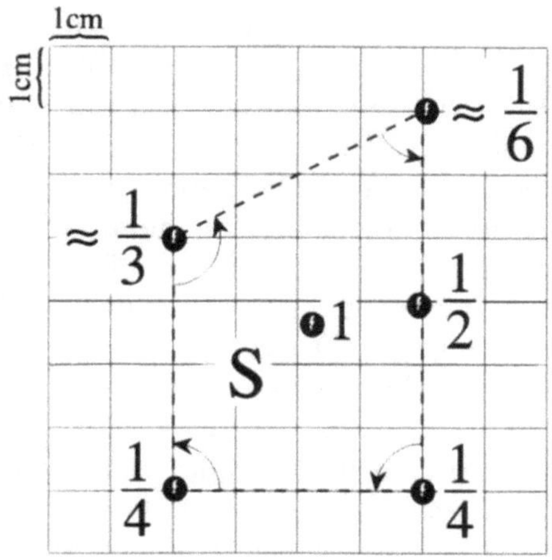

● = MW Antennas

$$n = \frac{1}{6} + \frac{1}{2} + \frac{1}{4} + \frac{1}{4} + \frac{1}{3} + 1 = 2{,}5$$

$$S = 20\ \text{cm}^2$$

$$\Rightarrow X = 2{,}8\ \text{cm}$$

Fig. 15.9. Definition of implant quality according to LEVENDAG et al. (1993). The "mean spacing" (*X*) is defined as square root of the central implant plane (*S*), which is perpendicular to the main direction of the implant, divided by the number of implanted applicators (*n*). Each of the heating applicators is given a specific weight, depending on its position within the implant. All applicators within the boundary of *S* have a weight 1, while applicators at the boundary of *S* are weighted less depending upon the angle under which the neighboring intersections are viewed

15.8.2 Treatment Quality

Appropriate *thermal data* can only be collected if the following conditions are met: (a) a large number of thermal sensors relative to the target volume; (b) thermal sampling at each sensor at intervals of no more than 1 min (minimum of 60 data points per sensor and hour); (c) thermometry in all critical sites, including tumor center and periphery and surrounding normal tissues; (d) thermometry evaluation not only with respect to time, but also with respect to location and characteristics of the individual heating curve; and (e) consideration of the position of the thermal sensors with respect to the heating characteristics and specific position of the HT applicators, e.g., thermometry within catheters containing HT applicators or not. Unfortunately, most series lack detailed information in this latter regard and only a few studies have reported the actual number of afterloading catheters implanted and temperature points independently measured.

Our study has tried to set a standard in this respect (SEEGENSCHMIEDT et al. 1994a–c). Thermal mapping procedures have been used in other studies and in clinical situations where only a few catheters have been implanted in order to expand the spatial temperature information (LEOPOLD et al. 1992). In addition, algorithms and interpolation procedures in respect of the thermal data have been developed to obtain a much more realistic idea of the actual thermal inhomogeneity and to compute the correct intratumoral thermal distribution, which should allow better prediction of the treatment outcome (OLESON et al. 1989).

Obviously, a high number of thermal sensors per target volume increases the probability of recording lower intratumoral temperatures (CORRY et al. 1988). The same is true for a low density of HT applicators. Therefore the quality of heating and thermal data can be improved if the number of HT applicators and/or the number of thermal sensors is increased, as outlined in Fig. 15.10. For example, in our study an average of 18 independent sites (range 6–42) were monitored within the treatment volume (mean tumor diameter: 69 cm^3), and an average of ten sensors (range: 3–20) were located in the tumor center and periphery (SEEGENSCHMIEDT et al. 1994a–c). The "spatial density"of our thermal data matrix was probably far better as compared to many other external and interstitial HT techniques, but this is still far from the ideal distribution of "one thermometry sensor per cubic centimeter" as suggested by STROHBEHN (1991). In future trials it is critical that the temporal and especially the spatial resolution of thermal data be improved, but in the longer term noninvasive thermometry may overcome this problem.

Interestingly in one study the different thermal characteristics were studied for measurements within catheters containing HT applicators and within catheters reserved for thermometry only (LEVENDAG et al. 1993). While the $T\text{mean}_{\text{mean}}$ inside catheters containing IHT applicators varied between 40.9° and 45.7°C, the $T\text{mean}_{\text{mean}}$ inside thermometry catheters was lower at 37.1°–39.6°C. It was found that the thermal profile across the implant volume was very inhomogeneous and characterized by low minima in between the HT applicators, and that the minimum temperatures increased with decreasing spacing of the HT applicators. This study clearly demonstrated the close correlation of implant quality and heating or thermal quality.

This finding is supported by our study (SEEGENSCHMIEDT et al. 1994a–c), in which even relatively low minimum tumor temperatures cor-

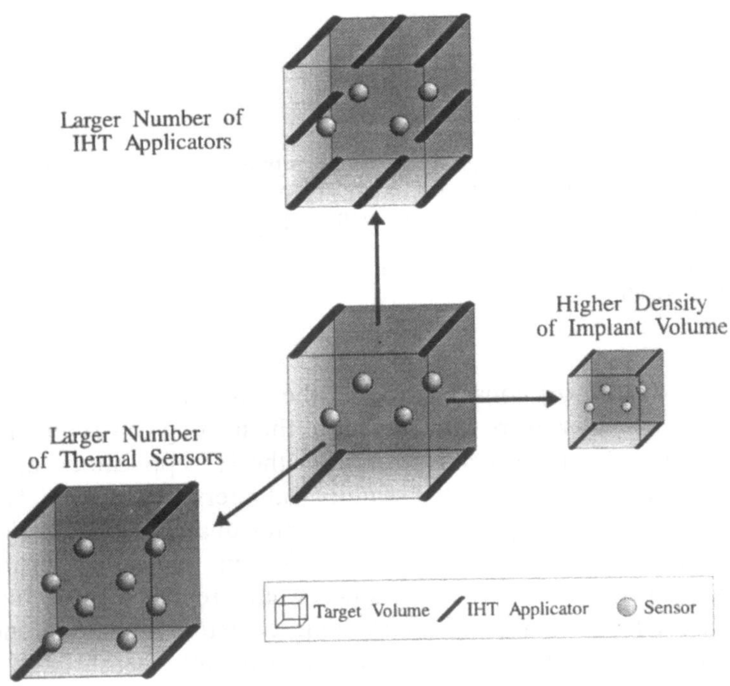

Fig. 15.10. Options to improve the quality of heating and thermal data for IHT: (a) by increasing the number of heating applicators (*upper box*); (b) by increasing the implant density per volume (*right box*); and (c) by increasing the number of thermal sensors within the target volume (*left box*)

related with treatment outcome. The reasons for the low temperatures were twofold: (a) invasive thermometry was strictly performed outside the HT sources and at locations most likely to record low temperatures; (b) many tumor sensors were employed (one sensor per 8 cm³), which increased the probability of recording low temperatures. In contrast, in most other series thermometry was performed inside or close to the HT applicators, thereby missing a potential lower minimum temperature. A way of demonstrating the thermal quality of a whole clinical series is shown in Fig. 15.11, which depicts the distribution of the percentage range of two selected thermal parameters exceeding a specific index temperature.

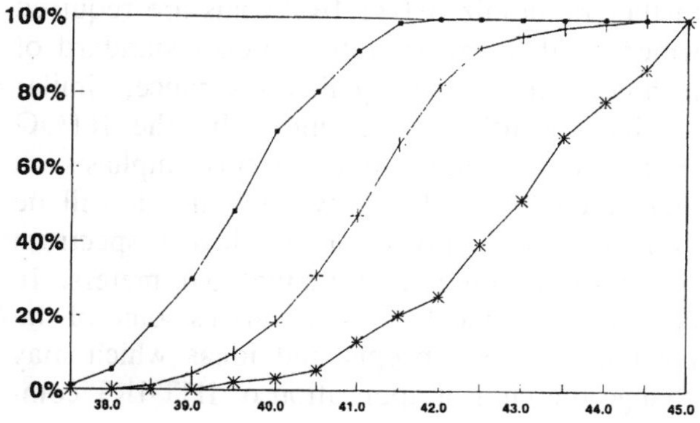

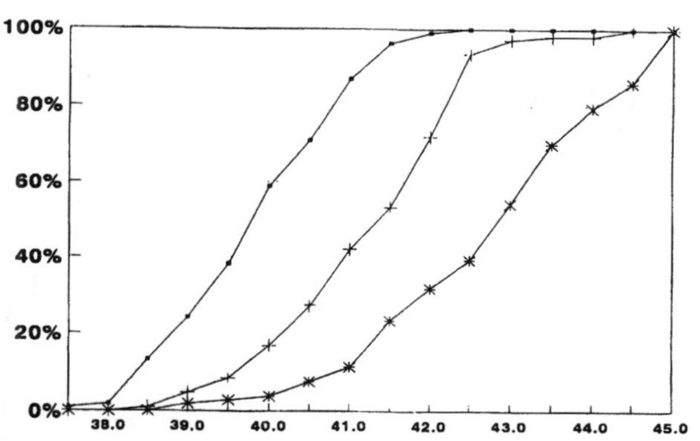

Fig. 15.11. **A** Cumulative distribution of three thermal index tumor parameters, T_{90} (mean: 39.8° ± 1.0°C), and T_{50} (mean: 41.2° ± 1.2°C), and T_{10} (mean: 43.2° ± 2.0°C) in a clinical series of 90 malignant lesions treated with combined 915-MHz MW IHT and interstitial and/or external beam RT (data derived from SEEGENSCHMIEDT et al. 1994c). **B** Cumulative distribution of three thermal tumor parameters, $T_{min(av)}$ (mean: 40.0° ± 1.1°C), T_{mean} (mean: 41.4° ± 1.2°C) and $T_{max(av)}$ (mean: 43.1° ± 2.0°C), in a clinical series of 90 malignant lesions treated with combined 915-MHz MW IHT and interstitial and/or external beam RT (data derived from SEEGENSCHMIEDT et al. 1994c)

Another approach to define the quality of heating was proposed by the group at Dartmouth Medical College. A hyperthermia Equipment performance rating was proposed which was based on the percentage of the tumor area exceeding an index temperature of 43°C over a fixed time period (PAULSEN et al. 1985). While this parameter applied well in phantom studies, its prognostic value has not yet been fully proven by clinical implementation in human tumor sites (COUGHLIN et al. 1991).

In conclusion, it is emphasized that invasive thermometry techniques are still inappropriate to monitor the whole tumor volume exactly, and that many factors compromise the quality of thermal data, including the number and location of thermometry sensors and the spatial and temporal resolution of measurements (CORRY et al. 1988). Unless a standardized HT data format (SAPARETO and CORRY 1989) is adapted for IHT and uniformly applied by all clinical users, interinstitutional comparisons of thermometry data and clinical parameters will continue to be very difficult.

15.9 Future Perspectives for Interstitial Thermoradiotherapy

Despite several insufficiencies in the past, technical and clinical research has shown that combined IHT-IRT is a versatile and safe method for treating confined implantable tumors at almost any site. Moreover, it has been clearly shown that IHT and IRT follow similar technical and clinical principles, which greatly facilitates their combined application: (a) *optimal targeting* of thermal and radiation dose to the tumor volume with adequate sparing of normal tissues; (b) *homogeneous dose distribution* of the radiation and thermal dose within the target volume; (c) induction of *completely different effects* as compared to fractionated external beam RT alone.

As IHT is compatible with most IRT procedures, IHT-IRT can be applied as an effective adjunct to external RT. Its cytotoxic potential is almost complementary to the RT effects at both the cellular and the environmental level (LEEPER 1985; REINHOLD and ENDRICH 1986; SONG 1984). Combined IHT-IRT is adaptable to various tumor sites, but is presently only applied for tumors that are poorly managed by standard treatments (KAPP 1986; OVERGAARD 1989). As each IHT technique has specific advantages, the IHT method of choice needs to be carefully selected.

Although the clinical practice of IHT-IRT has already undergone considerable evolution, further improvements are required. Targets of ongoing and future research include the following topics:

1. Biological, biochemical, biomolecular, and physiological studies regarding the radio-sensitizing effects of HT on LDR or HDR IRT
2. Assessment of different TERs for various tumor models, thermotolerance, and the influence of physiological tissue characteristics
3. Improvement of IHT technology (e.g., individual power steering, radial and longitudinal control of power deposition)
4. Improvement of thermometry methods (e.g., automatic thermal mapping) and development of noninvasive thermometry methods (e.g., microwave radiometry)
5. Thermal modeling and treatment control for all IHT techniques
6. Implementation of more user-friendly hard- and software components like screen- or mouse-controlled menus, integrated treatment planning, and prospective thermal data analysis
7. Design of multicenter prospective randomized trials which are controlled for specific tumor types and sites as well as specific IHT techniques and which employ a high quality assurance standard.

Presently two randomized phase I/II studies comparing IRT alone with combined IRT-IHT await final analysis: the RTOG 84-19 study and the ESHO 4-86 protocol. In a preliminary analysis of the RTOG protocol no benefit for the IHT-IRT arm was observed (EMAMI et al. 1991), but the trial was performed with old equipment, poor invasive thermometry documentation, and practically no specified quality assurance. Thus, further randomized IHT-IRT trials are required which need to incorporate a higher standard of technical and clinical quality assurance, similar to that recently recommended by the RTOG (EMAMI et al. 1991). Without this emphasis on quality control and quality assurance it will be impossible to control for the broad spectrum of critical tumor and treatment parameters. In conclusion, Table 15.21 summarizes some of the most attractive concepts and ideas which may change the clinical application of IHT-IRT completely in the future.

Table 15.21. Future concepts and ideas for clinical applications of IHT-IRT

Treatment techniques	
Surface-cooled interstitial heating applicators	
Axial and longitudinal power deposition control	
Automatic remote controlled IHT systems	
Treatment prescription	
Simultaneous heat and radiation application	
Short-term rapid scanning and long-duration application	
Treatment control	
Thermal modeling of all tissue components	
Individual preplanning for all IHT techniques	
Implementation of noninvasive thermometry	
Automatic feedback control of each IHT applicator	
On-line tumor imaging during heat application	
Prospective multicenter protocols	
Classic Design:	IRT alone versus combined IHT-IRT
Investigational:	PDR-IRT alone versus combined PDR-IRT plus continuous low-temperature IHT (41°C)
Investigational	HDR-IRT alone versus combined HDR-IRT and short-term high-temperature IHT (45°–47°C)
Investigational:	IHT combined with systemic or regional chemotherapy

PDR, pulsed dose rate
HDR, high dose rate

15.10 Summary

- IHT is defined by the placement of HT applicators directly into the tissue to be heated. In comparison to external HT methods it is expected to allow more homogeneous and selective heating of the tumor and much better sparing of normal tissues.
- There is a well-established biological and clinical rationale for the combined application of IHT and IRT: The observed thermal enhancement ratios (TERs) in experimental in vivo and in vitro studis range from 1.1 to 6.5. With an increasing RT dose rate the TER is maintained or even increased, and even continuously applied moderate HT of 39°–41°C has been shown to enhance simultaneous LDR RT.
- Careful treatment planning is required to achieve an optimal radiation dose distribution, and homogeneous "thermal dose" distribution within the implant. Specific implant recommendations have been developed for the different IHT techniques. There are guidelines for the implementation of invasive thermometry, which should be performed at the center of the implant, at the center of each subarray of three or four heating probes, at the tumor periphery, and in the surrounding normal tissues.
- The choice of the applied IHT technique for a particular tumor situation depends on availability, tumor site and volume, implant accessibility, and specific tissue and perfusion characterisics. Available IHT techniques fall into the following groups: microwave, radiofrequency, ferromagnetic, and hot source. Each of them has specific advantages and disadvantages.
- The applied treatment prescriptions vary considerably between different IHT-IRT studies not only with regard to the prescribed RT dose parameters, but also with respect to the "thermal dose" and the specific details of the HT treatment: IHT can be combined with either interstitial or external RT or both. The treatment prescription also depends on the tumor type and the extent of the pretreatment.
- So far almost 1300 patients have been treated with combined IHT-IRT and have been reported in clinical studies. Patients suffering from locally advanced or recurrent tumors of the head and neck, breast and chest-wall, pelvis, extremities, and brain have been the best candidates for the treatment.
- The reported overall and complete response (CR) rates vary depending upon the applied IHT technique and the treated tumor site: Head and neck tumors have an overall CR rate of 65%, while the overall CR rates of breast and chest wall lesions and colorectal lesions are 60%; the lowest CR rate is found for gynecological tumors of the pelvis (50%).
- The overall reported treatment toxicity rates are not considerably higher than those observed after IRT alone and range from 10% for breast and chest wall lesions to 20% for all other lesions. The toxicity is usually not exactly specified in each study.
- Although many intra-institutional phase I–II studies have indicated excellent tumor response rates and low treatment toxicity, the only randomized multicenter study (RTOG 84-19) has failed to show an advantage of combined IHT-IRT, probably due to poor technical equipment, insufficient thermometry, and lack of quality assurance.
- In large clinical series prognostic parameters have been determined, including patient- (age), tumor- (type, site, and volume) and treatment-related factors (RT dose, thermal variables). Among the treatment parameters, minimum tumor temperatures have been found to correlate with tumor response, while maximum temperatures correlate with treatment toxicity. In multivariate logistic regression analyses, only tumor volume, RT dose, and thermal parameters have been confirmed as independent prognostic parameters.
- Quality assurance is an absolute requirement in future IHT-IRT clinical trials, as both the quality of the implant and the IHT-IRT treatment have been found to impact on the treatment outcome. Specific quality assurance guidelines for IHT have recently been defined by the RTOG (Emami et al. 1991).
- Despite the fact that the clinical practice of IHT-IRT has evolved so far, further research is essential. The biological background of the heat-radiation interaction requires greater elucidation and further technical progress is essential, but the most important task is to perform a new randomized prospective study comparing IRT alone with combined IHT-IRT, while observing all the known quality assurance criteria. Only when such a study yields a positive

result will the role of interstitial thermoradiotherapy be fully established.

Acknowledgments. This work was supported by the following grants: Deutsche Krebshilfe e.V. (Dr. Mildred Scheel Stiftung) grant no. 300-402-521/6; Deutsche Forschungsgemeinschaft (DFG) grant no. Fi 371/2-1 and no. Se 525/4-2; Sophie-Wallner-Stiftung, Universität Erlangen-Nürnberg.

References

American Cancer Society (1993) Cancer facts and figures 1993. American Cancer Society, Atlanta

Aoyagi Y, Kanehira C, Kobori K, Hayakawa Y, Mochizuki S, Harada N (1989) Clinical experience with microwave interstitial hyperthermia. In: Sugahara T, Saito M (eds) Hyperthermic oncology 1988, vol 1. Taylor & Francis, London, pp 601–603

Arcangeli G, Overgaard J, Gonzalez-Gonzalez D, Shrivastava PN (1988) Hyperthermia trials. Int J Radiat Oncol Biol Phys 14: s93–s109

Arian-Schad KS, Leitner H, Stuecklschweiger G, Handl-Zeller L, Hackl A (1992) Interstitial warm-water hyperthermia combined with iridium 192-HDR implantation: principle, practical application and first clinical experiences. In: Handl-Zeller L (ed) Interstitial hyperthermia. Springer, Berlin Heidelberg New York, pp 171–182

Aristizabal SA, Oleson JR (1984) Combined interstitial irradiation and localized current field hyperthermia: results and conclusions from clinical studies. Cancer Res (suppl) 44: 4757s–4760s

Armour EP, Wang Z, Corry PM, Martinez AA (1991) Sensitization of rat 9L gliosarcoma cells to low dose rate irradiation by long duration 41°C hyperthermia. Cancer Res 51: 3088–3095

Armour EP, Wang Z, Corry PM, Martinez AA (1992) Equivalence of continuous and pulsed simulated low dose rate irradiation in 9L gliosarcoma cells at 37°C and 41°C. Int J Radiat Oncol Biol Phys 22: 109–114

Astrahan MA, Ligget P, Petrovich Z, Luxton G (1987) A 500 kHz localized current field hyperthermia system for use with ophthalmic plaque radiotherapy. Int J Hyperthermia 3: 423–432

Astrahan MA, Luxton G, Sapozink MD, Petrovich Z (1988) The accuracy of temperature measurement from within an interstitial microwave antenna. Int J Hyperthermia 4: 593–608

Atkinson WJ, Brezovich IA, Chakraborty DP (1984) Usable frequencies in hyperthermia with thermal seeds. IEEE Trans Biomed Eng 31: 70–75

Au KS, Cetas TC, Shimm DS, et al. (1989) Interstitial ferromagnetic hyperthermia and brachytherapy: preliminary report of a phase I clinical trial. Endocuriether Hypertherm Oncol 5: 127–136

Bagshaw MA, Ben-Yosef R, Fessenden P, et al. (1993) Combined interstitial irradiation and hyperthermia in the treatment of prostatic cancer. In: Gerner EW, Cetas TC (eds) Hyperthermic oncology 1992, vol 2. Arizona Board of Regents, Tucson, pp 363–366

Bedwinek JM, Fineberg B, Lee J, Ocwieza M (1981) Analysis of failures following local treatment of isolated local regional recurrence of breast cancer. Int J Radiat Oncol Biol Phys 7: 581–585

Ben-Hur E, Elkind MM, Bronk BV (1974) Thermally enhanced radiosensitivity of cultured Chinese hamster cells; inhibition of repair of sublethal damage and enhancement of lethal damage. Radiat Res 58: 38–51

Berdov B, Menteshasvili G (1990) Thermoradiotherapy of patients with locally advanced carcinoma of the rectum. Int J Hyperthermia 8: 33–43

Bicher HI, Wolfstein RS, Fingerhut AG, Frey HS, Lewinsky BS (1985a) An effective fractionation regime for interstitial thermoradiotherapy – preliminary clinical results. In: Overgaard J (ed) Hyperthermic oncology 1984, vol 1. Taylor & Francis, London, pp 575–578

Bicher HI, Moore DW, Wolfstein RS (1985b) A method for interstitial thermoradiotherapy. In: Overgaard J (ed) Hyperthermic oncology 1984, vol 1. Taylor & Francis, London, pp 595–598

Bichler K, Strohmaier W, Steimann J, Flüchter SH (1990) Hyperthermia in urology. In: Gautherie M (ed) Interstitial, endocavitary and perfusional hyperthermia: methods and clinical trials. Springer, Berlin Heidelberg New York, pp 43–58

Bolmsjö M, Seegenschmiedt MH (1989) Improved software for interstitial hyperthermia. In: Proceedings of the 37th RRS/9th NAHG Annual Meeting, Seattle, WA (USA), March 18–23, p 49[Bg-10]

Borrego JC, Martinez A, Corry PM, Clarke DH, Gersten D, Edmundson G, Leslie J (1990) Combined interstitial thermoradiotherapy for advanced or recurrent pelvic neoplasia. Int J Radiat Oncol Biol Phys 19 (suppl): 203 (abstract)

Brenner DJ, Hall EJ (1991) Conditions for the equivalence of continuous to pulsed low dose rate brachytherapy. Int J Radiat Oncol Biol Phys 20: 181–190

Brezovich IA, Meredith RF (1989) Practical aspects of ferromagnetic thermoseed hyperthermia. Radiol Clin North Am 27: 589–602

Brezovich IA, Atkinson WJ, Lilly BM (1984) Local hyperthermia with interstitial techniques. Cancer Res (suppl) 44: 4752s–4756s

Brezovich IA, Lilly BM, Meredith RF, Weppelmann B, Henderson RA, Brawner WR, Salter MM (1990) Hyperthermia of pet animal tumours with self regulating ferromagnetic thermoseeds. Int J Hyperthermia 6: 117–130

Budihna M, Lesnicar H, Handl-Zeller L, Schreier K (1992) Animal experiments with interstitial water hyperthermia. In: Handl-Zeller L (ed) Interstitial hyperthermia. Springer, Berlin Heidelberg New York, pp 155–164

Burton C, Hill M, Walker AE (1971) The RF thermoseed – a thermally self regulating implant for the production of brain lesions. IEEE Trans Biomed Eng 18: 104–109

Chan KW, Chou CK, McDougall MA, Luk KH (1988) Perturbation due to the use of catheters with non-perturbing thermometry probes. Int J Hyperthermia 4: 699–702

Chive M (1990) Use of microwave radiometry for hyperthermia monitoring and as basis for thermal dosimetry. In: Gautherie M (ed) Methods of hyperthermia control. Series, Clinical thermology; Subseries, Thermotherapy, vol 3. Springer, Berlin Heidelberg New York, pp 113–128

Colacchio TA, Coughlin CT, Taylor J, Douple E, Ryan T, Crichlow RW (1990) Intraoperative radiation therapy and hyperthermia: morbidity from this combined treatment modality for unresectable intra-abdominal carcinomas. Arch Surg 125: 370–375

Colacchio TA, Ryan T, Coughlin CT, Douple EB, Strohbehn JW (1993) Combined intraoperative thermoradiotherapy for abdominal malignancies: the Dartmouth experience. In: Seegenschmiedt MH, Sauer R (eds) Interstitial and intracavitary thermoradiotherapy, Springer, Berlin Heidelberg New York, pp 319–331

Corry PM, Jabboury K, Kong JS, Armour EP, McCraw FJ, LeDuc T (1988) Evaluation of equipment for hyperthermia treatment of cancer. Int J Hyperthermia 4: 53–74

Corry PM, Martinez AA, Armour EP, Edmundson G (1992) Simultaneous hyperthermia and brachytherapy with remote afterloading. In: Martinez AA, Orton CG, Mould RF (eds) Brachytherapy HDR and LDR. Nucletron, Veenendaal, Netherlands, pp 193–204

Corry PM, Gersten D, Langer S, Martinez AA (1993) Thermobrachytherapy: requirements for the future. In: Seegenschmiedt MH, Sauer R (eds) Interstitial and intracavitary thermoradiotherapy. Medical radiology series. Springer, Berlin Heidelberg New York, pp 373–380

Cosset JM (1990) Interstitial hyperthermia. In: Gautherie M (ed) Interstitial, endocavitary and perfusional hyperthermia. Methods and clinical trials. Springer, Berlin Heidelberg New York, pp 1–41

Cosset JM, Brule JM, Salama AM, Damia E, Dutreix J (1982) Low-frequency (0.5 MHz) contact and interstitial techniques for clinical hyperthermia. In: Gautherie M (ed) Biomed thermology, Liss, New York, pp 649–657

Cosset JM, Dutreix J, Gerbaulet A, Damia E (1984a) Combined interstitial hyperthermia and brachytherapy: Institute Gustave Roussy experience. In: Overgaard J (ed) Hyperthermic oncology, vol 1. Taylor & Francis, London, pp 587–590

Cosset JM, Dutreix J, Dufour J, Janoray P, Damia E, Haie C (1984b) Combined interstitial hyperthermia and brachytherapy: Institute Gustave Roussy technique and preliminary results. Int J Radiat Oncol Biol Phys 10: 307–312

Cosset JM, Dutreix J, Haie C, Gerbaulet A, Janoray P, Dewars JA (1985) Interstitial thermoradiotherapy: A technical and clinical study of 29 implantations performed at the Institute Gustave Roussy. Int J Hyperthermia 1: 3–13

Cosset JM, Dutreix J, Haie C, Mabire JP, Damia E (1986) Technical aspects of interstitial hyperthermia. Recent Results Cancer Res 101: 56–60

Coughlin CT (1990) Clinical hyperthermic practice: interstitial heating (chapter 7). In: Fields SB, Hand JW (eds) An introduction to the practical aspects of clinical hyperthermia. Taylor & Francis, London, pp 172–184

Coughlin CT (1992) Prospects for interstitial hyperthermia. In: Urano M, Douple E (eds) Hyperthermia and oncology, vol 3. Interstitial hyperthermia. VSP, Utrecht, pp 1–10

Coughlin TC, Strohbehn (1989) Interstitial thermoradiotherapy. Radiol Clin North Am 27: 577–588

Coughlin CT, Douple EB, Strohbehn JW, Eaton WL, Trembly BS, Wong TZ (1983) Interstitial hyperthermia in combination with brachytherapy. Radiology 148: 285–288

Coughlin CT, Wong TZ, Strohbehn JW, Colacchio TA, Sutton JE, Belch RZ, Douple EB (1985) Intraoperative interstitial microwave-induced hyperthermia and brachytherapy. Int J Radiat Oncol Biol Phys 11: 1673–1678

Coughlin CT, Ryan TP, Stafford JH (1991) Interstitial thermoradiotherapy: Dartmouth experience 1981–1990. In: Chapman JD, Dewey WC, Whitmore GF (eds) Radiation research: a twentieth century perspective, vol 1. Academic Press, San Diego, p 386 (abstract)

Coughlin CT, Wong TZ, Ryan TP, Jones EL, Crichlow RW, Spiegel PK, Jeffery R (1992) Interstitial microwave-induced hyperthermia and iridium brachytherapy for the treatment of obstructing biliary carcinomas. Int J Hyperthermia 8: 157–171

Crezee J, Mooibroek J, Lagendijk JJW (1993) Thermal model verification in interstitial hyperthermia. In: Seegenschmiedt MH, Sauer R (eds) Interstitial and intracavitary thermoradiotherapy, Springer, Berlin Heidelberg New York, pp 147–153

Cummings BJ (1992) Anal canal. In: Perez CA, Brady LW (eds) Principle and practice of radiation oncology. Lippincott, New York, pp 1015–1024

Denman DL, Elson HR, Lewis G, Breneman J, Clausen CL, Dine J, Aron BS (1988a) The distribution of power and heat produced by interstitial microwave antenna arrays. I. Comparative phantom and canine studies. Int J Radiat Oncol Biol Phys 14: 127–137

Denman DL, Foster A, Lewis G, et al. (1988b) The distribution of power and heat produced by interstitial microwave antenna arrays. II. The role of antenna spacing and insertion depth. Int J Radiat Oncol Biol Phys 14: 537–545

Deurloo IKK, Visser AG, Ruifrok ACC, Lakeman RF, Rhoon van GC, Levendag PC (1989) Radiofrequency interstitial hyperthermia: a multicentric program of quality assessment and clinical trials. In: Sugahara T, Saito M (eds) Hyperthermic oncology 1988, vol 1. Taylor & Francis, London, pp 874–875

Deurloo IKK, Visser AG, Morawski M, Geel van CAFJ, Levendag PC (1991) Application of a capactive-coupling interstitial hyperthermia system at 27 MHz: study of different applicator configurations. Phys Med Biol 36: 119–132

Deutsch M, Parsons JA, Mittal BB (1986) Radiation therapy for local-regional recurrent breast carcinoma. Int J Radiat Oncol Biol Phys 12: 2061–2065

Dewhirst MW, Sim DA (1986) Estimation of therapeutic gain in clinical trials involving hyperthermia and radiotherapy. Int J Hyperthermia 2: 165–178

Dewhirst MW, Sim DA, Sapareto S, Connor WG (1984) The importance of minimum tumour temperature in determining early and long-term reponse of spontaneous pet animal tumours to heat and radiation. Cancer Res (suppl) 44: 43s–50s

Diederich CJ, Hynynen KH (1993) Ultrasound technology for interstitial hyperthermia. In: Seegenschmiedt MH, Sauer R (eds) Interstitial and intracavitary thermoradiotherapy. Springer, Berlin Heidelberg New York, pp 55–62

Doss JD (1975) Use of RF fields to produce hyperthermia in animal tumors. In: Robinson JE (ed) Proceedings of the International Symposium on cancer therapy by hyperthermia and radiation. American College of Radiology, Washington DC, pp 226–227

Doss JD, McCabe CW (1976) A technique for localized heating in tissue: an adjunct to tumor therapy. Med Instrum 10: 16–21

Dunlop PRC, Dickinson RJ, Hand JW, Munro AJ, Vallis KA (1986) Early experience with combined interstitial hyperthermia and brachytherapy. Br J Radiol 59: 525–527

Dijk van JDP, Wieringen van N, Nieuwenhuys GJ, Koenis F, Koedooder C (1993) Ferromagnetic techniques for interstitial hyperthermia. In: Seegenschmiedt MH, Sauer R (eds) Interstitial and intracavitary thermoradiotherapy, Springer, Berlin Heidelberg New York, pp 49–53
Emami B (1992) Interstitial thermoradiotherapy in the treatment of malignant tumors. In: Urano M, Douple E (eds) Hyperthermia and oncology, vol 3. Interstitial hyperthermia. VSP, Utrecht, pp 199–219
Emami B, Perez CA (1985) Interstitial thermoradiotherapy: an overview. Endocurie Hypertherm Oncol 1: 35–40
Emami B, Marks JE, Perez CA, Nussbaum GH, Leybovich L, von Gerichten D (1984) Interstitial thermoradiotherapy in the treatment of recurrent residual malignant tumors. Am J Clin Oncol 6: 699–704
Emami B, Perez CA, Leybovich L, Straube W, von Gerichten D (1987) Interstitial thermoradiotherapy in the treatment of malignant tumours. Int J Hyperthermia 3: 107–118
Emami B, Stauffer P, Dewhirst MW, et al. (1991) RTOG quality assurance guidelines for interstitial hyperthermia. Int J Radiat Oncol Biol Phys 20: 1117–1124
Emami B, Grigsby PW, Cardenes H, Straube W, Myerson RJ, Perez CA (1992a) Interstitial thermoradiotherapy in malignant tumors: long term results. In: Gerner EW (ed) Hyperthermic oncology 1992, vol 1. Arizona Board of Regents, Tucson, 492 (abstract)
Emami B, Myerson RJ, Cardenes H, et al. (1992b) Combined hyperthermia and irradiation in the treatment of superficial tumors: results of a prospective randomized trial of hyperthermia fractionation (1/wk versus 2/wk). Int J Radiat Oncol Biol Phys 24: 145–152
Emami B, Scott C, Perez CA, et al. (1993) Phase III study of interstitial thermoradiotherapy compared with interstitial radiotherapy alone in the treatment of recurrent or persistent human tumors: a prospectively controlled randomized study by the Radiation Therapy Oncology Group. Int J Radiat Oncol Biol Phys 27(suppl): 155
Engin K, Tupchong L, Waterman FM, Nerlinger RT, Hoh LL, McFarlane JD, Leeper DB (1993) Thermoradiotherapy with combined interstitial and external hyperthermia in advanced tumours in the head and neck with depth ⩾3 cm. Int J Hyperthermia 9: 645–654
Engler MS, Dewhirst MW, Winget JW, Oleson JR (1987) Automated temperature scanning for hyperthermia treatment planning. Int J Radiat Oncol Biol Phys 13: 1377–1382
Eppert V, Trembly BS, Richter HJ (1991) Air cooling for an interstitial microwave array hyperthermia antenna: theory and experiment. IEEE Trans Biomed Eng 36: 977–986
Fabre JJ, Chive M, Dubois L, et al. (1993) 915 MHz microwave interstitial hyperthermia. Theoretical and experimental aspects with temperature control by multifrequency radiometry. Int J Hyperthermia 9: 433–444
Feldmann HJ, Molls M, Heinemann HG, Romanowski R, Stuschke M, Sack H (1993) Thermoradiotherapy in locally advanced deep seated tumors – thermal parameters and treatment results. Radiother Oncol 26: 38–44
Field SB, Morris CC (1983) The relationship between heating time and temperature: its relevance to clinical hyperthermia. Radiother Oncol 1: 179–183
Fietkau R (1992) Brachytherapy for head and neck tumours. SELECTRON Brachytherapy J, suppl 3, pp 3–14
Fietkau R, Weidenbecher M, Spitzer W, Sauer R (1991) Temporary and permanent brachycurietherapy in advanced head and neck cancer – the Erlangen experience. In: Sauer R (ed) Interventional radiation therapy: techniques – brachytherapy, Springer, Berlin Heidelberg New York, pp 159–169
Fietkau R, Grabenbauer GG, Seegenschmiedt MH (1993) Rationale for interstitial thermoradiotherapy for tumors in the head and neck region. In: Seegenschmiedt MH, Sauer R (eds) Interstitial and intracavitary thermoradiotherapy, Springer, Berlin Heidelberg New York, pp 163–178
Finger PT, Packer S, Svitra PP, Paglione R, Chess J, Albert DM (1984) Hyperthermic treatment of intraocular tumors. Arch Ophthalmol 102: 1477–1481
Finger PT, Packer S, Paglione R, Gatz JF, Ho TK, Bosworth JL (1989) Thermoradiotherapy of choroidal melanoma: clinical experience. Ophthalmology 96: 1384–1388
Forsyth K, Deshmukh, R, DeYoung DW, Dewhirst MW, Cetas TC (1985) Recent experience in pet animals with hyperthermic therapy in the head and neck induced with inductively-heated ferromagnetic implants. In: Overgaard J (ed) Hyperthermic oncology 1984, vol 1. Taylor & Francis, London, 599–602
Frazier OH, Corry PM (1984) Induction of hyperthermia using implanted electrodes (1984) Cancer Res (suppl) 44: 4864s–4866s
Garcia DM, Nussbaum GH, Fathman AE, Drzymala RE, Bleyer M, DeFord JA, Welsh D (1992a) Simultaneous chronic LDR interstitial radiotherapy and condutive interstitial hyperthermia treatment of recurrent prostatic tumors. In: Gerner EW (ed) Hyperthermic oncology 1992, vol 1. Arizona Board of Regents, Tucson, p 386
Garcia DM, Nussbaum GH, Fathman AE, et al. (1992b) Concurrent iridium-192 brachytherapy and long-duration, conductive interstitial hyperthermia for the treatment of recurrent carcinoma of the prostate. Endocurie Hypertherm Oncol 8: 151–158
Gautherie M (1989) Interstitial hyperthermia: state of the art and prospects. In: Sugahara T, Saito M (eds) Hyperthermic oncology 1988, vol 2. Taylor & Francis, London 63–68
Gautherie M, Cosset JM, Gerard JP, Horiot JC, Ardiet JM, El Akoum H, Alperovitch A (1989) Radiofrequency interstitial hyperthermia: a multicentric program of quality assessment and clinical trials. In: Sugahara T, Saito M (eds) Hyperthermic oncology 1988, vol 2. Taylor & Francis, London 711–714
van Geel CAJF, Visser AG, van Hooije CMC, van den Aardweg GJMJ, Kolkman-Deurloo IKK, Kaatee SJP, Levendag PC (1994) Interstitial hyperthermia and radiotherapy of a rat rhabdomyosarcoma; effects of sequential treatment and consequences for clonogenic repopulation. Int J Hyperthermia 10: 835–844
Gerard JP, Romestaing P, Ardiet JM, De Laroche G, Montbaron X, Sentenac I, Cosset JM (1992) Interstitial hyperthermia. General overview and preliminary results. In: Urano M, Douple E (eds) Hyperthermia and oncology, vol 3. Interstitial hyperthermia. VSP, Utrecht, pp 221–230
Gerner EW, Oval J, Manning MR, Sim DA, Bowden GT, Hevezi J (1983) Dose rate dependence of heat radiosensitization. Int J Radiat Oncol Biol Phys 9: 1401–1404
Goffinet DR, Prionas SD, Kapp DS, et al. (1990) Interstitial 192-iridium flexible catheter radiofrequency hyper-

thermia treatment of head and neck and recurrent pelvic carcinomas. Int J Radiat Oncol Biol Phys 18: 199–210

Gonzalez Gonzalez DG, van Dijk JDP, Blank LECM (1988) Chestwall recurrences of breast cancer: results of combined treatment with radiation and hyperthermia. Radiother Oncol 12: 95–103

Gottlieb CF, Hagman MJ, Babij TM, Abitbol AA, Levin AA, Houdek PV, Schwade JG (1990) Interstitial microwave hyperthermia applicators having submillimeter diameter. Int J Hyperthermia 6: 707–714

Gottschalk S (1899) Zur Behandlung des ulcerierenden-inoperablen Cervixcarcinoms. Zbl Gynäkol 23: 79–80

Grigsby PW, Emami B (1993) Interstitial thermoradiotherapy for pelvic tumors: the Washington University experience. In: Seegenschmiedt MH, Sauer R (eds) Interstitial and intracavitary thermoradiotherapy. Medical Radiology Series. Springer, Berlin Heidelberg New York, pp 265–270

Hahn GM (1992) Brachytherapy and hyperthermia: biological rationale. In: Handl-Zeller L (ed) Interstitial hyperthermia. Springer, Berlin Heidelberg New York, pp 1–10

Hall EJ (1985) The biological basis for endocurietherapy. Endocuriether Hypertherm Oncol 1: 141–152

Hall EJ (1988) Hyperthermia (chapter 14). In: Hall EJ (ed) Radiobiology for the radiologist, Lippincott, Philadelphia, pp 293–329

Hand JW (1987) Heat delivery and thermometry in clinical hyperthermia. In: Streffer C (ed) Hyperthermia and the therapy of malignant tumors. Springer, Berlin Heidelberg New York. Recent Results Cancer Research 104: 1–23

Hand JW (1990) Biophsics and technology of electromagnetic hyperthermia. In: Gautherie M (ed) Methods of external hyperthermic heating. Springer, Berlin Heidelberg New York, pp 1–59

Hand JW (1992) Physical aspects of interstitial hyperthermia. In: Handl-Zeller L (ed) Interstitial hyperthermia, Springer, Berlin Heidelberg New York, pp 51–76

Hand JW, Lagendijk JJW, Bach Andersen J, Bolomey JC (1989) Quality assurance guidelines for ESHO protocols. Int J Hyperthermia 5: 421–428

Handl-Zeller L (1992) Interstitial hyperthermia, 1st edn. Springer, Berlin Heidelberg New York

Handl-Zeller L (1993) Clinical experience of interstitial thermoradiotherapy using hot water perfusion techniques. In: Seegenschmiedt MH, Sauer R (eds) Interstitial and intracavitary thermoradiotherapy. Springer, Berlin Heidelberg New York, pp 211–221

Handl-Zeller L, Handl O (1992) Simultaneous application of combined interstitial high- or low-dose rate irradiation with hot water hyperthermia. In: Handl-Zeller L (ed) Interstitial hyperthermia, Springer, Berlin Heidelberg New York, pp 165–170

Handl-Zeller L, Menapace R (1992) A hot water hyperthermia system for use with ophthalmic plaque therapy. In: Gerner EW (ed) Hyperthermic oncology 1992, vol 1. Arizona Board of Regents, Tucson, p 494

Handl-Zeller L, Kärcher KH, Schreier K, Handl O (1987a) Beitrag zur Optimierung interstitieller Hyperthermiesysteme. Strahlenther Onkol 163: 460–463

Handl-Zeller L, Kärcher KH, Lesnicar H, Budihna M, Schreier K (1987b) Newly developed liquid heated interstitial hyperthermia system KHS-9/W 18. Int J Hyperthermia 3: 567 (abstract)

Handl-Zeller L, Arian-Schad K, Stücklschweiger G (1992) Review on clinical experiences using hot water. Hypertherm Bull 9: 64–67

Harisiadis L, Sung D, Kessaris N, Hall EJ (1978) Hyperthermia and LDR irradiation. Radiology 129: 195–198

Hilaris BS, Henschke UK (1985) General principles and techniques of interstitial brachytherapy. In: Hilaris BS (ed) Handbook of interstitial brachytherapy. Publishing Sciences, Acton, MA, pp 61–86

Hiraoka M, Jo S, Dodo Y, Ono K, Takahashi M, Nishida H, Abe M (1984) Clinical results of radiofrequency hyperthermia combined in the treatment of radioresistant cancers. Cancer 54: 2898–2904

Hynynen K, Davis KL (1993) Small cylindrical ultrasound sources for induction of hyperthermia via body cavities or interstitial implants. Int J Hyperthermia 9: 263–274

Inoue T, Masaki N, Ozeki S, Ikeda H, Nishiyama K, Matayoshi Y, Kozuka T (1989) Clinical experience of interstitial hyperthermia combined with external radiation using MA-251 interstitial applicator. In: Sugahara T, Saito M (eds) Hyperthermic oncology 1988, vol 1. Taylor & Francis, London, pp 598–600

Iskander MF, Tumeh AM (1989) Design optimization of interstitial antennas. IEEE Trans Biomed Eng 36: 238–246

James BJ, Strohbehn JW, Mechling JA, Trembly BS (1989) The effect of insertion depth on the theoretical SAR patterns of 915 MHz dipole antenna arrays for hyperthermia. Int J Hyperthermia 5: 733–747

Jones EL (1993) Biological rationale of interstitial thermoradiotherapy. In: Seegenschmiedt MH, Sauer R (eds) Interstitial and intracaviary thermoradiotherapy. Springer, Berlin Heidelberg New York, pp 3–15

Jones EL, Douple EB (1992) The biology of hyperthermia combined with low dose rate radiation. In: Urano M, Douple E (eds) Hyperthermia and oncology, vol 3. Interstitial hyperthermia. VSP, Utrecht, pp 135–154

Jones EL, Douple EB, Strohbehn J (1986) Thermal enhancement ratios for single and fractionated dose external beam radiotherapy combined with hyperthermia. In: Orphanoudakis SC (ed) Proceedings of the 12th Northeast Bioengineering Conference, New York. IEEE Press, Piscataway, NJ, pp 58–61

Jones EL, Lyons BE, Douple EB, Dain BJ (1989a) Thermal enhancement of low-dose irradiation in a murine tumour system. Int J Hyperthermia 5: 509–524

Jones EL, Lyons BE, Douple EB, Dain BJ (1989b) Response of a brachytherapy model using 125 Iodine in a murine tumor system. Radiat Res 118: 112–130

Joseph C, Astrahan M, Lipsett J, Archambeau J, Forell B (1981) Interstitial hyperthermia and interstitial iridium 192 implantation: a technique and preliminary results. Int J Radiat Oncol Biol Phys 7: 827–833

Kaplan I, Kapp DS, Bagshaw MA (1991) Secondary external beam radiotherapy and hyperthermia for local recurrence after 125-iodine implantation in adenocarcinoma of the prostate. Int J Radiat Oncol Biol Phys 20: 551–554

Kapp DS (1986) Site and disease selection for hyperthermia clinical trials. Int J Hyperthermia 2: 139–156

Kapp DS, Prionas SD (1992) Experience with radiofrequency local current field interstitial hyperthermia: biological rationale, equipment development, and clinical results. In: Handl-Zeller L (ed) Interstitial hyperthermia, Springer, Berlin Heidelberg New York, pp 95–120

Kapp DS, Barnett TA, Cox RS, Lee ER, Lohrbach A, Fessenden P (1991) Hyperthermia and radiation therapy of local-regional recurrent breast cancer: prognostic factors for response and local control of diffuse or nodular tumors. Int J Radiat Oncol Biol Phys 20: 1147–1164

Kapp KS, Kapp DS, Stücklschweiger G, Berger A, Geyer E (1994) Interstitial hyperthermia and high dose rate brachytherapy in the treatment of anal cancer: a phase I/II study. Int J Radiat Oncol Biol Phys 28: 189–199

Khan K, Thompson W, Karlsson U, Raju S (1992) Thermoradiotherapy of prostate cancer: a pilot study on 35 cases. In: Gerner EW (ed) Hyperthermic oncology 1992, vol 1. Arizona Board of Regents, Tucson, p 475

Kida Y, Kobayashi T, Tanaka T (1989) Local hyperthermia of brain tumor by implant heating system – preliminary clinical report. In: Sugahara T, Saito M (eds) Hyperthermic oncology 1988, vol 1. Taylor & Francis, London pp 393–394

Kobayashi T, Kida Y (1992) Interstitial hyperthermia of malignant brain tumors by an implant heating system using stereotactic techniques. Stereotact Funct Neurosurg 59: 123–127

Kobayashi T, Kida Y, Tanaka T, Kageyama N, Kobayashi H (1986) Magnetic induction hyperthermia for brain tumors using ferromagnetic implants with low Curie temperature. J Neuro-Oncol 4: 175–181

Kobayashi T, Kida Y, Tanaka T, Hattori K, Matsui M, Amemiya Y (1991) Interstitial hyperthermia of malignant brain tumors by implant heating system: clinical experience. J Neurooncol 10: 153–163

Kobayashi T, Kida Y, Tonai I, Matsui M (1992) Interstitial hyperthermia of malignant brain tumors and oral cancers by implant heating system (IHS). In: Gerner EW (ed) Hyperthermic oncology 1992, vol 1. Arizona Board of Regents, Tucson p 389 (abstract)

Kolotas C, Zamboglou N, Audretsch W, Muskalla K, Rezai M, Schnabel T, Schmitt G (1994) Interstitial hyperthermia and radiochemotherapy for breast cancer (chapter 19). In: Fietkau R, Mould F (eds) Brachytherapy state of the art in Germany. Nucletron, Veenendal, Netherlands, pp 163-171

Lagendijk JJW, Mooibroek J, Crezee J (1993) Future developments in respect of thermal modeling, treatment planning, and treatment control for interstitial hyperthermia. In: Seegenschmiedt MH, Sauer R (eds) Interstitial and intracavitary thermoradiotherapy. Springer, Berlin Heidelberg New York, pp 155–159

Lagendijk JJW, Visser AG, Crezee J, et al. (1995) Interstitial hyperthermia and treatment planning: the 27 MHz multi-electrode current source method. Nucletron-Odelft Veenendal, Activity Report No. 6: 83–90

Lam K, Astrahan M, Langholz B, Jepson J (1988) Interstitial thermoradiotherapy for recurrent or persistent tumours. Int J Hyperthermia 4: 259–266

Lee DJ, O'Neill MJ, Lam KS, Rostock R, Lam WC (1986) A new design of microwave interstitial applicators for hyperthermia with improved treatment volume. Int J Radiat Oncol Biol Phys 12: 2003–2008

Leeper DB (1985) Molecular and cellular mechanisms of hyperthermia alone or combined with other modalities. In: Overgaard J (ed): Hyperthermic oncology 1984, vol 1. Taylor & Francis, London 9–41

Leopold KA, Dewhirst MW, Samulski TV, et al. (1992) Relationships among tumor temperature treatment time and histopathological outcome using preoperative hyperthermia with radiation in soft tissue sarcomas. Int J Radiat Oncol Biol Phys 22: 989–998

Levendag PC, Visser AG, Deurloo IKK, van Rhoon GC, van Geel CAJF, van Hooiye C, Kaatee RSJP (1992) Interstitial radiation and/or interstitial hyperthermia in advanced and/or recurrent cancers in the head and neck: a pilot study. Hypertherm Bull 9: 70

Levendag PC, Kaatee RSJP, Visser AG, et al. (1993) Interstitial radiation and/or interstitial hyperthermia for advanced and/or recurrent cancers in the head and neck: a pilot study. In: Seegenschmiedt MH, Sauer R (eds) Interstitial and intracavitary thermoradiotherapy, Springer, Berlin Heidelberg New York, pp 233–239

Leybovich LB, Kurup RG (1993) Evaluation of microwave interstitial antennas in the phantom with varying cross-section. Int J Radiat Oncol Biol Phys 25: 105–112

Lin JC, Wang YJ (1987) Interstitial microwave antennas for thermal therapy. Int J Hyperthermia 3: 37–47

Linares LA, Nort D, Brenner H, et al. (1986) Interstitial hyperthermia and brachytherapy: a preliminary report. Endocuriether Hypertherm Oncol 2: 39–44

Lindholm CE, Kjellen E, Nilsson P, Hertzman S (1987) Microwave-induced hyperthermia and radiotherapy in human superficial tumours: clinical results with a comparative study of combined treatment versus radiotherapy alone. Int J Hyperthermia 3: 393–411

Luk KH (1992) Clinical application of interstitial hyperthermia. In: Urano M, Douple E (eds) Hyperthermia and oncology, vol 3. Interstitial hyperthermia. VSP, Utrecht, pp 155–180

Mack CF, Stea B, Kttelson JM, et al. (1992) Interstitial FM implants for the treatment of advanced and/or extracranial tumors. In: Gerner EW (ed) Hyperthermic oncology 1992, vol 1. Arizona Board of Regents, Tucson, p 367b

Mack CF, Stea B, Kittelson JM, et al. (1993a) Ferromagnetic implantation in extracranial neoplasms for interstitial thermoradiotherapy. In: Gerner EW, Cetas TC (eds) Hyperthermic oncology 1992, vol 2. Arizona Board of Regents, Tucson, pp 303–310

Mack CF, Stea B, Kittelson JM, et al. (1993b) Interstitial thermoradiotherapy with ferromagnetic implants for locally advanced and recurrent neoplasms. Int J Radiat Oncol Biol Phys 27: 109–115

Mackey MA (1993) In vitro effects and biological potential of long duration, moderate hyperthermia. In: Seegenschmiedt MH, Sauer R (eds) Interstitial and intracavitary thermoradiotherapy. Medical Radiology Series. Springer, Berlin Heidelberg New York, pp 21–29

Manning MR, Gerner EW (1983) Interstitial thermoradiotherapy. In: Storm FK (ed) Hyperthermia in cancer therapy. GK Hall, Boston, Mass. pp 467–477

Manning MR, Cetas TC, Gerner EW (1982a) Interstitial thermoradiotherapy. Monogr Natl Cancer Inst 61: 357–360

Manning MR, Cetas TC, Miller RC, Oleson JR, Conner WG, Gerner EW (1982b) Clinical hyperthermia: results of a phase I trial employing hyperthermia alone or in combination with external beam or interstitial radiotherapy. Cancer 49: 205–216

Marchal C (1992) Review on clinical experience using IHT-radiofrequency technique. Hypertherm Bull 9: 49–55

Marchal C (1993) Clinical experience of interstitial thermoradiotherapy using radiofrequency techniques. In: Seegenschmiedt MH, Sauer R (eds) Interstitial and intracavitary thermoradiotherapy. Medical Radiology

Series. Springer, Berlin Heidelberg New York, pp 187–192

Marchal C, Hofstetter S, Bey P, Pernot M, Gaulard ML (1985) Development of a new interstitial method of heating which can be used with conventional afterloading brachytherapy techniques using iridium-192. Strahlenther Onkol 161: 523–557

Marchal C, Nadi M, Hofstetter S, Bey P, Pernot M, Prieur G (1989) Practical interstitial method of heating operating at 27.12 MHz. Int J Hyperthermia 5: 451–466

Marchal C, Pernot M, Hofstetter S (1992) Clinical experience with different interstitial hyperthermia techniques. In: Handl-Zeller L (ed) Interstitial hyperthermia. Springer, Berlin Heidelberg New York, pp 121–134

Marchal C, Prevost B, Ardiet JM, Gerard JP, Cosset JM (1993) The French multicenter trial: results and conclusions. In: Seegenschmiedt MH, Sauer R (eds) Interstitial and intracavitary thermoradiotherapy. Medical Radiology Series. Springer, Berlin Heidelberg New York, pp 347–352

Marchosky JA, Babbs CF, Moran CJ, Fearnot NE, DeFord JA, Welsh DM (1990a) Conductive, interstitial hyperthermia: a new modality for treatment of intracranial tumors. In: Bicher HI (ed) Consensus on hyperthermia for the 1990s. Plenum Press, New York, pp 129–143

Marchosky JA, Moran CJ, Babbs CF (1990b) Hyperthermia catheter implantation and therapy in the brain. J Neurosurg 72: 975–979

Marchosky JA, Welsh DM, Horn BA, van Amburg AL (1992) Experience with long-duration interstitial hyperthermia and systemic BCNU in the treatment of recurrent malignant brain tumors. In: Gerner EW (ed) Hyperthermic oncology, vol 1. Taylor & Francis, London p 387 (abstract)

Martinez AA, Edmundson GK, Cox RS (1985) Combination of external beam irradiation and multiple-site perineal applicator (MUPIT) for treatment of locally advanced or recurrent prostatic, anorectal and gynecologic malignancies. Int J Radiat Oncol Biol Phys 11: 391–398

Martinez AA, Gersten D, Corry P (1993) Clinical rationale for interstitial thermoradiotherapy for gynecological tumors: review of clinical results and own experiences with continuous mild hyperthermia. In: Seegenschmiedt MH, Sauer R (eds) Interstitial and intracavitary thermoradiotherapy. Springer, Berlin Heidelberg New York, pp 179–185

Mechling JA, Strohbehn JW (1986) A theoretical comparison of the temperature distribution produced by three interstitial hyperthermia systems. Int J Radiat Oncol Biol Phys 12: 2137–2148

Mechling JA, Strohbehn JW, Ryan TP (1992) Three-dimensional theoretical temperature distribution produced by 915 MHz dipole antenna arrays with varying insertion depths in muscle tissue. Int J Radiat Oncol Biol Phys 22: 131–138

Mendecki J, Friedenthal E, Botstein C, Sterzer F, Paglione R, Nowogrodzki M, Beck E (1977) Microwave applicators for localized hyperthermia in the treatment of malignant tumors. J Bioeng 1: 511–518

Mendecki J, Friedenthal E, Botstein C, Sterzer F, Paglione R, Nowogrodzki M, Beck E (1978) Microwave induced hyperthermia in cancer treatment: apparatus and preliminary results. Int J Radiat Oncol Biol Phys 4: 1095–1103

Meridith RF, Brezovich IA, Weppelmann B, et al. (1989) Ferromagnetic thermoseeds: suitable for an afterloading interstitial implant. Int Radiat Oncol Biol Phys 17: 1341–1346

Merrick HW, Milligan AJ, Woldenberg LS, Ahuja RK, Dobelbower RR (1987) Intraoperative interstitial hyperthermia in conjunction with intraoperative radiation therapy in a radiation-resistant carcinoma of the abdomen: report on the feasibility of a new technique. J Surg Oncol 36: 48–51

Merrick HW, Milligan AJ, Greenblatt SH, Dobelbower RR (1988) Clinical experience with intraoperative interstitial hyperthermia and intraoperative radiation therapy. In: Abstracts of the 36th Annual Meeting of the Radiation Research Society, Philadelphia, April 16–21, 1988, p 45 (abstract)

Merry GA, Hale R, Zervas NT (1973) Induction thermocoagulation – a power seed study. IEEE Trans Biomed Eng 20: 302–303

Miller RC, Leith JT, Voemett RC, Gerner EW (1978) Effects of interstitial radiation therapy alone or in combination with localized hyperthermia on the response of a mouse mammary tumour. Radiat Res 19: 175–180

Milligan AJ, Merrick HW, Eltaki A (1992) Intraoperative hyperthermia. In: Urano M, Douple E (eds) Hyperthermia and oncology, vol 3. Interstitial hyperthermia. VSP, Utrecht, pp 259–274

Milligan AJ, Merrick HW, Dobelbower RR Jr (1993) In vivo intraoperative interstitial hyperthermia in the dog. In: Seegenschmiedt MH, Sauer R (eds) Interstitial and intracavitary thermoradiotherapy. Medical Radiology Series. Springer, Berlin Heidelberg New York, pp 31–34

Million RR, Cassisi N, Wittes RE (1985) Cancer of the head and neck. In: DeVita VT Jr, Heilman S, Rosenberg SA (eds) Cancer principles and practice of oncology. Lippincott, Philadelphia, pp 407–506

Mittal BB, Sathiaseelan V, Kies M (1990) Simultaneous localized 915 MHz external and interstitial microwave hyperthermia to heat tumors ≥3 cm depth. Int J Radiat Oncol Biol Phys 19: 669–675

Moidal RA, Wolfson SK, Selker R, Weine S (1976) Materials for selective heating in a radiofrequency electromagnetic field for combined chemothermal treatment of brain tumours. J Biomed Mater Res 10: 327–334

Molls M, Scherer E (1987) The combination of hyperthermia and radiation: clinical investigations. In: Streffer C (ed) Hyperthermia and the therapy of malignant tumors. Springer, Belin Heidelberg New York. Recent Results Cancer Research 104: 110–135

Mooibroek J, Crezee J, Lagendijk JJW (1993) Thermal modeling of vascular patterns and their impact on interstitial heating technology and temperature monitoring. In: Seegenschmiedt MH, Sauer R (eds) Interstitial and intracavitary thermoradiotherapy. Springer, Berlin Heidelberg New York, pp 131–137

Moorthy CR, Hahn EW, Kim JH, Feingold BS, Alifieri AA, Hilaris BS (1980) Improved response of a murine fibrosarcoma to interstitial radiation when combined with hyperthermia. Int J Radiat Oncol Biol Phys 6: 1386–1387

Moorthy CR, Hahn EW, Kim JH, Feingold BS, Alifieri AA, Hilaris BS (1984) Improved response of a murine fibrosarcoma (Meth-A) to interstitial radiation when combined with hyperthermia. Int J Radiat Oncol Biol Phys 10: 2145–2148

Mori M, Sugimachi K, Matsuda H (1991) Preoperative hyperthermochemoradiotherapy for patients with rectal cancer. In: Sekiba K (ed) Hyperthermic Oncology in Japan 90. Asahi Print, Okayama, pp 109–110

Müller RG (1991) Brachytherapy techniques. In: Sauer R (ed): Interventional radiation therapy: techniques – brachytherapy. Springer, Berlin Heidelberg New York, pp 35–51

Myerson RJ, Perez CA, Emami B, Straube W, Kuske R, Leybovich L (1990) Tumor control in long-term survivors following superficial hyperthermia. Int J Radiat Oncol Biol Phys 18: 1123–1129

Nakagawa K, Akanuma A, Hasezawa K, Takahshi N, Karasawa K, Muta N, Iio M (1989) Interstitial radiofrequency hyperthermia. II. merits and limitations in clinical application. Jpn J Hypertherm Oncol 5: 171–179

NCRP Report 67 (1981) Radiofrequency electromagnetic fields: properties, quantities and units, physical interactions and measurements. National Council on Radiation Protection and Measurements, Washington DC

Neyzari A, Cheung AY (1985) A review of brachyhyperthermia approaches for the treatment of cancer. Endocuriether/Hyperthermia Oncol 1: 257–264

Nishimura Y, Hiraoka M, Akuta K, et al. (1992) Hyperthermia combined with radiation therapy for primarily unresectable and recurrent colorectal cancer. Int J Radiat Oncol Biol Phys 23: 759–768

Oleson JR, Cetas TC (1982) Clinical hyperthermia with RF currents. In: Nussbaum GH (ed) Physical aspects of hyperthermia. American Institute of Physics, New York, pp 280–366

Oleson JR, Manning MR, Sim DA, et al. (1984a) In: Vaeth JM (ed) A review of the University of Arizona human clinical hyperthermia experience. Front Radiat Ther Oncol 18: 136–143

Oleson JR, Sim DA, Manning MR (1984b) Analysis of prognostic variables in hyperthermia treatment of 161 patients. Int J Radiat Oncol Biol Phys 10: 2231–2239

Oleson JR, Dewhirst MW, Harrelson JM, Leopold KA, Samulski TV, Tso CY (1989) Tumor temperature distributions predict hyperthermia effect. Int J Radiat Oncol Biol Phys 16: 559–570

Oleson JR, Samulski TV, Leopold KA, Clegg ST, Dewhirst MW, Dodge RK, George SL (1993) Sensitivity of hyperthermia trial outcomes to temperature and time: implications for thermal goals of treatment. Int J Radiat Oncol Biol Phys 25: 289–297

Overgaard J (1989) The current and potential role of hyperthermia in radiotherapy. Int J Radiat Oncol Biol Phys 16: 535–549

Overgaard M, Overgaard J, Sell A (1984) Dose-response relationship for radiation therapy of recurrent, residual, and primarily inoperable colorectal cancer. Radiother Oncol 1: 217–225

Pahlman L, Glimelius B, Ginman C, Graffman S, Adalsteinsson A (1985) Preoperative irradiation of primarily non-resectable adenocarcinoma of the rectum and rectosigmoid. Acta Radiol Oncol 24: 35–39

Papadopoulos D, Kimler BF, Estes NC, Durham FJ (1989) Growth delay effect of combined interstitial hyperthermia and brachytherapy in a rat solid tumor model. Anticancer Res: 45–47

Papillon J (1990) Effectiveness of combined radio-chemotherapy in the management of epidermoid carcinoma of the anal canal. Int J Radiat Oncol Biol Phys 19: 1217–1218

Parsons JT, McCarty PJ, Rao PV, Mendenhall NB, Million RR (1990) On the definition of local control. Int J Radiat Oncol Biol Phys 18: 705–706

Partington BP, Steeves RA, Su SL, Paliwal BR, Dubielzig RR, Wilson JW, Brezovich IA (1989) Temperature distributions, microangiographic and histopathologic correlations in normal tissue heated by ferromagnetic needles. Int J Hyperthermia 5: 319–327

Paulsen KD (1990) Calculation of power deposition patterns in hyperthermia. In: Gautherie M (ed) Methods of external hyperthermic heating. Springer, Berlin Heidelberg New York, pp 57–117

Paulsen KD, Strohbehn JW, Lynch DR (1985) Comparative theoretical performance of two types of regional hyperthermia systems. Int J Radiat Oncol Biol Phys 11: 1659–1671

Perez CA, Emami B (1989) Clinical trials with local (external and interstitial) irradiation and hyperthermia. Current and future perspectives. Radiol Clin North Am 27:525–542

Perez CA, Bauer M, Edelstein S (1986a) Impact of tumor control on survival in carcinoma of the lung treated with irradiation. Int J Radiat Oncol Biol Phys 12: 539–547

Perez CA, Kuske RR, Emami B, Fineberg B (1986b) Irradiation alone or combined with hyperthermia in the treatment of recurrent carcinoma of the breast in the chestwall: a nonrandomized comparison. Int J Hyperthermia 2: 179–187

Perez CA, Kuske RR, Camel HM (1988) Analysis of pelvic tumor control and impact on survival in carcinoma of the uterine cervix treated with radiation therapy alone. Int J Radiat Oncol Biol Phys 14: 613–621

Perez CA, Emami B, Nussbaum G, Sapareto S (1992) Hyperthermia. In: Perez CA, Brady LW (eds) Principles and practice of radiation oncology, 2nd edn. Lippinoctt, Philadelphia, pp 396–446

Persy JF (1916) Heat in the treatment of carcinomas of the uterus. Surg Gynecol Obstet 22: 77–79

Peschke P, Hahn EW, Wolber G (1993) In vivo experiments using interstitial radiation and hyperthermia. In: Seegenschmiedt MH, Sauer R (eds) Interstitial and intracavitary thermoradiotherapy. Medical Radiology Series. Springer, Berlin Heidelberg New York, pp 13–20

Petrovich Z, Baert V (1993) Intracavitary thermoradiotherapy for various tumor sites. In: Seegenschmiedt MH, Sauer R (eds) Interstitial and intracavitary thermoradiotherapy. Springer, Berlin Heidelberg New York, pp 311–317

Petrovich Z, Langholz B, Lam K, Luxton G, Cohen D, Jepson J, Astrahan M (1989) Interstitial microwave hyperthermia combined with iridium-192 radiotherapy for recurrent tumors. Am J Clin Oncol 12: 264–268

Phromratanapongse P, Seegenschmiedt MH, Karlsson UL, et al. (1990): Initial results of phase I/II interstitial thermo-radiotherapy for primary advanced and local recurrent tumors. Am J Clin Oncol 13: 259–268

Prevost B, de Cordoue-Rohart S, Mirabel X, Camart JC, Fabre JJ, Sozanski, Chive M (1993) 915 MHz microwave interstitial hyperthermia. III. Phase II clinical results. Int J Hyperthermia 9: 455–462

Prionas SD, Kapp DS (1992) Quality assurance for interstitial radiofrequency-induced hyperthermia. In: Handl-Zeller L (ed) Interstitial hyperthermia. Springer, Berlin Heidelberg New York, pp 77–94

Prionas SD, Fessenden P, Kapp DS, Goffinet DR, Hahn GM (1989) Interstitial electrodes allowing longitudinal control of SAR distributions. In: Sugahara T, Saito M

(eds) Hyperthermic oncology 1988, vol 2. Taylor & Francis, London pp 707–710
Prionas SD, Bagshaw MA, Kapp DS, Goffinet DR, Smitt M, Ben-Yosef R, Fessenden P (1992) Thermometry of interstitial radiofrequency-induced hyperthermia given in conjunction with brachytherapy for the treatment of carcinoma of the prostate. In: Gerner EW (ed) Hyperthermic oncology 1992, vol 1. Arizona Board of Regents, Tucson, p 477 (abstract)
Prionas SD, Kapp DS, Goffinet DR, Ben-Yosef R, Fessenden P, Bagshaw MA (1994) Thermometry of interstitial hyperthermia given as an adjuvant to brachytherapy for the treatment of carcinoma of the prostate. Int J Radiat Oncol Biol Phys 28: 151–162
Puthawala AA, Syed AMN, Khalid MA, Rafie S, McNamara CS (1985) Interstitial hyperthermia for recurrent malignancies. Endocuriether Hypertherm Oncol 1: 125–131
Puthawala AA, Syed AMN, Eads DL, Gillin L, Gates TC (1988) Limited external beam and interstitial 192-iridium irradiation in the treatment of carcinoma of the base of tongue: a ten-year experience. Int J Radiat Oncol Biol Phys 14: 839–848
Puthawala AA, Syed AMN, Rafie S, McNamara CS (1990) Interstitial hyperthermia and interstitial irradiation (thermoradiotherapy) in the treatment of recurrent and/or persistent head and neck cancers. Endocuriether Hypertherm Oncol 6: 203–210
Raaphorst GP, Heller DP, Bussey A, Ng CE (1994) Thermal radiosensitization by 41°C hyperthermia during low dose-rate irradiation in human normal and tumour cell lines. Int J Hyperthermia 10: 263–270
Radiation Therapy Oncology Group (1984) Acute and late radiation morbidity scoring (2 tables). Written communication, RTOG, Philadelphia
Radiation Therapy Oncology Group (1986) RTOG # 84-19. A randomized phase III study of interstitial thermoradiotherapy, 43°C compared with interstitial radiotherapy alone in the treatment of recurrent and persistent tumors. Written communication, RTOG, Philadelphia
Rafla S, Tchelebi M, Youssef E, Parikh K, Salloum N (1988) The treatment of advanced recurrent pelvic tumors by interstitial hyperthermia and brachytherapy – a promising approach. In: Abstracts of the 36th Annual Meeting of the Radiation Research Society, Philadelphia, April 16–21, 1988, p 46 (abstract)
Rafla S, Parikh K, Tchelebi M, Youssef E, Selim H, Bishay S (1989) Recurrent tumors of the head and neck, pelvis and chestwall: treatment with hyperthermia and brachytherapy. Radiology 172: 845–850
Reinhold HS, Endrich B (1986) Tumour microcirculation as a target for hyperthermia. Int J Hyperthermia 2: 117–137
Roos D, Hugander A (1988) Microwave interstitial applicators with improved longitudinal heating patterns. Int J Hyperthermia 4: 609–615
Ryan TR (1991) Comparison of six microwave antennas for hyperthermia treatment of cancer: SAR results for single antennas and arrays. Int J Radiat Oncol Biol Phys 21: 403–413
Ryan TR (1993) Methods of thermal modeling and their impact on interstitial hyperthermia treatment planning. In: Seegenschmiedt MH, Sauer R (eds) Interstitial and intracavitary thermoradiotherapy. Medical Radiology Series. Springer, Berlin Heidelberg New York, pp 95–116
Ryan TR, Mechling JA, Strohbehn JW (1990) Absorbed power deposition for various insertion depths for 915 MHz interstitial dipol antenna arrays: experiment versus theory. Int J Radiat Oncol Biol Phys 19: 377–387
Sapareto SA, Dewey WC (1984) Thermal dose determination in cancer therapy. Int J Radiat Oncol Biol Phys 10: 787–796
Sapareto SA, Corry PM (1989) A proposed standard format for hyperthermia freatment data. Jnt J Radiat Oncol Biol Phys 16: 613–627
Sapozink MD (1986) The application of thermal dose in clinical trials. Int J Hyperthermia 2: 157–164
Sapozink MD, Palos B, Goffinet DR, Hahn GM (1983) Combined continuous ultra-low dose rate radiotherapy and radiofrequency hyperthermia in the C3H mouse. Thermal dose determination in cancer therapy. Int J Radiat Oncol Biol Phys 9: 1357–1365
Sathiaseelan V, Leybovich L, Emami B, Stauffer PR, Straube W (1991) Characteristics of improved microwave interstitial antennas for local hyperthermia. Int J Radiat Oncol Biol Phys 20: 531–539
Satoh T, Stauffer PR (1988) Implantable helical coil microwave antenna for interstitial hyperthermia. Int J Hyperthermia 4: 497–512
Schlienger M, Krzisch C, Pene F, et al. (1989) Epidermoid carcinoma of the anal canal treatment results and prognostic variables in a series of 242 cases. Int J Radiat Oncol Biol Phys 17: 1141–1151
Schorcht J (1994) Radiothermotherapy of cervical carcinoma. In: Fietkau R, Mould F (eds) Brachytherapy state of the art in Germany. Nucletron, Veenendal, Netherlands pp 81–87
Schreiber DP, Overett TK, Schneider MJ (1992) Interstitial brachytherapy and hyperthermia for both primary and recurrent tumors. Endocurie Hypertherm Oncol 8: 61–69
Schreier K, Budihna M, Lesnicar H, et al. (1990) Preliminary studies of interstitial hyperthermia using hot water. Int J Hyperthermia 6: 431–444
Seegenschmiedt MH (1993) Clinical experience of interstitial thermoradiotherapy using microwave techniques. In: Seegenschmiedt MH, Sauer R (eds) Interstitial and intracavitary thermoradiotherapy. Medical Radiology Series. Springer, Berlin Heidelberg New York, pp 193–210
Seegenschmiedt MH, Sauer R (1989) Methoden und klinische Ergebnisse der interstitiellen Thermoradiotherapie. Strahlenther Onkol 165: 360–368
Seegenschmiedt MH, Sauer R (1992) The current role of interstitial thermoradiotherapy. Strahlenther Onkol 168: 119–140
Seegenschmiedt MH, Vernon CC (1993) Clinical considerations for the design and conduct of hyperthermia clinical trials. In: Seegenschmiedt MH, Sauer R (eds) Interstitial and intracavitary thermoradiotherapy. Medical Radiology Series. Springer, Berlin Heidelberg New York, pp 353–372
Seegenschmiedt MH, Visser AG (1991) Quality assurance for interstitial hyperthermia. Hypertherm Bull 5: 85–91
Seegenschmiedt MH, Sauer R, Herbst M, Thiel H-J, Fietkau R, Brady LW, Karlsson UL (1989a) Interstitial hyperthermia for head and neck tumors: treatment planning and quality assurance (QA). In: Sugahara T, Saito M (eds) Hyperthermic oncology 1988, vol 2. Taylor & Francis, London, pp 524–527
Seegenschmiedt MH, Karlsson UL, Sauer R, et al. (1989b) Superficial chestwall recurrences of breast cancer:

prognostic treatment factors for combined radiation therapy and hyperthermia. Radiology 173: 551–558
Seegenschmiedt MH, Brady LW, Sauer R (1990a) Interstitial thermoradiotherapy: review on technical and clinical aspects. Am J Clin Oncol 13: 352–363
Seegenschmiedt MH, Sauer R, Fietkau R, Brady LW, Karlsson UL (1990b) Primary advanced and local recurrent head & neck tumors: effective management with interstitial thermoradiotherapy. Radiology 176: 267–274
Seegenschmiedt MH, Sauer R, Brady LW, Karlsson UL (1992) Clinical practice of interstitial microwave hyperthermia combined with iridium-192 brachytherapy. In: Handl-Zeller L (ed) Interstitial hyperthermia, Springer, Berlin Heidelberg New York, pp 95–120
Seegenschmiedt MH, Sauer R, Fietkau R, Iro H, Brady LW (1993a) Interstitial thermoradiotherapy for head and neck tumors: results of a phase 1–2 study. In: Seegenschmiedt MH, Sauer R (eds) Interstitial and intracavitary thermoradiotherapy. Medical Radiology Series. Springer, Berlin Heidelberg New York, pp 241–256
Seegenschmiedt MH, Sauer R, Fietkau R, Iro H, Brady LW (1993b) Interstitial thermoradiotherapy for pelvic tumors: a cooperative phase 1–2 study. In: Seegenschmiedt MH, Sauer R (eds) Interstitial and intracavitary thermoradiotherapy. Medical Radiology Series. Springer, Berlin Heidelberg New York, pp 271–288
Seegenschmiedt MH, Martus P, Grabenbauer GG, Fietkau R, Erb J, Iro H, Wigand ME, Sauer R (1994a) Clinical experience with interstitial thermoradiotherapy for localized head and neck tumors. Tumordiagn Ther 15: 63–72
Seegenschmiedt MH, Martus P, Erb J, Fietkau R, Sauer R (1994b) Radiothermotherapy of head and neck tumours. In: Bruggmoser G, Mould RF (eds) Brachytherapy review. Freiburg Oncology Series Monograph 1. Medical Physics Publishing, Madison, pp 194–203
Seegenschmiedt MH, Martus P, Fietkau R, Iro H, Brady LW, Sauer R (1994c) Multivariate analysis of prognostic parameters using interstitial thermoradiotherapy (IHT-IRT): tumor and treatment variables predict outcome. Int J Radiat Oncol Biol Phys 29: 1049–1063
Shimm DS, Cetas TC, Buechler D, et al. (1989b) Inductively heated, thermoregulating FM seeds for interstitial thermoradiotherapy. In: Sugahara T, Saito M (eds) Hyperthermic oncology 1988, vol 1. Taylor & Francis, London, pp 594–595
Shimm DS, Cetas TC, Buechler D, et al. (1989b) Inductively heated, thermoregulating FM seeds for interstitial thermo-radiotherapy. In: Sugahara T, Saito M (eds) Hyperthermic oncology 1988, vol 1. Taylor & Francis, London, pp 594–595
Shimm DS, Kittelson J, Oleson JR, Aristizabal SA, Barlow LC, Cetas TC (1990) Interstitial thermoradiotherapy. Thermal dosimetry and clinical results. Int J Radiat Oncol Biol Phys 18: 383–387
Shimm DS, Kittelson J, Stea B (1992) Interstitial thermoradiotherapy. The University of Arizona experience. In: Urano M, Douple E (eds) Hyperthermia oncology, vol 3. Interstitial hyperthermia. VSP, Utrecht, pp 181–198
Sneed PK, Matsumoto K, Stauffer P, Fike JR, Smith V, Gutin PH (1986) Comparative thermal dosimetry of interstitial microwave and radiofrequency-LCF hyperthermia. Int J Radiat Oncol Biol Phys 12: 1887–1897
Sneed PK (1993) Interstitial thermoradiotherapy for brain tumors. In: Seegenschmiedt MH, Sauer R (eds) Interstitial and intracavitary thermoradiotherapy. Springer, Berlin Heidelberg New York, pp 289–295
Song CW (1984) Effect of local hyperthermia on bloodflow and microenvironment. Cancer Res (suppl) 44: 4721s–4730s
Spiro IJ, McPherson S, Cook JA, Ling CC, DeGraff W, Mitchell JB (1991) Sensitization of low dose rate irradiation by nonlethal hyperthermia. Radiat Res 127: 111–114
Stauffer PR (1990) Techniques for interstitial hyperthermia. In: Field SB, Hand JW (eds) An introduction to the practical aspects of clinical hyperthermia. Taylor & Francis, London, pp 344–370
Stauffer PR (1991) Interstitial hyperthermia: evolving technologies. In: Chapman JD, Dewey WC, Whitmore GF (eds) Radiation research: a twentieth century perspective. Academic Press, San Diego, pp 906–911
Stauffer PR (1992) Interstitial technology development: have we responded to the clinical needs? In: Gerner EW, Cetas TC (eds) Hyperthermic oncology 1992. Taylor & Francis, London, pp 237–240
Stauffer PR, Cetas TC, Fletcher AM, DeYoung D, Dewhirst MW, Oleson J, Roemer RB (1984) Observations on the use of ferromagnetic implants for inducing hyperthermia. IEEE Trans Biomed Eng 31: 76–90
Stauffer PR, Sneed PK, Suen SA, Satoh T, Matsumoto K, Fike JR, Phillips TL (1989) Comparative thermal dosimetry of interstitial microwave and radiofrequency-LCF hyperthermia. Int J Hyperthermia 5: 307–318
Stea B, Cetas TC, Cassady JR, et al. (1989) Interstitial thermoradiotherapy of brain tumors: preliminary results of a phase I clinical trial. Int J Radiat Oncol Biol Phys 19: 1463–1471
Stea B, Shimm D, Kittelson J, Cetas TC (1992a) Interstitial hyperthermia with ferromagnetic seed implants: preliminary results of a phase I clinical trial. In: Handl-Zeller L (ed) Interstitial hyperthermia. Springer, Berlin Heidelberg New York, pp 95–120
Stea B, Kittelson J, Cassady JR, et al. (1992b) Treatment of malignant gliomas with interstitial irradiation and hyperthermia. Int J Radiat Oncol Biol Phys 24: 657–667
Stea B, Shimm DS, Cetas TC (1993) Clinical experience of interstitial thermoradiotherapy using ferromagnetic implants. In: Seegenschmiedt MH, Sauer R (eds) Interstitial and intracavitary thermoradiotherapy. Springer, Berlin Heidelberg New York, pp 223–30
Steger (1993) Laser technology for interstitial hyperthermia. In: Seegenschmiedt MH, Sauer R (eds) Interstitial and intracavitary thermoradiotherapy. Springer, Berlin Heidelberg New York, pp 63–74
Steeves RA, Murray TG, Moros EG, Boldt HC, Mieler WF, Paliwal BR (1992) Concurrent ferromagnetic hyperthermia and 125 brachytherapy in a rabbit choroidal melanoma model. Int J Hyperthermia 8: 443–449
Streffer C (1988) Aspects of metabolic change after hyperthermia. In: Issels RD, Wilmanns W (eds) Application of hyperthermia in the treatment of cancer. Springer, Berlin Heidelberg New York, Recent Results Cancer Research 107: 7–16
Streffer C, van Beuningen D (1987) The biological basis for tumor therapy by hyperthermia and radiation. In: Streffer C (ed) Hyperthermia and the therapy of malignant tumors. Springer, Berlin Heidelberg New York, Recent Results Cancer Research 104: 24–70

Strohbehn JW (1987) Interstitial techniques for hyperthermia. In: Field SB, Franconi C (eds) Physics and technology of hyperthermia, Martinus Nijhoff, Amsterdam, pp 211–240

Strohbehn JW (1991) An engineer looks at hyperthermia. In: Dewey W, Edington M, Fry RJM, Hall EJ, Whitmore GF (eds) Radiation research – a twentieth- century perspective, vol 2. Academic Press, San Diego, pp 14–25

Strohbehn JW, Paulsen KD, Lynch D (1989) Numerical Modelling of SAR and temperature in 1992: where we might be. In: Sugahara T, Saito M (eds) Hyperthermic oncology 1988, vol 2. Taylor & Francis, London, pp 770–773

Stücklschweiger G, Arian-Schad KS, Handl-Zeller L, Leitner H, Poier E, Hackl A (1991) Interstitielle Ir-192-Afterloadingtherapie mit sequentieller Warmwasserhyperthermie. Strahlenther Onkol 167: 98–104

Stücklschweiger G, Arian-Schad KS, Kapp DS, Handl-Zeller L, Hackl A (1993) Analysis of temperature distributions of interstitial hyperthermia using hot water system. Int J Radiat Oncol Biol Phys 26: 891–895

Suit HD (1982) Potential for improving survival rates for the cancer patient by increasing the efficacy of treatment of the primary lesion. Cancer 50: 1227–1231

Suit HD, Westgate SJ (1986) Impact of improved local tumor control on survival. Int J Radiat Oncol Biol Phys 12: 453–458

Sundararaman S, Denman DL, Legoretta RA, et al. (1990) The modification of specific absorption rates in interstitial microwave hyperthermia via tissue-equivalent material bolus. Int J Radiat Oncol Biol Phys 19: 677–685

Surwit EA, Manning MR, Aristizabal SA, Oleson JR, Cetas TC (1983) Interstitial thermoradiotherapy in recurrent gynecological malignancies. Gynecol Oncol 15: 95–102

Tarczy-Hornoch P, Lee ER, Sokol JL, Prionas SD, Lohrbach AW, Kapp DS (1992) Automated mechanical thermometry probe mapping systems for hyperthermia. Int J Hyperthermia 8: 543–554

Taylor LS (1978) Electromagnetic syringe. IEEE Trans Biomed Eng 25: 303–304

Taylor LS (1980) Implantable radiators for cancer therapy. IEEE Proc 68: 142–149

Tohnai I, Goto Y, Hayashi Y, Kaneda T, Kobayashi T, Kida Y, Matsui M (1990) Interstitial hyperthermia for cancer of the tongue using an implant heating system. Jpn J Hypertherm Oncol 6: 450–561

Tohnai I, Goto Y, Hayashi Y, Kaneda T, Kobayashi T, Kida Y, Matsui M (1992) The hyperthermochemotherapy of oral cancer using an implant heating system to provide interstitial hyperthermia. In: Gerner EW (ed) Hyperthermic oncology 1992, vol 1. Arizona Board of Regents, Tucson, p 493 (abstract)

Tompkins DT, Partington BP, Steeves RA, Bartholow SD, Paliwal BR (1992) Effect of implant variables on temperatures achieved during ferromagnetic hyperthermia. Int J Hyperthermia 8: 241–251

Trembly BS, Wilson AH, Sullivan MJ, Stein AD, Wong TZ, Strohbehn JW (1986) Control of the SAR pattern within an interstitial microwave array used for hyperthermia. IEEE Trans Microwave Theory Tech 34: 568–571

Trembly BS, Wilson AH, Harvard JM, Sabatakakis K, Strohbehn JW (1988) Comparison of power deposition by in phase 433 and phase modulated 915 MHz interstitial antenna array hyperthermia systems. IEEE Trans Microwave Theory Tech 36: 908–916

Trembly BS, Douple EB, Hoopes PJ (1991) The effect of air cooling on the radial temperature distribution of a single microwave hyperthermia antenna in vivo. Int J Hyperthermia 7: 343–354

Trembly BS, Ryan TP, Strohbehn JW (1992) Physics of microwave hyperthermia. In: Urano M, Douple E (eds) Hyperthermia and oncology, vol 3. Interstitial hyperthermia. VSP, Utrecht, pp 11–98

Tumeh AM, Iskander MF (1989) Performance comparison of available interstitial antennas for microwave hyperthermia. IEEE Trans Microwave Theory Tech 37: 1126–1133

Tupchong L, Nerlinger RE, Waterman FM (1988) Combined use of external beam radiation and interstitial heat for advanced recurrent head and neck carcinomas. In: Abstracts of the 36th Annual Meeting of the Radiation Research Society, Philadelphia, April 16–21, 1988, p 42 (abstract)

Vaupel P, Kallinowski F, Kluge M (1988) Pathophysiology of tumors in hyperthermia. In: Issels RD, Wilmanns W (eds) Application of hyperthermia in the treatment of cancer. Springer, Berlin Heidelberg New York, Recent Results Cancer Research 107: 65–75

Visser AG, Kaatee RSJP (1993) Technical quality assurance for interstitial hyperthermia. In: Seegenschmiedt MH, Sauer R (eds) Interstitial and intracavitary thermoradiotherapy. Springer, Berlin Heidelberg New York, pp 341–345

Visser AG, Deurloo IKK, Levendag PC, Ruifrok ACC, Cornet B, van Rhoon GC (1989) An interstitial hyperthermia system at 27 MHz. Int J Hyperthermia 5: 265–276

Visser AG, Deurloo IKK, van Geel CAJF, van Rhoon GC, Levendag PC (1991) Evaluation of a capacitive-coupling interstitial hyperthermia system. Selectron Brachytherapy Journal 5: 114–119

Vora NL, Luk KH (1993) Interstitial thermoradiotherapy for pelvic tumors: the City of Hope experience. In: Seegenschmiedt MH, Sauer R (eds) Interstitial and intracavitary thermoradiotherapy. Medical Radiology Series. Springer, Berlin Heidelberg New York, pp 257–264

Vora NL, Forell B, Joseph C, Lipsett JA, Archambeau J (1982) Interstitial implant with interstitial hyperthermia. Cancer 50: 2518–2523

Vora NL, Shaw S, Forell B, Desai K, Archambeau J, Pezner RD, Lipsett JA, Covell J (1986) Primary radiation combined with hyperthermia for advanced (stage III - IV) and inflammatory carcinoma of breast. Endocuriether Hypertherm Oncol 2: 101–106

Vora NL, Luk KH, Forell B, et al. (1988) Interstitial local current field hyperthermia for advanced cancers of the cervix. Endocuriether Hypertherm Oncol 4: 97–106

Vora NL, forell B, Luk KH, Pezner RD, Desai KR, Lipsett JA, Wong JYA (1989) Interstitial thermoradiotherapy in recurrent and advanced carcinoma of malignant tumors: seven years experience. In: Sugahara T, Saito M (eds) Hyperthermic oncology 1988, vol 1. Taylor & Francis, London pp 588–590

Westermark F (1898) Über die Behandlung des ulcerierenden Cervixcarcinoms mittels konstanter Wärme. Zbl Gynäkol 22: 1335–1339

Wong JYC, Vora NL, Chou CK, et al. (1988) Intracatheter hyperthermia and iridium-192 radiotherapy in the treatment of bile duct carcinoma. Int J Radiat Oncol Biol Phys 14: 353–359

Wong TZ (1992) Microwave hyperthermia for benign prostatic hyperplasia and adenocarcinoma of the prostate. In: Urano M, Douple e (eds) Hyperthermia and oncology, vol 3. Interstitial hyperthermia. VSP, Utrecht, pp 221–230

Wong TZ, Ryan TP, Strohbehn JW, Jones KM (1989) A phase-coherent interstitial microwave antenna array hyperthermia system. In: Sugahara T, Saito M (eds) Hyperthermic oncology 1988, vol 1. Taylor & Francis, London, pp 894–895

World Health Organisation (1979) Handbook for reporting results of cancer treatment. WHO Offset Publication no 48, WHO, Geneva, Switzerland

Yabumoto E, Suyama S (1985) Interstitial radiofrequency hyperthermia in combination with external beam radiotherapy. In: Overgaard J (ed) Hyperthermic oncology 1984, vol 1. Taylor & Francis, London, pp 579–582

Yabumoto E, Suyama S, Show K, Yamazaki T (1989) A phase I clinical trial of radiofrequency interstitial hyperthermia combined with external radiotherapy. In: Sugahara T, Saito M (eds) Hyperthermic oncology 1988, vol 1. Taylor & Francis, London, pp 591–593

You Q-S, Wang R-Z, Suen G-Q, Yan F-C, Gao Y-J, Cui S-R, Zhao J-H, Zhao T-Z, Ding L (1993) Combination of preoperative radiation and endocavitary hyperthermia for rectal cancer: long term results of 44 patients. Int J Hyperthermia 9: 19–24

van der Zee J, Treurniet-Donker AD, The SK, et al. (1988) Low dose reirradiation in combination with hyperthermia: a palliative treatment for patients with breast cancer recurring in previously irradiated areas. Int J Radiat Oncol Biol Phys 15: 1407–1413

Zhang Y, Joines WT, Oleson JR (1991) Prediction of heating patterns of a microwave interstitial antenna array at various insertion depths. Int J Hyperthermia 7: 197–207

16 Clinical Practice of Intracavitary Thermoradiotherapy

Z. PETROVICH, P. DEBICKI, M.A. ASTRAHAN, and L. BAERT

CONTENTS

16.1 Introduction

During the past 15 years intracavitary heating techniques have emerged as useful new methods of applying hyperthermia in the management of carefully selected cancer patients. The selection process begins with the identification of patients who present with locally advanced cancer arising in a wall of a natural body cavity or those with tumors immediately adjacent to a wall of such a cavity. A common example of the former is carcinoma of the esophagus while the latter is represented by carcinoma of the prostate. Due to a limited radial power deposition, intracavitary hyperthermia (ICHT) can be successfully applied only in patients with *relatively small tumors*. Generally, tumors considered for treatment with ICHT should not exceed 2 cm in radial dimension while they may be considerably larger in longitudinal dimension (ASTRAHAN et al. 1989a,b, 1991a,b). In patients with tumors exceeding 2 cm in radial dimension, hyperthermic temperatures (>42°C) can only be obtained at the periphery of the lesion with the use of a two-antenna ICHT system (DEBICKI et al. 1992).

Application of ICHT in oncology, with rare exceptions (STAWARZ et al. 1993), should be limited to its role as an adjuvant treatment used in combination with radiotherapy and/or chemotherapy. The use of hyperthermia alone in the treatment of cancer is known to result in a low incidence of local tumor control (PEREZ et al. 1990). Additionally, patients considered for ICHT should have a life expectancy of more than 3 months and locally advanced tumors with a propensity for local recurrence following radiotherapy and or chemotherapy.

The main advantage of applying ICHT is the unique ability to treat deep-seated tumors without the problems and complexity associated with the use of deep regional hyperthermia (PETROVICH et al. 1989) or of considerably more invasive and complex interstitial hyperthermia (PEREZ et al. 1990). A major benefit of the use of ICHT is the possibility of applying this technique in sites inaccessible to other hyperthermia modes, such as in the case of carcinoma of the esophagus.

In addition to the use of ICHT in oncology there has been a major interest in applying it as a single modality in patients with benign prostatic hyperplasia (BPH) (PETROVICH et al. 1993a). Treatment of BPH patients with transurethral microwave hyperthermia (TUHT) resulted in major subjective and objective benefit in two-thirds of the patients with moderate to severe prostatism. This was accomplished in poor surgical risk patients for whom the useful therapeutic

Z. PETROVICH, MD, Professor and Chairman, Department of Radiation Oncology, Kenneth Norris Jr. Cancer Hospital and Research Institute, 1441 Eastlake Avenue, Room 34, P.O. Box 33804, Los Angeles, CA 90033-0804, USA
P. DEBICKI, MD, Department of Radiation Oncology, Kenneth Norris Jr. Cancer Hospital and Research Institute, 1441 Eastlake Avenue, Room 34, P.O. Box 33804 Los Angeles, CA 90033-0804, USA
M.A. ASTRAHAN, MD, Department of Radiation Oncology, Kenneth Norris Jr. Cancer Hospital and Research Institute, 1441 Eastlake Avenue, Room 34, P.O. Box 33804, Los Angeles, CA 90033-0804, USA
L. BAERT, MD, Professor and Chairman, Department of Urology, University of Leuven, St. Pieter's Hospital, Brusselsestraat 69, B-3000 Leuven, Belgium

options were very limited (PETROVICH and BAERT 1991). The treatment tolerance was good and no severe late toxicity was reported (PETROVICH et al. 1993a).

16.2 Treatment Technique

16.2.1 Clinical Treatment Approach

ICHT can be applied in most clinical situations without anesthesia, using only mild sedation. Due to a sharp temperature falloff, the precise placement of a hyperthermia applicator is of critical importance. Tumor volume is defined with the use of physical examination and various imaging modalities. An appropriate intracavitary applicator is selected. Since radial power deposition increases with the increase in the diameter of the applicator, the largest diameter applicator usable in a given clinical situation is selected (Fig. 16.1). The selected applicator is then placed into the assigned body cavity against the tumor and its position is verified. Depending on the site treated, this placement verification is accomplished with fluoroscopy, orthogonal radiographs, or ultrasound. Once the applicator position is found to be satisfactory, the treatment can be initiated. A typical ICHT treatment is given for 60 min at the steady state temperature level. The number of treatments varies widely, depending on the site treated and the primary treatment modality. Patients treated with episcleral plaque thermoradiotherapy usually receive a single 45-min hyperthermia treatment (PETROVICH et al. 1991; FINGER 1992). Patients treated with brachytherapy and ICHT for carcinoma of the esophagus receive two or more hyperthermia treatments each of 60 min duration (LI et al. 1982; MAEHARA et al. 1992). Protocols used for the treatment of carcinoma of the prostate of BPH use five or more ICHT treatments, given once or twice per week.

16.2.2 Temperature Monitoring

No ICHT should be administered without careful temperature monitoring throughout each treatment. Systems computing temperature only by using various algorithms based on applied power levels are grossly inaccurate and should not be used in clinical practice. In our opinion, at least two nonperturbing temperature sensors are required. One of these temperature sensors can remain stationary, while the other is used for the purpose of manual or automated thermal mapping. The temperature should be monitored continuously and recorded at least every 2 min. Temperature mapping should be obtained at least 3 times during each 60-min treatment. To increase the safety of the ICHT procedure, temperature mapping every 10 min is recommended. In the event of thermometry system failure during any part of an ICHT session, the treatment must be immediately discontinued.

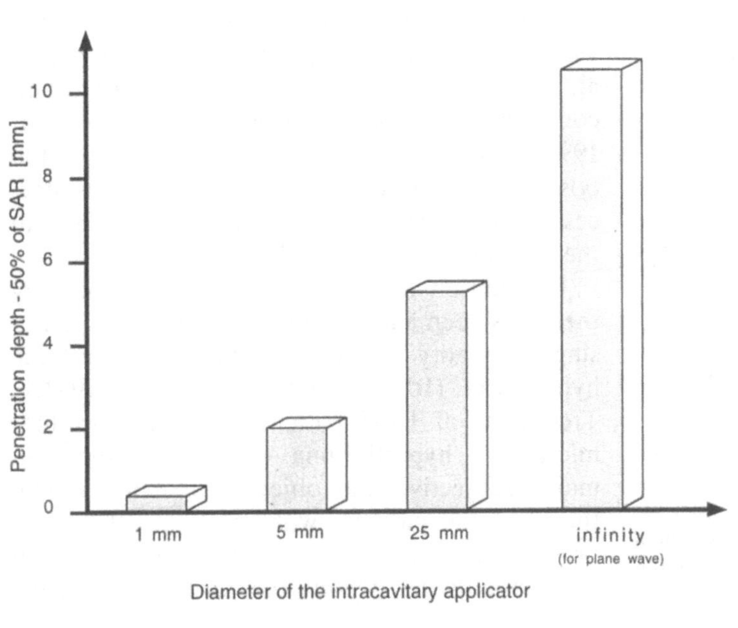

Fig. 16.1. Demonstration of a sharp increase in the depth of the 50% SAR level with the increase in the diameter of intracavitary applicator

Due to anatomical constraints in most patients treated with ICHT only surface temperature monitoring is possible. The surface temperature will always be the highest temperature recorded in any given clinical situation (ASTRAHAN et al. 1991a; DEBICKI et al. 1992). Patients treated with ICHT using a dual applicator system with phase steering require one or more interstitial temperature sensors in addition to the two sensors for each intracavitary applicator (DEBICKI et al. 1992).

16.2.3 General Features

The use of ICHT has various disadvantages and advantages. The disadvantages are:

1. A lack of interstitial (intratumoral) temperature monitoring in most clinical situations
2. Limited radial power deposition
3. Sharp radial temperature falloff resulting in temperature inhomogeneity through the volume of interest

The advantages are:

1. It is a relatively simple technique
2. It is minimally invasive
3. It can be performed without anesthesia
4. Most procedures can be performed on an outpatient basis
5. The technique is reproducible with accurate applicator placement for each treatment
6. Good treatment tolerance
7. No severe acute toxicity or serious late complications
8. An ability to treat deep-seated tumors where other hyperthermia techniques would be difficult or impossible to apply
9. It is easy to combine with irradiation and/or chemotherapy

16.3 Special Clinical Applications

16.3.1 Gastrointestinal Tumors

ICHT has been frequently utilized in patients with gastrointestinal (GI) malignancy, with the esophagus being the most frequently treated primary site (LI et al. 1982; KOCHEGAROV et al. 1981).

16.3.1.1 Carcinoma of the Esophagus

Management of tumors of the esophagus challenges the skills of GI oncologists. Although there has been a dramatic increase in resectability rates, long-term survival rates remain low (<20%) (LI 1982). An additional problem is a high incidence of local tumor recurrence in the esophagus following surgical resection and/or radiotherapy (PETROVICH and BAERT 1993). Recurrent tumors in the esophagus frequently cause distressing signs and symptoms of esophageal obstruction, which greatly diminish the patient's quality of life.

In the early 1980s promising results of clinical trials with the use of ICHT combined with irradiation stimulated interest in further rapid development in this area of hyperthermia (KOCHEGAROV et al. 1981; LI et al. 1982). These trials suggested increased local tumor control in patients treated with intracavitary thermoradiotherapy as compared to those treated with radiotherapy alone. Extensive laboratory and clinical studies including histological examination of the esophageal wall exposed to heat established sound principles for ICHT of the esophagus (LI et al. 1987, 1988, 1989). Several intracavitary microwave applicators have been developed (ASTRAHAN et al. 1989a,b; LIU et al. 1991). These applicators showed predictable and symmetrical power deposition. There was a limited radial penetration with the 50% SAR line being 6–8 mm from the applicator surface (ASTRAHAN et al. 1989; LIU et al. 1991). Some ICHT applicators were designed to be used with intracavitary radiotherapy (ASTRAHAN et al. 1989a,b; PETROVICH et al. 1988).

A major problem with the use of ICHT of the esophagus is a lack of interstitial temperature measurements with a total reliance on the use of intracavitary temperature sensors. We measured interstitial temperature during esophageal ICHT in a patient undergoing thoracotomy for carcinoma of the esophagus. With the patient under general anesthesia thoracotomy was performed in the usual fashion and a specially developed helical applicator (BSD Medical, Salt Lake City, Utah, USA) was placed into the esophagus against the tumor. This applicator was designed to fit within the esophageal applicator for low dose rate brachytherapy (Selectron-LDR Nucletron Co., Leersum, The Netherlands). Hyperthermia was given at 915 MHz with a BSD-300 system (BSD Medical, Salt Lake City, Utah, USA) and a 35 W power level. Temperature was controlled at the applicator surface at 46.5°C (Fig. 16.2). Interstitial and intracavitary temperatures were measured with nonperturbing Bowman-type sensors. Intratumoral temperatures were measured in five sites. The temperatures ranged from a maximum of 43.5°C in the center of the tumor (Fig. 16.2) to a minimum of 39°C at the tumor apex. These interstitial temperature measurements showed that it is possible to obtain hyperthermic temperatures (>42°C) in a case of carcinoma of the esophagus with the use of an intracavitary microwave applicator. However, this case should not be extrapolated to all malignant esophageal lesions.

Multiple clinical trials with the use of ICHT combined with radiotherapy and/or chemotherapy have been reported from Japan, China, and Russia (Goldobenko et al. 1987; Kochegarov et al. 1981; Sugimachi et al. 1988; Matsuda et al. 1992; Kai et al. 1988; Maehara et al. 1992). All of these trials have demonstrated benefit of ICHT in terms of increase in local tumor control and better survival as compared to the patients receiving radiotherapy alone.

It is of particular interest to study histological specimens in patients with carcinoma of the esophagus treated with *preoperative* intracavitary thermoradiochemotherapy (Sugimachi et al. 1992; Matsufuji et al. 1988; Ueo and Sugimachi 1990). These studies showed a statistically significant increase in the number of specimens without viable tumor cells in patients receiving thermoradiochemotherapy as opposed to those treated with preoperative chemoradiotherapy alone. In addition there was a statistically signiicant long-term survival advantage of the ICHT-treated patients (Matsufuji et al. 1988; Ueo and Sugimachi 1990). ICHT of the esophagus has been very well tolerated without major acute or severe late toxicity. See Chap. 6 for details on the treatment outcomes.

16.3.1.2 Carcinoma of the Rectum

Tumors of the rectum constitute common and important lesions. Excellent long-term survival rates have been obtained in surgically treated patients with tumors confined to the rectal wall. Patients with locally advanced lesions, although frequently resectable, have a high incidence of tumor recurrence (Petrovich and Baert 1993).

In order to reduce the incidence of tumor recurrence in these patients with locally advanced rectal carcinoma, preoperative or postoperative radiotherapy has been recommended. Additionally in patients with T4N0M0 lesions adjuvant

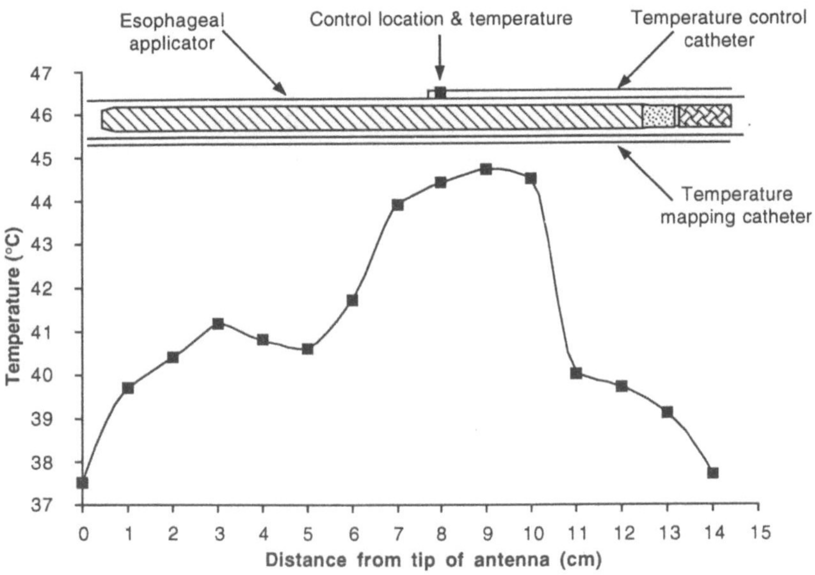

Fig. 16.2. Schematic representation of intraoperative temperature measurements with the use of an intraesophageal helical antenna. The applicator surface temperature was controlled at 46.5°C. Interstitial temperatures were measured in the tumor and across the esophageal wall from the applicator. The temperatures ranged from a minimum of 39°C at the upper pole of the tumor to a maximum of 43.5°C in the center of the tumor. The normal tissue temperature outside of the tumor was 36°C

preoperative therapy has been sought to downstage the lesion and allow for complete resection of the tumor. Both of the above groups of patients may also benefit from adjuvant thermoradiotherapy.

Laboratory studies have helped to establish the thermosensitivity of the rectum. It has been shown that the rectum is more sensitive to hyperthermia than the esophagus in terms of both acute and late complications. However, a temperature ≤43°C appears to be well tolerated without serious acute or late sequelae (Li et al. 1988, 1989).

In clinical trials, ICHT combined with external beam radiotherapy in patients with locally advanced rectal carcinoma showed a significant increase in local tumor control and an increase in long-term survival (Berdov and Menteshashvili 1990; Mori et al. 1991). In a prospective randomized trial of 115 T4N0M0 patients treated with preoperative thermoradiotherapy vs patients receiving preoperative irradiation alone, the 5-year survival was 36% for the former and 7% for the latter group ($P < 0.05$) (Berdov and Menteshashvili 1990).

16.3.1.3 Other Gastrointestinal Tumors

ICHT with brachytherapy or with external beam radiotherapy has been uncommonly used as a treatment for tumors of the GI tract other than carcinoma of the esophagus or rectum (Petrovich and Baert 1993; Wong et al. 1988), e.g., bile duct tumors. The relative paucity of data on ICHT of the bowel and biliary tree is primarily due to difficult access to the site to be treated.

16.3.2 Diseases of the Genitourinary Tract

Over the past 15 years carcinoma of the bladder and of the prostate has been the subject of numerous ICHT phase I–II clinical trials. The reported results suggested a benefit of this treatment in terms of increased local tumor control. However, more clinical work needs to be done to assess the influence of ICHT on long-term survival.

16.3.2.1 Carcinoma of the Prostate

Carcinoma of the prostate (CaP) is the most common malignant tumor seen in American males. Long-term survival rates in excess of 80% have been obtained with surgery or radiotherapy in T1 and T2 tumors (Bagshaw 1985; Duncan et al. 1993). However, treatment results in patients with T3 and T4N0M0 tumors were, as expected, not as good as in patients with tumors confined to the prostatic capsule.

In recent years a controversy has arisen regarding the efficacy of definitive radiotherapy in patients with CaP. The reported incidence of residual cancer following a curse of prostatic irradiation has varied widely from a minimum of approximately 20% to a maximum of more than 90% (Prestidge et al. 1993; Kabalin et al. 1989; Scardino et al. 1986). The true incidence of positive biopsy following irradiation is not known, but it appears to be closer to 20% than to 90%. The above controversy has resulted in an increased interest in the use of other adjuvant therapies, including the implementation of additional hyperthermia.

A study using deep regional hyperthermia combined with radiotherapy showed its effectiveness in patients with locally advanced and/or recurrent CaP (Petrovich et al. 1991; Petrovich and Baert 1991). However, a difficulty with the use of deep regional hyperthermia is the need for a stable performance of the cardiovascular system, which in patients with CaP frequently presents a problem. In this context ICHT has become an attractive treatment option in spite of the very limited radial power deposition seen with the use of this hyperthermia mode.

Yerushalmi et al. (1982) reported an excellent long-term palliative effect in 15 locally advanced cases of CaP treated with a transrectal microwave applicator at 2450 MHz without cooling. No temperature data were provided in this study.

More recently, 44 patients with locally advanced CaP were treated with transrectal microwave hyperthermia at 915 MHz using a water-cooled applicator. Temperatures were monitored in the rectum and urethra and ranged from 41° to 44°C. A total of six to ten treatments were given on a once or twice a week schedule (Servadio and Leib 1991). The authors reported good results in terms of palliation and local tumor control. This study, however, is difficult to evaluate since nearly all patients received simultaneous pelvic irradiation and/or hormonal treatment. Similar good treatment results with the use of transrectal microwave hyperthermia have been reported in a study of 46 stage D_1 and D_2 CaP patients. An excellent palliative benefit was noted, which lasted for at least 24 months (Montorsi et al. 1992). Stawarz et al. (1993) reported treatment results in 15 patients treated with six transrectal microwave treatments and followed for at least 5 years. The authors found an excellent and long-lasting palliative effect, with 5 of the 15 treated patients surviving more than 5 years, including three who had no evidence of CaP at the last follow-up. It is of importance to note that 2 of the 15 treated patients had complete regression of distant metastatic disease for 5 years or longer. This interesting finding was additionally investigated by studies of cell-mediated immunity (Szmigielski et al. 1991; Stawarz et al. 1993) and needs to be confirmed in further clinical trials.

Transrectal ultrasound hyperthermia combined with external beam irradiation has been under study at the University of Arizona for patients with stage C_2 or D_1 CaP (Fosmire et al. 1993). Good temperature data were obtained. In 90% of treatments, tolerance was good or fair and no serious complications were reported.

Strohmaier et al. (1991) treated 20 CaP patients preoperatively with transrectal microwave hyperthermia. Intraprostatic temperatures of 42°–43°C were obtained. Histological examination of prostatectomy specimens obtained 1–2 weeks following completion of ICHT showed edema, hyperemia, and white cell infiltrates of the prostate but no tumor necrosis.

The simultaneous use of newly designed transrectal and transurethral microwave applicators has been under study at the University of Southern California. Ultimately, detailed interstitial temperatures were performed in six patients. A transrectal applicator alone was able to heat the prostate to >42°C within 2 cm of the rectal wall, while transuretharal applicators alone were heating periurethral prostatic tissue to >42°C within 6 mm of the urethral wall (Debicki et al. 1992). In either case the highest temperatures were measured next to each applicator with a subsequent steep temperature falloff. However, energizing both applicators simultaneously resulted in a different heating pattern. This was particularly apparent with an appropriate phase " steering" technique. The highest temperatures were measured in the center of the prostate rather than next to the urethra or rectum (Debicki et al. 1992). Based on these studies a phase I–II clinical trial was initiated using a dual-applicator system ICHT combined with pelvic irradiation in patients with locally advanced prostate carcinoma. Figure 16.3 demonstrates this temperature distribution with the combined use of transrectal and transurethral applicators. The following parameters were used in these calculations of power deposition: microwave frequency, 915 MHz; applied power of the transurethral applicator, 15 W; applied power of the transrectal applicator, 45 W.

16.3.2.2 Carcinoma of the Bladder

A number of phase I–II clinical trials have been conducted in patients with locally advanced transitional cell carcinoma of the bladder using a multidisciplinary therapeutic approach. These trials utilized a combination of thermoradiochemotherapy and were conducted primarily in Japan, Germany, and Italy (Kubota et al. 1984; Bichler et al. 1989; Matsui et al. 1991; Rigatti et al. 1991). The interpretation of the achieved treatment results reported from these trials is rather difficult. There appears to be a significant increase in the response rate in patients treated with regimens containing hyperthermia combined with radiochemotherapy as compared to those receiving radiotherapy alone. Treatment tolerance was reported to be very good and no serious complications were observed. There is a need for prospective randomized trials to assess the effectiveness of adjuvant hyperthermia in patients with locally advanced transitional carcinoma of the bladder.

16.3.2.3 Benign Prostatic Hyperplasia

Benign prostatic hyperplasia is a very common disease affecting a large number of older males. Considerable controversy exists as to the time of possible therapeutic interventions in BPH patients. In a recently reported study moderate to severe obstructive symptoms were seen in 13% of males from 40 to 49 years of age and in 28% of males older than 70 years (Chute et al. 1993). It has been estimated that 25% of all male patients in the United States will require treatment for BPH during their lifetime.

The treatment of choice for BPH is considered to be transurethral resection of the prostate (TURP). The procedure is performed in the United States on nearly 400 000 patients annually. Treatment morbidity of importance has been reported in approximately 20% of surgically treated BPH

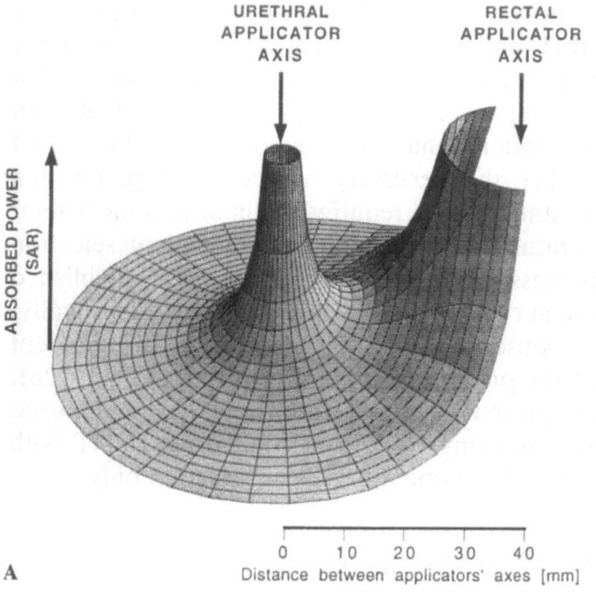

A

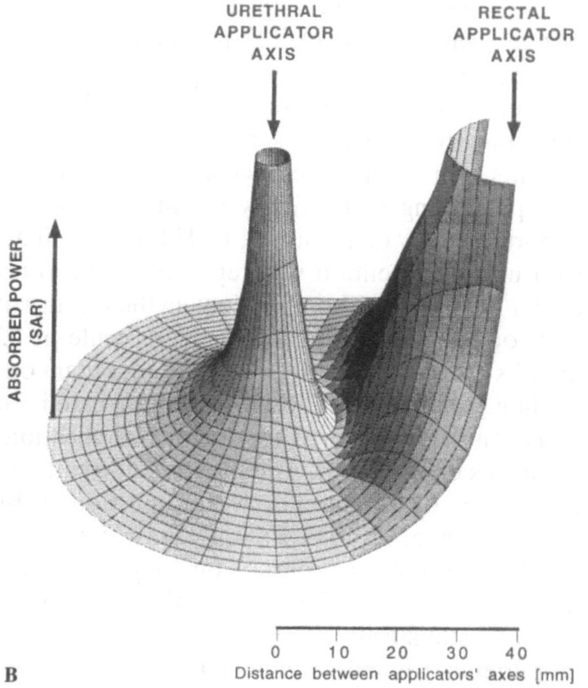

B

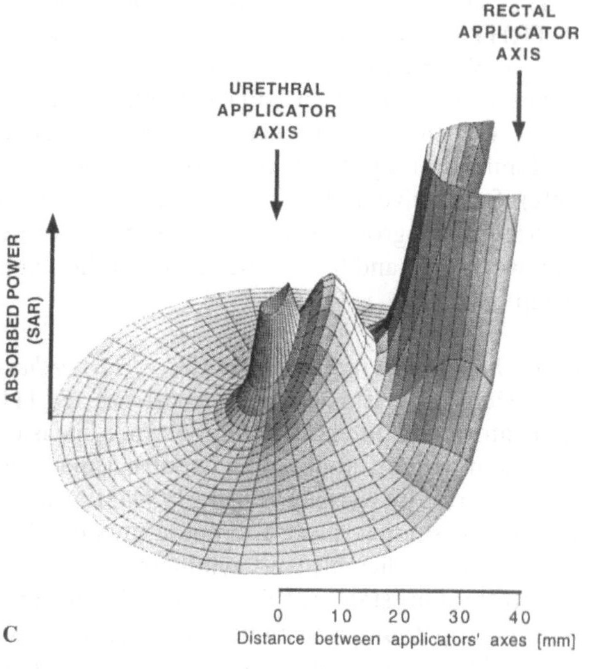

C

Fig. 16.3A–C. Calculated power deposition with simultaneous use of transrectal and transurethral microwave applicators. Both applicators were driven at 915 MHz. The applied power of the transrectal applicator was 45 W, and that of the transurethral applicator, 15 W. **A** Both applicators were operated as *incoherent* sources. Note a sharp increase in SAR next to each applicator and a decrease in SAR 10–15 mm from each antenna. **B** Similar pattern of power deposition as in **A**, with both applicators operated as *coherent* sources with destructive interference. **C** Both applicators were operated as *coherent* sources with constructive interference. Note a broad peak of increased power deposition between the applicators

patients (Roos et al. 1989). Because of this relatively high treatment morbidity associated with surgical resection there has been growing interest in the development of a less invasive but equally effective treatment for BPH. Therefore ICHT has been under intensive study in the treatment of this disease since the early 1980s. Nowadays ICHT for BPH can be applied transrectally or transurethrally or both.

16.3.2.3.1 Transrectal Hyperthermia (TRHT). The first report on the use of TRHT was published by Yerushalmi et al. (1985). A total of 29 patients with high surgical risks and moderate to severe of BPH were treated with a 2450-MHz TRHT system. An average of 12 treatments, each of 60 min, were given on an outpatient basis, without any sedation or anesthesia. Excellent subjective and objective benefit was reported in nearly all patients. This included especially 8 of the 11 patients presenting with urinary retention. Another important study on the use of TRHT in 72 patients with urinary retention was reported by LINDNER et al. (1990a). At 1 month following the treatment 50% of patients were catheter free, while at 12 months post-treatment 40% had spontaneous voiding. Of the 435 TRHT patients treated for BPH, only 27 (6%) had treatment complications (LINDNER et al. 1990b). These excellent treatment results in BPH patients were questioned by STROHMAIER et al. (1990) and STAWARZ et al. (1991). The former group of investigators found no effectiveness of TRHT while the latter group showed statistically significant, better results in patients treated with TUHT than in those receiving TRHT. KAPLAN et al. (1992) reported a good (>41.5°C ± 1°C) temperature distribution in the prostate in 15 BPH patients treated with TRHT. These investigators recommended the use of TRHT as an effective treatment for urinary outflow obstruction caused by BPH.

The use of TRHT in BPH patients was compared with the sham procedure in a prospective randomized study of 68 patients (ZERBIB et al. 1992). Subjective and objective response rates in the treatment group were 68% and 53%, while they were 33% and 0%, respectively, in the sham group.

16.3.2.3.2 Transurethral Microwave Hyperthermia. Heating characteristics of various TUHT applicators and interstitial temperature measurements in patients undergoing hyperthermia have been reported by ASTRAHAN et al. (1989a, 1991a,b). The above studies showed temperatures of 42°C distributed predictably and symmetrically in the periurethral prostate, within 6 mm of the urethral wall. Histopathological studies of patients receiving TUHT demonstrated a sharply demarcated zone of hemorrhagic necrosis limited to the immediate periurethral prostate in a pattern predicted by the reported interstitial temperature measurements (BAERT et al. 1990; LAUWERYNS et al. 1991). Ultimately, healing of the necrotic zone took place and the resulting scar tissue retracted the urethra, permitting a decrease in urinary outflow obstruction.

In two phase I studies of 36 high surgical risk BPH patients major subjective and objective improvement was noted in more than 70% (SAPOZINK et al. 1990; BAERT et al. 1990). In subsequent phase I–II studies with the use of TUHT the necessary number of hyperthermia treatments, the required optimal treatment temperature, and the appropriate patient selection process for hyperthermia have been established (BAERT et al. 1991, 1992, 1993). Additionally, response to TUHT was found to be independent of the prostate volume (PETROVICH et al. 1992a). At present a phase III prospective randomized trial is being conducted comparing TUHT with surgical treatment versus observation only.

16.3.3 Gynecological Tumors

Patients with locally advanced carcinoma of the cervix and vagina are particularly suitable for the use of adjuvant ICHT. Heating characteristics of several intracavitary microwave applicators for cervical and vaginal tumors have been reported (ZHONG et al. 1990; LI et al. 1991; RYAN et al. 1992). A maximum temperature of 51.5°C was reported on the applicator surface, with an average temperature of 46.0°C ± 2.1°C at the center of the cervical carcinoma and an average of 44.5°C ± 0.8°C at its periphery (LI et al. 1991). The same investigators also reported a good treatment tolerance in 28 of the 30; treated patients.

The use of combined interstitial microwave hyperthermia with ICHT antennae placed in a modified vaginal obturator permitted an improved temperature distribution in a larger tumor volume (RYAN et al. 1992).

In a prospective randomized trial of 50 patients with stage II and III carcinoma of the cervix, treated with an ICHT/radiotherapy combination versus radiotherapy alone, significantly better tumor control was noted in the group receiving ICHT (SHARMA et al. 1990). The treatment was well tolerated and during a minimum follow-up period of 18 months no additive or late toxicity of ICHT was recorded. Clinical results in patients with locally advanced tumors are shown in Table 16.1.

16.3.4 Tumors of Other Sites

Few case reports are available on the treatment of patients with recurrent carcinoma of trachea or

Table 16.1. Selected clinical results with intracavitary hyperthermia for locally advanced tumors

Site treated	Investigator	N	Treatment	HT°C	Effects	% Survival		
						2 ys	5 ys	Median
Esophagus	Ueo and Sugimachi 1990	62	HT[1] – CT[2] + RT[3] + Surg	42.5–44		50	43	
		121	CT – RT + Surg			27	15	
		31	HT – CT – RT	42.5–44		15		
		83	CT – RT			1		
	Sugimachi et al. 1992	27	HT – CT – RT + Surg	42.5–44	27% no ca in surg. specimen			
		26	CT – RT + Surg		8% no ca in surg. specimen			
	Matsufugi et al. 1988	16	Surg			0		
		38	RT – CT + Surg			16		
		10	HT – CT – RT + Surg	42–45		34		
Rectum	Berdov 1990	56	HT – RT + Surg	42–43	CR[4] 54%		36	
		59	RT + Surg		CR[5] 34%		7	
	Montorsi et al. 1992	44	Transrectal HT	43.5	Improved quality of life at 2 ys in 80% patients.			
Prostate	Servadio 1991	44	Transrectal HT – RT	41–44	"Improvement in most patients"			
	Petrovich et al. 1993	15	Transcrectal HT	43	Major long term palliative benefit in 53% of patients			
Bladder	Matsui et al. 1991	56	HT – CT – RT	42–43	CR 45% PR 37%			
Cervix	Sharma et al. 1990	25	HT – RT	42–43	"No increase in complications improved local tumor control"			
		25	RT					
Benign prostatic hyperplasia	Petrovich et al. 1993	36	Transurethral HT	44–45	Major improvement in >70% patients			

[1] Hyperthermia [2] Chemotherapy [3] Radiotherapy [4] Complete response [5] Partial response

nasopharynx managed with a combination of ICHT and brachytherapy or teletherapy (Petrovich and Baert 1993; Zhong et al. 1990).

An important application of thermoradiotherapy is in its use in the management of uveal melanoma (Finger 1992; Petrovich et al. 1992b; Petrovich and Baert 1993). The treatment is given using a specially designed episcleral gold plaque, which contains radioactive isotope, usually iodine-125. The same modified episcleral plaque may also serve as a radiofrequency radiator. The use of adjuvant hyperthermia has permitted a substantial radiation dose reduction, resulting in a lower incidence of treatment complications while at the same time maintaining a high incidence of local tumor control (see Chap. 13 for details).

16.4 Conclusions

Intracavitary hyperthermia has emerged as an important adjuvant treatment in selected patients with tumors of the esophagus, prostate, vagina and cervix, rectum, and eye. However, the evaluation of treatment outcome in many published reports presents a major problem. There is a lack of sufficiently detailed data on patients and tumors, making the interpretation of results very difficult. Many reports lack sufficient temperature data. It is a strong feeling of the authors that such reports should not be accepted for publication as they may be misleading and are of very limited scientific value.

ICHT is also useful in the treatment of certain benign tumorous diseases. It is becoming a major nonsurgical treatment for patients with BPH. It also may be of interest to study ICHT in patients with chronic nonbacterial prostatitis refractory to the standard treatments.

16.5 Summary

Advantages of ICHT

- Predictable temperature distribution: $T \geqslant 42°C$ is easy to obtain and easy to maintain
- Minimally invasive technique: Reproducible and relatively easy applicator insertion
- Good to excellent treatment tolerance: Low incidence of early and late treatment complications
- Suitable for treatment with radiotherapy of recurrent or locally advanced primary tumors (esophagus, prostate, vagina, cervix, rectum and eye)
- Effective as a single modality treatment for benign prostatic hyperplasia, prostadynia and chronic nonbacterial prostatitis refractory to standard therapy

Disadvantages of ICHT

- Limited radial power deposition
- The need for invasive interstitial thermometry
- Requirement for highly selected patients with tumors arising from or adjacent to natural body cavities such as: esophagus, rectum, urethral etc.

References

Astrahan MA, Sapozink MD, Cohen D, et al. (1989a) Microwave applicator for transurethral hyperthermia of benign prostatic hyperplasia. Int J Hyperthermia 5: 283–296

Astrahan MA, Sapozink MD, Luxton G, Kampp T, Petrovich Z (1989b) A technique for combining microwave hyperthermia with intraluminal brachytherapy of the esophagus. Int J Hyperthermia 5: 37–51

Astrahan MA, Ameye F, Oyen R, Willemen P, Baert L, Petrovich Z (1991a) Interstitial temperature measurements during transurethral microwave hyperthermia. J Urol 145: 304–308

Astrahan MA, Imanaka K, Jozsef G, Ameye F, Baert L, Sapozink MD, Petrovich Z (1991b) Heating characteristics of a helical microwave applicator for transurethral hyperthermia of benign prostatic hyperplasia. Int J Hyperthermia 7: 141–155

Baert L, Ameye F, Willemen P, et al. (1990) Transurethral microwave hyperthermia for benign prostatic hyperplasia: preliminary clinical and pathological results. J Urol 144: 1383–1387

Baert L, Willemen P, Ameye F, Petrovich Z (1991) Treatment response with transurethral microwave hyperthermia in different forms of benign prostatic hyperplasia. Prostate 18: 315–320

Baert L, Ameye F, Pike M, Willemen P, Astrahan MA, Petrovich Z (1992) Transurethral hyperthermia for BPH patients with retention. J Urol 147: 1558–1561

Baert L, Ameye F, Pike M, Petrovich Z (1994) Optimization of transurethral Hyperthermia: number of treatments. Urology 43: 567–571

Bagshaw MA (1985) Potential for radiotherapy alone in prostatic cancer. Cancer 55: 2079–2085

Berdov BA, Menteshashvili GZ (1990) Thermoradiotherapy of patients with locally advanced carcinoma of the rectum. Int J Hyperthermia 6: 881–890

Bichler KH, Fluchter SH, Steimann J, Strohmaier WL (1989) Combination of hyperthermia and cytostatics in the treatment of bladder cancer. Urol Int 44: 10–14

Chute CG, Panser LA, Girman CJ, et al. (1993) The prevalence of prostatism: a populationbased survey of urinary symptoms. J Urol 150: 85–89

Debicki P, Astrahan MA, Ameye F, et al. (1992) Temperature steering in the prostate by simultaneous transurethral and transrectal hyperthermia. Urology 40: 300–307

Duncan W, Warde P, Catton CN, et al. (1993) Carcinoma of the prostate: results of radical radiotherapy (1970–1985). Int J Radiat Oncol Biol Phys 26: 203–210

Finger PT (1992) Microwave plaque thermoradiotherapy for choroidal melanoma. Br J Ophthalmol 76: 358–364

Fosmire H, Hynynen K, Orach GW, et al. (1993) Feasibility and toxicity of transrectal ultrasound hyperthermia in the treatment of locally advanced adenocarcinoma of the prostate. Int J Radiat Oncol Biol Phys 26: 253–259

Goldobenko GV, Durnov LA, Knysh IV, et al. (1987) Experience in the use of thermoradiotherapy of malignant tumors. Med Radiol 32: 30–35

Kabalin JN, Hodge KK, McNeal JE, et al. (1989) Identification of residual cancer in the prostate following radiation therapy: role of transrectal ultrasound guided biopsy and prostate specific antigen. J Urol 142: 326–331

Kai H, Matsufuji H, Okudaira Y, Sugimachi K (1988) Heat, drugs and radiation given in combination is palliative for unresectable esophageal cancer. Int J Radiat Oncol Biol Phys 14: 1147–1152

Kaplan SA, Shabsigh R, Saldo K, Olsson CA (1992) Prostatic and periprostatic temperature measurements in patients treated with transrectal thermal therapy (local intracavitary microwave hyperthermia). J Urol 147: 1562–1565

Kochegarov AA, Maratkhodzhazv NK, Alimorazov SA (1981) Hyperthermia in the combined treatment of esophageal cancer patients. J Sov Oncol 2: 17–22

Kubota Y, Shuin T, Miura T, Nishimura R, Fukushima S, Takai S (1984) Treatment of bladder cancer with a combination of hyperthermia radiation and bleomycin. Cancer 53: 199–202

Lauweryns J, Baert L, Vandenhove J, Petrovich Z (1991) Histopathology of prostatic tissue after transurethral hyperthermia. Int J Hyperthermia 7: 221–230

Li DJ (1990) Present status on treatment of esophageal cancer in China. Int J Radiat Oncol Biol Phys 18: 477–484

Li DJ, Wang CQ, Qiu SL, Shao LF (1982) Intraluminal microwave hyperthermia in the combined treatment of esophageal cancer. A preliminary report of 103 patients. Natl Cancer Inst Mongr 61: 419–421

Li DJ, Zhou SL, Qiu SL, Qiao SJ (1987) thermodamage, thermosensitivity and thermotolerance of normal swine esophagus. Int J Hyperthermia 3: 141–151

Li DJ, Qiu SL, Zhou SL, Liu HL (1988) Acute heat injury to the normal swine rectum. Int J Hyperthermia 4: 191–201

Li DJ, Qiu SL, Zhou SL (1989) Late heat damage in normal swine rectum: a comparison of thermosensitivity of rectum and esophagus. Int J Hyperthermia 5: 717–724

Li DJ, Chou CK, Luk KH, et al. (1991) Design of intracavitary microwave applicators for the treatment of uterine cervix carcinoma. Int J Hyperthermia 7: 693–701

Lindner A, Braf Z, Lev A, et al. (1990a) Local hyperthermia of the prostate gland for the treatment of benign prostatic hypertrophy and urinary retention. Br J Urol 65: 201–203

Lindner A, Siegel YI, Saranga R, et al. (1990b) Complications in hyperthermia treatment of benign prostatic hyperplasia. J Urol 144: 1390–1392

Liu RL, Zhang EY, Gross EJ, Cetas TC (1991) Heating pattern of helical microwave intracavitary esophageal applicator. Int J Hyperthermia 7: 577–586

Maehara Y, Kuwano H, Kitamura K, et al. (1992) Hyperthermochemo-radiotherapy for esophageal cancer (review). Anticancer Res 12: 805–810

Matsuda H, Tsutsui S, Morita M, et al. (1992) Hyperthermo-chemo-radiotherapy as a definitive treatment for patients with early esophageal carcinoma. Am J Clin Oncol (CCT) 15: 509–514

Matsufuji H, Kuwano H, Hidenobu K, et al. (1988) Preoperative hyperthermia combined with radiotherapy and chemotherapy for patients with incompletely resected carcinoma of the esophagus. Cancer 62: 889–894

Matsui K, Takebayashi S, Watai K, et al. (1991) Combination radiotherapy of urinary bladder carcinoma with chemohyperthermia. Int J Hyperthermia 7: 19–26

Montorsi F, Guazzoni G, Colombo R, et al. (1992) Transrectal microwave hyperthermia for advanced prostate cancer: long term clinical results. J Urol 148: 342–345

Mori M, Sugimachi K, Matsuda H, et al. (1991) Preoperative hyperthermochemoradiotherapy for patients with rectal cancer. In: Sekiba K (ed) Hyperthermic Oncology, 1990. Asahi Print, Okayama, Japan, pp 109–110

Ohno S, Morita M, Tsutsui S, et al. (1990) Correlation between hyperthermoradiosensitivity and clinical effect in carcinoma of the esophagus. Surg Gynecol Obstet 171: 472–476

Perez CA (1990) International consensus meeting on hyperthermia. Final report. Int J Hyperthermia 6: 837–877

Petrovich Z, Baert L (1991) Hyperthermia in the management of benign and malignant tumors of the prostate. In: Sekiba K (ed) Hyperthermic oncology, 1990. Asahi Print, Okayama, Japan, pp 1–10

Petrovich Z, Baert LV (1993) Intracavitary thermoradiotherapy for various tumor sites. In: Seegenschmiedt MH, Sauer R (eds) Interstitial and intracavitary thermoradiotherapy. Springer, Berlin Heidelberg New York pp 311–317

Petrovich Z, Astrahan MA, Lam K, Tildon T, Luxton G, Jepson J (1988) Intraluminal thermoradiotherapy with teletherapy for carcinoma of the esophagus. Endocurietherapy Hyperthermia Oncol 4: 155–161

Petrovich Z, Langholz B, Gibbs FA, et al. (1989) Regional hyperthermia for advanced tumors: a study of 353 patients. Int J Radiat Oncol Biol Phys 16: 601–607

Petrovich Z, Emami B, Kapp DS, et al. (1991) Regional hyperthermia in patients with recurrent genitourinary cancer. Am J Clin Oncol 14: 472–477

Petrovich Z, Ameye F, Pike M, Boyd S, Baert L (1992a) The relationship of response to transurethral hyperthermia and prostate volume in BPH patients. Urology 40: 317–321

Petrovich Z, Astrahan MA, Luxton G, Green R, Langholz B, Liggett PE (1992b) Episcleral plaque thermoradiotherapy in patients with choroidal melanoma. Int J Radiat Oncol Biol Phys 23: 599–603

Petrovich Z, Ameye F, Baert L, et al. (1993a) New trends in the treatment of benign prostatic hyperplasia and carcinoma of the prostate. Am J Clin Oncol 16: 187–200

Petrovich Z, Astrahan MA, Luxton G, et al. (1993b) Primary malignant melanoma of the uvea: radioactive plaque therapy and other treatment modalities. In: Alberti WE, Sagerman RH (eds) Radiotherapy of intraocular and orbital tumors. Springer, Berlin Heidelberg New York, pp 31–44

Prestidge BR, Kaplan I, Cox RS, Bagshaw MA (1993) The clinical significance of a positive post-irradiation prostatic biopsy without metastases. Int J Radiat Oncol Biol Phys 24: 403–408

Rigatti P, Lev A, Colombo R (1991) Combined intravesical chemotherapy with Mitomycin C and local bladder microwave-induced hyperthermia as a preoperative therapy for surgical bladder tumors. A preliminary clinical study. Eur Urol 20: 204–210

Roos NP, Wennberg JE, Malenka DJ, et al. (1989) Mortality and reoperation after open and transurethral resection of the prostate for benign prostatic hyperplasia. N Engl J Med 320: 1120–1124

Ryan TP, Taylor JH, Coughlin CT (1992) Interstitial microwave hyperthermia and brachytherapy for malignancies of the vulva and vagina. I Design and testing of modified intracavitary obturator. Int J Radiat Oncol Biol Phys 23: 189–199

Sapozink MD, Boyd SD, Astrahan MA, et al. (1990) Transurethral hyperthermia for benign prostatic hyperplasia: preliminary clinical results. J Urol 143: 944–950

Scardino PT, Frankel JM, Wheeler TM, et al. (1986) The prognostic significance of post-radiation biopsy results in patients with prostatic cancer. J Urol 135: 510–516

Servadio C, Leib Z (1991) Local hyperthermia for prostate cancer. Urology 38: 307–309

Sorbe B, Roos DI, Karlsson LG (1990) The use of microwave induced hyperthermia in conjunction with afterloading irradiation of vaginal carcinoma. A preliminary report. Acta Oncol 29: 1029–1033

Sharma S, Sandhu APS, Patel FD (1990) Side effects of local hyperthermia: results of a prospective randomized clinical study. Int J Hyperthermia 6: 279–285

Stawarz B, Szmigielski S, Ogrodnik J, Astrahan MA, Petrovich Z (1991) A comparison of transurethral and transrectal microwave hyperthermia in poor surgical risk BPH patients. J Urol 146: 353–357

Stawarz B, Zielinski H, Szmigielski S, et al. (1993) Transrectal hyperthermia as a palliative treatment for advanced adenocarcinoma of the prostate and a study of cell mediated immunity. Urology 41: 548–553

Strohmaier WL, Bichler KH, Flüchter SH, Wilbert DM (1990) Local microwave hyperthermia of benign prostatic hyperplasia. J Urol 144: 913–917

Strohmaier WL, Bichler KH, Bocking A, Flüchter SH (1991) Histological effects of local microwave hyperthermia in prostatic cancer. Int J Hyperthermia 7: 27–33

Sugimachi K, Matsuda H, Ohno S, Fukuda A, Matsuoka H, Mori M, Kuwano H (1988) Long term effects of hyperthermia combined with chemotherapy and irradiation for the treatment of patients with carcinoma of the esophagus. Surg Gynecol Obstet 169: 319–323

Sugimachi K, Kitamura K, Baba K, et al. (1992) Hyperthermia combined with chemotherapy and irradiation for patients with carcinoma of the esophagus – a prospective randomized trial. Int J Hyperthermia 8: 289–295

Szmigielski S, Sobczynski J, Sokolska G, Stawarz B, Zielinski H, Petrovich Z (1991) Effects of local prostatic hyperthermia on human NK and T-cell function. Int J Hyperthermia 7: 869–880

Ueo H, Sugimachi K (1990) preoperative hyperthermo-chemo-radiotherapy for patients with esophageal carcinoma or rectal carcinoma. Semin Surg Oncol 6: 8–13

Wong JYC, Vora NL, Chou CK, et al. (1988) Intracavitary hyperthermia and iridium-192 radiotherapy in the treatment of bile duct carcinoma. Int J Radiat Oncol Biol Phys 14: 353–359

Yerushalmi A, Servadio C, Leib Z, et al. (1982) Local hyperthermia for treatment of carcinoma of the prostate. A preliminary report. Prostate 3: 623–630

Yerushalmi A, Fishelowitz Y, Singer D, et al. (1985) Localized deep microwave hyperthermia in the treatment of poor operative risk patients with benign prostatic hyperplasia. J Urol 133: 873–876

Zerbib M, Steg A, Conguy S, et al. (1992) Localized hyperthermia versus the sham procedure in obstructive benign hyperplasia of the prostate: a prospective randomized study. J Urol 147: 1048–1052

Zhong QR, Chou CK, McDougall JA, et al. (1990) Intracavitary hyperthermia applicators for treating nasopharyngeal and cervical cancer. Int J Hyperthermia 6: 997–1004

17 Clinical Practice of Intraoperative Thermoradiotherapy

T.A. Colacchio and T.P. Ryan

CONTENTS

T.A. Colacchio, MD, Professor of Surgery, Section of General Surgery, Dartmouth-Hitchcock Medical Center, Lebanon, NH 03756, USA
T.P. Ryan, MS, Section of General Surgery, Dartmouth-Hitchcock Medical Center, Lebanon, NH 03756, USA

17.1 Introduction

Despite the increasing use of multimodality therapy, locally advanced and recurrent abdominal malignancies (in particular, pancreatic and colorectal) continue to be the cause of significant cancer-related morbidity and mortality.

17.1.1 Pancreatic Cancer

An estimated 27700 Americans will develop pancreatic carcinoma this year (Boring et al. 1993), and 90% will succumb within 1 year. At the time of surgery 85%–90% of malignancies are unresectable, yet nearly half of this patient group will have only local or regional disease (Aston and Longmire 1973; Tepper 1976, Levine et al. 1978; Wilson and Block 1974). Even in the patients undergoing surgical resection, 5-year survival rates are only 10%–20% (Connolly and Dawson 1987; Trede 1985; Fortner 1984; Sindelar 1989; Cameron and Christ 1991). Radiation therapy has been shown to have a definite effect on disease control but little impact on survival (Dobelbower 1981; Rich 1985; Haslom 1973; Shipley et al. 1980; Whittington et al. 1981), whereas the Gastrointestinal Tumor Study Group showed an improved median survival from 5.5 to 12.5 months in patients without distant metastases receiving high-dose radiotherapy (RT) and 5-fluorouracil (5-FU) (GITSG 1988). With the limitations of normal tissue tolerance, several centers in the United States and Japan have reported the use of an *intraoperative radiotherapy boost* (IORT) in the management of pancreatic cancer (Shipley et al. 1984; Roldan et al. 1988; Gunderson et al. 1987; TUCKSON 1988; ABE 1987; HOEKSTRA et al. 1988; SINDELAR 1988). Despite varying techniques, initial reports noted some improvement in local control, but there was no significant increase in cure rates. This was reinforced by the multi-institutional trial (RTOG 8505) of external beam radiotherapy (EBRT) plus 5-FU in conjunction with IORT in patients with unresectable nonmetastatic pancreatic cancers. Of the 51 analyzed patients the median survival was 9 months and the 18-month actuarial survival was 9% (TEPPER et al. 1991). Two other reports of IORT in patients with unresected pancreatic primaries from Japan and Spain have corroborated these poor clinical results (ABE et al. 1991; CALVO and SANTOS 1991). Nevertheless, encouraging data included a series from Japan of patients undergoing a combination of extended radical resection plus IORT, and this group (14 patients) had a 5-year survival of 33.3% (HIRAOKA et al. 1990). In an attempt to maximize the possible resectability of these patients and gain the added advantage of combination therapy, there have been two recent reports of trials using *neoadjuvant chemoradiation with IORT ± resection* in locally advanced pancreatic cancer. In one (EVANS et al. 1992), 23 of 28 patients underwent exploration following chemoradiation and 17 of these were able to undergo resection (61%). In the second (JESSUP et al. 1993), only 2 of the 14 patients completing the neoadjuvant therapy were able to undergo resection. Nevertheless, both these reports demonstrated advanced regional disease as the cause for unresectability in a large portion of the unresected cases: 3 of 11 and 5 of 12 respectively. Based on these preliminary data, RTOG 9102 was begun as a phase III study to evaluate the benefit of adding IORT to chemoradiation in nonmetastatic, unresectable cases.

17.1.2 Colorectal Cancer

In contrast to pancreatic carcinoma, cancer of the colon and rectum is the most common visceral cancer in the United States, with 152000 new cases anticipated this year (BORING et al. 1993). Early-stage lesions are effectively treated with surgery, and recently reported trials with levamisole and 5-FU (GREM 1991) have demonstrated an improvement in disease-free survival and overall survival of 47%–63% and 55%–71% respectively for patients with node-positive primary disease. Despite this, regional recurrence is a major problem, with rates approaching 50%–80% following surgery alone for rectal cancer (BENOTTI 1987; TEPPER 1987; EISENBERG 1982). The adjuvant use of EBRT either pre- or postoperatively has markedly decreased the local recurrence in stage B2, C, and D rectal and rectosigmoid cancers (TEPPER 1987; ROSCUIT 1975; STEVENS 1976; RIDER 1975; GUNDERSON 1980; EMAMI 1982; PILEPICH 1978). However, the high RT doses required to control local disease increase the complication rates (WANG 1962), and patients who do not undergo complete resection have a poor survival rate (KLIGERMAN 1975; TEPPER 1983; WITHERS 1977). Uncontrolled pelvic recurrence causes tremendous morbidity and the results with systemic chemotherapy have generally been poor (EINHORN and WILLIAMS 1984).

This dilemma has led to renewed enthusiasm for IORT (GOLDSON 1981), which is currently being utilized in the United States to provide a "boost" dose in conjunction with surgical resection and EBRT. In a large clinical series of patients with locally advanced colorectal carcinomas (TEPPER et al. 1986; WILLETT et al. 1991a,b) who received preoperative EBRT plus IORT, the group having a complete resection (microscopic residual) had a 4-year suvival rate of 79%, as compared to 44% in those with a partial resection. and only 27% in those with unresected tumors. These reports highlight the relationship between the completeness of surgical resection and outcome; nevertheless, they stress that even completely resected lesions still have local recurrences. Similar survival rates and difficulties with local recurrence have been reported in the Mayo Clinic series (GUNDERSON et al. 1988), and the preliminary results of RTOG-8508 have been presented and once again demonstrate that the amount of local disease remaining determines both frequency of local recurrence and survival, with 22% of patients with microscopic disease failing locally and dying of their disease (LANCIANO 1990).

17.1.3 Rationale for and Principles of Intraoperative Hyperthermia

The above results show that despite the aggressive approach of combination IORT, surgical resection, and EBRT to control local disease recurrence in pancreatic and colorectal carcinomas, a major cause of failure with these modalities continues to be a lack of local disease control, even in those patients able to undergo complete surgical resections. As a result, the use of hyperthermia in combination with radiation therapy is a logical next step to investigate for these cancers. The biological rationale for hyperthermia as a cancer treatment has been well described by numerous workers (HAHN 1982). Several recent series have reported a benefit of adding hyperthermia to other treatment modalities for both superficial and intra-abdominal tumors. Nonrandomized series have generally reported an improvement in local control in those patients who received hyperthermia and suggest: (a) the relative tolerance of adjacent normal tissue (LYNG et al. 1991; JO et al. 1989); (b) that previous EBRT (BORNSTEIN and ZOURAJIAN 1992), the average maximum tumor temperature, and the number of treatments per field (KAPP et al. 1992) affect complications; (c) that available technology is inadequate (ARCICASA and FRANCHIN 1992); and (d) that multiple hyperthermia treatments do not improve outcome, but effective local control can be achieved with a single "good" treatment (ENGIN 1993; MYERSON 1990; OLESON 1989). In addition, the final report of the randomized trial, RTOG 8104 (PEREZ et al. 1991), states that although there was no overall advantage in the hyperthermia arm, further analysis revealed that tumors <3 cm and patients receiving >29 Gy had an increase in complete responses and time to relapse in the hyperthermia arm. However, they also noted that only 42% of lesions <3 cm and 31% of those >3 cm received adequate therapy (i.e., ≥29 Gy and 42.5°C for at least 45 min).

The major equipment development efforts in hyperthermia have concentrated on noninvasive devices, with the majority of techniques for delivering hyperthermia having been designed for treating superficial tumors. Regional hyperthermia systems have been the principal approach used to try to treat deep-seated tumors, and include capacitive type heating systems, concentric coils, and annular phased arrays (KATO 1985; OLESON 1986; SAPOZINK 1985; SAMULSKI 1987). Three recent reports from Japan have described attempts to use radiofrequency (RF) capacitive heating devices to treat patients intra-abdominally with pancreatic, colorectal and biliary carcinomas. Although no significant improvements in outcome were noted, each of these underscored the difficulties of obtaining adequate thermometry, and the inability of the current technology to effectively treat these deep-seated tumors (NISHIMURA et al. 1992; YAMADA et al. 1992a,b; HAMAZOE et al. 1991).

These studies once again emphasize the importance of designing hyperthermia equipment that can bring the *entire tumor volume to therapeutic temperatures* without overheating normal tissue, and provide the background for this invasive therapeutic approach. The advantage of the *intraoperative approach* is the ability to localize the radiation and the hyperthermia to the tumor volume and hence have much better control over the dose. The disadvantage is that *only a single dose* can be administered; however, it is quite possible that a single "adequate" dose is all that is required.

Treating the patient in the operating room with applicators placed in direct contact with the tumor mass with no intervening layers of skin, subcutaneous fat, or viscera eliminates many of the problems associated with noninvasive systems. Unfortunately, commercial multielement ultrasound systems are very bulky (SAMULSKI et al. 1990a) and are thus unsuitable for intraoperative use; in addition, they typically have unsophisticated control software.

17.1.4 Techniques for Intraoperative Hyperthermia

The three techniques employed for intraoperative hyperthermia have utilized either ultrasound, microwaves, or RF capacitive techniques. Interstitial hyperthermia in catheters that are implanted in the tumor during surgery have been previously reported (COUGHLIN et al. 1983, 1985, 1988) using a minimally invasive procedure with interstitial microwave arrays (TREMBLY et al. 1982; RYAN 1991a,b; RYAN et al. 1991c, 1992b, 1993, 1994). The Dartmouth experience with 42 patients with lesions in vaginal, bile duct, brain, lung, and pelvic sites utilized arrays of 4–15 microwave antennas. Inherent problems included localizing tumor margins along multiple catheters and treatment planning in an array with multiple trajectories and with catheters that may bend (COUGHLIN et al. 1985). The opportunity for direct visualization of the tumor volume in the operating room (OR) makes it possible to use a direct contact, sterilizable ultrasound applicator which has the capability of various depths of penetration.

The third technique uses RF capacitive heating with direct skin contact (YAMADA et al. 1992a,b; KATO and ISHIDA 1993; HAMAZOE et al. 1991) and placement of thermocouples during surgery. However, these latter approaches were originally designed for superficial treatments and all of these systems present physical and logistical problems which limit their utility in the OR environment.

Historically, a variety of techniques have been used for deep heating targeted from the surface. These include RF capacitive heating (KATO and ISHIDA 1993; YAMADA et al. 1992a,b; NISHIMURA et al. 1992) and deep regional heating with microwaves (FELDMANN et al. 1993). Power deposition in three dimensions with ultrasound can be controlled by utilizing either mechanically or electrically scanned focused systems. Stationary deep heating ultrasound was developed by FESSENDEN et al. (1984). Mechanically scanned focused ultrasound systems were developed by LELE (1983) and HYNYNEN et al. (1987), using focused elements that can create a traveling focal region when moved. These systems have the ability to heat deep targets below the skin surface with noraml tissue overlaying. The systems are relatively complex and bulky, require scan speeds and patterns that have to be determined beforehand, have thermal ripple related to scan speed and thermal time constants (CAIN and UMEMURA 1986), and complicate the patient–applicator interface. These systems are not applicable in intraoperative procedures that limit access to the treatment site (i.e., pancreas, liver, or pelvis). In addition, the treatment volume may take longer to heat up and temperature probe placement may fail to capture the maximum temperature (HARRISON and BALEER-KUBICZEK 1986).

Focused ultrasound with electrically scanned applicators has been described (DKICKINSON 1984; OCHELTREE et al. 1984; IBBINI and CAIN 1990; HARRISON and BALZER-KUBICZEK 1986; CAIN and UMEMURA 1986; BENKESER et al. 1987, 1989). Electronically phased arrays of ultrasound elements rapidly move the focal point around in three dimensions. The drawbacks are the large number of elements, amplifiers, and phasing circuits (OCHELTREE et al. 1984) required. In addition, these systems have never been used clinically and would be too bulky for intraoperative use.

The major impediments to achieving good temperature distributions with noninvasive hyperthermia systems are: (a) lack of direct access to the tumor; (b) low-frequency electromagnetic (EM) energy penetrated deeply but cannot be focused on the tumor; (c) ultrasound energy has problems with air–tissue interfaces and bone; (d) difficulty in implanting enough thermometry in the awake patient to provide sufficient feedback for control; and (e) patient discomfort. Intraoperative hyperthermia (IOHT) eliminates most of the problems associated with deep-heating from outside of the body:

Specifications for an *ideal hyperthermia system* require devices that can raise the tumor tissue to the range of 43°–55°C without overheating normal tissue. Early systems for superficial or deep-seated tumors consisted of single-element applicators for delivering the power, and hence the clinician had few means for controlling the temperature distribution throughout the tumor. Recent clinical studies that have reported more detailed information on temperature variability in the tumor (CORRY et al. 1982) hve shown that virtually all devices produced temperature distributions far from ideal. Quantitative measures of the effectiveness of a device to heat a tumor have been created and it has been shown that for a wide range of devices, only about 50% of the intratumoral points were reported above 43°C (OLESON 1989; KAPP et al. 1988), although some groups have argued that in the tumor volume, the percentage that will be above 43°C will be far lower (EDELSTEIN-KESHET and DEWHIRST 1989). Scanning ultrasound systems reported by HYNYNEN et al. (1990) were able to raise only 20%–60% of the intratumoral points to 42.5°C, and only 20% of the treatments had 70% of the intratumoral points above 43°C. Three recent reports from Japan have described attempts to use RF capacitive heating devices to treat patients intra-abdominally with pancreatic, colorectal, and biliary carcinomas. Although no significant improvements in outcome were noted, each of these underscored the difficulties of obtaining adequate thermometry, and the inability of the current technology to effectively treat these deep-seated tumors (NISHIMURA et al. 1992; YAMADA et al. 1992a,b; HAMAZOE et al. 1991).

Thus, we have been developing applicators to target IOHT treatments for a number of years (COLACCHIO et al. 1989, 1990; RYAN et al. 1986, 1992a; RYAN 1991a). Initially, we adapted our cylindrical single element ultrasound applicators which were designed for superficial hyperthermia treatments to be used intraoperatively. However, because IOHT imposes different constraints on the applicator design in terms of size and sterilizability, we have been developing applicators based on an array of square ultrasound elements (RYAN et al. 1991a). Due to variability in tumor size, shape, and location, arrays of different shapes and sizes of applicators are required. In addition, we are exploring an array of steerable applicators whose elements are swept over an arc (RYAN et al. 1993). This applicator is designed to be quite compact for the IOHT setting. We have shown in simulations that at fixed angles it is possible to direct power into or out of regions under the applicator with planar, unfocused elements (RYAN et al. 1993). The simulations show fixed angles as snapshots of the fields in time, as the elements swivel back-and-forth every second. The computer control could easily cause the elements to swivel along circles, ellipses, or squares or in an "X" pattern.

17.2 Physics and Engineering for Intraoperative Hyperthermia

17.2.1 Applicator Design

The intraoperative ultrasound applicator was designed to meet the following specifications:

1. Applicator easily assembles for rapid insertion of 1-, 2-, or 3-MHz elements in the sterile field
2. Expandable latex membrane to conform to tumor surface
3. Completely immersible housing with watertight RF connection
4. Inlet/outlet ports for circulating water located adjacent to RF cable to allow easier placement in deep body cavities
5. A range of applicator sizes with a total maximal applicator height of 4.0 cm.

The applicator went through three stages of development. The third-generation design is shown in Fig. 17.1. The applicator shell is machined from a single block of aluminum with a recessed threaded water inlet and outlet ports as shwon. The RF coaxial cable is fed through a waterproof connector that also serves as a shock cord. The piezoelecctric (PZT) crystal (C5800, Valpey-Fisher, Framingham, Mass.) is air-backed and firmly edge-clamped to ensure watertightness. A latex covering over the open face insures against blood contamination of the crystal and internal transducer wall. The exterior surface is smoothly

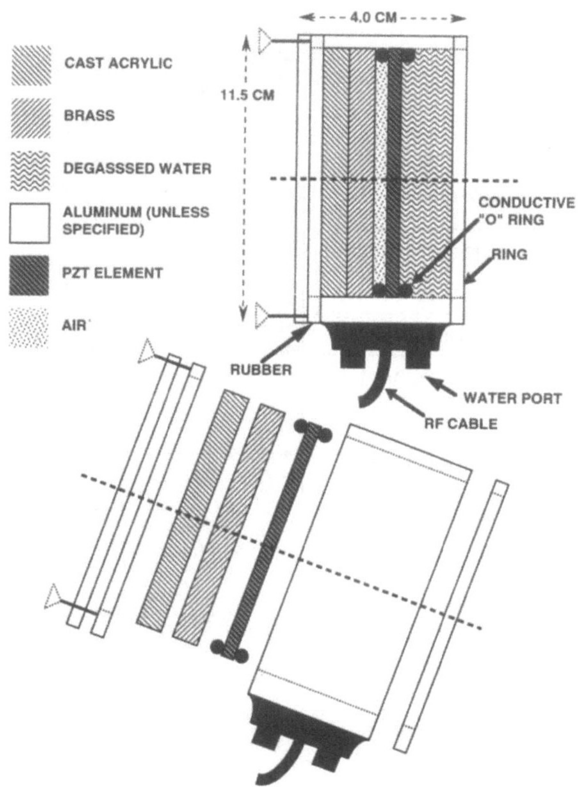

Fig. 17.1. Diagram of the design of the immersible, intraoperative ultrasound transducer. The 1-, 2-, or 3-MHz PZT ceramic is inserted into the applicator during surgery. The entire assembly is sterilized before surgery and assembled just prior to insertion into the patient

polished and coated with a protective sealer to assist in cleanup. The transducer is assembled during surgery with the appropriate ultrasound element to achieve the desired heating depth.

17.2.2 Power Delivery

Initially we used a single-channel ultrasound source (RYAN et al. 1992a) with 400 W capability. This power level was sufficient for single-element transducers with sizes up to 10.0 cm diameter. Recently, to address the multielement transducer requirements, a multichannel system has been designed and constructed (Fig. 17.2). This system is divided between the digital controller (16 channels/board) that controls amplitude and phase to each channel, and the power modules (one channel/module) that amplify the signal for the individual elements. This technology was shared by the group at the University of Michigan under Charles Cain. To interface with this controller

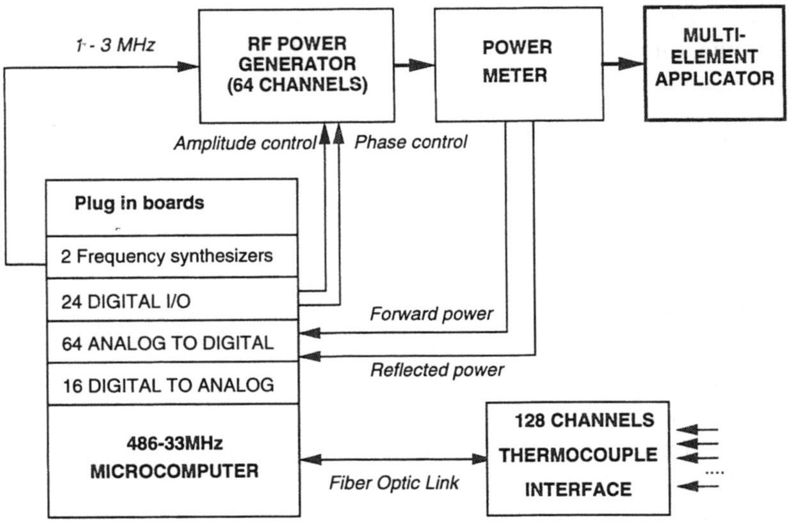

Fig. 17.2. Ultrasound hyperthermia treatment system. Temperature data collection, frequency synthesis, and RF amplifiers (amplitude and phase) are all under computer control

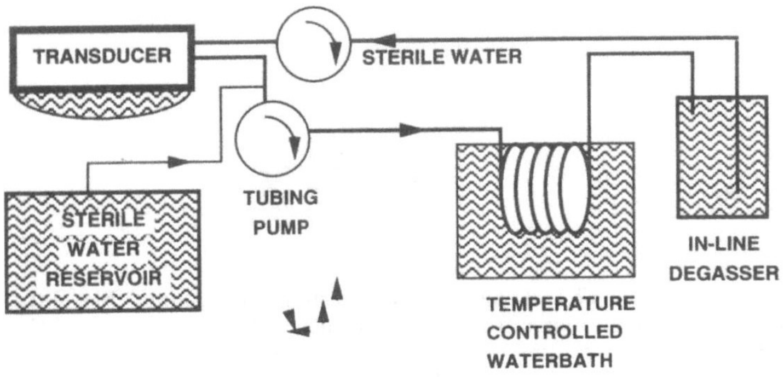

Fig. 17.3. Sterile, constant-volume, circulating water system. The temperature of the degassed, circulating water is controlled for surface cooling. An in-line degasser continuously removes any microbubbles due to cavitation

board, we designed a board to supply up to 100 W/channel over 0.5–4.0 MHz.

17.2.3 Water Circulation System

A sterile water circulation system was used in the OR (Fig. 17.3). The sterile, degassed water provided cooling of the ultrasound applicator as well as surface cooling of the tissue in contact with the applicator. A path for ultrasound with nearly the same acoustic impedance as tissue was also provided by the temperature-controlled water. Temperature was monitored both at the water inlet and at outlet locations in the transducer. An in-line degasser in the most recent system removes any microbubbles resulting from cavitation. There is also a bubble trap that will remove any bubbles from the circulation volume. The system has a constant volume which is adjustable.

17.2.4 Thermometry Placement

Thermometry sites were selected in order to monitor the deepest and lateral tumor margins and superficial sites as recommended by the Radiation Therapy Oncology Group (RTOG). Any adjacent normal tissue structures that could not be removed from the field were also carefully instrumented with thermocouples. A thermocouple was mounted inside the waterbath to monitor circulating water coolant temperature. The water inlet and outlet temperatures of the transducer were also monitored. Power was switched off briefly at intervals to record the effects of ultrasound-induced artifacts on the thermocouples.

17.2.5 Operating Room Preparation

The applicator was ethylene oxide sterilized with the PZT elements in a separate holder to insure against breakage in handling. The PZT elements were prone to crack if left in place in an aplicator with only one face exposed to ambient temperature and pressure. Also, the extent of residual tumor to be treated following resection dictated the element frequency and size and thus the appropriate and individualized assembly was done in the OR.

After discussion with the surgeon regarding the extent of the residual tumor mass, the applicator size was chosen from the 6-, 8-, or 10-cm-diameter bodies and assembled with the applicator element appropriate for the tumor thickness. The assembly was done with sterile tools by the engineer who assisted with the pretreatment preparation.

After assembly of the ultrasound transducer, the sterile water lines were connected, the entire system was filled with sterile water, and air was evacuated through the bubble trap. Flow rate, temperature, and volume of the coolant were controlled. Once the system was assembled, the tubing that was inserted into the tubing pump could be handled in a nonsterile manner since the internal sterility of the lines was maintained. At this time, the end of the sterile coaxial cable was fed to the RF amplifier, and the transducer was tuned to the resonant frequency. The transducer was then run at 100 W for 30 min to cavitate any microbubbles contained in the closed-volume circulating system. This procedure was done in parallel with the ongoing surgical procedure.

17.2.6 Transducer Selection Criteria

Since ultrasound plane waves attenuate in tissue with a frequency dependence, optimum depth of penetration can be extended by using a lower frequency PZT element. Our ultrasound applicator shells were assembled during the surgical procedure to best match the intended treatment depth and cross-sectional area of the tumor. Consideration was also given to the size of the applicator regarding access into the body cavity for placement over the tumor. Prior to assembly of the transducer in the OR and after most of the surgical resection was completed, the surgeon carefully measured the intended heating volume. The appropriate applicator shell (total applicator diameter = 4.0, 6.0, 8.0, or 10.0 cm element size +1.5 cm in wall thickness) was selected and inserted into the patient to check for optimal fit. If the tumor's surface diameter was ≤5.0 cm, the 6.0-cm-diameter applicator was used. If the diameter was in the range of 5.5–7.0 cm or ≥7.5 cm then the 8.0- and 10.0-cm applicators were used, respectively. Following the size selection, the PZT element appropriate for the depth was selected.

As a guide for frequency selection, the optimal frequency was calculated according to the intended depth of heating:

$$f = \frac{1}{2Az},$$

where f = frequency (MHz), A = attenuation coefficient (dB/cm per MHz), and z = depth of penetration (cm).

The attenuation coefficient was assumed to be the same in skin, fat, muscle, and tumor (Dickinson 1984). For depths ≤1.0 cm or ≥3.0 cm, 3.0-cm or 1.0-MHz elements were used, respectively. Within the range of 1.0–3.0 cm, the 2.0-MHz element was used. After determining the applicator shell size and frequency of the element, the applicator was assembled and sealed from the environment in preparation for complete immersion into the surgical field.

17.2.7 Quality Assurance

Quality Assurance (QA) is critical in the OR due to the fact that everything must be calibrated and tested at least 24 h before surgery. Also, all items are packaged and sterilized and only opened in the sterile field shortly before use. Special efforts were made to shorten setup time in the OR so as not to extend the length of surgery. The QA efforts in IOHT are divided into three categories.

1. *Water circulation system*. A thorough check for leaks is made before sterilization to prevent system contamination by bodily fluids, and vice versa.

2. *Applicator acoustic tests*. A nondegradable, acoustic absorbing phantom is used (Ryan 1991b).

3. *Thermometry*. Before each treatment, a waterbath is set up with a precision thermistor and the clinical thermocouples. The precision thermistor is referenced to an National Bourd of Standurds (NBS)-traceable calibration specification that is accurate to ±0.002°C. The temperature of the bath is run from 20°C to 75°C with data measured every 5 s (roughly every 0.1°C) and recorded and plotted at 0.5°C intervals. Corrections are applied to each channel by a polynomical fit of each channel of measured data to the refer-

ence data. After each treatment, the thermometry probes are disinfected, visually inspected, and automatically calibrated over the 10°–65°C range against a precision thermistor. Before each treatment, the probes will be rechecked at 43°C and then gas sterilized.

17.2.8 Acoustic Power Tests

For acoustic power tests, a smooth layer of sound absorbing rubber was placed on an electronic balance immersed in degassed water. The applicator was then positioned in the water parallel to the absorbing rubber. The scale resolution was 0.01 g and the reflection coefficient was less than 0.05 at 1.0 MHz. The speed of sound in the 23°C water was 1490 m/s and the conversion factor of 14.6 W/g was used to relate acoustic power output to the force applied to the scale by the acoustic beam. These tests were administered by the Hyperthermia Physics Center staff during a QA visit to our institution.

17.2.9 Ultrasonic Field Intensity Measurement Tests

Ultrasound applicator testing was done in a 60 × 35 × 48 cm tank filled with degassed, deionized water and lined with absorbing rubber. Acoustic measurements were made with a needle hydrophone (NTR Systems model TNU001A, Seattle, Wash.), with a 0.6-mm-diameter, 28-μm PVDF sensing element. The hydrophone was moved around the tank by a computer-controlled, three-dimensional positioning system fabricated by us with a positional accuracy of 0.042 mm. Measurements were made in the tank and referenced to precision calibration measurements made by the manufacturer at our request at the frequencies of 1, 2, and 3 MHz. Tests were made in the x- and y-directions, in planes parallel to the ultrasound element and either 1.0 or 5.0 cm from the applicator face. Tests in the z-direction, orthogonal to the applicator face, were also done. All tests measured acoustic pressure in 0.5-mm steps and averaged 100 readings per location. Hydrophone scans were plotted as normalized intensity with acoustic intensity (dB) = 10 × log(I/I_o), where I is the measured intensity at a point and I_o is the maximum intensity along the scan. Intensity is the measured pressure squared. The half-power (3 dB) beam width was also calculated from the measured data and appears in the intensity plots.

17.2.10 Thermometry System

A compact 128-channel thermocouple thermometry system was built for placement adjacent to the operating table. To simplify connection to the patient, the self-contained unit includes an isolation transformer and transmits the temperature data through a fiber optic digital link. Each channel was calibrated against an NBS traceable thermistor and with a linear correction term: (a) drift ≤ 0.04° ± 0.02°C in 100 measurements over 90 min; (b) accuracy over the range of 10°–65°C within 0.2°C, specifically within 0.1°C at 43°C; (c) channel interchangeability (one probe in several channels) or probe interchangeability in a single channel did not introduce additional errors. Thermal conduction errors have been addressed previously (Ryan et al. 1989). Artifacts were measured (Ryan et al. 1992a) according to RTOG guidelines and were within the specified ±0.5°C (Waterman et al. 1991) for ultrasound hyperthermia, including viscous and absorption heating, and thermal conduction. We use the following steps to minimize artifacts: (a) probes are made of stainless steel to reduce absorption heating; (b) thermocouple sizes are 21 gauge needles to minimize scatter; (c) no common wires for the triple-junction thermocouples are used to minimize thermoelectric junction error; and (d) right-angled probes are used to minimize viscous heating since the sensors are parallel to the direction of propagation. The reference used is a precision thermistor (Thermometrics model D774, Edison, NJ) accurate to ±0.002°C and NBS traceable.

For measurement artifacts in ultrasound hyperthermia, four types are addressed: (a) viscous heating of the thermometry probe; (b) absorption heating if the probe material absorbs ultrasound energy differently than the surrounding medium; (c) reflection or scattering due to the presence of the probe; and (d) conduction errors along metallic components.

For fixed temperature points temperatures are measured by right-angled needle thermocouples with distances of bend-to-tip of 1.0–6.0 cm to accommodate various tumor depths. These probes are custom made to our specifications as noted above to minimize artifacts with the probe axis parallel to the direction of ultrasound propagation. Temperature artifact is determined for each sensor from thermal washout at the end of each treatment at the location of the point of maximum temperature. The linear portion of the decay curve is extrapolated to the time of power off (WATERMAN 1990). Recent standards proposed by the Hyperthermia Quality Assurance Committee (WATERMAN et al. 1991) recommend multiplying this value by 1.5 because of the underestimation of the artifact with this technique. After each treatment, the thermometry probes are disinfected, visually inspected, and automatically calibrated over the 10°–65°C range against a precision thermistor. Before each treatment, the probes will be rechecked at 43°C and then ethylene oxide sterilized.

17.2.11 Treatment Analysis

The treatment system collects data every 5 s including: (a) 128 temperature channels; (b) forward and reflected power to each ultrasound element; (c) target minimum and maximum temperatures for each channel; and (d) percentage that each probe is affected by each element. Upon commencement of the treatment, the following are displayed: (a) thermal dose and average temperature for each channel; (b) the power to each element; (c) percent of all measured points in tumor ≥43°C; (d) T_{50} (temperature exceeded by 50% of all measured points in tumor); and (e) T_{90}. Plots of index temperature versus percent of points ≥ index temperature are plotted for each patient. We also estimate the HEP rating (percentage of volume ≥43°C) for each set of patients (pancreatic and colorectal).

17.2.12 Control Algorithm

Fixed source hyperthermia systems with multiple applicator elements and multiple temperature probes require determining to what degree each thermal probe is affected by each ultrasound source. The control algorithm used in this project is novel and has been presented elsewhere (HARTOV 1991; HARTOV et al. 1993a). Our requirements were: (a) to recognize the probe-element dependencies automatically; (b) to compensate for blood flow variations or movement; and (c) to control simple (one probe affects one element) as well as complex cases (several probes affect one element or one probe is affected by several elements). An adaptive multiple-input multiple-output controller was developed to either attempt to raise temperatures to target values or attempt to keep temperatures within a specified range. The applicators were characterized in water utilizing a hydrophone measurement system, in phantoms, in perfused organs (liver and kidney), and in vivo (dog). This design provided adequate power to heat up to 6 cm deep and the mosaic element arrangement greatly improved our ability to control the power delivery more evenly.

The algorithm underwent extensive testing in simulations and experiments with perfused organs (Fig. 17.4), in vivo (dog) and superficial patient treatments. Results show that the algorithm performs well (HARTOV et al. 1993a) if sufficient power is available. The algorithm uses data from the previous 4 min of treatment to evaluate the probe/element dependencies and is able to recognize changes within 2 min although it cannot track faster changes such as respiratory motion. It can readjust itself in the face of sudden changes, such

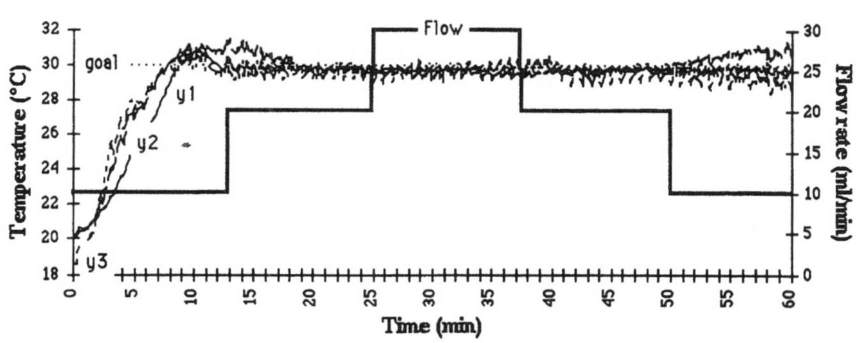

Fig. 17.4. *y1*, *y2*, and *y3* are temperature probes at three locations in the kidney. Although perfusion was changed several times during the experiment, the algorithm maintained probe temperatures

as rotating the applicator 90°C. Although this algorithm was developed for our intraoperative application, an adapted form has shown good results with an array of microwave applicators at Stanford University (ZHOU and FESSENDEN 1993).

17.2.13 Computer Modeling

We performed simulations on a computer to obtain field profiles for a given element arrangement. Software was developed to compute acoustic fields in nonlossy media by computing the field values at selected points based on source points arrangement. The source points constitute a discretized representation of the source elements, and the field points consist of the set of points in front of the applicator at which the field is to be computed. The source is discretized so that three points per wavelength are used to compute the filed. The actual distance between the points is a function of the frequency to be simulated. The field computations consist of summing the contributions of the individual source points to the acoustic pressure at he current field point using the following expression:

$$P(x) = \sum_{j=1}^{N} P_j \frac{\exp(-ikr_j)}{r_j}$$

where x is a generalized coordinate, r is the source to field point distance, k is the wave number $(2p/l)$, i is the imaginary unity, and P_j includes the source velocity term and any constant associated with the medium.

17.3 Methods: Clinical Study Design for Intraoperative Hyperthermia

17.3.1 Patient Selection

For our phase I trial, we chose to select those patients with recurrent and large untrsetable intra-abdominal carcinomas, primarily pancreatic and colorectal. The treatment protocol was reviewed and approved by the institution's Institution Review Board (IRB). Patients having received previous EBRT and those with solid organ metastases were eligible if their expected survival was >3 months. In addition, we decided to use IOHT only in patients with measurable residual disease (generally greater than 2 cm thick) in which temperature monitoring was feasible, and thereby eliminated those patients with minimal or microscopic residual disease. As a result of these criteria we have seleted out a population of patients with the *worst overall prognosis* from among those who would be eligible for the future phase II trials of this combination treatment modality. Patients who were felt to be eligible for this protocol had the treatment explained thoroughly, and following sufficient discussion, they all signed an informed consent. Nineteen patients have been treated with combination IORT with IOHT. Ten have had coloreatal cancer recurrences, seven have had unresectable primary pancreatic cancers, and, in addition, we have treated one gastric and one endometrial cancer. The patients' demographic, tumor size, treatment details, and follow-up data are shown in Tables 17.1–17.3.

Table 17.1. IORT and IOHT: colorectal cancer experience

Pt.	Sex	Age	Tumor volume (cc)	Metastatic disease[a]	IORT dose (cGy)	Temperature probes	Thermal dose[b]		Follow-up (months)
							Max.	Min.	
P.P.	M	49	360	No	1200	3	3955	0	16.5
H.R.	M	73	729	Yes	1700	10	5×10^5	0	5.0
A.W.	M	63	108	No	1750	6	2533	29	25
J.E.	M	70	48	Yes	1750	4	359	1	10.5
W.V.	M	60	144	No	1750	6	463	0	4.5
M.S.	F	43	188	Yes	1750	7	1×10^4	37	18
W.W.	M	57	84	No	1750	6	9486	37	37
J.E.	M	57	65	No	1750	12	117	2	16
F.R.	M	70	173	No	1500	17	1715	0	21.5
W.P.	M	77	72	No	1500	12	69	0	22.5

[a] Present at time of treatment
[b] Equivalent minutes at 43°C

Table 17.2. IORT and IOHT: pancreatic cancer experience

Pt.	Sex	Age	Tumor volume (cc)	Metastatic disease[a]	IORT dose (cGy)	Temperature probes	Thermal dose[b] Max.	Thermal dose[b] Min.	Follow-up (months)
B.D.	M	55	243	No	1750	6	1599	51	22
R.F.	F	81	71	No	1750	4	962	147	5.5
B.M.	F	59	289	No	1750	4	295	–	0.5
V.S.	M	61	500	Yes	1750	6	694	230	3
R.P.	M	49	175	No	1500	9	120	0	7
V.R.	F	59	252	Yes	1500	14	698	0	0.5
P.B.	F	62	245	Yes	1500	11	4214	3	5.5

[a] Present at the time of treatment
[b] Equivalent minutes at 43°C

Table 17.3. IORT and IOHT: other malignancies

Pt.	Sex	Age	Tumor volume (cc)	Metastatic disease[a]	IORT dose (cGy)	Temperature probes	Thermal dose[b] Max.	Thermal dose[b] Min.	Follow-up (months)
R.M.[c]	M	61	361	Yes	1500	6	343	122	4
E.E.[d]	F	65	320	No	1750	8	491	0	12.5

[a] Present at the time of treatment
[b] Equivalent minutes at 43°C
[c] Primary: gastric
[d] Primary: endometrial

17.3.2 Surgery

All patients underwent exploratory laporotomy at which time their tumors were exposed and biopsied, and adherent or involved structures overlying or adjacent to the tumor were either resected, retracted, or defunctionalized. The tumors were debulked whenever possible in an attempt to minimize the residual disease and to achieve a maximum diameter of 10 cm and a maximum thickness of 5 cm. The surface of the tumor was thereby exposed and the IORT and IOHT treatments were performed. Following this, the necessary bypasses, resections, etc. were performed and the operation was completed.

17.3.3 Radiotherapy

A Phillips RT 305 orthovoltage (300 kvp) x-ray machine, installed in one of the operating suites, was used to deliver intraoperative radiation therapy. The beam has a half-value layer (HVL) of 3.8 mmCu, which requires relatively little shielding for the room. A full complement of cones were fashioned with both 25 and 30 cm focal skin distance (FSD). Cone diameters range from 4 to 10 cm and have 0°, 15°, or 30° bevel angles. It was felt that tumors with a thickness of up to 5 cm would be satisfactorily treated with 300 kvp x-rays. Generally, the dose of radiation was determined by the thickness of the tumor, i.e., tumors >2 cm thick received 17.5 Gy while tumors <2 cm received 15 Gy. Treatment times ranged from 15 to 25 min, and there were no tumors which were inaccessible to placement of the IORT cones. A summary of the IORT doses used is shown in Tables 17.1–17.3. Of the 19 IORT/IOHT patients, have received either pre- or postoperative EBRT. Of the remaining eight, five refused additional therapy and three expired before having recovered sufficiently to begin therapy.

17.3.4 Hyperthermia Treatment

Following the IORT, all 19 patients then received an IOHT treatment. This was delivered using either a 6.0- or 10-cm single-element ultrasound transducer with either a 1-, 2-, or 3-MHz piezoelectric crystal. Therapeutic temperatures (>42°C) were achieved and maintained for 60 min in each IOHT treatment. The power required to attain these temperatures ranged from 70 to 180 W. Thermometry sites were selected in order to monitor the deepest and lateral tumor margins, and superficial sites as recommended by the RTOG and documented by WATERMAN et al. (1991). Any adjacent normal tissue structures that could not be removed from the field were also carefully instrumented with thermocouples. For temperature measurements, customized 21 gauge stainless steel needle thermocouples were fabricated (Sensortek, Clifton, N.J.) with 90° bends for precise depth placement. These triple-junction probes had sensors at the tip, halfway between the tip and bend, and 2.0 mm from the bend for superficial measurements. Flexible, bare-ended microthermocouples were placed superficially or implanted into tissue by placing and removing a 17 gauge needle, leaving the flexible probe in the tissue. The flexible and 90° triple thermocouple probes were then pulled out after the treatment. A thermocouple was mounted inside the waterbath to monitor circulating water coolant temperature. The water inlet and outlet temperatures of the transducer were also monitored. Power was switched off briefly every 10 min to record the effects of ultrasound-induced artifacts on the thermocouples.

The number of temperature points within each tumor and the thermal doses for the 19 IOHT patients are shown in Tables 17.1–17.3. A schematic representation of the locations of these points within the tumor volume of two of the patients is shown in Figs. 17.5 and 17.6. In addition, Fig. 17.7 shows a thermal map done of one patient across the center of the tumor, at a depth of 0.5 cm from the surface.

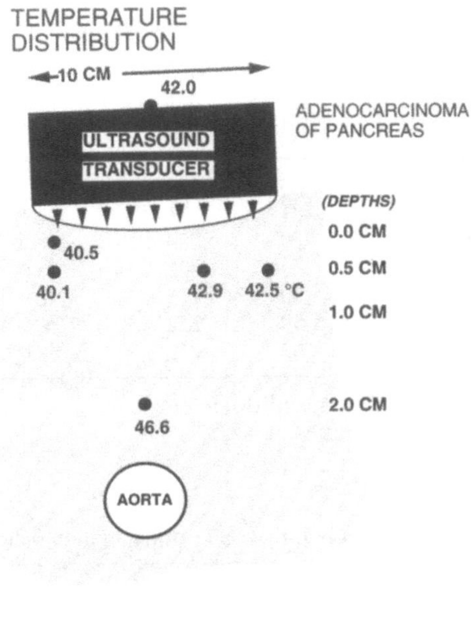

Fig. 17.6. Temperature distribution in a plane orthogonal to the applicator face. Tumor measured 9 × 9 × 3 cm and was in the pancreas. Deepest tumor margin along the central axis abutted the aorta

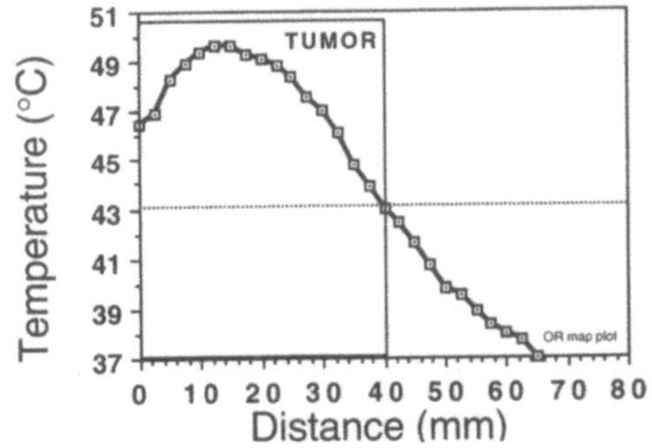

Fig. 17.7. Temperature map through the entire tumor during surgery. The temperature mapping track is pictured in Fig. 17.5. All points in the tumor are ⩾43°C

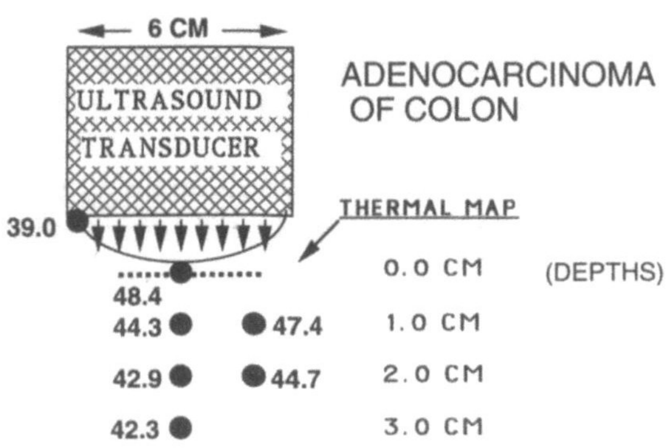

Fig. 17.5. Temperature distribution in a plane orthogonal to the applicator face. A thermal map was made along the *dotted line* and appears in Fig. 17.7. Tumor dimensions measured 4 × 4 × 3 cm (deep)

17.4 Results of the Dartmouth Experience

17.4.1 Intraoperative Hyperthermia Treatment Analysis

Right-angled thermocouples made it possible to meausre temperatures at exact depths during the intraoperative ultrasound treatments. Figure 17.5 shows the distribution of fixed points in a plane orthogonal to the applicator front face. In this case, the applicator housed a 6.0-cm PZT ceramic operating at 1.0 MHz. The tumor was 4 cm × 4 cm × 3 cm (deep). The temperature at the tumor margin along a central axis was 42.3°C, with the superficial central tumor temperature averaging 48.4°C at an intensity over the applicator surface of 2.26 W/cm^2 (net forward power/applicator element area). A thermal map was made along the dotted line, and the resultin temperature distribution is shown in Fig. 17.7. The tumor boundaries are demarcated by the box. In most of the tumors in the IOHT series, temperature mapping was not feasible. Figure 17.6 shows another treatment with a tumor of 9 cm × 9 cm × 3 cm (deep), with the aorta underlying the deepest tumor boundary. A 10.0-cm transducer was used with a 1.0-MHz crystal, and the temperature distribution is shown in the figure.

The results of analysis of temperatures attained in the IOHT patients are shown in Table 17.4. A comparison was made with the outpatient (i.e., Clinic) series of patients undergoing 64 superficial treatments using the same applicators applied externally. A comparison was also made between fixed position probes and mapping probes which were scanned through the tumor. The average maximum and minimum temperatures sustained throughout the entire 60-min heat treatments were 45.4° and 39.7°C in the Clinic series and 46.6°C and 39.8°C in the IOHT series, respectively. The higher maximum temperature in the IOHT series was statistically significant ($P < 0.011$), whereas the minimum temperature difference was not ($P = 0.971$). The overall average of all fixed temperature points was 42.0°C in the Clinic and 43.0°C in the IOHT series. The difference was found to be statistically significant ($P < 0.0002$). All statistical analyses were based on Student's unpaired *t*-test.

Table 17.5 extends the comparison to the analysis of T_{90} and T_{50}. T_{90} is the temperature that 90% of all measured temperatures are greater than or equal to. The T_{90} value is higher in the IOHT series than in the Clinic series (39.2° vs 38.8°C), as is the T_{50} value (42.9° vs 41.9°C). In fact, 50% of all fixed measurement points measured in the IOHT series were ⩾43.0°C, while only 30% were ⩾43.0°C for the Clinic series.

The average intensity in IOHT was 30% higher than in the Clinic series ($P < 0.003$). Tables 17.4 and 17.5 compare the same values of T_{90}, T_{50}, and average temperatures when mapping points are used as a measure of the Clinic series treatments. Maps were made at 2.0- or 5.0-mm intervals in orthogonal hollow needles. The T_{90} was raised slightly when comparing fixed measurement points to mapped points for the Clinic series. This is also demonstrated in Fig. 17.8, which plots index temperature versus percentage of points ⩾ the index temperature. There is good overlap for the two types of analysis.

Table 17.4. Mean maximum and minimum temperatures (°C) by series

Series	T_{max} ± SD	Range	T_{min} ± SD	Range	No.	T_{all} ± SD	No.
Clinic:							
Fixed points	45.4 ± 2.8	39.3–52.2	39.7 ± 1.5	36.2–43.2	64	42 ± 2.6	691
Mapping points	44.7 ± 2.4	40.5–52.9	40 ± 1.5	36.9–43.0	54	41.5 ± 1.9	1457
Intraoperative:							
Fixed points	46.6 ± 3.1	43.0–56.0	39.8 ± 1.8	36.0–43.2	19	43 ± 3.2	133

Table 17.5. Mean temperature distribution, power, and tumor volume by series

Series	T_{90} (°C)	T_{50} (°C)	Percentage points	No rxs.	Power density ± SD	Range (W/cm^3)	Volume (cm^3)	Range	No.
Clinic:									
Fixed points	38.8	41.9	29.6	64	1.14 + 0.47	0.4–2.6	127	5.4–640	64
Mapping points	39.6	42.1	37.1	64					
Intraoperative:									
Fixed points	39.2	42.9	49.6	19	165 + 0.98	0.6–5.0	231	48–1296	19

rxs,

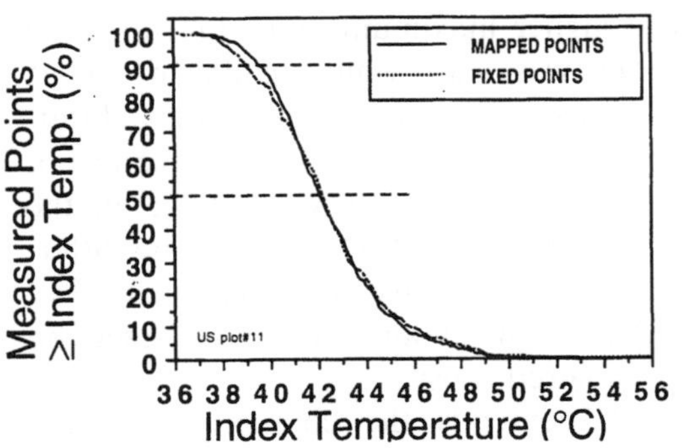

Fig. 17.8. Mapped versus fixed temperature points for 64 treatments in the Clinic series. T_{90} was 39.6°C and 38.8°C, respectively, for mapped and fixed points. T_{50} was 42.1°C and 41.9°C, respectively

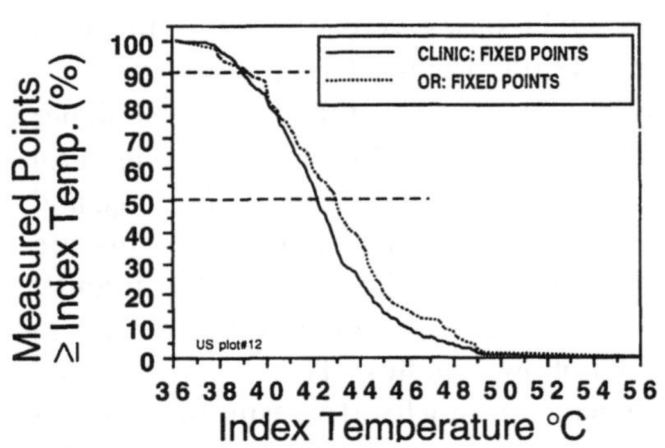

Fig. 17.9. Fixed temperature measurement for Clinic versus IOHT series. T_{90} was 38.8° and 39.2°C, respectively, for Clinic versus IOHT series. T_{50} was 41.9° and 42.5°C, respectively

Figure 17.9 illustrates the difference in distribution between the Clinic and IOHT fixed points. In the IOHT series, by using higher intensity, temperatures were elevated, as compared to the Clinic series.

Temperature artifacts were in the range of 0.1°–0.2°C, which is in agreement with a larger ultrasound clinical study by SAMULSKI et al. (1990a). Additionally, acoustic output of the 1.0-MHz transducers were within 10% of the RF net forward power readings, as verified by the Hyperthermia Physics Center.

17.4.2 Morbidity and Mortality

The morbidity and mortality rates are summarized in Table 17.6. Eleven patients have developed complications for an overall complication rate of 58%. These are summarized in Table 17.7 and include three with pelvic abscess, two cases of prolonged postoperative ileus, one case of partial bowel obstruction not requiring reoperation, and two cases of increased nerve paresis. In both of the latter cases, lumbosacral nerve paresis was demonstrated preoperatively, and they both returned to their baseline deficits within 3 months. In addition, one patients developed osteomyonecrosis of the left lateral abdominal wall 8 months following treatment in association with a regional recurrence. This required debridement and reconstruction. There have been no wound infections, delayed hemorrhages, new permanent neuropathies leading to motor deicits, skin burns, or enteric fistulae in association with the treatment fields.

There have been two postoperative deaths (within 30 days of surgery) in this series, for an

Table 17.6. IORT and IOHT for unresected and gross residual intra-abdominal carcinomas

Site	No.	Morbidity	Mortality
Colorectal	10	50%	0
Pancreas	7	57%	29%
Other	2	100%	0
Total	19	58	11%

Table 17.7. Complications of combined IOHT/IORT

Complication	Colorectal	Pancreatic	Other	Total
Adult respiratory distress syndrome	0	1	0	1
Small bowel ischemia	0	1	0	1
Pelvic abscess	3	0	0	3
Osteomyonecrosis	1	0	0	1
Prolonged ileus	0	2	0	2
Partial small bowel obstruction	0	0	1	1
Increased nerve paresis	1	0	1	2
Total (%)	5 (50)	4 (57)	2 (100)	11 (58)

operative mortality of 11%. The first was a patient with pancreatic cancer who developed evidence of progressive bowel ischemia along the distribution of the superior mesenteric artery 14 days following surgery, and who was noted to have patent measenteric vessels at autopsy. The second was a patient with pancreatic cancer who developed progressive respiratory distress beginning 15 days post surgery and 2 days following initiation of chemotherapy. This progressed to adult respiratory distress syndrome and was thought to be result of tumor necrosis. She expired from respiratory failure on postoperative day 19.

17.4.3 Patient Follow-up and Outcome

Despite the fact that this preliminary group of patients has had a dismal overall prognosis, we have been encouraged by the number of partial and complete responses to this therapy. The average tumor volume was large, with the mean volumes for the colorectal and pancreatic tumors being 197 cc and 254 cc respectively, and seven patients had solid organ metastases at the time of therapy.

Table 17.8 presents a summary of the patient follow-up data with a breakdown by primary tumor type. All the patients in this series have been followed until their death; overall survival ranged from 0.5 to 37 months with a mean of 12 months for the entire series. Colorectal cancer patients had a mean survival of 18 months (range 4.5–37 months), whereas pancreatic cancer patients had a mean survival of 6 months with a range of 0.5–22 months. All but three patients ultimately died of progression of their disease, with one patient each dying from overwhelming sepsis, progressive renal failure, and trauma resulting from an aoutomobile accident. Nine patients had a partial response to the treatment which was usually manifested by a marked decrease in symptomatology (i.e., pain). These responses lasted for a mean of 9.7 months (range of 5–18 months), with the majority of them being patients with colorectal cancer. In addition, there were three patients with complete responses in the field which lasted for 10.5–22 months. Two of these were colorectal patients and the third was a patient with a metastatic endometral carcinoma. Finally, seven patients had no response to this combination therapy, including five patients with pancreatic carcinoma, two of whom had perioperative deaths.

17.5 New Directions

17.5.1 Nerve Conduction/Electrophysiological Monitoring

Pain is frequently the cause for the premature cessation of a hyperthermia treatment and for the inability to achieve target temperatures. IORT and IOHT treatments allow for the retraction, defunctionalization, and/or resection with acceptable morbidity of essentially all intra-abdominal structures with known radiosensitivity except for peripheral nerves and retroperitoneal tissue (Colacchio et al. 1990). A significant advantage of intraoperative hyperthermia treatment is that the anesthetized patient does not perceive pain, and the treatment is more likely to achieve therapeutic temperatures. Howevr, the inability to perceive pain also allows the possibility for *inadvertant injury to normal structures* in the treatment field, especially nerve tissue. A few experimental studies have been published concerning the effects of heat on peripheral nerves (Sminia et al. 1991a; Wondergem et al. 1988; Froese et al. 1991; Hoogeveen 1993; Panjwani et al. 1991; DeVrind and Wondergem 1992), and neurotoxic effects of clinical hyperthermia in humans have been observed by several authors

Table 17.8. Summary of follow-up and outcome of therapy

Primary site	Survival[a], mean (range)	Partial response	Complete respoñe	No response	Dead of disease
Colorectal	18 (4.5–37)	6/10 (10 mos)[b]	2/10 (16.5 mos)[b]	2/10	7/10
Pancreatic	6 (0.5–22)	2/7 (11.5 mos)	0/7	5/7	7/7
Other	8 (4–12.5)	1/2 (4 mos)	1/2 (12 mos)	0/2	2/2
Total	12 (0.5–37)	9/19 (9.7 mos)	3/19 (15 mos)	7/19	16/19

[a] Expressed in months
[b] Mean duration of response shown within parentheses

(Ben-Yosef et al. 1992; Bull and Lees 1979; Scott et al. 1985); however, many of the patients studied had also received chemotherapy. Although nerve injury was not a significant complication in our pilot study, it was a relatively frequent cause for morbidity in the series of IORT patients reported by Sindelar and Kinsella (1993). The periphral nerve tolerance studies done by us have shown that there is a fairly sharp drop in tolerance of the nerve from 44° to 45°C, and this seems to have long-term sequelae. Our electrophysiology study of IOHT to the sciatic nerve showed significant decreases in conduction velocity and action potential amplitude after 1 h of IOHT for all treatment temperatures (Vujaskovic et al. 1993). The greatest conduction velocity decrease, below 40 m/s (normal < 50 m/s), was observed for temperatures of 45°C immediately after treatment. It is possible that the reason for our lack of neurological morbidity in the phase I trial was in part a manifestation of our inability to effectively heat the large tumors in our series. Improved methods for hyperthermia delivery may increase the likelihood of nerve injury. The ability to adequately monitor the temperature along the entire course of a nerve within the field is often hampered by the presence of bone, muscle, and other structures. In addition, the sensitivity of the nerves in a given patient may vary from normal based on the addition, the sensitivity of the nerves in a given patient may vary from normal based on the amount and type of previous therapy, e.g., external beam radiation or neurotoxic chemotherapy. Therefore, a method of evaluating the effects of the hyperthermia treatment on the nerve while the treatment is actually occurring would allow for changes to be made in time to avert irreversible injury. The real-time analysis of *evoked sciatic nerve potentials* can be used to monitor critical parameters of peripheral nerve function and to determine points t which serious nerve damage would occur if the treatment procedure continued without alterations. Electrophysiological monitoring of somatosensory nerve patterns of conductivity is routinely done (Grundy et al. 1982; Chiappa and Ropper 1982; McPherson et al. 1985; Veilleux et al. 1987) to monitor potential injury during spinal stabilization surgery. We plan to perform real-time monitoring of these nerves during the hyperthermia treatment, so that the ability to identify patterns of change in electrophysiology which predict irreversible damage may then be adapted to allow monitoring of normal tissue (i.e., nerve) acute toxicity during the clinical treatments.

17.5.2 Concentric Ring Applicator

We have developed an ongoing interest in radial power control after performing an extensive analysis of our single-element ultrasound treatments (Ryan et al. 1986). By dividing the tumor into concentric rings and applying a temperature to each ring from temperature map information, the distribution of weighted temperature over the tumor volume was analyzed. It was found that the outer margins with the greatest volume had the lowest temperatures. Directing power to the outer margin became a goal of our development.

A 10-cm circular planar PZT transducer, the same size as our previous designs (Ryan et al. 1986; Colacchio et al. 1989, 1990), was modified by etching concentric circles on one surface of a PZT ceramic to create four rings (Ryan et al. 1991b). The 10-cm-diameter transducer had four active rings and an unenergized center. The transducer housing ws designed to be completely immersed in fluid, suitable for IOHT. The transducer was resonant at 1.0 MHz and was tested in water tank. A comparison between a single 10-cm element and the concentric ring modification with all rings at equal power density showed performance to be nearly identical. In vivo experiments in canine thigh verified the phantom predictions as individual rings were energized. Theoretical intensity calculations were made and compared favorably to water tank test results. Clinical hyperthermia treatments for chest wall and head and neck tumors showed that the temperature distribution was highly modifiable by adjusting power to individual rings while holding the transducer stationary (Ryan et al. 1991b,e). Automated temperature mapping parallel to the transducer face was used to compare a single-element applicator to the concentric ring applicator in clinical treatments on the same lesion. The concentric ring applicator was radially adjustable and found to be advantageous in lowring central peak temperatures and flattening the temperature distribution in tumors. A comparison between the single-element clinical and OR series showed that when pain is removed as a treatment-limiting factor, higher central tumor temperatures are possible and more of the tumor volume achieves therapeutic temperatures. The concentric ring design improves temperature distribution such that the higher central temperatures will not be necessary. No distinct central peak temperatures were observed in eight patients treated. Only those rings necessary to cover the tumor are energized, thus creating a virtual transducer size of 4.0–10.0 cm.

Figure 17.10 shows results using the concentric ring and the single-element applicators (10 cm, 1.0 MHz) on the same tumor. Power to the outer ring was adjusted to bring tumor margins up to therapeutic levels. This applicator reduced central peak temperatures. In addition, the central peak was eliminated, as seen in Fig. 17.10, where the 49°C peak decreases to 43.2°C and the temperature varies from 40.1° to 43.2°C, versus 39° to 49°C for a single-element applicator.

17.5.3 2 × 2 Element Applicator

In our multielement applicators that are composed of single, square elements, a modular design is utilized (Fig. 17.11). This design basically uses a separate housing for each PZT element that provides power, air backing, RF shielding, and water cooling. Prototype multielement designs are created using a computer-aided design program that ultimately operates a computer-driven milling machine. The milling machine takes a single solid block of brass or stainless steel, and completes the piece without human intervention.

A patient was treated in our clinical series with our conventional 10.0-cm ultrasound applicator

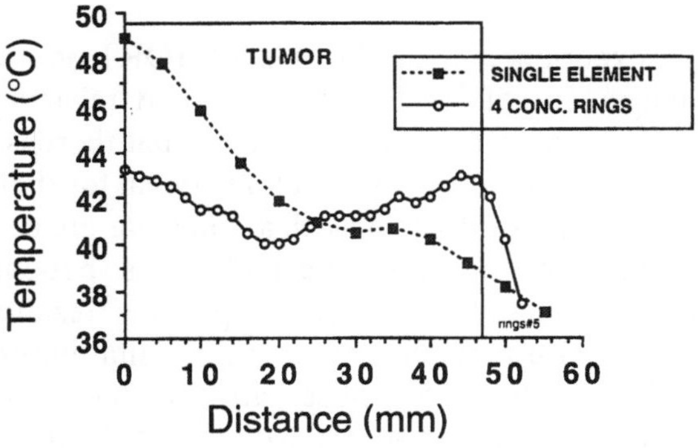

Fig. 17.10. Comparison of temperature distributions between single-element and concentric ring, four-element applicators on the same lesion. The highest temperatures were reduced and the lower temperatures raised by use of the concentric ring applicator. Temperatures were based on pullback measurement data

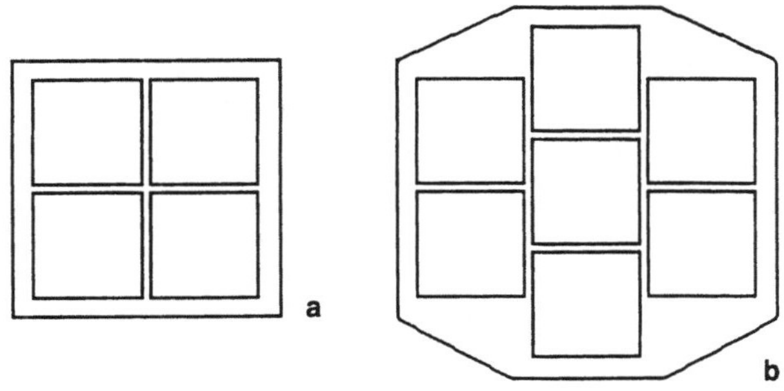

Fig. 17.11a,b. Four- and seven-element ultrasound applicators. Each 3 × 3 cm square element is interchangeable and under individual power control

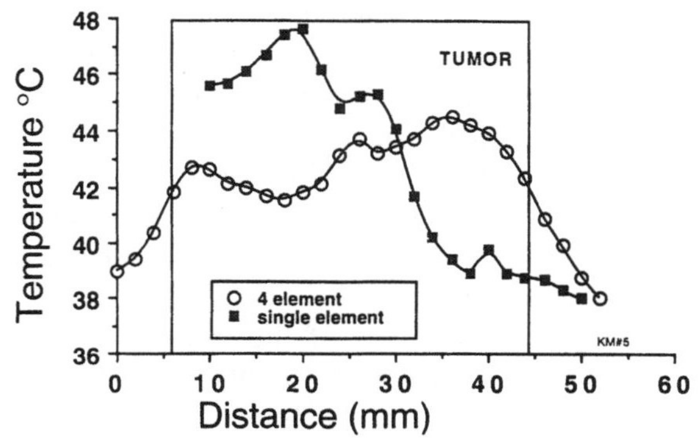

Fig. 17.12. Single-element versus multielement applicators on the same tumor. Temperature mapping was done at 2.0-mm intervals during the treatment. Single-element results show the characteristic high central peak. Four-element results (mapped across two of the elements) show the lessening of the central peak

(Ryan et al. 1992a). Power levels of 100–150 W were required for therapeutic temperatures. The maximum temperature was 47.5°C (as seen in Fig. 17.12). The next treatment used the new multielement applicator in a 2 × 2 configuration (Fig. 17.11a) with 3-cm-square elements at 1.0 MHz (Ryan et al. 1991a). Identical needle placement between treatments was assured by tattooing the needle entrance and exit locations. For the pullback shown in the plot, the elements directly in place over the needle were at 18 and 16 W, respectively. The temperature varied from 39°C to 47.5°C with the single element and from 41.5° to 44.2°C with the 2 × 2 element applicator. The high temperature central peak was eliminated with the multielement applicator. It was found that the size and shape of the 2 × 2 applicator made it suitable for these patients when the standard clinical designs were not. Thus it was also demonstrated that for intraoperative treatments where single-element applicators had major limitations in the ability to distribute power adequately (RYAN et al. 1992a), these shortcomings could be overcome by the use of multielement applicators.

17.5.4 Seven-Element Applicator

Figure 17.11b shows a seven-element design, but since the individual element holders are modular and self-contained, they are applicable to any shape or configuration of square, rectangular, or elliptical applicators (HARTOV 1991, 1993b). Conductive "O" rings above and below the elements provide electrical contact as well as watertight placement. An individual element is easy to replace if it does not pass QA checks or if damaged. The RF connections and water hoses are on the same side for ease of placement inside the patient. The bolus conforms to the surface of the treatment field.

Computer simulations of the intensity profile were made with all the elements excited at he same power level, except the center element, which was off. The results appear in Fig. 17.13.

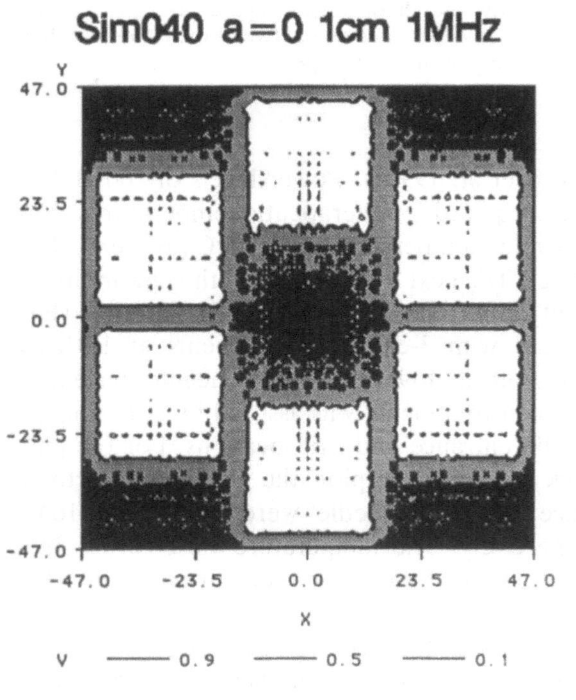

Fig. 17.13. Computed acoustic field intensity profile on a plane parallel to the applicator, 5 cm away. All elements are excited at the same power level except the one in the center, which is off

Note the six active regions due to the collimated beams of the six elements that were on at equal power.

17.5.5 Swivel Element Applicator

A novel, movable beam prototype ultrasound applicator was built and tested. Each element was 3 × 3 cm, individually powered by stepper motors, and swiveled ±45° once per second about its axis in its own housing. Power to the element could be varied as it moved. Beam steering experiments were done in a water tank and computer simulations were made. Computed results closely matched the measured results in the water tank. These experiments showed that the single elements have highly collimated beams that are appropriate for beam steering under computer control. The applicator can treat regions larger than its physical size by pointing the beams outward. This design has the potential to aim the ultrasound beams at cold spots and smooth otherwise uneven temperature profiles by controlling power as each element moves. There are a variety of scan paths that could be programmed for each element (concentric rings, spirals, zigzags) and some previous work done at the Univ. of Arizona (HYNYNEN et al. 1987) with scanned, focused systems has shown that a doughnut shaped scan with two concentric circles has been useful clinically as well as a raster scan (back-and-forth). Power modulation during the scan is also possible.

17.5.6 "Near-Field Hyperthermia" for Minimal Residual Disease

The experience with the use of IORT in the management of locally advanced and recurrent colorectal cancer has demonstrated that there is a benefit in both local control and survival for these patients. In addition, it is clear that the greatest increment in efficacy is achieved for those patients with minimally or microscopically residual disease, with a much smaller incremental improvement in efficacy for those patients with grossly residual disease. However, even with only microscopically residual disease, there is still local recurrence rate of ≥20%, and this rises sharply with the increase in the amount of residual disease. Therefore, it is reasonable to conclude that patients with minimal residual disease would present the best opportunity for cure with the addition of IOHT. Regional heating approaches are less well adapted for this situation since their ability to focus and specify the precise limits of energy deposition are considerably less than that which is feasible with the intraoperative approach. In addition, this scenario increases the probability that normal thermally sensitive structures will be in the hyperthermia field. Finally, beneficial effects have been shown theoretically for adding control of surface cooling as a means of achieving better temperature distribution in tissue (Dhar and Sinha 1989). Thus, the development and testing of methods for the intraoperative delivery of "near-field," shallow-depth heating to the residual tumor beds following complete or near-complete surgical resection could have a significant impact on the long-term survival and local control of these tumors. The realization of this capability will require not only the adaptation of the current applicators but also more extensive and precise thermometry.

17.5.7 Noninvasive Thermometry

New efforts in the field noninvasive thermometry (Paulsen et al. 1991, 1994) have shown some interesting preliminary results (Moskowitz et al. 1994). These techniques incorporate an impedance measurement system (Ryan et al. 1991d) that inputs current into contact electrodes and measures the resultant voltages. The recording electrode array has been found to be compatible with superficial heating applicators (Moskowitz et al. 1994). This technique could easily be incorporated into the intraoperative multielement applicator since control of power in two dimensions is available. This could potentially enable more precise treatment field mapping and configuration, but would create new challenges for the application of an effective computer control algorithm.

17.6 Discussion

Locally advanced intra-abdominal carcinomas are significant clinical problems which are relatively resistant to conventional modes of therapy. Some improvement in local control has been achieved with adjuvant radiotherapy. However, normal tissue tolerances make it difficult to deliver sufficient doses of EBRT to irradicate residual disease. Intraoperative radiation therapy has allowed the delivery of "boost" doses of radiation to the residual tumor in these cases. However, this has been most successful in patients with only microscopic residual disease. Those patients with gross residual and primarily unresectable disease still have unacceptably high rates of local recurrence despite the use of IORT. This latter situation is particularly suited for the use of hyperthermia in combination with radiation and surgery.

Numerous techniques have been investigated to alter the Gaussian-shaped temperature distribution induced by single-element, unfocused applicators in ultrasound hyperthermia. Harrison and Balcer-Kubiczek (1986) used elaborate electrode shaping of the crystal face by etching the conductive surface to change the intensity distribution across the applicator, and facilitate more uniform heating. Pounds and Britt (1984) found that for a single transducer, a small change in frequency dramatically altered the sound field distribution and thus suggested frequency wobbling.

Although the above features assist in flattening the temperature distribution, the beam size of unfocused, single-element applicators does not necessarily match the treatment dimensions. Since the spatial distribution of ultrasonic energy is inflexible and fixed within the treatment field, it cannot be modified to adapt to local changes in blood perfusion or discomfort that may occur during patient treatments. Although the agreement between measured and computed intensity profiles is fairly good (Ryan et al. 1991b), the irregularity of the measured patterns may be attributed to imperfections such as composition of thickness variations of the crystal, as compared to an ideal plane transducer with a uniform velocity profile at its surface. In addition, points of pressure in the back and on the edges of the crystal which are needed to make electrical contact and isure a watertight fit will affect the velocity profile of the transducer. Also, theory assumes a free-boundary model with freely vibrating elements, neglecting the effects of mechanical damping due to the attached neighboring elements (Underwood et al. 1987). This damping decreases acoustic output of the element near the edges and smooths out the intensity variations. The theory computations exhibit a sharp secondary peak along the central axis, whereas the experimental results show central axis profiles that are rounded or bilobed with a minimum at $r = 0$.

Direct contact superficial ultrasound aplicators applied intraoperatively have advantages over other hyperthermia systems available that will effectively heat the deep-seated tumors presented by this group of patients. The advantage of the intraoperative approach is the ability to localize the radiation and the hyperthermia to the tumor volume and hence have much better control over the dose. The principal disadvantage is that only a single dose is administered. Since these treatments are to be administered to patients under general anesthesia, the combination of IORT with IOHT raises specific concerns regarding its effect on certain normal tissue structures such as central and peripheral nerves which cannot be retracted or defunctionalized, since irreversible injury could lead to significant morbidity. A number of reports address the effects of IORT on normal issues, including the spinal cord and nerves (HOEKSTRA et al. 1988; TEPPER 1983; GUNDERSON et al. 1988; SINDELAR 1982a,b; SINDELAR et al. 1983; SINDELAR and KINSELLA 1993; KINSELLA et al. 1988, 1985, 1991; POULAKOS et al. 1988; ANG et al. 1983; HOPEWELL 1975; LEITH and DEWYNGAERT 1981; HOOPES 1987; MASTAGLIA et al. 1976; VAN DER KOGEL 1977, 1980; WHITE and HORNSEY 1980; BECK and GILLETTE 1987; LAVEY 1992; POWERS 1992; LO 1991; GILLETTE 1988). There are also reports with experimental data on the effects of hyperthermia on normal tissues (MARTINEZ 1983; RIES et al. 1988; WONDERGEM et al. 1988; FAJARDO 1984; ELIASSON et al. 1986; ELKON 1980; HUME et al. 1983; FROESE et al. 1991; HOOGEVEEN 1993; SMINIA et al. 1991a; PANJWANI et al. 1991; DEVRIND and WONDERGEM 1992). Finally, there are several reports which describe the effects of combinations of radiation and hyperthermia on these structures (HAVEMAN 1986; WONDERGEM 1986; 1987, WONDERGEM and HAVEMAN 1987b; MILLER 1976; ABE 1985; CRILE 1963; VUJASKOVIC and GILLETTE 1993; GOFFINET et al. 1977; SMINIA 1985, et al. 1991b).

We have reviewed the results of our phase I trial of IORT plus IOHT in 19 patients with unresectable intra-abdominal cancers (COLACCHIO et al. 1990). In that series, the complication rate and treatment-related mortality were found to be similar to those reported by groups treating similar patients with IORT alone, and the complication rate was less than the 84% reported by NISHIMURA et al. (1992) in patients receiving combination IORT/HT therapy. The addition of IOHT to the IORT is expected to produce an enhancement of the normal tissue damage (HUME 1982; BAKER and SAGER 1983; WONDERGEM and HAVEMAN 1983; LAW 1984, 1985; EMANI and PEREZ 1987; GILLETTE 1987), and whole-body hyperthermia (HT) (BULL 1984) has caused acute myelopathy in a few patients who had received neurotoxic drugs or external beam fractionated irradiation of the spinal cord (BARLOGIE and CORRY 1979; PARKS et al. 1979; DOUGLAS et al. 1981). It is therefore important to know both the tolerance of these critical normal tissues to IORT and to the combined IORT plus IOHT, in order to plan treatment fields and dosages, and also to interpret post-treatment changes in motor and sensory function both acutely and chronically.

A major difficulty in evaluating a phase I trial of this combined modality therapy is identifying an appropriate patient group for comparison of morbidity and mortality. There are now several reports of the use of IORT in the management of intra-abdominal (primarily colorectal and pancreatic) carcinomas. However, it is often difficult to identify those patients who had the same disease stage as in this trial (i.e., grossly unresectable, residual, recurrent, and primary disease) in order to make valid comparisons. Tables 17.9 and 17.10

Table 17.9. IORT for colorectal cancers: unresected/gross residual

Institution	No. of patients	Morbidity	Mortality
MGH (1983)	4	13%[a]	0
MGH (1984)	41	32%	0
NED (1984)	8	25%	0
MGH (1986)	11	45%[a]	0[a]
Mayo (1988)	2	35%[a]	2%[a]
NCl (1988)	4	100%	0

[a] Includes cases in addition to those reported

Table 17.10. IORT for pancreatic cancer: Unresected/gross residual

Institution	No. of patients	Morbidity	Mortality
NED (1984)	15	33%	6%
MGH (1987)	63	NR	NR
Kyoro (1987)	69	45%	1.4%
Mayo (1988)	44	40%	2%
NCI (1988)	16	25%	6%
NCI (1988)	33	NR	24%
Howard (1988)	19	74%	16%

NR, not reported
[a] Includes cases in addition to those shown

represent a summary of those cases from other published series with their morbidity and mortality data. For unresected and grossly residual colorectal carcinomas, most of the series in Table 17.9 have relatively small numbers of patients ranging from 2 to 11 (SINDELAR 1988; TEPPER et al. 1986; GUNDERSON et al. 1988; TEPPER et al. 1984; RICH et al. 1984). The largest series from the MGH (TEPPER et al. 1984) did not specify the amount of residual disease which was treated with IORT. In addition, the morbidity and mortality rates reported often include patients in addition to those described in the paper. Nevertheless, the morbidity rates range from 13% to 100% with a low mortality of 0%–20%. This is certainly consistent with the 50% morbidity and 0% mortality rates for colorectal cancer patients in this series.

There is somewhat less difficulty in identifying an appropriate group for comparison with pancreatic cancer, since most of the patients treated have unresectable primary disease. As shown in Table 17.10, the complication rate for these patients is generally higher, ranging from 25% to 74% (GUNDERSON et al. 1987; TUCKSON 1988; ABE 1987; HOEKSTRA et al. 1988; SINDELAR 1988; RICH 1985) and this is consistent with the morbidity rate in this series of 58%. The mortality is also considerably higher, ranging from 1.4% to 24%, and this is not significantly different from the mortality of 29% for the pancreatic cancer patients in this series. Of interest, there was a similar case of small bowel necrosis resulting in a postoperative death reported from the NCI series (HOEKSTRA et al. 1988).

Several reports with RF capacitive heating at 8.0 MHz have appeared in the literature. NISHIMURA et al. (1992) used RF capacitive heating in a clinical study (not intraoperative) and found the maximum, average, and minimum temperatures for 27 tumors to be 42.2°C, 41.3°C, and 40.3°C, respectively. A 5°C bolus between the applicator and subcutaneous fat was placed to avoid overheating the fat. In 54 of 201 sessions, only a single point was monitored. The $T_{min} >$ 42.0°C occurred in only 15/115 sessions. HAMAZOE et al. (1991) reported on 318 treatments with 39 patients; only 20 patients had tumor temperatures determined, and three reached 43°C or higher. The study by YAMADA et al. (1992a,b) compared 17 patients with pancreatic carcinoma who received IORT plus IOHT to a control group of 56 similar patients who were treated with IORT alone. There was no difference in the relief of pain between the two groups, but local control and survival were slightly better in the combined modality group. Most of the IORT/IOHT patients (15 of 17) also received EBRT, and some (8 or 17) had additional (three to four) RF capacitive hyperthermia treatments. Only three or four sites were measured for temperature during the IOHT treatments, and only 5 of the 17 patients had a measured temperature of >42°C at any location in the treatment field. The poor performance with this technology may be due to the fact that the SAR in fat may be ten times that in muscle. Thus surface cooling is required in order to heat deeper structures (KATO and ISHIDA 1993). Finally, one of the patients in the Yamada series suffered a severe burn of the subcutaneous fat.

In our series, 50% of all the measured temperature sites (average of seven sites per patient) were ⩾43°C. In all OR treatments at least one temperature measurement site averaged ⩾43.0°C. With the first few patients, the treatments were power-limited since only a 100-W RF generator was available, providing 1.3 W/cm^2 with the largest applicator. A replacement generator capable of 400 W provided more than sufficient intensity at 5.2 W/cm^2. Even at these levels, however, the mechanism of damage is presumed to be "thermal" (FRIZZELL 1988; BORRELLI et al. 1981), rather than "cavitational." The electroacoustic efficiency for PZT elements at 1.0 MHz is typically around 90% (BENKESER et al. 1989), and our results fall within this range.

During some of the procedures, the applicator was forced into a tight cavity provided by the surgeon and could not be optimally positioned. In other cases, thermal protection of normal tissue structures that could not be removed from the treatment field limited the applied power. Each channel of thermometry was assigned a maximum allowable temperature, and power was automatically adjusted so that this limit was not exceeded.

When pain is removed as a treatment limitation, maximum temperature, T_{90}, and T_{50} each increase. This is shown in the comparison between the 19 patient series in the OR and the 43 patient Clinic series (64 treatments) with the same type of applicator. The T_{90} increased from 38.8°C to 39.2°C, and T_{50} increased from 41.9°C to 42.9°C. For fixed measurement points when comparing the Clinic and IOHT series, respectively. Although the T_{90} and T_{50} were greater in the IOHT series than in the Clinic series, the single-element applicator is still severely limited in performance even if adequate power is available. In addition, some tumor dimensions exceeded the applicator's capability and thus the 10 cm circular shape was a limitation. CORRY et al. (1987) reported a series which achieved a $T_{90} = 41.4°C$ and $T_{50} = 45.7°C$ for superficial ultrasound in the awake patient. SAMULSKI et al. (1990b) reported a series of 147 treatments with $T_{50} = 40.5°C$ and $T_{90} = 38.5°C$ in which pain rather than temperature was often the limiting factor. It appears that a multielement applicator would be the best way to improve performance (CAIN and UMEMURA 1986; RYAN et al. 1991a) in the setting of intraoperative hyperthermia treatments where access to the treatment site is constrained.

Patient tolerance may be gauged by the maximum temperature at a fixed measurement site averaged over the 60 min treatment. In the OR, where adjacent tissue preservation rather than pain becomes a limiting factor, the range of power density was 0.58–4.95 W/cm^2. In the clinic with the single-element applicator, the average maximum temperature for 48 treatments was 44.5°C. In the OR, the average maximum was 46.6°C, for 19 treatments. Also, the highest recorded average temperature was 56°C in the OR. In the series with single-element applicators in the clinic, the maximum average temperature at a fixed location and the maximum pullback temperature were identical, 44.5°C for 48 treatments. The multielement applicator experience is not extensive enough at this time to draw conclusions; however, we feel the limitation in rise of temperature values is due to the limitations of the single-element applicator (RYAN et al. 1992a).

The difficulties in the placement of thermometry deep in body cavities were evaluated in the OR and underwent a series of refinements. Initially, microthermocouples were placed in the tumor inside of 17 gauge, open needles. The needles were then slowly withdrawn with the microthermocouples remaining in tissue. The exact final placement was difficult to ascertain with this technique and there was a danger of the thermocouple lead being moved, thereby dislodging the sensor. The next step was to instrument the same hollow needles with two or three microthermocouples with 1–2 cm separation, which was decided at the time of implant. The final step was to have needle thermocouples custom-fabricated with fixed sensor locations and 90° bends. These allowed precise depth of penetration and alignment and insured an exact spacing bwteen sensors. The 21 gauge sensors were also much smaller in diameter than the 17 gauge needles used previously. We currently have a selection of right-angled, needle thermocouples with lengths after the bend of 10–60 mm. All of these probes have three sensors, located at the tip, halfway along the bend, and 2.0 mm before the bend for superficial measurements.

17.7 Conclusions

Although the use of hyperthermia as part of a multimodality approach for cancer treatment has not been shown in prospective, randomized trials to result in improved survival, the weight of the available evidence would clearly support a positive effect. The ongoing dilemma continues to be the *shortcomings of the available equipment to adequately and reproducibly heat a tumor mass to the previously determined target temperature*. This situation is especially true for intra-abdominal tumors, and it is in this setting that an invasive, intraoperative approach offers the most likely opportunity for success. The series which have been reviewed have demonstrated the feasibility of this approach, but have underscored the continued need for improved technological development for heat delivery. In addition, it is our belief that the focus for hyperthermia as part of the multimodality approach needs to shift more towards minimal residual disease, even though this setting presents additional technical challenges. It will be in this latter category of patients (analogous to and expanding upon the therapeutic advantages achieved with IORT) that the addition of IOHT to the multimodal treatment plan will have the greatest likelihood of improving local control and long-term survival. It is in this area that researchers in the field of hyperthermia need to concentrate their efforts if this modality is to secure a lasting role in the cancer treatment armamentarium.

17.8 Summary

- Intraoperative radiotherapy continues to be a useful component of the multimodality treatment of advanced intra-abdominal carcinomas
- Recent prospective randomized European clinical trials have demonstrated the efficacy of combined therapy with radiotherapy and hyperthermia

- Intra-abdominal tumors are difficult to treat with hyperthermia due to the problems of inadequate thermometry and inability of external equipment to effectively raise the temperature
- Intraoperative hyperthermia offers a viable solution to these difficulties
- Further development of hyperthermia equipment will be required to allow the performance of multi-institutional trials to verify its efficacy

References

Abe M (1985) Review; localized hyperthermia and radiation in cancer therapy. Int J Radiat Oncol Biol Phys 47: 347–359

Abe M (1987) intraoperative radiotherapy in carcinoma of the stomach and pancreas. World J Surg 11: 459–464

Abe M, Shibamoto Y, Ono K, et al. (1991) Intraoperative radiation therapy for carcinoma of the stomach and pancreas. Front Radiat Ther Oncol 25: 258–269

Ang KK, Vander Kogel AJ, et al. (1983) The effect of small irradiation doses on the rat spinal cord: the concept of partial tolerance. Int J Radiat Oncol Biol Phys 9: 1487–1491

Arcicasa M, Franchin G, et al. (1992) Hyperthermia in clinical practice: preliminary results and current problems in the treatment of 21 patients. Tumori 78: 262–265

Aston SJ, Longmire WP (1973) Pancreaticoduodenal resection. Arch Surg 106: 813–817

Baker DG, Sager H (1983) The response of previously irradiated skin to combinations of X-radiation and ultrasound-induced hyperthermia. Radiat Res 96: 367–373

Barlogie B, Corry PM (1979) Total body hyperthermia with and without chemotherapy for advanced human neoplasma. Cancer Res 39: 1481–1489

Beck ER, Gillette EL (1987) Peripheral neuropathies following experimental intraoperative radiotherapy. 8th Int Cong Radiat Res Edinburgh, Scotland

Benkeser PJ, Frizzell LA, Ocheltree KB, Cain CA (1987) A tapered phased array ultrasound transducer for hyperthermia treatments. IEEE Trans Ultrasonics Ferroelectrics Frequency Control 33: 446–453

Benkeser PJ, Frizzell LA, Goss SA, Cain CA (1989) Analysis of a multielement ultrasound hyperthermia applicator. IEEE Trans Ultrasonices Ferroelectrics Frequency Control 36: 319–325

Benotti PN (1987) Management of recurrent pelvic tumors. Arch Surg 122: 457–460

Ben-Yosef R, Sullivan DM, Kapp DS (1992) Peripheral neuropathy and myonecrosis following hyperhtermia and radiation therapy for recurrent prostatic cancer: correlation of damage with predicted SAR pattern. Int J Radiat Oncol Biol Phys 8: 173–185

Boring CC, Squirtes TS, Tong T (1993) Cancer statistics. CA 43: 7–26

Borrelli MJ, Bailey KE, Dunn F (1981) Early acoustic effects upon mammalian CNS structures. J Acoust Soc Am 69: 1514–1516

Bornstein BA, Zourajian PS (1992) Local hyperthermia, radiation and chemotherapy in patients with local regional recurrence of breast carcinoma. Int J Radiat Oncol Biol Phys 25: 79–85

Bull JMC (1984) A review of systemic hyperthermia. Front Radiat Ther Oncol 18: 171–176

Bull JMC, Lees D (1979) Whole body hyperthermia: a phase I trial of a potential adjuvant to chemotherapy. Ann Intern Med 90: 317–323

Cain CA, Umemura S-I (1986) Concentric-ring and sector-vortex phased-array applicators for ultrasound hyperthermia. IEEE Tran Microwave Theory Tech 34: 542–551

Calvo FA, Santos M (1991) Intraoperative radiation therapy in gastric and pancreatic carcinoma: a European experience. Front Radiat Ther Oncol 25: 270–283

Cameron JL, Crist DW (1991) Factors influencing survival after pancreaticoduodenectomy for pancreatic carcinoma. Am J Surg 161: 120–125

Chiappa KH, Ropper AH (1982) Evoked potentials in clinical medicine. N Engl J Med 9: 1140–1150 and 20: 1205–1211

Colacchio TA, Coughlin CT, Strohbehn JW, Stafford JH, Ryan TP, Douple EB, Crichlow RW (1989) Intraoperative radiation therapy and hyperthermia for unresectable intra-abdominal carcinomas. In: Sugahara T, Saito M (eds) Hyperthermic Oncology 1988, vol 1, summary papers. Taylor & Francis, London, pp 561–562

Colacchio TA, Coughlin CT, Taylor J, Douple EB, Ryan T, Crichlow RW (1990) Intraoperative radiation therapy and hyperthermia. Arch Surg 125: 370–375

Connolly MM, Dawson PJ (1987) Survival in 1001 patients with carcinoma of the pancreas. Ann Surg 206: 366–373

Corry PM, Barlogie B, Tilchen EJ, Armour EP (1982) Ultrasound induced hyperthermia for the treatment of human superficial tumors. Int J Radiat Oncol Biol Phys 8: 1225–1229

Coughlin CT, Douple EB, Strohbehn JW, Eaton WL, Trembly BS, Wong TZ (1983) Interstitial microwave-induced hyperthermia in combination with brachytherapy. Radiology 148: 285–288

Coughlin CT, Wong TZ, Strohbehn JW, Colacchio TA, Sutton JE, Belch, RZ, Douple EB (1985) Intraoperative interstitial microwave-induced hyperthermia and brachytherapy. Int J Radiat Oncol Biol Phys 11: 1673–1678

Coughlin CT, Strohbehn JW, Ryan TP, Roberts DW, Colacchio TA, Douple EB (1988) Interstitial hyperthermia for deep-seated malignancies. In: Sugahara T, Saito M (eds) Hyperthermic oncology 1988, vol 1, summary papers. Taylor & Francis, London, pp 596–597

Crile G (1963) The effects of heat and radition on cancers implanted in the feet of mice. Cancer Res 23: 372–380

Devrind HH, Wondergem J (1992) Hyperthermia induced damage to rat sciatic nerve assessed in vivo with functional methods and electrophysiology. J Neurosci Methods 45: 164–174

Dhar PK Sinha DK (1989) Optimal temperature control in hyperthermia by artificial surface cooling. Int J Systems Sci 20: 2275–2282

Dickinson RJ (1984) An ultrasound system for local hyperthermia using scanned focused transducers. IEEE Trans Biomed Eng 31: 120–125

Dobelbower RR (1981) Current radiotherapeutic approaches to pancreatic cancer. Cancer 47: 1729–1733

Douglas MA, Parks LC, Bebin J (1981) Sudden myelopathy secondary to therapeutic total-body hyperthermia after spinal-cord irradiation. N Engl J Med 10: 583–585

Edelstein-Keshet L, Dewhirst MW (1989) Characterization of tumour temperature distributions in hyperthermia based on assumed mathematical forms. Int J Hyperthermia 5: 757–777

Einhorn LH, Williams SD (1984) Combination chemotherapy with platinum (P) plus 5-FU in metastatic colorectal carcinoma. Proc Am Soc Clin Oncol (abstr) 3: 133

Eisenberg B (1982) Carcinoma of the colon and rectum. Cancer 49: 1131–1134

Eliasson SG, Monafo WW, et al. (1986) Differential effects of in vitro heating of rat sciatic nerve branches and spinal roots. Exp Neurol 93: 57–66

Elkon D (1980) Response of mouse kidney to hyperthermia. Arch Pathol Lab Med 104: 153–158

Emami B, Perez CA (1987) Combination of surgery, irradiation and hyperthermia in treatment of recurrences of malignant tumors. Int J Radiat Oncol Biol Phys 13: 611–613

Emami B (1982) Effect of preoperative irradiation on resectability of colorectal carcinomas. Int J Radiat Oncol Biol Phys 8: 1295–1299

Engin K (1993) Randomized trial of one versus two hyperthermia treatments per week in patients with superficial tumors. Int J Hyperthermia 9: 327–340

Evans DB, Rich TA, Byrd DR, et al. (1992) Preoperative chemoradiation and pancreaticoduodenectomy for adenocarcinoma of the pancreas. Arch Surg 127: 1335–1339

Fajardo LF (1984) Pathologic effects of hyperthermia in normal tissues. Cancer Res 44: 4826–4835

Feldmann HJ, Molls M, Krumpelmann S, Stuschke M, Sack H (1993) Deep regional hyperthermia: comparison between the annular phased array and the sigma-60 applicator in the same patients. Int J Radiat Oncol Biol Phys 26: 111–116

Fessenden P, Lee ER, Anderson TL, Strohbehn JW, Meyer JL, Samulski TV, Marmor JB (1984) Experience with a multi-transducer ultrasound system for localized hyperthermia of deep tissues. IEEE Trans Biomed Eng 32: 126–135

Fortner JG (1984) Regional pancreatectomy for cancer of the pancreas, ampulla, and other related sites; tumor staging and results. Ann Surg 199: 418–425

Frizzell LA (1988) Threshold dosages for damage to mammalian liver by high intensity focused ultrasound. IEEE 35: 578–581

Froese G, Das RM, Dunscombe PB (1991) The sensitivity of the thoracolumbar spinal cord of the mouse to hyperthermia. Radiat Res 125: 173–180

Gastrointestinal Tumor Study Group (1988) Treatment of locally unresectable carcinoma of the pancreas: comparisons of combined modality therapy to chemotherapy alone. J Natl Cancer Inst 80: 751–755

Gillette EL (1987) Response of oral canine carcinomas to heat and radiation. Int J Radiat Oncol Biol Phys 13: 1861–1867

Goffinet DR, Choi KY, Brown JM (1997) The combined effects of hyperthermia and ionizing radiation on the adult mouse spinal cord. Radiat Res 72: 238–245

Goldson AL (1981) Past, present and prospects of intraoperative radiotherapy. Semin Oncol 3: 59–64

Grem JL (1991) Adjuvant treatment of node positive colon carcinoma with levamisole and 5-fluorouracil. Oncology 5: 63–74

Grundy BL, Nash CL, Brown RH (1982) Deliberate hypotension for spinal fusion: prospective randomized study with evoked potential monitoring. Can J Anaesth 29: 452–462

Gunderson LL (1980) Residual, inoperable or recurrent colorectal cancer. Am J Surg 139: 518–525

Gunderson LL, Martin JK, Kvols LK, et al. (1987) Intraoperative and external beam irradiation =/–5-FU for locally advanced pancreatic cancer. Int J Radiat Oncol Biol Phys 13: 319–329

Gunderson LL, Martin JK, Beart RW, et al. (1988) Intraoperative and external beam irradiation for locally advanced colorectal cancer. Ann Surg 207: 52–60

Hahn GM (1982) Hyperthermia and cancer. Plenum Press, New York

Hamazoe R, Maeta M, Murakami A, Yamashiro H, Kaibara N (1991) Heating efficiency of radiofrequency capacitive fhyperthermia for treatment of deep-seated tumors of the peritoneal cavity. J Surg Oncol 48: 176–179

Harrison GH, Balcer-Kubiczek EK (1986) Single-transducer electrode design for beam shaping in biomedical ultrasound. IEEE Trans Ultrasonics Ferroelectrics Frequency Control 33: 265–272

Hartov A (1991) Multiple element intraoperative ultrasound hyperthermia system. PhD Thesis, Dartmouth College

Hartov A, Ryan TP, Strohbehn JW, Colacchio TA, Hoopes PJ (1992) A new type of controller for a multiple source hyperthermia system. In: Gerner E (ed) Hyperthermic oncology 1992, vol 1. Arizona Board of Regents, Tucson, A2, p 234

Hartov A, Colacchio TA, Strohbehn JW, Ryan TP, Hoopes PJ (1993a) Performance of an adaptive MIMO controller for a multiple-element ultrasound hyperthermia system. Int J Hyperthermia 9: 563–579

Hartov A, Ryan TP, Colacchio TA, Strohbehn JW (1993b) Multiple element intraoperative ultrasound applicator. Abstract North Am Hyperthermia Soc Dallas, Texas, p 14

Haslom J (1973) RT in the treatment of unresectable carcinoma of the pancreas. Cancer 32: 1341–1345

Haveman J (1986) Enhancement of radiation effect by heat. In: Angherlieri LJ, Roberts J (eds) Hyperthermia in cancer treatment CRC Press, Boca Raton Fl. pp 169–282

Hiraoka T, Uchino R, Kanemitsu K et al. (1990) Combination of intraoperative radiation and resection of cancer of the pancreas. Int J Pancreatol 1: 201–207

Hoekstra HJ, Restrepo C, Kinsella TJ, et al. (1988) Histopathologic effects of intraoperative radiotherapy on pancreas and adjacent tissues: a postmortem analysis. J Surg Oncol 37: 104–108

Hoogeveen JF (1993) Heat shock proteins in thermotolerant rat sciatic nerves. Int J Hyperthermia 9: 361–368

Hoopes P (1987) Intraoperative radiation of the canine abdominal aorta and vena cava. Int J Radiat Oncol Biol Phys 13: 715–722

Hopewell J (1975) The effects of dose and field size on late radiation damage to the rat spinal cord. Int J Radiat Oncol Biol Phys 28: 325–333

Hume SP (1982) Increased hyperthermal response of previously irradiated mouse intestine. Br J Radiol 55: 438–443

Hume SP, Matigold JCL, Michalowski A (1983) The effect of local hyperthermia on nonproliferative compared with proliferative epithelial cells of the mouse intestinal mucosa. Radiat Res 94: 252–262

Hynynen K, Roemer R, Anhalt D, Johnson C, Xu ZX, Swindell W, Cetas T (1987) A scanned, focused, multiple transducer ultrasonic system for localized hyperthermia treatments. Int J Hyperthermia 3: 21–35
Hynynen K, Shimm D, Anhalt D (1990) Temperature distributions during clinical scanned, focused ultrasound hyperthermia treatments. Int J Hyperthermia 6: 891–900
Ibbini MS, Cain CA (1990) The concentric-ring array for ultrasound hyperthermia: combined mechanical and electrical scanning. Int J Hyperthermia 6: 401–419
Jessup JM, Steele g, Mayer RJ, et al. (1993) Neoadjuvant therapy for unresectable pancreatic carcinoma. Arch Surg 128: 559–564
Jo S, Hiraoka M, Akuta K, et al. (1989) Histopathologic changes of human tumors following thermoradiotherapy. Int J Radiat Oncol Biol Phys 17: 1265–1271
Kapp DS, Fessenden P, Samulski TV, et al. (1988) Stanford University institutional report-phase I evaluation of equipment for hyperthermic treatment of cancer. Int J Hyperthermia 4: 75–116
kapp DS, Cox RS, Fessenden P, et al. (1992) Parameters predictive for complications of treatment with combined hyperthermia and radiation therapy. Int J Radiat Oncol Biol Phys 22: 999–1008
Kato H, Ishida T (1993) present and future status of non invasive selective deep, heating using RF in hyperthermia. Med Biol Eng Comput 31: s2–s11
Kato H (1985) Deep heating characteristics of an RF capacitive heating device. Int J Hyperthermia 1: 15–28
Kinsella TJ (1985) Tolerance of peripheral nerve to intraoperative radiotherapy (IORT): clinical and experimental studies. Int J Radiat Oncol Biol Phys 11: 1579–1585
Kinsella TJ, Sindelar WF, Deluca AM, et al. (1988) Tolerance of the canine bladder to intraoperative radiation therapy: an experimental study. Int J Radiat Oncol Biol Phys 14: 939–946
Kinsella TJ, Deluca AM, Barnes M, et al. (1991) Threshold dose for peripheral neuropathy following IORT in a large animal model. Int J Radiat Oncol Biol Phys 20: 697–701
Klingerman MM (1975) Preoperative radiation therapy in rectal cancer. Cancer 36: 61–95
Lanciano N (1990) A phase I/II study of intraoperative radiation therapy in advanced unresectable or recurrent carcinoma of the rectum: a RTOG study. Annual Int IORT Meeting
Lavey RS (1992) The effect of hyperfractionation on spinal cord response to radiation. Int J Radiat Oncol Biol Phys 24: 6881–6886
Law M (1984) A long-term effect of x-rays on thermal sensitivity of the mouse ear. Br J Radiol 57: 729–731
Law M (1985) Thermal enhancement of radiation damage in previously irradiated skin. Br J Radiol 58: 161–167
Leith JT, Dewyngaert JK (1981) Radiation myelopathy in the rat. Int J Radiat Oncol Biol Phys 7: 1673–1677
Lele PP (1983) Physical aspects and clinical studies with ultrasound hyprthermia. In: Storm FC (ed) Hyperthermia in cancer therapy. Medical Hall Boston, pp 333–367
Levine G, Remine WH, Hermann RE, et al. (1978) Cancer of the pancreas. Am J Surg 135: 185–191
Lo Y (1991) The effects of single dose radiation on mouse spinal cord. Int J Radiat Oncol Biol Phys 22: 57–63
Lyng H, Monge OR, Bohler PJ, et al. (1991) Relationships between thermal-dose and tissue and vascular damage after thermoradiotherapy of locally advanced breast cancer. Int J Hyperthermia 7: 403–415
Martinez A (1983) Thermal sensitivity and thermotolerance in normal porcine tissues. Cancer Res 43: 2072–2075
Mastaglia FL, McDonald WI, Watson JV, et al. (1976) Effects of x-irradiation on the spinal cord: an experimental study of the morphological changes in central nerve fibres. Brain 99: 101–122
McPherson RW, Mahla M, Johnson R, et al. (1985) Effects of enflurane, isoflurane and nitrous oxide on somatosensory evoked potentials during fentanyl anesthesia. Anaesthesiology 62: 626–633
Miller RC (1976) Potentiation of radiation myelitis in rats by hyperthermia. Br J Radiol 49: 895–896
Moskowitz MJ, Ryan TP, Paulsen KD (1994) Complete temperature field estimation using kHz-range electrical inverse profiling methods. II. Experimental system design and phantom heating results. Int J Hyperthermia 10: 229–247
Myerson RJ (1990) Tumor control in long term survivors following superficial hyperthermia. Int J Radiat Oncol Biol Phys 18: 1123–1129
Nishimura Y, Hiraoka M, Akuta K, et al. (1992) Hyperthermia combined with radiation therapy for primarily unresectable and recurrent colorectal cancer. Int J Radiat Oncol Biol Phys 23:759–768
Ocheltree KB, Benkeser PJ, Frizzell LA, Cain CA (1984) An ultrasonic-phased array applicator for hyperthermia. IEEE Trans Sonics Ultrasonics 31: 526–531
Oleson JR (1986) The role of magnetic induction techniques for producing hyperthermia. In: Anghileri LJ, Robert J (eds) Hyperthermia in cancer treatment vol II. CRC Press, Boca Raton Fl., pp 141–154
Oleson JR Tumor temperature distributions predict hyprthermia effect. Int J Radiat Oncol Biol Phys 16: 559–570
Oleson JR (1993) Sensitivity of hyperthermia trial outcomes to temperature and time: implications for thermal goals of treatment. Int J Radiat Oncol Biol Phys 25: 289–297
Panjwani GD, Mustafa NK, Muhailan A, et al. (1991) Effect of hyperthermia on somatosensory evoked potentials in the anesthetized rat. Electroencephalogr Clin Neurophysiol 80: 384–391
Parks LC, Minaberry D, Smith DP, Neely WA (1979) Treatment of far advanced bronchogenic carcinoma by extracorporeally induced systemic hyperthermia. Thorac Cardiovsc Surg 78: 883–892
Paulsen KD, Moskowitz MJ, Ryan TP (1991) A combined invasive-noninvasive conductivity profile reconstruction approach for thermal imaging in hyperthermia. Proceedings of the international conference of the IEEE Engineering in Medicine and Biology Society, IEEE press Piscataway, NJ, pp 323–324
Paulsen KD, Moskowitz MJ, Ryan TP (1994) Complete temperature field estimation using kHz-range electrical inverse profiling methods. I. Reconstruction algorithm and simulated currents. Int J Hyperthermia 10: 209–229
Perez CA, Pajak T, Emami B, et al. (1991) Randomized phase III study comparing irradiation and hyperthermia with irradiation alone in superficial measurable tumors. Am J Clin Oncol 14: 133–141
Pilepich M (1978) Preoperative irradiation of primarily unresectable colorectal carcinoma. Cancer 42: 1077–1081
Poulakos L, Elwell JH, Osbourne JW, et al. (1988) Intraoperative irradiation in a rat model: histopathologic

changes in irradiated segments of duodenum. J Surg Oncol 38: 130–135
Pounds DW, Britt RH (1984) Single ultrasonic crystal techniques for generating uniform temperature distributions in homogeneously perfused tissues. IEEE Trans Sonics Ultrasonics 31: 482–490
Powers BE (1992) Pathology of radiation injury to the canine spinal cord. Int J Radiat Oncol biol Phys 23: 539–549
Rich TA (1985) Radiation therapy for pancreatic cancer: eleven year experiment, JCRT. J Can Assoc Radiat 11: 759–763
Rich TA, Cady B, McDermott WV, et al. (1984) Orthovoltage intraoperative radiotherapy. A new look at an old idea. Int J Radiat Oncol Biol Phys 10: 1957–1965
Rider W (1975) Is the Miles' operation neceassary for the treatment of rectal cancer? J Can A Rad 26: 167–175
Ries MC, Milligan AJ, Merrick HW, et al. (1988) Biochemical and cellular effects of radiofrequency induced interstitial hyperthermia on normal canine liver. Int J Radiat Oncol Biol Phys 14: 529–536
Roldan GE, Gunderson LL, Nagorney DM, et al. (1988) External beam versus intraoperative and external beam irradiation for locally advanced pancreatic cancer. Cancer 61: 1110–1116
Roscuit B (1975) Preoperative irradiation for carcinoma of the rectum and rectosigmoid: report of a national veterans administration randomized study. Cancer 35: 1597–1602
Ryan TP (1991a) Comparison of six microwave antennas for hyperthermia treatment of cancer: SAR results for single antennas and arrays. Int J Radiat Oncol Biol Phys 21: 403–413
Ryan TP (1991b) Techniques for heating brain tumors with implanted microwave antennas. In: Heiter GL (ed) IEEE MTT-S international microwave symposium digest, IEEE Press, Piscataway, NJ, pp 791–794
Ryan TP (1993) Methods of thermal modelling and their impact on interstitial hyperthermia treatment planning. In: Seegenschmiedt HM, Sauer R (eds) Medical Radiology-Diagnostic imaging and radiation oncology: interstitial and intracavitary thermo-radiotherapy. Springer Berlin Heidelberg New York, pp 95–116
Ryan TP, Coughlin CT, Stafford JH, Lyons BE, Strohbehn JW, Douple EB (1986) Temperature analysis of ultrasound-induced hyperthermia in patients with superficial tumors. North American Hyperthermia Group Annual Meeting, Las Vegas, NV (abstract)
Ryan TP, Samulski TV, Lyons BE, Lee E, Holdren D, Fessenden P, Strohbehn JW (1989) Thermal conduction effects associated with temperature measurements in proximity to radiofrequency electrodes and microwave antennas. Int J Radiat Oncol Biol Phys 16: 1557–1564
Ryan TP, Colacchio TA, Coughlin CT, Hartov A (1991a) Analysis of hyperthermia treatments: single vs multiple-element applicators. Proceedings of the International Conference of the IEEE Engineering in Medicine and Biology Society, vol 13. IEEE Press, Piscataway, NJ, pp 181–182
Ryan TP, Hartov A, Colacchio TA, Coughlin CT, Stafford JH, Hoopes PJ (1991b) Analysis and testing of a concentric ring applicator for ultrasound hyperthermia with clinical results. Int J Hyperthermia, 7: 587–603
Ryan TP, Hoopes PJ, Taylor JH, Strohbehn JW, Roberts DW, Douple EB, Coughlin CT (1991c) Experimental brain hyperthermia: techniques for heat delivery and thermometry. Int J Radiat Nocol Biol Phys 20: 739–750
Ryan TP, Paulsen KD, Moskowitz MJ (199d) The Dartmouth electrical impedance tomography system for thermal imaging. Proceedings of the International Conference of the IEEE Engineering in Medicine and Biology Society, IEEE Press, Piscataway, NJ, pp 321–322
Ryan TP, Wikoff R, Hoopes PJ (1991e) An automated temperature mapping system for use in ultrasound or microwave hyperthermia. J Biomed Eng 13: 348–354
Ryan TP, Colacchio TA, Douple EB, Coughlin CT (1992a) Techniques for intraoperative hyperthermia with ultrasound: the Dartmouth experience with 19 patients. Int J Hyperthermia 8: 407–421
Ryan TP, Taylor JH, Coughlin CT (1992b) Interstitial microwave hyperthermia and brachytherapy for malignancies of the vulva and vagina. I. Design and testing of a modified intracavitary obturator Int J Radiat Oncol Biol Phys 23: 189–199
Ryan TP, Hartov A, Colacchio TA (1993) Steerable-beam therapeutic ultrasound for superificial heat treatments. Proceedings of the International Conference of the IEEE Engineering in Medicine and Biology Society, IEEE Press, Piscataway, NJ, pp 198–199
Ryan TP, Trembly BS, Roberts DW, Strohbehn JW, Coughlin CT (1994) Dartmouth brain hyperthermia. I. Interstitial microwave antenna array techniques. Int J Radiat Oncol Biol Phys (submitted)
Samulski TV (1987) Heating deep-seated eccentrically shaped tumors with an annular array system: a comparitive clinical study using two annular array configurations. Int J Radiat Oncol Biol Phys 13: 83–94
Samulski TV, Grant WJ, Oleson JR, Leopold KA, Dewhirst MW, Vallario P, Blivin J (1990a) Clinical experience with a multi-element ultrasonic hyperthermia system: analysis of treatment temperatures. Int J Hyperthermia 6: 909–922
Samulski TV, Fessenden P (1990b) Spiral microstrip applicators: technical design and clinical performance. Int J Radiat Oncol Biol Phys 18: 233–242
Sapareto SA, Dewey WC (1984) Thermal dose determination in cancer therapy. Int J Radiat Oncol Biol Phys 10: 787–800
Sapozink MD (1985) A comparison of deep regional hyperthermia from an annular array and a concentric coil in the same patients. Int J Radiat Oncol Biol Phys 11: 179–190
Scott RS, Clay L, Storey KV, Johnson JR (1985) Transient microwave induced neurosensory reactins during superficial hyperthermia treatment. Int J Radiat Oncol Biol Phys 11: 561–566
Shaw EG, Gunderson LL (1990) Peripheral nerve and ureteral tolerance to intraoprative radiation therapy: clinical and dose-response analysis. Radiother Oncol 18: 247–255
Shipley WU, Nardi GL, Cohen AM, et al. (1980) Iodine 125 implant and external beam irradiation in patients with localized pancreatic carcinoma. A comparative study to surgical resection. Cancer 45: 709–714
Shipley WU, Wood WC, Tepper JE, et al. (1984) Intraoperative electron beam irradiation for patients with unresectable pancreatic carcinoma. Ann Surg 200: 289–296
Sindelar WF (1989) Clinical experience with regional pancreatectomy for adenocarcinoma of the pancreas. Arch Surg 124: 127–132
Sindelar W (1982a) Tolerance of retroperitoneal structures to intraoperative irradiation. Ann Surg 196: 601–608

Sindelar WF (1982b) Tolerance of bile duct to intraoperative irradiation. Surgery 92: 533–540
Sindelar WF, Morrow BM, Travis EL, et al. (1983) Effects of intraoperative electron irradiation in the dog on cell turnover in intact and surgically anastomosed aorta and intestine. Int J Radiat Oncol Biol Phys 9: 523–532
Sindelar WF, Hoekstra H, Restrepo C, Kinsella TJ (1986) Pathological tissue changes following intraoperative radiotherapy. Am J Clin Oncol 9: 504–509
Sindelar WF (1988) Surgical approaches and techniques in intraoperative radiotherapy for intra-abdominal, retroperitoneal, and pelvic neoplasms. Surgery 103: 247–256
Sindelar WF, Kinsella TJ (1993) IORT in retroperitoneal sarcomas. Arch Surg 128: 402–410
Smini P (1985) A microwave heating technique for the rat spinal cord; thermometry and first results on the acute effects of hyperthermia on cervical spinal cord. Strahlentherapie 161: 550
Sminia P, Haveman J, Koedooder C (1991a) Effects of hyperthermia applied to previously irradiated cervical spinal cord in the rat. Radiother Oncol 2: 60–67
Sminia P, Haveman J, Jansen W, et al. (1991b) Hyperthermia promotes the incidence of tumors following x-radiation of the rat cervical cord region. Int J Radiat Biol 60: 833–845
Sporn MB, Roberts AB (1992) Transforming growth factor-B: recent progress and new challenges. J Cell Biol 119: 1017–1021
Stevens K (1976) Preoperative radiotherapy for adenocarcinoma of the recto sigmoid. Cancer 37: 2866–2874
Strohbehn JW (1985) Summary of physical and technical studies. In: Overgaard J (ed) Hyperthermic Oncology 1984, vol 2. Taylor and Francis, London, pp 353–369
Strohbehn JW (1991) An engineer looks at hyperthermia. Robinson Award Lecture, 9th International Congress in Radiation Research. Toronto. Congress Proceedings pp 14–25
Strohbehn JW, Mechling J (1986) Interstitial techniques for clinical hyperthermia. In: Hand J, James J (eds) Handbook of techniques for clinical hyperthermia. Research Studies Press, Letchworth, Herts, England, pp 210–287
Strohbehn JW (1986) Use of finite element method in computerized thermal dosimetry. In: Hand J, James J (eds) Handbook of techniques for Clinical Hyperthermia. Research Studies Press, Letchworth, Herts England, pp 383–451
Tepper J (1976) Carcinoma of the pancreas. Review of MGH experience from 1963–1973. Cancer 37: 1519–1524
Tepper J (1983) tolerance of canine anastomoses to intraoperative irradiation. Int J Radiat Oncol Biol Phys 9: 987–992
Tepper JE, Gunderson LL, Orlow E, et al. (1984) Complications of intraoperative radiotheropy. Int J Radiat Oncol Biol Phys 10: 1831–1839
Tepper JE, Cohen AM, Wood WC, et al. (1986) Intraoperative electron beam radiotherapy in the treatment of unresectable rectal cancer. Arch Surg 121: 421–423
Tepper JE (1987) Postoperative radiation therapy of rectal cancer. Int J Radiat Oncol Biol Phys 13: 5–10
Tepper JE, Noyes D, Krall JM (1991) Intraoperative radiation therapy of pancreatic carcinoma: a report of RTOG-8505. Int J Radiat Oncol Biol Phys 21: 1145–1149
Trede M (1985) The surgical treament of pancreatic carcinoma. Surgery 97: 28–35
Trembly BS, Strohbehn JW, deSieyes DC, Douple EB (1982) Hyperthermia induced by an array of invasive microwave antennas. Monogr Natl Cancer Inst 61: 497–499
Tuckson W (1988) Intraoperative RT for patients with carcinoma of the pancreas. Ann Surg 207: 648–654
Underwood HR, Burdette EC, Ocheltree KB, Magin RL (1987) A multi-element ultrasonic hyperthermia applicator with independent element control. Int J Hyperthermia 3: 257–267
Vander Kogel AJ (1977) Radiation tolerance of the rat spinal cord: time-dose relationships. Radiology 122: 505
Vander Kogel AJ (1980) Mechanisms of late radiation injury in the spinal cord. In: Myer R, Withers HR (eds) Radiation biology in cancer research. Raven Press New York, pp 461–470
Veilleux M, Daube JR, Cucchiara RF (1987) Monitoring of cortical evoked potentials during surgical procedures of the cervical spine. Mayo Clin Proc 62: 256–264
Vujaskovic Z, Gillette SM, et al. (1993) Effects of intraoperative radiotherapy (IORT) on sciatic nerve. Radiation and Oncology 30: 133–139
Vujaskovic Z, Mcchesney-Gillette S, Powers BE, et al. (1994) Effects of intraoperative hyperthermia on peripheral nerves: neurologic and electrophysiologic studies. Int J Hyperthermia 10: 41–49
Wang C (1962) Role of RT in the management of carcinoma of sigmoid, rectosigmoid, rectum. Radiology 79: 1–5
Waterman FM (1990) Determination of the temperature artifact during ultrasound hyperthermia. Int J Hyperthermia 6: 131–142
Waterman FM, Dewhirst MW, Fessenden P, et al. (1991) RTOG quality assurance guidelines for clinical trials using hyperthermia administered by ultrasound. Int J Radiat Oncol Biol Phys 20: 1099–1107
White A, Hornsey S (1980) Time dependent repair of radiation damage in the rat spinal cord after x-rays and neutrons. Eur J Cancer 16: 957
Whittington R, Dobelbower RR, Mohiuddin M, et al. (1981) Radiotherapy of unresectable pancreatic carcinoma. A six year experience with 104 patients. Int J Radiat Oncol Biol Phys 7: 1639–1644
Willett CG, Shellito PC, Tepper JE, et al. (1991a) Intraoperative electron beam radiation therapy for recurrent locally advanced rectal or rectosigmoid carcinoma. Cancer 67: 1504–1508
Willett CG, Shellito PC, Tepper JE, et al. (1991b) Intraoperative electron beam radiation therapy for primary locally advanced rectal and rectosigmoid carcinoma. J Clin Oncol 9: 843–849
Wilson SM, Block GE (1974) Periampullary carcinoma. Arch Surg 108: 539–544
Withers H (1977) Postoperative RT for adenocarcinoma of the rectum and rectosigmoid. Int J Radiat Biol Phys 2: 1069–1074
Wondergem J, Haveman J (1983) The response of previously irradiated mouse skin to heat alone or combined with irradiation: influence of thermotolerance. Int J Radiat Oncol Biol Phys 44: 539–552
Wondergem J, Haveman J (1987) The effect of previous treatment on the response of mouse feet to irradiation and hyperthermia. Radiother Oncol 10: 253–261
Wondergem J (1986) Effects of hyperthermia and x-irradiation on mouse stromal tissues. Int J Radiat Oncol Biol Phys 50: 65–76

Wondergem J, Haveman J, Schol E, et al. (1987) Influence of prior heat treatment on the effects of heat alone or combined with x-rays on mouse stromal tissues. Int J Radiat Oncol Biol Phys 51: 81–90

Wondergem J, Haveman J, Rusma NP, et al. (1988) Effects of local hyperthermia on the motor function of the rat sciatic nerve. Int J Radiat Biol 53: 429–438

Yamada S, Takai Y, Nemoto K, et al. (1992a) Intraoperative radiation therapy combined with hyperthermia for pancreatic cancer. Int J Oncol 1: 795–798

Yamada S, Takai Y, Nemoto K, et al. (1992b) Intraoperative radiation therapy combined with hyperthermia against for pancreatic carcinoma. Tohoku J Exp Med 166: 397–401

Zhou L, Fessenden P (1993) Automation of temperature control for large-array microwave surface applicators. Int J Hyperthermia 9: 479–490

18 Clinical Practice of Whole-Body Hyperthermia: New Directions

J.M.C. BULL

CONTENTS

18.1 Introduction

Whole-body hyperthermia (WBH) is a modality that was developed to treat disseminated cancer (LARKIN et al. 1977; PETTIGREW et al. 1974a,b). It is generally used in combination with chemotherapy (BULL et al. 1987, 1992b; ENGELHARDT et al. 1982, 1990; KOGA et al. 1985; PAGE et al. 1992a; ROBINS et al. 1993), and less frequently with radiation; although therapies combining WBH with cytokines also promise to become effective anticancer treatments (ANJUM and FLEISCHMANN 1992; DOLEIRE et al. 1992; GEEHAN et al. 1993; MAKINO et al. 1993a; ROBINS et al. 1989; TAPAZAGLOU et al. 1990). In addition to its major application to treat metastatic disease, WBH may be useful with chemotherapy as a neoadjuvant or adjuvant treatment. WBH can also be used in combination with local or regional heating techniques. Used as an auxiliary to local heating techniques, systemic hyperthermia can increase the basal core body temperature, thereby boosting the overall median tumor temperature level targeted by the local hyperthermia device (THRALL et al. 1990). This supplementary application of WBH combined with local-regional hyperthermia creates a more homogeneous and higher temperature within tumors as part of multimodality therapies using radiation or chemotherapy (THRALL et al. 1990). In noncancerous medical settings, WBH may prove additionally useful as an adjuvant to antibiotics to treat of infectious disease resistant to standard antibiotics (ADAMS 1993). Moderate heat, "fever," increases the cytotoxicity of host leukocytes and also enhances cytokine-induced response to bacterial, viral, fungal, or parasitic infections. Although controversial, WBH has been used as a single modality to treat AIDS-related Kaposi's sarcoma (ALONSO et al. 1992).

In clinical and veterinary practice, normal tissue tolerance limits the WBH temperature to a maximum of 41.8°–42°C (BULL et al. 1979; PAGE et al. 1987). For a time, the temperature ceiling of 41.8°–42°C was thought to pose a severe limitation to the useful application of WBH in cancer therapy. As experience with local-regional tech-

J.M.C. BULL, MD, Division of Oncology, The University of Texas at Houston Medical School, University of Texas, P.O. Box 20708, 6431 Fannin Road, Houston, TX 77225, USA

niques to induce hyperthermia matured, it became obvious that the induction of hyperthermia in the 41.8°–42°C temperature range is therapeutically effective (DEWHIRST et al. 1984; OLESON et al. 1989, 1993) when combined with either radiation (STEEVES et al. 1987) or chemotherapy (HERMAN et al. 1982). The 41.8°–42°C temperature limit actually exceeds the median tumor temperature induced by currently available local-regional hyperthermia induction devices used to treat tumors greater than 1 cm in diameter or tumors in any body regions deeper than the subcutaneous tissue (ENGIN et al. 1994a; OLESON et al. 1993; THRALL et al. 1990).

Inspired by Armour's preclinical and clinical applications of long-duration lower temperatures used in local-regional heat and combined with radiation (ARMOUR et al. 1991, 1993), new interest is developing in WBH therapies that rely on the induction of lower WBH temperatures in the range of 40°–41°C that are maintained over prolonged durations (6–24 h) in a combined modality setting using chemotherapy and/or cytokines (SAKAGUCHI et al. 1994d). This new WBH application harks back to Coley's historical use of bacterial toxins (Coley's toxins) to induce fever and induce tumor response in cancer patients with sarcoma and melanoma (COLEY 1893; NAUTS 1975).

While the studies of LIENARD et al. (1992) are of regional isolated limb perfusion treatment, not WBH, they are quite relevant to WBH. These investigators have made very effective use of heated limb perfusion combined with melphalan and two cytokines, recombinant human tumor necrosis factor-α (TNF) and recombinant human interferon-γ to treat patients with soft tissue sarcoma and melanoma of the extremities. They observed a greater than 90% complete durable response in these patients. While TNF may not be safely combined clinically with WBH at this time, both recombinant human interferon-α and interferon-γ may be combined investigationally with WBH in the clinic (ROBINS et al. 1989; TAPAZOGLOU et al. 1990). It may also be quite important that WBH itself induces the endogenous production of cytokines (DOLEIRE et al. 1993; NEVILLE and SAUDER 1988). Endogenously produced interferons, TNF, interleukins, and myelostimulants may well be components of antitumor as well as infectious disease response to WBH.

18.2 Methods of Heat Induction

There are three general methods of inducing WBH (BULL 1983, 1984). All three techniques to induce systemic hyperthermia rely to some extent on the heat produced by normal body metabolism to increase the core body temperature (BULL 1984; ROBINS and NEVILLE 1986; VAN DER ZEE et al. 1987).

18.2.1 Use of Bacterial Toxins

An important historical method of inducing systemic hyperthermia was developed by W.C. Coley. Coley injected bacterial toxins that produced fevers of prolonged duration (COLEY 1893; NAUTS 1975, 1982). His use of bacterial toxins induced complete and durable tumor regressions that have been well documented by Nauts (NAUTS et al. 1953; NAUTS 1982). Although Coley was the first to administer bacterial products to induce fever, tumor regression associated with fever was first described by W. BUSCH (1866), and 20 years later by BRUNS (1888). These nineteenth century physicians published descriptions of two patients with cancer who developed an incidental bacterial infection with erysipelas. Complete tumor regressions were associated with the prolonged high fevers accompanying the bacterial infections. Although immunologists argue that such tumor responses are secondary to toxin-induced cytokines, hyperthermia investigators regard the cancer responses to be secondary to prolonged systemic temperature elevation. Our understanding of tumor biology and immunology today suggests that elevated systemic temperatures and cytokine induction may act synergistically to induce the antitumor response (GEEHAN et al. 1993). The method of inducing WBH is based on exogenous pyrogens and uses bacterial or other exogenous protein or chemical compounds injected subcutaneously, intramuscularly, or intravenously to trigger the normal immune and neuromuscular systems to produce a fever, thus elevating the systemic temperature. Unfortunately, the response of an individual patient to bacterial endotoxins, proteins, or chemicals is not completely uniform or predictable. The regulation and control of fevers stimulated by a foreign protein show considerable variation in individual patients, and fevers are also imperfectly controlled by the therapist. Thus, at least today, this type of WBH induction is not practical.

18.2.2 Extracorporeal Heating of Blood

A second WBH induction method involves extracorporeal heating of the blood. This method was first described by Parks (PARKS et al. 1979; PARKS and SMITH 1983), who modified extracorporeal blood diversion methods developed for open heart surgery. The Parks' technique involves cannulating the femoral artery and vein, forming an arteriovenous shunt that can be connected to an extracorporeal heat exchange unit. This methodology was developed to cool the heart during cardiac bypass surgery (PARKS and SMITH 1983). The heated blood is returned to the systemic circulation and relatively rapidly increases body core temperature both by direct diffusion and by supplementing metabolic heat. Initially, extracorporeal heating appeared to be the most rapid means of inducing the target WBH temperature as well as later cooling the patient. An average-sized patient (70 kg) may be heated to 42°C within an hour, and following treatment can be cooled to below 40°C within 30 min (PARKS and SMITH 1983). Unfortunately, because this technique induces alterations in the coagulation system, the extracorporeal heating method also may be the most invasive and dangerous technique of WBH induction. Extracorporeal heating of the blood activates the coagulation cascade, acutely causing thrombocytopenia. It can be associated with hyper- and hypocoagulable states and, therefore, with potential complications of bleeding or thrombosis. These complications occur more frequently with extracorporeal heating of the blood than with the other WBH induction methods (BULL 1984).

18.2.3 Epidermal Heating Methods

The third and most commonly used means of inducing WBH transfers heat from an external source to the body core by using the patient's skin surface area as a heat transfer (BULL 1984). Like the extracorporeal heating technique, the epidermal heating methods all supplement the intrinsic heat produced by body metabolism. These heating methods have a greater requirement to block evaporative heat loss for efficiency, compared to WBH induction using either exogenous pyrogens or the extracorporeal blood heating method. An historical, yet effective heating technique involved immersion of the patient in warm wax (PETTIGREW et al. 1974b). Other methods use warm water (LOSHEK et al. 1981; SELKER et al. 1983), heated air (VAN DER ZEE et al. 1983), heated water blankets (BARLOGIE et al. 1979; HERMAN et al. 1988; LARKIN et al. 1977), or heated water suits (BULL et al. 1979) to induce systemic temperature elevation. A newer technique developed by ROBINS et al. (1985) employs radiant heat and a humidified closed environment. Because the humidified warm chamber does not allow body cooling by perspiration, the radiant heat method is the most rapid noninvasive technique to induce WBH. To heat a 70-kg patient to a core temperature of 41.8°–42°C using this device typically takes 60–90 min. The other epidermal heating methods are somewhat slower and usually require 120–180 min to achieve a core temperature of 41.8°–42°C. Increasing the insulation of the patient diminishes heat loss and decreases the time required to reach the target temperature. To a lesser extent, the patient's own metabolic heat generation and body mass or size influence the time needed to achieve this temperature. If prior to WBH induction a subject is inadvertently allowed to cool to 36.0°C, as can easily occur in an air-conditioned treatment area, target temperature induction may commonly be delayed by an additional hour or more. Such inadvertent pretreatment cooling remains a nontrivial influence on the WBH induction time, although pre-treatment is a minor problem with the radiant heat device with it's humidified chamber.

18.3 Toxicities of Whole-Body Hyperthermia

The toxicities of WBH used as a single modality to 41.8°–42.0°C are largely cardiovascular in nature because of heat-induced high cardiac output (LEES et al. 1982; PAGE et al. 1987). WBH to 41.8°–42.0°C can also induce disequilibrium of the coagulation system (BULL et al. 1982; KLAUBERT et al. 1988; STROTHER et al. 1986). Systemic heat elevation can induce a *capillary leak syndrome* (BULL et al. 1982). The heat-induced vascular endothelial changes (FAJARDO et al. 1985) that lead to capillary leak syndrome are thought to be, at least in part, mediated by TNF (KILBOURNE et al. 1990). The capillary leak syndrome is usually observed as an innocuous peripheral edema (TONNESEN et al. 1987), but can become a serious complication if it progresses to pulmonary edema (BULL et al. 1982; STARK et al. 1985). While WBH-induced pulmonary edema usually becomes clinically evident in a setting of advanced pulmonary metastases, it may be induced in normal lungs if excessively generous quantities of intravenous fluid are administered during or immediately following the treatment (BULL et al. 1992a). While it is a temptation to administer large quantities of intravenous fluid during and immediately following WBH because heat-induced hypotension occurs (LEES et al. 1982), a cautious use of vasopressors rather than large amounts of intravenous fluid is strongly recommended (CRONAU et al. 1984).

An acute, albeit transient and usually mild, *thrombocytopenia* follows all WBH procedures. WBH-induced thrombocytopenia (BULL et al. 1978; GERARD et al. 1984; STROTHER et al. 1986) occurs secondary to heat-induced endothelial changes in the microvasculature (FAJARDO et al. 1985). Platelets attach to the endothelium altered by elevated temperature. WBH-induced endothelial derangement may result from endogenous cytokine induction, particularly of TNF and interleukin (MAKINO et al. 1993b; NEVILLE and SAUDER 1988). Although transient, a mild *coagulopathy* may complicate the invariable acute thrombocytopenia that accompanies WBH (BULL et al. 1978; STROTHER et al. 1986). Uncommonly, a hypercoagulable state can develop in the immediate period following WBH therapy. Patients with advanced adenocarcinoma are particularly vulnerable to low-grade disseminated intravascular coagulation (ROHNER et al. 1966; SACK et al. 1977). Hypercoagulable states are a component of cancer-associated (particularly adenocarcinoma) paraneoplastic syndrome (SPERO et al. 1980). As described above, the most severe acute transient thrombocytopenia observed following a WBH treatment follows the extracorporeal blood heating method used to induce systemic hyperthermia (PARKS and SMITH 1983).

Hyperthermia affects both normal and tumor tissue response to anesthetic, sedative, and local anesthetic drugs. The anesthetic agents used to sedate or anesthetize the patient, therefore, have an important influence on both the toxicity and the antitumor efficacy of the WBH procedure (CRONAU et al. 1984; LEES et al. 1980). For example, because lidocaine alters cell membrane fluidity, it makes cells more susceptible to heat-induced damage (YATVIN 1977; YATVIN et al. 1979). Administration of lidocaine intravenously during WBH treatments is used to improve the WBH-induced antitumor effect (ROBINS et al. 1984). Clearly, using systemic lidocaine during WBH reduces the risk of heat-induced seizures (CRONAU et al. 1984). Anesthetic agents also interact with chemotherapy agents and thus change heat-enhanced drug-induced toxicity of thermochemotherapy (WONDERGEM et al. 1988b, 1993). Wondergem et al. found that Nembutal anesthesia increased cisplatin-induced toxic side-effects at 37.0°C and at WBH to 41.5°C for 120 min. The toxicities included acute renal tubular dysfunction and diarrhea. On the other hand, a combination anesthetic consisting of ketamine, xylazine, and acepromazine reduced the acute renal toxicity at both normothermic and WBH temperatures, whereas the inhalation anesthetic halothane had only a minor influence on cisplatin-induced renal tubular dysfunction (WONDERGEM et al. 1988b). These anesthetic interactions with cisplatin may be mediated by an effect on blood flow to the kidneys. As well as affecting the consciousness level and neurological function, anesthetic agents combined with heat alter the systemic and tumor microvascular endothelium (HALL et al. 1988; TAKAHASHI et al. 1991). Because anesthetic agents significantly alter heat- and chemotherapy-induced toxicity as well as antitumor effects (ROBINS et al. 1984; WONDERGEM et al. 1988b, 1993), it is imperative to standardize the anesthetic agent, their concentrations within whole-body hyperthermia regimens.

18.4 Thermochemotherapy

A combined modality therapy using WBH with chemotherapy has an intuitive appeal because the two systemic modalities can interact in an additive or synergistic mode to increase antitumor effect. A positive interaction of hyperthermia with chemotherapy was first demonstrated in vitro by Hahn (HAHN 1978; HAHN and STRANDE 1976; BRAUN and HAHN 1975) and others (ALBERTS et al. 1980; BARLOGIE et al. 1980; HERMAN 1983; HERMAN et al. 1984; MEYN et al. 1979). An indication that hyperthermia could overcome drug resistance in cells drew considerable interest (HERMAN et al. 1981; WALLNER et al. 1986). In vivo antitumor effects of thermochemotherapy were also observed (DAHL 1983; HONESS and BLEEHEN 1982; MARMOR et al. 1979; MELLA 1985). Unfortunately, while in vivo WBH animal studies (BABA et al. 1989; MELLA 1985) demonstrated enhanced antitumor effects of chemotherapy combined with systemic temperatures between 41° and 42°C, they also revealed increased toxicity (HINKELBEIN et al. 1988). While WBH does not add unusual, previously unknown toxicities to an individual chemotherapeutic agent, it does increase the unique drug-associated normal tissue toxicity of specific chemotherapy agents (BABA et al. 1991; HONESS and BLEEHEN 1985b; OHNO et al. 1991, 1993; WONDERGEM et al. 1988a, 1991). In clinical WBH, heat-enhanced drug-specific toxicity may be the greatest barrier to be overcome if the general application of systemic thermochemotherapy is to be achieved (GERARD et al. 1983; KIM et al. 1979b). It is not the antitumor effect, but rather the therapeutic index, that is of utmost importance when WBH is combined with chemotherapy. The ways to reduce heat enhancement of normal tissue toxicities are:

1. To alter the schedule and time of the combination of heat and drugs
2. To add a protective agent
3. To use a drug analog with a different toxicity specturm

Animal studies suggest that offset times, e.g., nonconcomitant exposures to drug and WBH, reduce heat-enhanced drug-induced toxicity while still retaining an increased antitumor effect (though this effect is less than that achieved with simultaneous administration of heat and drug) (BABA et al. 1989). As described above, other options include use of a protective agent (BABA et al. 1991) or a drug analog with a different toxicity spectrum (OHNO et al. 1991). Preliminary studies also suggest that the use of long-duration low systemic hyperthermia temperatures (between 40.0° and 41.0°C for more than 4 h) in combination with chemotherapy is associated with increased antitumor effect without increasing chemotherapy-induced drug toxicity (SAKAGUCHI et al. 1994d).

Interestingly, WBH appears to enhance those chemotherapy drug-induced toxicities that are organ-unique, e.g., cisplatin-induced renal proximal tubular dysfunction, or doxorubicin-induced cardiotoxicity, more than chemotherapy-induced bone marrow toxicity (OHNO et al. 1993). A lower temperature in the bone marrow compared with more vulnerable, "warmer" critical organs such as the kidney, liver, and heart may explain the relatively minimally enhanced in vivo bone marrow toxicity following thermochemotherapy. THRALL et al. (1986), using a radiant heat system to induce WBH, found that the temperature within the bone marrow in dogs heated with a radiant heating device was lower than temperatures in other critical organs. Another explanation is that WBH protects bone marrow from radiation-induced myelosuppression (SHEN et al. 1991). Additionally, O'HARA et al. (1991a,b) have shown that hyperthermia induces thermotolerance in both myeloprogenitor cells and myeloid stromal cells. Also, thermotolerance is known to reduce drug-induced cytotoxicity, and heat induces thermotolerance in myeloid cells (MIVECHI and LI 1988). A third explanation for the less-than-expected heat enhancement of drug-induced myelosuppression is that WBH induces the endogenous release of myelostimulatory cytokines that act to offset drug or radiation-induced myelosuppression (DOLEIRE et al. 1993; NETA and OPPENHEIM 1991; SHEN et al. 1991). These endogenous signals stimulate TNF production, and also stimulate other inflammatory cytokines: the interleukins (e.g., IL-1, IL-6, IL-8), multiple colony-stimulating factors (CSFs), interferons (IFNs), and TGF-β. Moreover, TNF itself stimulates the production of myelostimulatory cytokines (NETA et al. 1992).

In what is now considered a classical reference, Hahn described several characteristic in vitro patterns of hyperthermic interaction with drugs. The classes of drugs that show linear increases in cytotoxicity with increases in temperature are the alkylating agents and the bifunctional alkylating agents, e.g., the nitrosoureas, and cisplatin (HAHN 1982). Drugs that show an in vitro threshold effect to heat, e.g., are interactive only above 42.0°C, are anthracyline agents, bleomycin (HAHN 1982), and actinomycin D (DONALDSON et al. 1978; HAR-KEDAR 1975; YERUSHALMI 1978). Some preclinical studies do suggest that threshold heat interactions with these drugs may not be as prominent in vivo as in vitro, and that supra-additive cytotoxicity occurs at temperatures of 42°C and below (BABA et al. 1991).

18.5 Alkylating Agents

Early in vivo studies demonstrated a more than additive effect of hyperthermia and the prototype alkylating agent, nitrogen mustard, in vitro and in vivo (BRETT and SCHLOERB 1962; BRONK et al. 1973; SUZUKI 1967). BEN-HUR and ELKIND (1974) also described an increase in the cytotoxicity of the monofunctional alkylating agent methyl methanesulfonate at temperatures greater than 41.0°C. These investigators suggested that heat enhances alkylating agent-induced cytotoxicity by increasing DNA single strand breaks and slowing repair of DNA damage (Ben-Hur and Elkind 1974; Bronk et al. 1973). Johnson and Pavelec (1973) studied the in vitro cytotoxicity of thio-TEPA over 37.0°–43.0°C and found a linear increase in cell kill with an increase in temperature between 40.0° and 43.0°C.

18.5.1 Cyclophosphamide

Because cyclophosphamide must be metabolized to become cytotoxic, in vitro studies with heat and this drug are somewhat confusing. In vivo studies, however, combining cyclophosphamide with 42.5°C local hyperthermia, showd a significant reduction in the TCD_{50} (Hazan et al. 1981; West et al. 1980; Yerushalmi and Hazan 1979). Using cyclophosphamide combined with local WBH at 41.0°C for 40 min in mice, Honess and Bleehen found that tumor growth delay was significantly increased, although the bone marrow toxicity was concomitantly increased such that there was no improvement in the therapeutic index. Because of myeloid toxicity, these investigators found no increase in therapeutic gain when combining hyperthermia with other alkylating agents: BCNU, CCNU, chlorambucil, and cisplatin (Honess and Bleehen 1982, 1985b). In their studies melphalan was the only alkylating agent combined with local-regional heat or WBH that induced a positive therapeutic ratio (Honess and Bleehen 1985a,b).

18.5.2 Melphalan

Melphalan shows increased cytotoxicity with heat in vitro at temperatures of 40.5°–44.0°C (Giovanella et al. 1970; Goss and Parsons 1977; Neumann et al. 1985; Zupi 1984). Several investigators found significant increases in the TCD_{50} combining melphalan with local regional hyperthermia at temperatures of 42.5°–44°C in vivo (Honess and Bleehen 1985b; Joiner et al. 1982). In contrast to their rather discouraging experience when combining other alkylating agents with heat, Honess and Bleehen (1982, 1985a) observed an increased therapeutic index when they combined melphalan with WBH.

In the clinic, melphalan has shown excellent efficacy in melanoma and sarcoma of the extremities when administered with isolated heated limb perfusion (Ghussen et al. 1988; Stehlin et al. 1975, 1979). When using isolated heated limb perfusion, a greatly decreased dose of melphalan reaches the systemic circulation and therefore the dose to the bone marrow is at least a log lower than with systemic administration of the drug. Unfortunately, in a phase I clinical WBH study treating 33 tumor-bearing pet dogs, Page et al. (1991) found that the maximum tolerated dose (MTD) of melphalan was actually decreased by a factor of 1.9 when it was administered simultaneously with WBH, compared to the MTD of melphalan as a single agent.

18.5.3 Nitrosoureas

1-3-Bis(2-chloroethyl)-1-nitrosourea (BCNU), CCNU, and methyl-CCNU all demonstrate a linear enhancement in cytotoxicity with increasing in vitro temperatures (Hahn 1978; Herman 1983; Marmor 1979). Heat-enhanced cytotoxicity of BCNU was also demonstrated in vivo with temperatures of 43.0°–44.0°C and greater by a number of investigators using transplantable murine tumors (Dahl and Mella 1982; Joiner et al. 1982; Li and Hahn 1984; Twentyman et al. 1978). No increase in the cytotoxicity induced by CCNU or BCNU when combined with WBH of 41.0°C was observed in the Lewis lung carcinoma (Rose et al. 1979) or in nude mice transplanted with human colon carcinoma xenografts (Osieka et al. 1978). Although Honess and Bleehen (1982, 1985b) observed an increased antitumor response when either BCNU or CCNU was administered concomitantly with 41.0°C WBH, they saw no therapeutic gain because of enhanced bone marrow toxicity.

Sixteen patients with a variety of neoplasms were treated with BCNU in a reduced dose combined simultaneously with 40.5°–41.9°C. There were no remarkable tumor responses and toxicity was significant with thrombocytopenia, liver function abnormalities, and a polyneuropathy (Selkev et al. 1983). On the other hand, in a phase II study of patients with metastatic soft tissue and osteosarcoma who had all been heavily pretreated with chemotherapy, BCNU combined simultaneously with WBH to 41.8°–42.0°C for 2 h did show clinical efficacy. In this report one remarkable patient was observed to have very long-term stabilization (>4 years) of chondrosarcoma metastatic to the lung (BULL et al. 1992b).

18.6 Platinum Agents

18.6.1 Cisplatin

Cisplatin has been one of the most effective chemotherapy drugs to be combined with heat. It has been administered concomitantly with WBH in vivo preclinically as well as clinically. BARLOGIE et al. (1980) and FISHER and HAHN (1982) found synergistic cytotoxicity in Chinese hamster cells in culture. Like the alkylating agents, cisplatin shows a linear increase in cytotoxicity with increasing temperature. Mild hyperthermia, in the temperature ranges relevant to WBH from 41° to 42°C, potentiates cisplatin-induced cytotoxicity in human osteosarcoma cells and fibroblasts (YAMANE et al. 1986) as well as in human acute lymphoblastic leukemia cells in vitro (COHEN and ROBINS 1987). MEYN et al. (1980) and later HERMAN (1983) found that hyperthermia in the range of 42°–43°C increased the number of DNA adducts and decreased the rate of adduct elimination. Of considerable relevance to clinical oncology, WALLNER et al. (1986) and HERMAN et al. (1988) found that hyperthermia reduced the drug resistance of cells intrinsically resistant to cisplatin. The in vitro heat-induced increase in cisplatin-induced cytotoxicity closely predicted the in vivo antitumor activity of cisplatin thermochemotherapy. By quantitating the clonogenicity of both normal bone marrow cells and P388 lymphocytic leukemia cells using a spleen colony culture technique after in vivo heating of the limbs of mice, ALBERTS et al. (1980) demonstrated a 100-fold increase in cisplatin-induced cytotoxicity at a temperature of 42°C. A similar enhancement of the in vivo antitumor of cisplatin by local hyperthermia was described by MELLA (1985). BABA et al. (1989) found that WBH at 41.5°C for 2h significantly enhanced the cisplatin-induced tumor growth delay of a rat fibrosarcoma.

When cisplatin is combined simultaneously with WBH in vivo, however, cisplatin-induced renal toxicity is significantly increased in the rat (MELLA et al. 1987; WONDERGEM et al. 1988a). Wondergem et al. found that the cisplatin thermal enhancement ratio was 2.1–2.7 when it was combined concomitantly with WBH to 41.5°C for 120min. Saline diuresis decreased cisplatin-induced toxicity at 37°C but did not reduce renal tubular dysfunction at 41.5°C (WONDERGEM et al. 1988b). The increased renal toxicity seen in rats was foreshadowed by clinical observations in patients made earlier by GERARD et al. (1983). In addition to acute toxicity, WBH also significantly enhanced chronic renal toxicity induced by cisplatin (STREBEL et al. 1991; WONDERGEM et al. 1994). Interestingly, in dogs, the enhancement of cisplatin-induced renal toxicity by WBH may be somewhat less pronounced than that in rat and man. The most thorough analysis of WBH enhancement of cisplatin-induced toxicity has been a clinical study in tumor-bearing dogs performed by PAGE et al. (1992b). These investigators found in this nonrandomized study of 54 tumor-bearing dogs supported with vigorous saline hydration, that the maximal tolerated dose of cisplatin that induced acute toxicity (renal toxicity, myelosuppression and respiratory distress) when administered at 42.0°C WBH temperature was 54.6 mg/m^2, compared to 73.6 mg/m^2 for cisplatin given as a single agent. When estimating chronic renal toxicity, the maximal tolerated dose of cisplatin with WBH was 46.4 mg/m^2, compared to 70.0 mg/m^2 for cisplatin alone. The thermal dose modifying factor was 1.35 for acute toxicity and 1.5 for acute and chronic toxicity.

Using a rat model, BABA et al. (1989) found that heat-enhanced, cisplatin-induced renal toxicity could be significantly reduced by altering the timing of the cisplatin dose in relation to the administration schedule of WBH. This modification in the timing and scheduling improved the specific therapeutic efficacy, because a supra-additive antitumor activity of the thermochemotherapy was retained. These investigators found that cisplatin administered approximately 4h after WBH gave the greatest specific therapeutic efficacy, with an approximately threefold increase in efficacy. However, therapeutic efficacy was increased over cisplatin alone, even if the cisplatin dose was administered 12–30 min prior to WBH or 30 min to 6h after the WBH treatment. The greatest normal tissue toxicity occurred with cisplatin administered during WBH. WBH did not enhance either acute or chronic cisplatin-induced renal toxicity if the drug was given before or after WBH (BABA et al. 1989).

Another way to improve the therapeutic index is to use a protective agent to decrease WBH-enhanced cisplatin-induced renal toxicity to acceptable limits without impairing the heat-enhanced antitumor effect of cisplatin (Bull et al. 1988). Yet another approach to improve the therapeutic index substitutes a nonrenal toxic platinum analog, carboplatin, for cisplatin (Ohno et al. 1991; Robins et al. 1993; Strebel et al. 1991).

18.6.2 Carboplatin

Tapazaglou, Cohen, and Robins et al. showed that when hyperthermia was combined simultaneously with carboplatin in vitro it significantly enhanced the latter's cytotoxicity (Cohen and Robins 1990; Cohen et al. 1989; Tapazoglou et al. 1988). Unlike cisplatin, carboplatin alone does not induce renal or neurological toxicity; however, also unlike cisplatin, carboplatin causes acute myelosuppression (Perry et al. 1986). Because, however, WBH-enhanced myelosuppression is less profound than WBH enhancement of renal and cardiac toxicity (Ohno et al. 1993), carboplatin can be effectively administered simultaneously with WBH in vivo, whereas in man and dog, cisplatin must be administered either before or after hyperthermia to reduce renal toxicity to an acceptable level (Baba et al. 1994). Carboplatin administered simultaneously in vivo with WBH has a significantly greater therapeutic index than cisplatin administered with WBH (Ohno et al. 1991). Robins et al. (1993) reported a phase I protocol combining carboplatin with WBH in 30 patients. Significantly, they were able to administer as much as 575 mg/m^2 carboplatin simultaneously with WBH during the WBH plateau of 41.8°–42.0°C, although at this level, myelotoxicity was profound (grade IV). The investigators encountered no renal toxicity and recommended a carboplatin dose of 400–480 mg/m^2 to be used in combination with WBH. It is noteworthy that this dose is higher than the standard 300–350 mg/m^2 dose of carboplatin administered at normal body temperature (Robins et al. 1993). In this study they observed five patients with complete or partial tumor responses: two complete responses in patients with advanced ovarian cancer, one complete response in a patient with a neuroendocrine tumor of the gastrointestinal tract, and partial responses in one patient with pancreatic and one with small-bowel cancer.

18.6.3 Other Platinum Agents

The second-generation platinum drug tetrachloroplatinum(II) shows heat-enhanced cytotoxicity both in vitro and in vivo (Epelbaum et al. 1992). Herman et al. (1990) synthesized and tested the cytotoxicity of a number of unique second-generation platinum compounds complexing tetrachoroplatinum(II) to positively charged nuclear dyes. With many of these complexes, as with cisplatin and carboplatin, heat-enhanced antitumor acitivity is maximized if the drug and heat are administered concomitantly, although several of them showed greatest activity enhancement at 43.0°C if administered 5 h before heat in vitro (Kusumoto and Teicher 1993). Combining the hypoxic cell sensitizer, etanidazole, with each of five of these complexes and WBH to 42.0°C for 60 min caused supra-additive tumor growth delay in subcutaneous tumors and reduced the numbers of lung metastases of the Lewis lung tumor in a mouse model (Teicher et al. 1992).

18.7 Anthracycline Antibiotics

18.7.1 Doxorubicin

Hyperthermia has been found to increase doxorubicin-induced cytotoxicity in a number of tumor and normal cell lines in vitro. Hahn and Strande (1976) showed that Chinese hamster cells had increased doxorubicin cytotoxicity at 43°C. Hahn (1978) found that doxorubicin's interaction with heat exhibited a threshold function; there was no in vitro enhancement of doxorubicin-induced cytotoxicity until the temperature exceeded 42°C, while at temperatures above 42°C, cytotoxicity increased in a linear manner with increased heat duration. At 42°C doxorubicin-induced cytotoxicity is increased in L1210 leukemia (Block et al. 1975), mouse leukemia (Muzuno et al. 1980), the BT_4C neurogenic tumor (Dahl 1982), and human melanoma and Burkitt's lymphoma (Oshnoshi 1985). Of considerable interest, a temperature of 42°C also enhanced doxorubicin-associated cytotoxicity in a doxorubicin-resistant cell line with MDR-type drug resistance (Bates and Mackillop 1986). On the other hand, Hahn and Strande (1976) reported that Chinese hamster ovary cells became refractory to doxorubicin after heating for 30 min at 43°C. Using rats, Wondergem et al. (1991) found that WBH enhanced doxorubicin-induced toxicity only if combined simultaneously or if administered after doxorubicin exposure: If WBH was administered prior to doxorubicin administration, no enhancement in doxorubicin-enhanced cytotoxicity was seen. While a supra-additive cytotoxicity of doxorubicin was observed when it was combined simultaneously with WBH to 41.5°C for 120 min in rats, doxorubicin-induced glomerulonephritis also increased significantly (WONDERGEN et al. 1991). In rats, unlike man, glomerulonephritis is a major dose-limiting acute and chronic toxicity induced by doxorubicin (WONDERGEM et al. 1991). This toxicity, as in doxorubicin-induced cardiomyopathy, is thought to be caused by oxidative damage. The renal and cardiac toxicity is associated with doxorubicin, not WBH, although WBH enhances the doxorubicin-induced toxicity. BABA et al. (1991), by using the chelating agent ICRF 127, significantly reduced the WBH-enhanced doxorubicin-induced glomerulonephritis and cardiotoxicity. WBH also enhanced the doxorubicin-induced myelosuppression; however, the myelosuppression was not as drug dose-limiting as the treatment-induced glomerulonephritis (WONDERGEM et al. 1991).

Using a radiant heat device, NOVOTNEY et al. (1992) treated 15 dogs with high-grade lymphomas in a phase I study of doxorubicin administered concurrently with WBH to 42.0°C for 90 min. The investigators found no treatment-related toxicity at 12 mg/m^2, but one dog demonstrated premature ventricular cardiac contractions at a doxorubicin dose of 24 mg/m^2, and two of eight dogs (25%) developed treatment-related toxicities at a dose of 30 mg/m^2. One dog developed severe myelosuppression and one dog showed cardiac toxicity documented as a decreased ejection fraction. Partial responses of short duration occurred in all three dogs treated with WBH + 12 mg/m^2 of doxorubicin. Four dogs treated with WBH + 24 mg/m^2 doxorubicin were documented to have complete tumor responses lasting 150–200 days, while eight dogs treated with WBH + 30 mg/m^2 doxorubicin experienced complete responses lasting a mean duration of 241 days.

As a follow-up to Novotney's protocol, a randomized clinical trial in pet dogs with high-grade lymphoma was conducted by PAGE et al. (1992a). The phase III trial combining WBH concomitantly with doxorubicin demonstrated a trend toward increased disease-free survival in dogs treated with the systemic thermochemotherapy compared to doxorubicin alone. Although clinically there was no indication of an increase in doxorubicin-induced cardiomyopathy, autopsy results did suggest an increase in myocardial cell degeneration in dogs treated with doxorubicin combined simultaneously with WBH.

During careful clinical observations of a patient, KIM et al. (1979b) observed that WBH combined concomitantly with doxorubicin was associated with acute cardiac arrhythmia, whereas neither WBH nor doxorubicin alone induced a change in heart rate. The WBH/doxorubicin-induced arrhythmia was associated with increased serum catecholamine levels (KIM et al. 1979a).

GERARD et al. (1984) treated 11 patients with soft tissue sarcoma with WBH to 41.8°–43.0°C for 2 h concurrently with both doxorubicin (45 mg/m^2) and cyclophosphamide 1000 mg/m. They reported two complete and two partial responses in five patients with either liposarcomas and leiomyosarcomas. The investigators reported cardiac toxicity, cardiac arrhythmias, anasarca, nausea, vomiting, diarrhea, myalgias, reversible neuropathy, skin burns, hypotension, hyperglycemia, and hypophosphatemia. They also described acute thrombocytopenia as well as liver enzyme elevations lasting 1 week after therapy. The study indicates that seven patients were treated to peak WBH temperatures of 42.2°–43.0°C for 2 h. One must hypothesize that an error was made in thermometry, for if patients were indeed treated to 43°C core temperature for 2 h, it is remarkable there were no treatment-related deaths.

18.7.2 Mitoxantrone

While mitoxantrone, an anthracene dye derivative of doxorubicin, has like its parent, shown increased cytotoxicity in vitro when combined with temperatures greater than 42.0°C (HERMAN et al. 1992; WANG et al. 1987). Neither in vivo studies nor clinical studies have as yet been reported.

18.8 Bleomycin

BRAUN and HAHN (1975) found that heat in vitro enhanced bleomycin-induced cytotoxicity in Chinese hamster cells at temperatures between 42.0° and 43.0°C. The observations were confirmed in a number of cell lines by a number of investigators (HAR-KEDAR 1975; HERMAN 1983;

Marmor et al. 1979; Morgan and Bleehen 1980; Roizin-Towle and Hall 1982; Urano et al. 1988). On the other hand, Kano et al. (1988) found that temperatures of 40.0°C enhanced bleomycin killing in both bleomycin-sensitive and bleomycin-resistant Chinese hamster V79 cells and in mouse leukemia cells.

WBH to 41.5°C concomitantly combined with bleomycin significantly increased the in vivo antitumor effect in a rat model; however, normal tissue toxicity was also signficantly increased, such that no WBH enhancement of the therapeutic index resulted (Ohno et al. 1991). The bleomycin analog liblomycin did not induce as much oxygen radical damage to normal tissue and did not induce the severe toxicity elicited by bleomycin. Combining liblomycin with WBH gave an enhanced therapeutic index (Ohno et al. 1991). To date, protective agents or alternative scheduling of the two agents has not been tested.

18.9 Antimetabolites

18.9.1 5-Fluorouracil

In the past 5-Flurorouracil (5-FU) and 5-FU analogs were generally found either not to be interactive or to be minimally interactive when combined simultaneously with hyperthermia in vitro (Adwankar and Chitnis 1984; Giovanella et al. 1970; Joshi and Barendsen 1984; Mizuno et al. 1980; Tsumura et al. 1988). More recently, however, Kido et al. (1991) found that if cells were exposed to 5-FU prior to exposure to heat, 5-FU-induced cytotoxicity was increased in vitro. Using the Ward colon cancer subcutaneously implanted in Fischer rats, Sakaguchi et al. found that if 5-FU was given by continuous i.v. infusion, with the administration ending 24 h prior to a WBH treatment of 42.0°C, the antitumor effect was significantly increased (Sakaguchi et al. 1994b). This combination significantly increased apoptosis and necrosis in a 5-FU-sensitive colon cancer, and also signficantly increased the number of complete responses (Sakaguchi et al. 1994b).

18.9.2 Methotrexate

Methotrexate has shown an increased in vitro activity when tested in specific cell lines (Herman et al. 1981), but not all cell lines demonstrated increased cytotoxicity to methotrexate at 43°C in vitro (Hahn and Shiu 1983), and a positive cytotoxic interaction was not demonstrated in vivo at 42°C (Muckle and Dickson 1973). There are no reports of either in vitro or in vivo methotrexate interaction with simultaneously administered heat at WBH temperatures of 42°C or below. It may be that methotrexate, like 5-FU, will show a synergistic interaction with moderate hyperthermia if administered using an optimized schedule.

Two other antimetabolites, cytosine arabinoside and PALA (phosphoracetyl aspartate), did not shown enhanced cytotoxicity when administered simultaneously with hyperthermia.

18.10 Drugs Interfering with Microtubular Function

Neither vincristine (Mizuno et al. 1980; Rose et al. 1979) nor vinblastine (Giovanella et al. 1970; Neumann et al. 1985) has demonstrated heat enhancement of cytotoxicity either in vitro or in vivo at WBH temperatures of 41.5°–42.0°C. As in the case of the clinically useful vinca alkaloids, the heat interactions of etoposide (VP-16) and taxol have not been sufficiently tested to describe their activity with hyperthermia in vitro or in vivo, although preliminary in vitro studies suggest that taxol administered concurrently with heat is not interactive in the temperature ranges relevant to WBH (Sakaguchi et al. 1993).

18.11 Investigative Chemotherapy Agents

18.11.1 Lonidamine

Lonidamine is an investigational anticancer agent that induces cytotoxicity by inhibiting glycolysis and respiration so that cellular energy store (ATP) levels are reduced. It also alters membrane transport (Kim et al. 1984) and inhibits DNA synthesis (Chitnis et al. 1986). Kim et al. found that temperatures from 41.0° to 42.0°C potentiated the cytotoxicity of lonidamine in vitro. Robins et al. (1990) completed a phase I trial of WBH to 41.8°–42.0°C and used a dose of 360 mg/m^2 as the highest dose of lonidamine to be combined with WBH. Lonidamine also potentiates the cytotoxicity of doxorubicin given in combination with heat (Chitnis and Adwankar 1986), as well as that of radiation, and has been used in a clinical trial with total-body irradiation for lymphomas and other B-cell neoplasms (ROBINS 1991).

18.11.2 *α-Difluoromethylornithine*

α-Difluoromethylornithine (DFMO) inhibits ornithine decarboxylase. Heat has been found to enhance its cytotoxicity, and a preliminary clinical study of WBH with DFMO showed meaningful responses of liver and lung metastases in patients with metastatic melanoma (CROGHAN et al. 1990).

18.12 Cytokines

WBH induces endogenous cytokines, e.g., the interferons, tumor necrosis factors, interleukins, myeloid growth factors, and other cytokines, within the host (DOLEIRE et al. 1993; NEVILLE and SAUDER 1988). Additionally, interesting preclinical studies as well as several clinical studies suggest useful antitumor activity of exogenous cytokines combined with WBH.

18.12.1 *Interferons*

YERUSHALMI et al. (1982) using an in vivo mouse model, demonstrated a synergy for interferon-α combined with hyperthermia. In vivo studies with B16 melanoma in mice have shown that interferon-α combined with WBH has an additive antitumor effect, whereas interferon-γ has a synergistic effect with WBH (ANJUM and FLEISCHMANN 1992). Clinical studies with interferon-α have combined it with a WBH temperature of less than the 41.8°–42.0°C. ROBINS et al. (1989) conducted a phase I trial of human recombinant interferon-α with WBH. Interferon was administered intramuscularly 1 h prior to induction of 40.5°C WBH for 75 min. Patients tolerated the interferon dose escalation to 10×10^6 units/m^2 without acute or long-term complications (some of the patients were followed up for 12 months). A pilot trial of eight patients with renal cell carcinoma using 3×10^6 units/m^2 of human recombinant interferon-α with WBH to 40.5°C for 75 min for 3–16 treatments was reported by TAPAZUGLOU et al. (1990). The patients developed toxicities expected of interferon-α alone, although one patient developed elevated liver transminase enzyme levels. There were no tumor regressions, although six patients achieved stable disease. Because of the minimal disease response, despite minimal toxicity, the investigators recommended no further investigation of the combination in patients with renal cell carcinoma.

Interferon-α alone, or with chemotherapy, is commonly used clinically on a daily or 3× weekly basis, but as yet no clinical study has been reported using interferon administered other than as a single bolus dose with WBH, and repeated 3–4 weeks later as a new cycle.

18.12.2 *Tumor Necrosis Factor*

Recombinant human tumor necrosis factor-α (TNF) has shown synergistic antitumor activity with hyperthermia in vitro (KLOSTERGAARD et al. 1991) and at least supra-additive antitumor activity when combined with WBH in vivo. Although in vivo TNF was not itself toxic to rats in doses as high as 10^7 units/kg, when TNF was combined with WBH (41.5°C for 2 h) in doses exceeding 1×10^6, it caused hypotension and a capillary leak syndrome (MAKINO et al. 1993b). Lower doses of TNF ($<10^6$ units/kg) did not induce toxicity in the rats, and TNF contributed to a supra-additive antitumor effect when combined with WBH and chemotherapy (SAKAGUCHI et al. 1994a). SRINIVASAN et al. (1990) injected TNF directly into RIF-1 tumors and found it to be supra-additive with 41.5°C hyperthermia. TNF caused acute toxicity to the tumor microvascular endothelium.

By far the most compelling clinical study to date, by LIENARD et al. (1992), treated patients with sarcoma and melanoma of the extremities with a combination of hyperthermic isolated limb perfusion to 40°–40.5°C and high-dose TNF (2–4 mg), interferon-γ, and melphalan. This multimodality regimen induced a >90% complete tumor response. The dose of TNF used by the investigators in the isolated limb perfusion was, however, tenfold higher ($>10^6$ units/kg) than would be tolerated using systemic administration of the TNF with or without WBH. Combination solely of TNF with hyperthermic isolated limb perfusion has been found to be only minimally effective in treating melanoma of the extremity (POSNEL et al. 1994).

18.12.3 Interleukin-1α

Interleukin-1α (IL-1α) 25 μg/kg combined with local hyperthermia at 42.5° and 43.0°C was studied in vivo using mice (SONG et al. 1993). The cytokine alone and hyperthermia alone each decreased tumor blood flow for more than 24 h. When IL-1α was combined with local hyperthermia, tumor growth delay, as well as animal survival, significantly increased, while tumor cell clonogenicity was significantly decreased compared to either modality alone. Unfortunately, temperature ranges relevant to WBH were not tested. On the other hand, SHEN et al. (1991) found that WBH to 40.0°C in vivo induced increased production of IL-1α and was associated with myeloprotection from total-body irradiation-induced granulocytopenia and reduced numbers of animal deaths.

18.13 Whole-Body Hyperthermia with Radiation

Hyperthermia and radiation have long been recognized to induce synergistic cytotoxicity both in vitro and in vivo when simultaneously combined. In the clinic, heat-radiation interaction has been positive generally in superficial tumors of a small size. In larger or deep-seated tumors, technical as well as physiological barriers have prevented induction of uniform temperatures much above 41°C. Simultaneous combinations of heat and radiation have usually been the most effective in vitro; however, clinically it has been impractical to administer radiation simultaneously with hyperthermia except when combining interstitial radiation (brachytherapy) and hyperthermia. There are practical problems of a logistical nature that hinder simultaneous combination of heat and radiation in the clinic, in addition to the technical barriers to achieving high temperatures throughout the tumor. As intimated above, despite the technical problems with local hyperthermia induction that have plagued this dual-modality therapy, the treatment of superficial lesions such as chest wall disease in breast cancer (ENGIN et al. 1993b; KAPP 1988) and head and neck tumors (ENGIN et al. 1993a, 1994b; VALDAGNI and AMICHETTI 1994) has been effective, as has brachytherapy combined with heat and external beam irradiation (SEEGENSCHMIEDT et al. 1994). The response to combination hyperthermia and radiation correlates with a small tumor volume as well as with minimum tumor temperature (DEWHIRST and SIM 1984; SEEGENSCHMIEDT et al. 1994). ENGIN et al. (1994a) found that in addition to tumor volume ($<20\,cm^3$) and superficial depth from the surface (<1.5 cm), low tumor extracellular pH (<7.2) was a good predictor of response to thermoradiotherapy.

With reference to systemic hyperthermia, the interactions of heat and radiation at temperatures compatible with WBH (less than 42.0°C) are well documented in vitro. Armour and co-workers have described studies using long-duration mild hyperthermia that are quite promising and have stimulated a clinical protocol combining long-duration interstitial mild hyperthermia with brachytherapy irradiation in patients with recurrent pelvic tumors (MARTINEZ et al. 1993).

Clinical investigations combining systemic hyperthermia with radiation go back to historical work of WARREN (1935), who combined diathermy-induced hyperthermia with radiation therapy and wrote about "moderate to marked" improvement in approximately 50% of patients with a variety of advanced cancers. The work was later updated by LEVIN and BLAIR (1978) using the wax immersion technique of PETTIGREW et al. (1974b) to induce systemic hyperthermia.

In a phase I study in dogs, MCCHESNEY et al. (1993) administered 2 h of 42.0°C WBH on days 1, 22, and 40 of a course of whole-thorax irradiation to 45 Gy in 1.5 fractions given 5 times weekly over 6 weeks. The addition of whole-thorax radiation to WBH did not appear to increase the toxicity of WBH, although the investigators documented a radiation-induced increase in the protein content of lung lavage.

ROBINS et al. (1988) have combine WBH and ionizing radiation to treat patients with inoperable non-small-cell lung cancer. They used radiant heat-induced WBH to 40.5°–41.0°C for 75 min. The WBH was given twice a week for the first 2 weeks of a 6-week (60 Gy) radiotherapy course, with the WBH induction beginning 10 min after radiation treatments. The therapy was well tolerated and partial responses were observed in five of six patients with bulky disease.

ROBINS et al. (1990) also reported a study combining total-body irradiation (TBI) with four courses of WBH to treat patients with indolent B-cell malignancies, nodular low-grade lymphoma, and chronic lymphocytic leukemia. Each TBI radiation treatment (12.5 cGy midplane dose) was followed by radiant heat-induced WBH to 41.8°C for 75 min. The investigators observed no increased toxicity from the WBH; in fact, WBH appeared to decrease TBI-induced thrombocytopenia. Of the eight patients treated with this protocol, three achieved a complete response and four, a partial response. The median survival was 52.5 months, with a median of 9.4 months to treatment failure. The WBH-associated reduction of radiation-induced thrombocytopenia was an important observation of this small clinical trial. The myeloprotective effect of WBH has also been described by Shen et al. (1991) in mice treated in vivo with WBH to 40.0°C 20 h prior to 9 Gy TBI. WBH protected 100% of the animals from an LD_{100} TBI dose. The WBH reduced the days of granulocytopenia induced by TBI. As described above, Shen et al. (1991) found that WBH induced increased production of interleukin-1, and attributed the myeloprotection to the increased levels of this cytokine.

18.14 Newer Aspects of Whole-Body Hyperthermia

18.14.1 Scheduling and Timing

It is generally accepted that WBH is an adjunctive antitumor modality, not for use by itself but rather in combination with either chemotherapy or cytokine therapy. In any treatment, but especially with two systemic treatments, the therapeutic index is a very important factor. In studies combining the majority of chemotherapy drugs as well as cytokines with WBH, the effect of timing and scheduling has not been considered. The timing and scheduling are likely to be critical in enhancing the therapeutic index. It is likely that the schedules, and a critical understanding of the timing of heat with the agents, will be highly specific to each class of agents, if not each individual agent. Preclinical WBH studies using a rat model (Baba et al. 1991) show that to increase the efficacy of cisplatin yet reduce the toxicity to an acceptable level, it is necessary to administer cisplatin either prior to or following WBH. Yet carboplatin, an analog of cisplatin, is a platinum agent that induces myelosuppression rather than renal toxicity. Unlike in the case of cisplatin, a superior therapeutic index is achieved when carboplatin is simultaneously combined with WBH (Ohno et al. 1991; Robins et al. 1993).

Using another analogy, the antimetabolite 5-FU did not demonstrate increased cytotoxicity when combined simultaneously with heat, yet recent studies demonstrate that WBH significantly enhances the 5-FU-induced antitumor effect if used 24 h following the administration of a continuous intravenous infusion of WBH (Sakaguchi et al. 1994). An understanding of the optimal timing of WBH with drug or cytokine may be more objectively achieved by examining the onset and timing of biological events induced by both WBH and the individual drugs, such as apoptosis and necrosis, in tumor as well as in normal tissue (Sakaguchi et al. 1994a).

18.14.2 Long-duration Low Temperatures

In the preclinical and clinical application of WBH as an anticancer modality, systemic hyperthermia at the highest possible tolerated temperature has been used. As previously described, the maximum tolerated systemic temperature level in the clinical situation has been demonstrated to be 42.0°C for a duration from 1 to 24 h (Bull et al. 1978; Pettigrew et al. 1974b). Yet recent preclinical studies suggest that lower systemic temperatures, more in keeping with fever levels occurring physiologically in response to infection, may be as efficacious as the maximally tolerated systemic temperatures when combined with chemotherapy (Mulcahy et al. 1987, 1988) and with cytokines (Geehen et al. 1993; Shen et al. 1994).

While clinical trials have not been reported, studies in tumor-bearing rats suggest that the use of prolonged mild temperature WBH (long-duration low temperatures of 40°C) is as effective as higher temperatures in achieving tumor response, but importantly the lower temperatures are not associated with either WBH-induced toxicity or WBH enhancement of drug-induced toxicities seen with the maximal WBH temperatures of 41.8°–42.0°C (Sakaguchi et al. 1994d). Looking at the heated isolated limb perfusion data of Lienard et al. (1992) and harking back to historical yet relevant observations of Busch (1888), Bruns (1866), and Coley (1893), it is likely that a combination of lower heat of long duration with cytokines and chemotherapy will lead to a significantly greater therapeutic index. Therefore it is anticipated that the role of WBH in cancer treatment will expand.

Many more in vivo and clinical trials need to be initiated to examine the optimal combination of WBH with the agents, yet it would appear that the future of WBH in combination with chemotherapy drugs, radiation, and cytokines is quite promising.

18.15 Summary

- WBH is induced by pyrogens, extra-corporeal heating of the blood or by external heating of the skin using heated wax, submersion in heated water, water suits and blankets or radiant heat.
- WBH increases the cytotoxicity of many chemotherapy agents, radiation and cytokines.
- Specific chemotherapy agents each may differ in interaction with systemic heat and the combination of agent and heat result in variable toxicity and antitumor effect.
- The increased cytotoxicity affects both tumor and normal tissue therefore to increase the therapeutic index a use of optimal scheduling and timing or protective agents is often imperative.
- It may be useful to examine biological endpoints such as heat-induced apoptosis and/or necrosis to better understand interactions of heat and other agents such as chemotherapy, cytokines and radiation in the use of whole body hyperthermia.
- There may be a therapeutic advantage in the use of long-duration-low-temperature heat combined with chemotherapy, radiation and cytokines.

References

Adams DB (1993) Systemic responses to challenge infection with Haemonchus contortus in immune Merino sheep. Vet Res Commun 17: 25–35

Adwankar MK, Chitnis MP (1984) Effect of hyperthermia alone and in combination with anticancer drugs on the viability of P388 leukemic cells. Tumori 70: 231–234

Alberts DS, Peng YM, Chen HSG, Moon TE, Cetas TC, Hoschele JD (1980) Therapeutic synergism of hyperthermia/cis-platinum in a mouse tumor model. J Natl Cancer Inst 65: 455–461

Alonso K, Pontiggia P, Nardi C, Sabato A, Cuppone-Curto F (1992) Systemic hyperthermia in the treatment of HIV-related Kaposi's sarcoma. A phase I study. Biomed Pharmacother 46: 21–24

Anjum A, Fleischmann WRJ (1992) Effect of hyperthermia on the antitumor actions of interferons. J Biol Regul Homeost Agents 6: 75–86

Armour EP, Wang ZH, Corry P, Martinez A (1991) Sensitization of rat 91 gliosarcoma cells to low dose rate irradiation by long duration 41°C hyperthermia. Cancer Res 51: 3088–3095

Armour EP, McEachern D, Wang Z, Corry PM, Martinez A (1993) Sensitivity of human cells to mild hyperthermia. Cancer Res 53: 2740–2744

Baba H, Siddik ZH, Strebel FR, Jenkins GN, Bull JMC (1989) Increased therapeutic gain of combined cis-diamminedichloro-platinum (II) and whole body hyperthermia by optimal heat scheduling in the rat. Cancer Res 49: 7041–7044

Baba H, Stephens LC, Strebel FR, Siddik ZH, Newman RA, Ohno S, Bull JMC (1991) Protective effect of ICRF-187 against normal tissue injury induced by adriamycin in combination with whole body hyperthermia. Cancer Res 51: 3559–3567

Baba H, Siddik ZH, Strebel FR, Jenkins GN, Bull JMC (1989) Increased therapeutic gain of combined cis-diamminedichloro-platinum (II) and whole body hyperthermia by optimal heat scheduling in the rat. Cancer Res 49: 7041–7044

Barlogie B, Corry PM, Yip E, et al. (1979) Total-body hyperthermia with and without chemotherapy for advanced human neoplasms. Cancer Res 39: 1481–1489

Barlogie B, Corry P, Drewinko B (1980) In vitro thermochemotherapy of human colon cancer cells with cis-dichlorodiammineplatinum (II) and mitomycin C. Cancer Res 40: 1165–1170

Bates DA, Mackillop WJ (1986) Hyperthermia, adriamycin transport, and cytotoxicity in drug-sensitive and -resistant Chinese hamster ovary cells. Cancer Res 46: 5447–5481

Ben-Hur E, Elkind M (1974) Thermal sensitization of Chinese hamster cells to methyl methanesulfonate: relation of DNA damage and repair to survival response. Cancer Biochem Biophys 1: 23–32

Block J, Harris P, Peale A (1975) Preliminary observations on temperature-enhanced drug uptake by leukemic leukocytes in vitro. Cancer Chemother Rep 59: 985–988

Braun J, Hahn GM (1975) Enhanced killing by bleomycin and 43°C hyperthermia and the inhibition of recovery from potentially lethal damage. Cancer Res 35: 2921–2927

Brett D, Schloerb P (1962) Intermittent hyperthermia on Walker 256 carcinoma. Arch Surg 85: 154–157

Bronk B, Wilkins R, Regan JD (1973) Thermal enhancement of DNA damage by an alkylating agent in human cells. Biochem Biophys Res Commun 52: 1064–1070

Bruns P (1888) Die Heilwirkung des Erysipels auf Geschwulste. In: Bruns P (ed) Beiträge zur klinischen Chirurgie, Mitteilungen aus der chirurgischen Klinik zu Tübingen. Verlag der H. Laupp'schen Buchhandlung, Tubingen, pp 28–30

Bull JMC (1983) Systemic hyperthermia: background and principles. In: Storm FK (ed) Hyperthermia in cancer therapy. GK Hall, Boston, Mass, pp 401–407

Bull JMC (1994) A review of systemic hyperthermia. A new therapy in the treatment of cancer. In: Vaeth JM (ed) Frontiers in radiation therapy and oncology. Karger, Basel, pp 171–177

Bull JMC, Lees DE, Schuette J, et al. (1978) Whole body hyperthermia – now a feasible addition to cancer treatment. Proc Am Soc Clin Oncol 14: 405

Bull JMC, Lees DE, Schuette WH, et al. (1979) Whole body hyperthermia: a phase-I trial of a potential adjuvant to chemotherapy. Ann Intern Med 90: 317–323

Bull JMC, Lees DE, Schuette W, Smith R, Glatstein E, DeVita V Jr (1982) Immunological and physiological responses to whole body hyperthermia. Monogr Natl Cancer Inst 61: 77–79

Bull JMC, Mansfield B, Cronau L (1987) Whole body hyperthermia with chemotherapy in the treatment of metastatic colon carcinoma. The 8th International Congress of Radiation Research 1: 328

Bull JMC, Strebel FR, Sunderland BA, Bulger RE, Edwards M, Siddik ZH, Newman RA (1988) *O*-[(*β*-hydroxyethyl)-rutoside]-mediated protection of renal injury associated with cis-diamminedichloroplatinum (II)/hyperthermia treatment. Cancer Res 48: 2239–2244

Bull JMC, Cronau L, Newman B, et al. (1992a) Chemotherapy resistant sarcoma treated with whole body hyperthermia (WBH) combined with 1-3 bis(2-chloroethyl)-1-nitrosourea (BCNU). Int J Hyperthermia 8: 297–305

Bull JMC, Cronau L, Bigham C, Weiss G, Tonnesen A (1992b) A phase II study of whole body hyperthermia (WBH) with mitomycin C (mito-C) and continuous intravenous (civ) 5-fluorouracil (5-FU) in colon cancer. Proceedings of the 83rd annual meeting of the American Association of Cancer Research 33: 1500

Busch W (1866) Uber den Einfluss welche heftigere Erysipelen zuweilig auf organisierte Neubildungenausüben. Verhandlungen Naturhist Preuss Rhein Westphal, Bonn 23: 28–30

Chitnis M, Adwankar M (1986) Potentiation of adriamycin cytotoxicity in P388 murine leukemia sensitive and resistant to adriamycin by use of lonidamine and hyperthermia. Tumori 72: 469–473

Chitnis M, Juvekar A, Adwankar M, Advani S (1986) Inhibition of DNA synthesis by lonidamine and hyperthermia in human chronic myeloid leukemia cells. Anticancer Res 6: 749–752

Cohen JD, Robins HI (1987) Hyperthermic enhancement of cis-diammine-1,1-cyclobutane dicarboxylate platinum (II) cytotoxicity in human leukemia cells in vitro. Cancer Res 47: 4335–4337

Cohen JD, Robins HI (1990) Thermal enhancement of tetraplatin and carboplatin in human leukemic cells in vitro. Int J Hyperthermia 6: 1013–1017

Cohen JD, Robins HI, Schmitt C (1989) Interactions of hyperthermia with carboplatin, cisplatin and etopside in human leukemia cells in vitro. Cancer Lett 44: 205–210

Coley WC (1893) The treatment of malignant tumors by repeated inoculations of erysipelis: with a report of ten original cases. Am J Med Sci 105: 487–511

Croghan M, Shimm D, Dean S, Booth A, Modaino M, Meyskins F, Gerner E (1990) Treatment of disseminated malignant melanoma with alpha-difluoromethylornithine (DFMO) and systemic hyperthermia (S delta). Proc Annu Meet Am Assoc Cancer Res 31: A1171

Cronau L, Bourke D, Bull JMC (1984) General anesthesia for whole body hyperthermia. Cancer Res 44: 4873s–4877s

Dahl O (1982) Interaction of hyperthermia and doxorubicin on a malignant neurogenic rat cell line (BT_4C) in culture. Monogr Natl Cancer Inst 61: 251–253

Dahl O (1983) Hyperthermic potentiation of doxorubicin and 4′-epi-doxorubicin in a transplantable neurogenic rat tumor (BT^4A) in BD IX rats. Int J Radiat Oncol Biol Phys 9: 203–207

Dahl O, Mella O (1982) Enhanced effect of combined hyperthermia and chemotherapy (bleomycin, BCNU) in a neurogenic rat tumour (BT_4A) in vivo. Anticancer Res 2: 359–364

Dewhirst MW, Sim DA (1984) Analysis of prognostic variables which influence early and long-term response of pet animal tumors to radiation alone and radiation plus heat. Front Radiat Ther Oncol 18: 1951–1961

Dewhirst M, Sim D, Sapareto S, Conner W (1984) The importance of minimum tumor temperature in determining early and long term responses of spontaneous canine and feline tumors to heat and radiation. Cancer Res 44: 43–50

dOleire F, Spriggs D, Bird A, Schmitt CL, Robins HI (1992) The interaction of alpha-tumor necrosis factor, melphalan and 41.8°C hyperthermia in L929 cells. Proc Annu Meet Am Assoc Cancer Res 34: A2163

dOleire F, Schmitt CL, Robins HI, Cohen JD, Spriggs D (1993) Cytokine induction in humans by 41.8 degrees C whole-body hyperthermia. Letter J Natl Cancer Inst 85: 833–834

Donaldson S, Gordon L, Hahn GM (1978) Protective effect of hyperthermia against the cytotoxicity of actinomycin D on Chinese hamster cells. Cancer Res Treat Rep 62: 1489–1495

Engelhardt R, Neumann H, von der Tann M, Lohr G (1982) Preliminary results in the treatment of oat cell carcinoma of the lung by combined application of chemotherapy (CT) and whole-body hyperthermia. In: Gautherie JM, Albert E (eds) Biomedical thermology, progress in clinical biological research. Liss, New York, pp 761–775

Engelhardt R, Muller U, Weth-Simon R, Neumann HA, Lohr GW (1990) Treatment of disseminated malignant melanoma with cisplatin in combination with whole-body hyperthermia and doxorubicin. Int J Hyperthermia 6: 511–515

Engin K, Tupchong L, Waterman F, Nerlinger R, Hoh L, McFarlane J, Leeper D (1993a) Thermoradiotherapy with combined interstitial and external hyperthermia in advanced tumours in the head and neck with depth > or = 3 cm. Int J Hyperthermia 9: 645–654

Engin K, Tupchong L, Waterman F, Komarnicky L, Mansfield C, Leeper D (1993b) "Patchwork" fields in thermoradiotherapy for extensive chest wall recurrences of breast carcinoma. Breast Cancer Res Treat 27: 263–270

Engin K, Leeper D, Thistlethwaite A, Tupchong L, McFarlane J (1994a) Tumor extracellular pH as a prognostic factor in thermoradiotherapy. Int J Radiat Oncol Biol Phys 29: 125–132

Engin K, Tupchong L, Waterman F, et al. (1994b) Thermoradiotherapy for superficial tumour deposits in the head and neck. Int J Hyperthermia 10: 153–164

Epelbaum R, Teicher B, Holden S, Ara G, Varsheny A, Herman T (1992) Interaction of D,L- and D-tetraplatin with hyperthermia in vitro and in vivo. Eur J Cancer 28A: 794–800

Fajardo LF, Schreiber AB, Kelly NI, Hahn GM (1985) Thermal sensitivity of endothelial cells. Radiat Res 103: 276–285

Fisher GA, Hahn GM (1982) Enhancement of cis-diamminedichloroplatinum (cis-DDP) cytotoxicity by hyperthermia. Monogr Natl Cancer Inst 61: 255

Geehan DM, Fabian DF, Lefor AT (1993) Immunotherapy and whole-body hyperthermia as combined modality treatment of a subcutaneous murine sarcoma. J Surg Oncol 53: 180–183

Gerard H, Egorin MJ, Whitacre M, van Echo DA, Aisner J (1983) Renal failure and platinum pharmacokinetics in

three patients treated with cis-diamminedichloroplatinum (I) and whole-body hyperthermia. Cancer Chemother Pharmacol 11: 162–166
Gerard H, van Echo DA, Whitacre M, et al. (1984) Doxorubicin, cyclophosphamide, and whole body hyperthermia for treatment of advanced soft tissue sarcoma. Cancer 53: 2585–2591
Ghussen F, Kruger I, Groth W, Stutzer H (1988) The role of regional hyperthermic cytostatic perfusion in the treatment of extremity melanoma. Cancer 61: 654–659
Giovanella B, Lohman W, Heidelberger C (1970) Effects of elevated temperatures and drugs on the viability of L1210 leukemia cells. Cancer Res 30: 1623–1631
Goss P, Parsons P (1977) The effect of hyperthermia and melphalan on survival of human fibroblast strains and melanoma cell lines. Cancer Res 37: 152–156
Hahn GM (1978) Interactions of drugs and hyperthermia in vitro and in vivo. In: Streffer C (ed) Proceedings of the international symposium on hyperthermia in cancer treatment. Urban and Schwarzenberg, Baltimore, pp 72–79
Hahn GM (1982) Hyperthermia and cancer. Plenum Press, New York
Hahn GM, Shiu E (1983) Effect of pH and elevated temperature on the cytotoxicity of some chemotherapeutic agents in Chinese hamster cells in vitro. Cancer Res 43: 5789–5781
Hahn GM, Strande D (1976) Cytotoxic effects of hyperthermia and adriamycin on Chinese hamster cells. J Natl Cancer Inst 57: 1063–1067
Hall J, Bull JMC, Cronau L (1988) Hypo- and hyperthermia in clinical auditory brain stem response measurement: two case reports. Ear Hear 4: 137–143
Har-Kedar I (1975) Effect of hyperthermia and chemotherapy in EMT6 cells. Proceedings of the international symposium on cancer therapy by hyperthermia and radiation. pp 91–93
Hazan G, Ben-Hur E, Yerushalmi A (1981) Synergism between hyperthermia and cyclophosphamide in vivo: the effect of dose fractionization. Eur J Cancer 6: 681–684
Herman TS (1983) Temperature dependence of adriamycin, cis-diamminedichloroplatinum (II), bleomycin, and 1,3-bis(2-chloroethyl)-1-nitrosourea cytoxocicity in vitro. Cancer Res 43: 365–369
Herman TS, Cress A, Sweets C, Gerner E (1981) Reversal of resistance to methotrexate by hyperthermia in Chinese hamster ovary cells. Cancer Res 41: 3840–3843
Herman TS, Zukoski CA, Anderson RM, et al. (1982) Whole-body hyperthermia and chemotherapy for treatment of patients with advanced, refractory malignancies. Cancer Treat Rep 66: 259–265
Herman TS, Henle K, Nagle W, Moss A, Monson T (1984) Effect of step-down heating on the cytotoxicity of adriamycin, bleomycin, and cis-diamminedichloroplatinum (II). Cancer Res 44: 1823–1826
Herman TS, Teicher BA, Collins LS (1988) Effect of hypoxia and pH on the cytotoxicity of four platinum complexes at normal and hyperthermic temperatures. Cancer Res 48: 2342–2347
Herman TS, Teicher BA, Pfeffer M, Khandekar V (1990) Interaction with hyperthermia of platinum complexes of triaminotriphenylmethane dyes. Int J Hyperthermia 6: 629–639
Herman TS, Teicher BA, Varsheny A, Khandekar V, Brann T (1992) Effect of hypoxia and acidosis on the cytotoxicity of mitoxantrone, bisantrene and amsacrine and their platinum complexes at normal and hyperthermic temperatures. Anticancer Res 12: 827–836
Hinkelbein W, Birmelin M, Menger D, Engelhardt R (1988) Toxic effects of irradiation or doxorubicin in combination with moderate whole-body hyperthermia on bone marrow in rats. Recent Results Cancer Res 109: 71–82
Honess D, Bleehen N (1982) Sensitivity of normal mouse marrow and RIF-1 tumour to hyperthermia combined with cyclophosphamide or BCNU: a lack of therapeutic gain. Br J Cancer 46: 236–248
Honess D, Bleehen N (1985a) Potentiation of melphalan by systemic hyperthermia in mice: therapeutic gain for mouse lung microtumours. Int J Hyperthermia 1: 57–68
Honess D, Bleehen N (1985b) Thermochemotherapy with cisplatinum, CCNU, BCNU, chlorambucil and melphalan on murine marrow and two tumours: therapeutic gain for melphalan only. Br J Radiol 58: 63–72
Johnson H, Pavelec M (1973) Thermal enhancement of thio-TEPA cytotoxicity. J Natl Cancer Inst 50: 903–908
Joiner M, Steel G, Stephens I (1982) Response of two mouse tumours to hyperthermia with CCNU or melphalan. Br J Cancer 45: 17–26
Joshi D, Barendsen G (1984) Hyperthermic modification of drug effectiveness for reproductive death of cultured mamalian cells. Indian J Exp Biol 22: 248–250
Kano E, Furukawa-Furuya M, Nitta K, et al. (1988) Sensitivities of bleomycin-resistant variant cells enhanced by 40°C hyperthermia in vitro. Int J Hyperthermia 4: 547–553
Kapp D (1988) Hyperthermia treatment (HT) of superficial malignancies. Sugatrara T, Saito M (eds) The 5th international symposium of hyperthermic oncology
Kido Y, Kuwano H, Maehara Y, Mori M, Matsuoka H, Sugimachi K (1991) Increased cytotoxicity of low-dose, long-duration exposure to 5-fluorouracil of V-79 cells with hyperthermia. Cancer Chemother Pharmacol 28: 251–254
Kilbourne R, Gross S, Jubran A, Adams J, Griffith O, Levi R, Lodato R (1990) NG-methyl-L-arginine inhibits tumor necrosis factor-induced hypotension: implications for the involvement of nitric oxide. Proc Natl Acad Sci USA 87: 3629–3632
Kim JH, Kim SH, Alfieri A, Young CS, Silvestrini B (1984) Lonidamine: a hyperthermic sensitizer of HeLa cells in culture and of the Meth-A tumor in vivo. Oncology 4: 30–35
Kim YD, Lake R, Lees DE, Schuette WH, Bull JMC, Weise V, Kopin IJ (1979a) Hemodynamic and plasma chatecholamine responses to hyperthermia cancer therapy in humans. Am J Physiol 237: H570
Kim YD, Lees DE, Lake CR, Whang-Peng J, Schuette W, Smith R, Bull JMC (1979b) Hyperthermia potentiates doxorubicin-related cardiotoxic effects. JAMA 24: 1816–1817
Klaubert W, Eisler K, Lange J, Wilmanns W (1988) Coagulation and fibrinogenolysis during whole-body hyperthermia. Recent Results Cancer Res 107: 205–208
Klostergaard J, Lu S, Tomasovic S (1991) Potentiation of TNF cytotoxicity by hyperthermia: comparative in vitro studies of TNF-α, TNF-γ, and TNF-S AM2. Lymphokine Res
Koga S, Maeta M, Shimizu N, et al. (1985) Clinical effects of total-body hyperthermia combined with anticancer chemotherapy for far-advanced gastrointestinal cancer. Cancer 55: 1641–1647
Kusumoto T, Teicher B (1994) Analysis of the interaction of seven platinum complexes with murine FSaII

fibrosarcoma in culture. 18th international congress of chemotherapy. Proc Annu Meet Am Assoc Cancer Res 35: A3803

Larkin JM, Edwards WS, Smith DE, Clark PJ (1977) Systemic thermotherapy: description of a method and physiologic tolerance in clinical subjects. Cancer 40: 3155–3159

Lees DE, Kim YD, Bull JMC, Whang-Peng J, Smith R, MacNamara TG (1980) Anesthetic management of whole body hyperthermia with and without chemotherapy. Anesthesiology 52: 418–428

Lees DE, Kim YD, Dubois M, Bull JMC, Smith R, Schuette WH, MacNamara TG (1982) Internal organ hypoxia during hyperthermia cancer therapy in humans. In: Dethlefsen L, Dewey WC (eds) Proceedings of the third international symposium on cancer therapy by hyperthermia, drugs and radiation. National Cancer Institute Monograph, Fort Collins, CO, pp 339–401

Levin W, Blair R (1978) Clinical experience with combined whole-body hyperthermia and radiation. In: Streffer C, van Beuningen D, Dietzel F (eds) Cancer therapy by hyperthermia and radiation. Urban and Schwarzenberg, Baltimore, pp 322–325

Li D, Hahn G (1984) Response of RIF tumors to heat and drugs: dependence on tumor size. Cancer Treat Rep 68: 1149–1151

Lienard D, Ewalenko P, Delmotte JJ, Renard N, Lejeune FJ (1992) High dose recombinant tumor necrosis factor alpha in combination with interferon gamma and melphalan in isolation perfusion of the limbs for melanoma and sarcoma. J Clin Oncol 10: 52–60

Loshek DD, Greenlaw RH, Doyle LA (1981) Whole body hyperthermia using a water circulator. Strahlentheroncol 157: 620–621

Makino M, Sakaguchi Y, Strebel FR, Jenkins G, Ohno S, Klostergaard J, Tomasovic S, Bull JMC, et al. (1993a) The importance of timing and sequence in using tumor necrosis factor (TNF) in a combination treatment with whole body hyperthermia (WBH) + carboplatin (CBDCA) in rats. Proceedings of the 84th meeting of the American Association for Cancer Research 34: 388 (2311)

Makino M, Stephens LC, Sakaguchi Y, Lodato RF, Strebel FR, Jenkins G, Bull JMC (1993b) Alteration in blood profile and tissue histopathology caused by tumor necrosis factor combined with whole body hyperthermia in rats. Proceedings of the 41st annual meeting of the Radiation Research society and the 13th annual meeting of the North American Hyperthermia Society. 29: 50

Marmor JB (1979) Interactions of hyperthermia and chemotherapy in animals. Cancer Res 39: 2269–2276

Marmor JB, Kozak D, Hahn G (1979) Effects of systemically administered bleomycin or adriamycin with local hyperthermia on primary tumor and lung metastases. Cancer Treat Rep 63: 1279–1290

Martinez A, Gersten D, Leslie J, Borrego C, Armour E, Corry P (1993) Interstitial thermobrachytherapy with continuous mild hyperthermia for the treatment of locally advanced or recurring pelvic malignancies. 41st annual meeting of the Radiation Research Society 41: 122 (S-12-4)

McChesney Gillette S, Dawson C, Scott R, et al. (1993) Whole-body hyperthermia combined with hyperfractionated irradiation of the thorax in dog: acute physiological response. Int J Hyperthermia 9: 369–382

Mella O (1985) Combined hyperthermia and cis-diamminedichloroplatinum in BD IX rats with transplanted BT_4A tumours. Int J Hyperthermia 1: 171–183

Mella O, Eriksen R, Dahl O, Laerum O (1987) Acute systemic toxicity of combined cis-diamminedichlorplatinum and hyperthermia in the rat. Eur J Cancer 23: 365–373

Meyn R, Corry P, Fletcher S, Demetriades M (1979) Thermal enhancement of DNA strand breakage in mammalian cells treated with bleomycin. Int J Radiat Oncol Biol Phys 5: 1487–1489

Meyn R, Corry P, Fletcher S, Demetriades M (1980) Thermal enhancement of DNA damage in mammalian cells treated with cisdiamminedichloroplatinum (II). Cancer Res 47: 4335–4337

Mivechi N, Li G (1988) Heat sensitivity, thermotolerance and profile of protein synthesis of human bone marrow progenitors. Cancer Res 48: 3630–3633

Mizuno S, Amagai M, Ishida A (1980) Synergistic cell killing by antitumor agents and hyperthermia in cultured cells. Jpn J Cancer Res 71: 471–478

Morgan J, Bleehen N (1980) A comparison of the interaction between hyperthermia and bleomycin on the EMT6 tumour as a monolayer or spheroids in vitro and in vivo. In: Arcangeli G, Mauro F (eds) Hyperthermia in radiation oncology. Masson, Milan, pp 165–170

Muckle D, Dickson J (1973) Hyperthermia (42°C) as an adjuvant to radiotherapy and chemotherapy in the treatment of the allogeneic VX2 carcinoma in the rabbit. Br J Cancer 27: 307–315

Mulcahy R, Gipp J, Tanner M (1987) Enhancement of misonidazole chemopotentiation by mild hyperthermia (41°C) in vitro and selective enhancement in vivo. Int J Radiat Biol 52: 57–65

Mulcahy R, Gipp J, Tanner M (1988) Sensitization of nitrosourea-resistant Mer+ human tumor cells to *N*′-(2-chloroethyl)-*N*-cyclohexyl-*N*-nitrosoruea by mild (41°C) hyperthermia. Cancer Res 48: 1086–1090

Muzuno S, Amagai M, Ishida A (1980) Synergistic cell killing by antitumor agents and hyperthermia in cultured cells. Jpn J Cancer Res 34: 397–406

Nauts HC (1975) Pyrogen therapy of cancer: a historical overview and current activities. Proc 1st international symposium on cancer therapy by hyperthermia and radiation. Wizenberg M, Robinson JE (eds) Proc of the International Symposium on Cancer There by Hyperthermia and Radiation. American College of Radiology Press, Baltrmore, MD 239–250

Nauts HC (1982) Bacterial pyrogens: beneficial effects on capycer patients. In: Gutherie JM, Albert E (eds) Biomedical thermology, progress in clinical biological research. Liss, New York, pp 687–696

Nauts HC, Fowler GA, Bogatko FH (1953) A review of the influence of bacterial infections and bacterial products (Coley's toxins) on malignant tumors in men. Acta Med Scand (suppl) 276: 1–103

Neta R, Oppenheim J (1991) Radioprotection with cytokines – learning from nature to cope with radiation damage. Cancer Cells 3: 391–396

Neta R, Perlstein R, Vogel S, Ledney G, Abrams J (1992) Role of interleukin 6 (IL-6) in protection from lethal irradiation and in endocrine responses to IL-1 and tumor necrosis factor. J Exp Med 175: 689–694

Neumann H, Fiebig H, Lohr G, Engelhardt R (1985) Effects of cytostatic drugs and 40.5°C hyperthermia on human bone marrow progenitors (CFU-C) and human clonogenic tumor cells implanted into mice. J Natl Cancer Inst 75: 1059–1066

Neville A, Sauder D (1988) Whole body hyperthermia (41–42°C) induces interleukin-1 in vivo. Lymphokine Res 7. 201–204

Novotney C, Page R, Macy D, et al. (1992) Phase I evaluation of doxorubicin and whole-body hyperthermia in dogs with lymphoma. J Vet Intern Med 6: 245–249

O'Hara M, Lin C, Leeper D (1991a) The thermal response and development of thermotolerance of the bone marrow stromal progenitor CFU-E. Exp Hematol 99: 1096–1100

O'Hara M, Pollard M, Xiong Q, Leeper D (1991b) The development of thermotolerance in bone marrow CFU-S during chronic hyperthermia. Exp Hematol 99: 878–881

Ohno S, Strebel FR, Siddik ZH, Stephens LC, Khokar A, Bull JMC (1991) The effect of carboplatin combined with whole body hyperthermia on normal tissue and tumor in rats. Cancer Res 51: 2994–3000

Ohno S, Strebel FR, Stephens LC, Siddik ZH, Makino M, Khokar AR, Bull JMC (1993) Haematological toxicity of carboplatin and cisplatin combined with whole body hyperthermia in rats. Br J Cancer 68: 469–474

Ohno S, Strebel FR, Stephens LC, Siddik ZH, Makino M, Bull JMC (1991) Effect of bleomycin or liblomycin Combined with whole body hyperthermia in tumor and normal tissue in rats. Droc 9th Internat Congress of Radiation Research, Toronto, Canada

Oleson JR, Dewhirst MW, Harrelson JM, Leopold KA, Samulski TV, Tso CY (1989) Tumor temperature distributions predict hyperthermia effect. Int J Radiat Oncol Biol Phys 16: 559–570

Oleson JR, Samulski TV, Leopold KA, Clegg ST, Dewhirst MW, Dodge RK, George SL (1993) Sensitivity of hyperthermia trial outcomes to temperature and time: implications for thermal goals of treatment. Int J Radiat Oncol Biol Phys 25: 289–297

Oshnoshi T, Ohnuma T, Beranek J, Holland J (1985) Combined cytotoxicity effect of hyperthermia and anthracycline antibiotics on human tumor cells. J Natl Cancer Inst 74: 275–281

Osieka R, Magin RL, Atkinson ER (1978) The effect of hyperthermia on human colon cancer xenografts in nude mice. In: Streffer C (ed) Cancer therapy by hyperthermia and radiation. Urban and Schwarzenberg, Munich, pp 287–290

Page RL, Meyer RE, Thrall DE, Dewhirst MW (1987) Cardiovascular and metabolic response of tumour-bearing dogs to whole body hyperthermia. Int J Hyperthermia 3: 513–525

Page RL, Thrall DE, Dewhirst MW, et al. (1991) Phase I study of melphalan and whole body hyperthermia in dogs with malignant melanoma. Int J Hyperthermia 7: 559–566

Page RL, Macy DW, Ogilvie GK, et al. (1992a) Phase III evaluation of doxorubicin and whole body hyperthermia in dogs with lymphoma. Int J Hyperthermia 8: 187–197

Page RL, Thrall DE, George SL, et al. (1992b) Quantitative estimation of the thermal dose-modifying factor for cis-dimminedichloroplatinum (CDDP) in tumour-bearing dogs. Int J Hyperthermia 8: 761–769

Parks LC, Minaberry D, Smith DP, Neely WH (1979) Treatment of far advanced bronchogenic carcinoma by extracorporeally induced systemic hyperthermia. J Thorac Cardiovasc Surg 28: 883–897

Parks LC, Smith GV (1983) Systemic hyperthermia by extracorporeal induction: techniques and results. In: Storm FK (ed) Hyperthermia in cancer therapy. C.K. Hall, Boston, Mass, pp 407–447

Perry DJ, Weiss RB, Creekmore SP, Micetich KC, Curt GA (1986) Carboplatin for advanced colorectal carcinoma: a phase II study. Cancer Treat Rep 70: 301–302

Pettigrew RT, Galt JM, Ludgate CM, Horn DB, Smith AN (1974) Circulatory and biochemical effects of whole body hyperthermia. Br J Surg 61: 727–730

Pettigrew RT, Galt JM, Ludgate CM, Smith AN (1974b) Clinical effects of whole body hyperthermia in advanced malignancy. BMJ 4: 679–682

Posner M, Lienard D, Lejeune F, Rosenfelder D, Kirkwood J (1994) Hyperthermic isolated limb perfusion (HILP) with tumor necrosis factor (TNF) alone for metastatic intransit melanoma. Proc ASCO 13: 396, 1351

Robins HI (1991) Combined modality clinical trials for favorable B-cell neoplasms: lonidamine plus whole body hyperthermia and/or total body irradiation. Semin Oncol 18: 23–27

Robins HI, Neville AJ (1986) Biology and methodology of whole-body hyperthermia. In: Angileri, Robert (eds) Hyperthermia in cancer treatment. CRC Press, Boca Raton, Fl., pp 183–206

Robins HI, Dennis W, Martin P, Sondel P, Yatvin M, Steeves R (1984) Potentiation of differential hyperthermic sensitivity of AKR leukemia and normal bone marrow cells by lidocaine or thiopental. Cancer 54: 2831–2835

Robins HI, Dennis WH, Neville AJ, et al. (1985) A nontoxic system for 41.8°C whole body hyperthermia: results of a phase I study using a radiant heat device. Cancer Res 45: 3937–3944

Robins HI, Longo WL, Steeves R, et al. (1988) A pilot study of whole body Hyperthermia and local irradiation for aduanced non-small cell lung cancer confined to the thorax. The International Journal of Radiation Oncology Biology & Physics 15: 427–431

Robins HI, Sielaff KM, Storer B, Hawkins MJ, Bofden EC (1989) Phase I trial of human lymphoblastoid interferon with whole body hyperthermia in advanced cancer. Cancer Res 49: 1609–1615

Robins HI, Longo W, Steeves R, et al. (1990) Adjunctive therapy (whole body hyperthermia) versus lonidamine to total body irradiation for the treatment of favorable B-cell neoplasms: a report of two pilot clinical trials and laboratory investigations. Int J Radiat Oncol Biol Phys 18: 909–920

Robins HI, Cohen JD, Schmitt CL, et al. (1993) Phase I clinical trial of carboplatin and 41.8°C whole body hyperthermia. J Clin Oncol 11: 1787–1794

Rohner R, Peior J, Sipple J (1966) Mucinous malignancies, venous thrombosis and terminal endocarditis with emboli: a syndrome. Cancer 19: 1805–1810

Roizin-Towle L, Hall E (1982) Interaction between hyperthermia and cytotoxic agents. NCI Monogr 61: 149–151

Rose WC, Veras G, Laster WRJ, Schabel FMJ (1979) Evaluation of whole-body hyperthermia as an adjunct to chemotherapy in murine tumors. Cancer Treat Rep 63: 1311–1325

Sack G, Levin J, Bell W (1977) Trousseau's syndrome and other manifestations of chronic disseminated coagulopathy in patients with neoplasms; clinical, pathologic and therapeutic features. Medicine

Sakaguchi Y, Stephens L, Danhauser L, Makino M, Strebel FR, Jenkins G, Bull JMC (1993) Enhancement of antitumor effect and induction of apoptosis by a combination of 5-fluorouracil and whole body hyperthermia in rats. Proc Am Assoc Cancer Res 34: 361(2151)

Sakaguchi Y, Stephens L, Kaneko T, Danhauser L, Strebel FR, Jenkins G, Bull JMC (1994a) Apoptosis and tumor response induced by 5-fluorouracil and whole body hyperthermia in rats. Proc 85th meeting of Am Assoc Cancer Res 35: 151(3352)

Sakaguchi Y, Stephens LC, Makino M, Danhauser LL, Strebel FR, Jenkins GN, Kaneko T, Bull JMC (1993b) Efficacy of prolonged intravenous infusion of 5-fluorouracil combined with hyperthermia in vivo: apoptosis and tumor response. Proc Amer Assoc Cancer Res 34: 361(2151)

Sakaguchi Y, Stephens LC, Makino M, Kaneko T, Strebel FR, Danhauser LL, Jenkins GN (1994c) Apoptosis and tumor response induced by 5-fluorouracil and whole body hyperthermia in vivo. Proc Amer Assoc Cancer Res 36: 151(3352)

Sakaguchi Y, Makino M, Kaneko T, et al. (1994d) Therapeutic efficacy of long-duration-low-temperature whole body hyperthermia when combined with tumor necrosis factor and carboplatin in rats. Cancer Res 54: 2223–2227

Seegenschmiedt MH, Martus P, Fietkau R, Iro H, Brady L, Sauer R (1994) Multivariate analysis of prognostic parameters using interstitial thermoradiotherapy (IHT-IRT): tumor and treatment variables predict outcome. Int J Radiat Oncol Biol Phys 29: 1049–1063

Selker RG, Jacobs S, Stoller R, Kristojik M, Randall M (1983) On the limits of human tolerance to whole body hyperthermia and simultaneous chemotherapy. Radiat Res 94: 550–555

Shen R, Hornback N, Shidnia H, Wu B, Lu L, Broxmeyer H (1991) Whole body hyperthermia: a potent radioprotector in vivo. Int J Radiat Oncol Biol Phys 20: 525–530

Shen R, Lu L, Young P, Shidnia H, Hornback N, Broxmeyer H (1994) Influence of elevated temperature on natural killer cell activity, lymphokine-activated killer cell activity and lectin-dependent cytotoxicity of human umbilical cord blood and adult blood cells. Int J Radiat Oncol Biol Phys 29: 821–826

Song CW, Lin J-C, Lyons JC (1993) Antitumor effect of interleukinla in combination with hyperthermia. Cancer Res 53: 324–328

Spero J, Lewis J, Hasiba U (1980) Disseminated intravascular coagulation: findings in 346 patients. Thromb Haemost 43: 28–34

Srinivasan J, Fajardo L, Hahn G (1990) Mechanism of antitumor activity of tumor necrosis factor alpha with hyperthermia in a tumor necrosis factor alpha-resistant tumor. J Natl Cancer Inst 82: 1904–1910

Stark P, Guthrie A, Bull J (1985) Thoracic radiographic changes after systemic hyperthermia for advanced cancer. Radiology 154: 55–58

Steeves RA, Robins HI, Miller K, Martin P, Schecterle L, Dennis W (1987) Interaction of whole-body hyperthermia and irradiation in the treatment of AKR mouse leukemia. Int J Radiat Biol 52: 935–947

Stehlin JJ, Giovanella B, de Ipolyi P, Muenz L, Anderson R (1975) Results of hyperthermic perfusion for melanoma of the extremities. Surg Gynecol Obstet 140: 339–348

Stehlin JJ, Giovanella B, de Ipolyi P, Anderson R (1979) Results of eleven years' experience with heated perfusion for melanoma of the extremities. Cancer Res 39: 2255–2257

Strebel FR, Ohno S, Stephens LC, Siddik ZH, Travis EL, Khokhar AR, Bull JMC (1991) Comparison of the acute and chronic normal tissue toxicities of cisplatin and carboplatin combined with WBH in rats. Dewey WC, Edington N, Fry RJM, Hall EJ, Whitmore GF (eds) The 9th international congress of radiation research 1991. Academic Press Inc., Sandigo

Strother S, Branham S, Bull JMC (1986) Activation of coagulation during therapeutic whole body hyperthermia. Thromb Res 43: 353–360

Suzuki K (1967) Application of heat to cancer chemotherapy - experimental studies. Nagoya J Med Sci 30: 1–21

Takahashi H, Tanaka R, Sekihara Y, Hondo H (1991) Auditory brainstem response during systemic hyperthermia. Int J Hyperthermia 7: 613–620

Tapazoglou E, Robins H, Cohen J, Khatana A, Schmitt C, Franken K, Sapareto SA (1990) The enhancement of cytotoxicity of carboplatin (CBDCA) by whole body hyperthermia (WBH) in murine AKR leukemia. 38th Ann Meeting of the Rad Res Soc 10th Ann Meeting of the North American Hyperthermia a Group 1990 26 (AN-5)

Teicher B, TSH, Menon K, Korbut T (1992) Whole-body hyperthermia as an adjuvant to treatment with platinum complexes with and without etanidazole in mice bearing the Lewis lung carcinoma or the FSaLL fibrosarcoma. Int J Hyperthermia 8: 783–794

Thrall DE, Page RL, Dewhirst MW, Meyer RE, Hoopes PJ, Kornegay JN (1986) Temperature measurements in normal and tumor tissue of dogs undergoing whole body hyperthermia. Cancer Res 46: 6229–6235

Thrall DE, Dewhirst MW, Page RL, Samulski TV, McLeod DA, Oleson JR (1990) A comparison of temperatures in canine solid tumours during local and whole-body hyperthermia administered alone and simultaneously. Int J Hyperthermia 6: 305–317

Tonnesen A, Marnock C, Bull JMC, Morgenweck C, Fallon K (1987) Sweating, hemodynamic responses, and thermal equilibration during hyperthermia in humans. J Appl Physiol 62: 1596–1602

Tsumura M, Yoshiga K, Takada K (1988) Endancement of antitumour effects of 1-helycarbamyl-5-fluorouracil combined with hyperthermia on Ehrlich ascites tumor in vivo and Nakahara-Fukuoka sarcoma cell in vitro. Cancer Res 48: 3977–3980

Twentyman P, Morgan J, Donaldson J (1978) Enhancement by hyperthermia of the effect of BCNU against the EMT6 mouse tumor. Cancer Treat Rep 62: 439–443

Urano M, Kahn J, Kenton LA (1988) Effect of bleomycin on murine tumour cells at elevated temperatures and two different pH values. Cancer Res 48: 615–619

Valdagni R, Amichetti M (1994) Report of long-term follow-up in a randomized trial comparing radiation therapy and radiation therapy plus hyperthermia to metastatic lymph nodes in stage IV head and neck patients. Int J Radiat Oncol Biol Phys 28: 163–169

van der Zee J, Van Rhoon GC, Wilce-Hooley JL, Faithfull NS, SRH (1983) Whole-body hyperthermia in cancer therapy: a report of a phase I–II study. Eur J Cancer 19: 1189–1200 van der Zee J, Faithfull NS, van Rhoon GC, Reinhold HS (1987) Whole body hyperthermia as a treatment modality. Nato Asi Ser E 127: 420–440

Wallner KE, DeGregario MW, Li GC (1986) Hyperthermic potentiation of cis-diamminedichloroplatinum (II) cytotoxicity in Chinese hamster ovary cells resistant to the drug. Cancer Res 46: 6242–6245

Wang B, Lumanglas A, Silva J, Ruszala-Mallon V, Durr F (1987) Effect of hyperthermia on the sensitivity of human colon carcinoma cells to mitoxantrone. Cancer Treat Rep 61: 831–836

Warren SL (1935) Preliminary study of the effect of artificial fever on hopeless tumor cases. Am J Roentgenol 33: 75–87

West K, Weber T, Grosfeld J (1980) Snergistic effect of hyperthermia, papaverine, and chemotherapy in murine neuroblastoma. J Pediatr Surg 15: 913–917

Wondergem J, Bulger R, Strebel FR, Newman R, Travis E, Stephens L, Bull JMC (1988a) Effect of cis-diamminedichloroplatinum (II) combined with whole body hyperthermia on renal injury. Cancer Res 48: 440–446

Wondergem J, Strebel FR, Siddik ZH, Newman R, Bull JMC (1988b) The effects of anesthetics on cisplatinum-induced toxicity at normal temperatures and during whole body hyperthermia: the influence of NaCl concentration of the vehicle. Int J Hyperthermia 4: 643–654

Wondergem J, Stephens LC, Strebel FR, et al. (1991) Effect of adriamycin combined with whole body hyperthermia on tumor and normal tissues. Cancer Res 51: 3559–3567

Wondergem J, Siddik ZH, Strebel FR, Bull JMC (1993) Effect of whole body hyperthermia on cis-diamminedichloroplatinum (II)-induced antitumor activity and tissue Pt-distribution: do anesthetics influence the therapeutic ratio? Eur J Cancer 29A: 549–554

Wondergem J, Strebel FR, Stephens LC, Siddik ZH, Bull JMC (1995) Chronic effect of whole body hyperthermia combined simultaneously with cis-diamminedichloroplatinum II on normal tissue in rats. Int J Hyperthermia 11: 37–49

Yamane T, Nakabayashi H, Ito S, Sumii H, Kawal A (1986) In vitro thermochemotherapy of human osteosarcoma cells with cis-dichlorodiammineplatinum (II). Hiroshima J Med Sci 35: 191–195

Yatvin M (1977) The influence of membrane liquid composition and procaine on hyperthermic death of cells. Int J Radiat Biol 32: 513–521

Yatvin M, Clifton K, Dennis W (1979) Hyperthermia and local anesthetics: potentiation of survival in tumor-bearing mice. Science 205: 195–196

Yerushalmi A (1978) Combined treatment of a solid tumour by local hyperthermia and actinomycin D. Br J Cancer 37: 327–832

Yerushalmi A, Hazan G (1979) Control of Lewis lung carcinoma by combined treatment with local hyperthermia anc cyclophosphamide: preliminary results. Isr J Med Sci 15: 462–463

Yerushalmi A, Tovey G, Gresser I (1982) Antitumor effect of combined interferon and hyperthermia in mice. Proc Soc Exp Biol Med 169: 412–415.

Zupi G, Badaracco G, Caraliere R, Natali PG, Greco C (1987) Influence of sequence on hyperthermia and drug Combination in Hyperthermic Oncology, Overquards (ed) Taylor and Francis Press, London vol 1: 429–432

19 Clinical Practice of Hyperthermic Extremity Perfusion in Combination with Radiotherapy and Chemotherapy

R. CAVALIERE, F. DI FILIPPO, F. CAVALIERE, S. CARLINI, M. SCHIRATTI, M. ANZÀ, R. GARINEI, A. CALLOPOLI, A. CAPUA, F.A. IMPIOMBATO, P. PERRI, and A. PSAILA

CONTENTS

19.1 History and Rationale

The technique of normothermic antiblastic perfusion was first introduced into clinical practice by Krementz in 1957 (KREMENTZ et al. 1958). This method permits temporary isolation of the tumor-bearing limb from the systemic circulation by means of an extracorporeal circuit. In this manner, high dosages of antineoplastic drugs (5–10 times greater than those administered systemically) can be administered into a restricted area, with high drug concentrations being achieved in the tumor and surrounding tissues.

The first case, treated at Charity Hospital in New Orleans, Louisiana, involved a 76-year-old patient with about 80 in-transit metastases in the lower left limb that had developed 2 years after the excision of a hip melanoma and groin dissection. In the days following the treatment, the neoplastic nodules began to disappear until complete regression was achieved some months later. The patient lived with no evidence of disease for 16 years and died at the age of 92 of other causes.

After this first remarkable success, many other patients were treated with *normothermic* antiblastic perfusion with positive results and the technique rapidly became widespread, particularly in the United States.

In the early 1960s, a research project conducted both in vitro and in vivo was initiated at the Institute of Biochemistry of the University of Rome and at the Regina Elena National Cancer Institute of Rome to study the effects of high temperatures (42°–43°C) on tumor cells. These studies showed that there is a selective sensitivity of tumors towards hyperthermia inasmuch as they are submitted to irreparable damage (by means of direct or indirect mechanisms, mediated by the modifications of the tumor microcirculation and microenvironment), while the healthy tissues are able to repair such sublethal damage produced by the heat (CAVALIERE et al. 1967).

Hyperthermia was first employed as an antitumor agent at the Regina Elena National Cancer Institute in 1964. From a technical point of view, Krementz's idea of *extracorporeal circulation* was employed, with a modification that consisted of the introduction of a heat exchanger into the circuit. The circulating blood, passing through the heat exchanger, was heated and, circulating in the limb, acted as a means of heat transfer, raising the tumor temperature to the preestablished level.

The hyperthermic perfusion, conducted for a period of 2–4 h at a tumor temperature of 42° and 43°C, provided good tumor response and a large amount of necrosis in the neoplastic sites. In some patients with limb melanomas in the locoregional spreading phase (stages II, IIIA, and IIIAB), complete responses and even subsequent cure

R. CAVALIERE, MD, F. DI FILIPPO, MD, F. CAVALIERE, MD, S. CARLINI, MD, M. SCHIRATTI, MD, M. ANZÀ, MD, R. GARINEI, MD, A. CALLOPOLI, MD, A. CAPUA, MD, F. AMBESI IMPIOMBATO, MD, P. PERRI, MD, A. PSAILA, MD, Istituto Regina Elena Per Lo Studio e La Cura Dei Tumori, 291, Viale Regina Elena, I-00161 Rome, Italy

were obtained. In patients affected with soft tissue or osteogenic sarcomas, the perfusion was followed by surgical removal of the remaining tumor bulk, in many cases avoiding amputation, which was the treatment of choice at that time.

At the end of the 1960s, Stehlin combined the two techniques, using *hyperthermia and the neoplastic agents by perfusion simultaneously*, and observed both greater tumor response and higher 5-year survival rates, rising from 22% with normothermic perfusion to 76% with hyperthermic antiblastic perfusion (HAP) in stage IIIA melanoma (Stehlin et al. 1969).

It was in this manner that HAP was born, and it rapidly spread to all of the major oncology institutions in the world. Thus far, more than 5000 patients have been treated with this technique. Thanks to the technological improvements, this treatment modality is not burdened by high morbidity and mortality rates.

The rationale for employing HAP resides in the following features:

1. The entire tumor-bearing limb and all the regional lymph nodes are involved in the treatment.
2. The temporary isolation of the limb from the systemic circulation permits the use of doses of antineoplastic drugs that are 5–10 times greater than those administered systemically without serious systemic toxic effects.
3. The administration of high doses of antineoplastic drugs directly into the tributary limb artery with continual regional circulation, without metabolization or loss to other systemic districts, provides a high local drug level and increased tumor drug uptake.
4. During the perfusion, heparin is usually employed: this has been proven to have not only an antimetastatic effect but also a direct antitumor effect.
5. During the extracorporeal circulation, high concentrations of pO_2, ranging between 200 and 300 mmHg, are employed, creating a sort of artificial hyperbaric chamber of the limb. The hyperoxygenation obtained not only potentiates the effects of the alkylating drugs but also has a direct antitumor effect.
6. Hyperthermia used during perfusional treatment can potentiate the tumoricidal effect of the drugs and possesses an antitumor activity per se. The simultaneous application of hyperthermia and drugs results in a synergistic activity and therefore in a possible therapeutic gain. Alternatively, the drugs employed enable an isoeffect to be achieved at a lower temperature (41°–42°C); this will entail only minor toxicity to the healthy tissues and therefore a higher therapeutic index is achieved.
7. The reduction of the tumor mass obtained after the perfusion often permits the performance of conservative rather than destructive surgery.

The rationale for employing HAP explains its therapeutic potential and its success in the treatment of limb tumors. Although this technique has been used for approximately 40 years in many oncological centers, it has not been completely standardized, especially with regard to the treatment parameters. The latter, strictly related to perfusion, may have an impact on the efficacy and toxicity of the treatment and will be illustrated and discussed, while the interactions between hyperthermia and chemotherapy will not be presented in detail (see elsewhere in this book). The clinical results of our own experience and those of others with adequate follow-up will be reported and discussed.

19.2 Treatment Technique

19.2.1 The Upper Limbs

The patient is placed in a supine position with the limb abducted at a 90° angle. The entire limb is prepared with Betadine, including the axilla, the upper third of the thorax, the shoulder, and the neck.

The skin incision is made from the clavicle to the deltoid pectoral groove. The spared cephalic vein is isolated and the large pectoral muscle is lowered, after resecting the insertion of the clavicular fibers and part of the sternal ones. The small pectoral muscle is resected in order to expose the first and second portions of the axillary vessels.

During the preparation of these vessels, frozen sections of enlarged nodes are carried out and, if pathological involvement is found, an axillary node dissection is performed.

All of the collateral vessels of the artery and axillary vein (the acromiothoracic, the small pectoral muscle, and the external mammary vessels) are temporarily isolated, including the subscapular vessels to reduce leakage.

Once the vessels have been prepared, the patient is given systemic heparin (150–200 IU/kg of body weight); after 2–3 min, the axillary vessels are clamped and cannulated with a 10–12 French catheter for the artery and a 12–14 French catheter for the vein, after making a transverse incision on the vessel wall (Fig. 19.1). The two catheters are secured with umbilical tape to prevent dislodgement during the perfusion. These are then connected to the previously primed extracorporeal circuit, composed of an oxygenator, a heat exchanger, and a pump (Fig. 19.2). The extracorporeal circulation begins at a minimum flow (30 ml/l of limb volume) that is gradually increased until it reaches an equilibrium based on the venous outflow so that the oxygenator level remains constant.

A tourniquet is applied to the root of the limb, anchored by two Steinmann pins, positioned in the trapezius muscle above and in the large dorsal muscle below the axilla, respectively. This blocks the superficial circulation and helps to restrict leakage to a minimum, normally monitored at the very beginning of the perfusion and before the drug administration. Radio-labelled albumin is then injected into the circuit and radioactivity is measured with a scanner, placed on the cardiac area. A 10% leakage rate is considered acceptable, while the perfusion should not be carried out if the value is higher, because of the risk of systemic toxicity.

The temperature of the heat exchanger at the start of the perfusion is 39°–40°C and it is raised until the desired tissue and tumor temperature is reached. For the upper limbs, needle thermocouples are inserted into the skin and muscles of the arm and forearm, into the neoplastic nodules, and into the arterial and venous line of the circuit near the catheters. The thermocouples are connected to a thermometer, able to read and record the temperature of the monitored sites for the entire duration of the treatment. A sort of "thermal map" of the perfused limb is therefore made, which is extremely important for monitoring both the healthy tissue (skin, subcutaneous fat, and muscles) and the tumor localizations in order to "steer" the treatment to gain the maximum therapeutic index.

The appropriate use of water-circulating blankets is extremely important: these must be

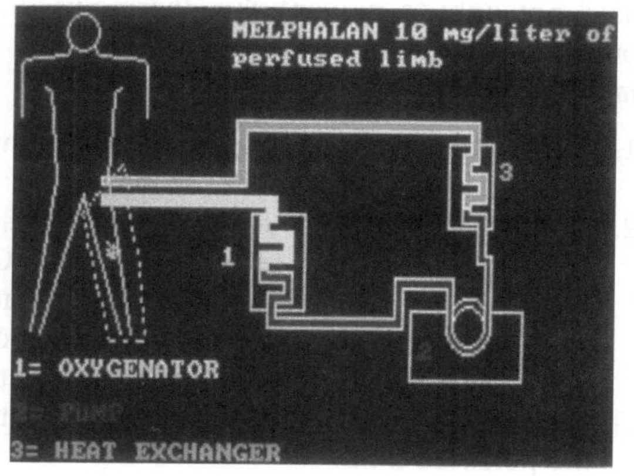

Fig. 19.2. Components of the extracorporeal circuit

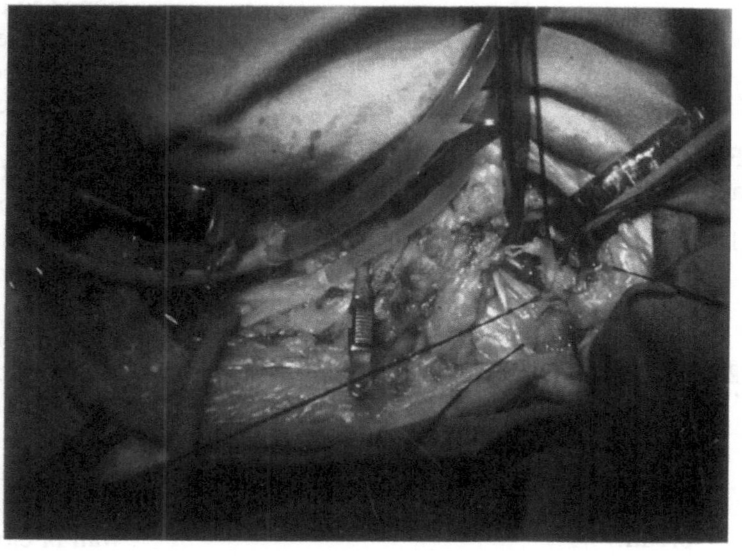

Fig. 19.1. Isolation and cannulation of the axillary vessels between the first and second portion

used not only to prevent skin thermodispersion but as an external source of heat, providing two important advantages:

1. Shorter times to reach the expected treatment tumor temperature (41.5°C or more)
2. During the treatment, the possibility of maintaining the perfusate temperature at 42°C or slightly lower, achieving a tumor temperature of more than 41.5°C within 20–30 min and, at the same time, maintaining the muscle temperature below 41.8°C, with minor toxicity in the perfused limb

Once the desired tumor temperature has been reached (40°C and 41.5°C, depending on preference of the different groups), the antineoplastic drug is introduced into the perfusional circuit. Sixty minutes after the introduction of the drug, the circuit is washed with saline solution and low molecular weight dextran to remove any residual drug and possible toxic products from the perfused limb. The washing is completed with the addition of 1 500 000 IU of aprotinine to the last liter that, in our experience, appears to reduce the post-treatment edema in the perfused limb.

After the washing, the arterial and venous catheters are removed and the vessel incisions are sutured with 4 and 5 zero prolene stitches for the artery and vein respectively. A drainage is positioned and the muscles, fascia, and skin are sutured without reconstructing the small pectoral muscle. The limb is wrapped with elastic bands to reduce postoperative edema. The patient is kept in forced diuresis for at least 48–72 h, while anticoagulants are administered up to the 8th–10th post-treatment day to avoid vascular morbidity.

19.2.2 The Lower Limbs

For the lower limbs, the more proximal, iliac approach is preferred for two principal reasons:

1. During the preparation of the iliac vessels, a retrocrural iliac-obturator lymphadenectomy is always performed, which permits a more definite staging of the disease.
2. The positioning of the cannula in the external iliac or common femoral artery permits treatment of the entire lower limb and the femoral lymph nodes, allowing potential "sterilization" of the entire area of possible neoplastic cell spread.

Obviously, these considerations are valid for patient with tumors localized in the thigh. For localizations below the knee, a more distal approach may be used in the case of soft tissue sarcomas. However, the femoral or popliteal vessels may be employed for a second or third perfusion in the event of disease relapse.

A groin dissection is made only when the nodes are clinically positive or if node involvement is revealed at frozen section examination. However, when necessary, a node dissection is performed at the end of the perfusional treatment, assuming the neoadjuvant role of perfusion.

The patient is placed in a supine position and the entire limb, including the buttock, hip and abdominal wall, is sterilized.

The iliac vessels are exposed by means of a transverse suprapubic skin incision, made from the pubis towards the anterosuperior iliac spine and deepened to reach the peritoneal sac. This is detached from the retroperitoneal structures and moved medially.

The common, external, and internal iliac vessels are now completely exposed. The collateral vessels of the artery and external iliac vein (the superficial and deep circumflex iliac and lower epigastric vessels) are ligated and sectioned.

The internal and external iliac vessels are isolated and surrounded by umbilical tape. Before clamping of these two vessels, the patient receives systemic heparin at the same dose employed for the upper limbs. A transverse arteriotomy and venotomy are carried out on the external iliac vessels, usually at 5–6 cm from the inguinal ligament and the arterial (16–18 French) and venous (18–20 French) cannulae are positioned so that the tip of the two catheters is in the common femoral vessels. (Fig. 19.3). The cannulae are secured with umbilical tape and connected to the extracorporeal circuit. Once the extracorporeal circulation has begun, a tourniquet is placed at the root of the limb, anchored to one or two Steinmann pins, inserted into the anterior superior iliac spine.

The procedures for the extracorporeal circulation are the same as those previously described for the upper limbs. Thermocouples are also inserted into the femoral nodes.

At the end of the perfusion, the circuit is washed, the internal iliac vessels are reopened, the external iliac vessel incisions are sutured, two drainage tubes are positioned, and the abdominal wall in closed in layers.

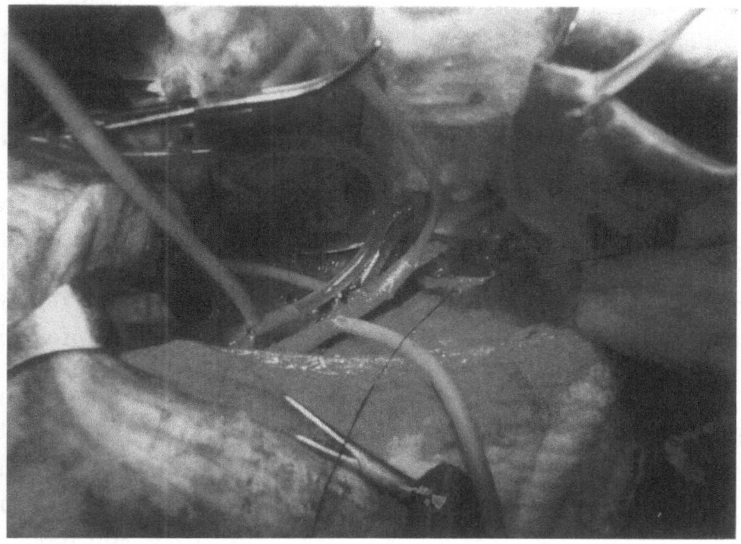

Fig. 19.3. Isolation and cannulation of the external iliac vessels

19.2.3 Parameters of the Perfusional Treatment

The parameters that most influence the safety and efficacy of HAP will be described in detail (Table 19.1).

19.2.3.1 Perfusate Composition and Volume Priming

The composition of the perfusate varies somewhat in the different centers that employ HAP. Most use a mixture of blood and saline solution with a hematocrit value of 25% for priming the extracorporeal circuit.

In experimental and clinical studies, GHUSSEN et al. (1984) demonstrated that the use of *whole blood* for priming provides a very low complication rate. The use of whole blood might also enhance the effectiveness of alkylating drugs by increasing the pO_2, because of increased oxygen transport. Moreover, the use of whole blood could provide a higher perfusate protein concentration, increasing the half-life of L-phenylalanine mustard (L-PAM) and its availability for tumor uptake (KREMENTZ et al. 1961; BRIELE et al. 1987). However, the risk of utilizing whole blood at high temperatures is directly related to red blood cell disruption and hemoglobinuria production. Further investigations are therefore warranted before employing whole blood in priming the extracorporeal circuit.

The volume used in priming must be not less than 1200–1500 ml as the injection of the cytotoxic drug into a lower volume might cause too high a peak concentration, enhancing limb toxicity (KLAASE et al. 1993).

Table 19.1. Therapeutic parameters

Perfusate composition and volume priming
Blood gas value
Flow rate and in flow pressure
Drug doses
Scheduling
Temperature levels

19.2.3.2 Blood Gas Value

It has been demonstrated that *high pO_2 values* potentiate the activity of alkylating agents and also produce a direct tumoricidal effect (DE COSSE 1966). During regional perfusion, a mixture of O_2 and CO_2 (95% and 5%) or pure O_2 is normally delivered to the perfusate by means of the oxygenator. The pH and the pO_2 values are usually maintained in a normal range (pH range: 7.35–7.50; pO_2 range: 100–200 mmHg).

A profound alkalosis in the limb must be avoided because the increased pH can reduce the cytotoxic effect of L-PAM, as demonstrated in vitro experiments (SCOTT et al. 1989).

19.2.3.3 Flow Rates and In-flow Pressure

A flow rate of 30 and 40 ml/min per liter (for the upper and lower limbs, respectively) provides a physiological blood gas value. However, FONTIJNE et al. (1985) demonstrated that pre-perfusion tissue oxygenation levels (measured by a transcutaneous pO_2 electrode) could only be obtained with flow rates at more than twice those mentioned above in animal experiments as well as in a clinical setting. Therefore, the flow rate during the perfusion must range between 60 and 80 ml/min per liter of limb volume and the perfusion pressure should be no more than 15 mmHg below the mean systemic pressure (FONTIJNE et al. 1985). This level guarantees a homogeneous drug distribution and avoids venous congestion; the latter could increase leakage, which mainly depends on the transfer by the venous system.

19.2.3.4 Drug Dose

To date, *L-PAM* is the most widely employed antineoplastic drug for treating limb melanoma. Different authors have employed dosages varying from 0.5 to 1.0 mg/kg of body weight for the upper limbs and from 1.0 to 2.0 mg/kg of body weight for the lower limbs (KREMENTZ et al. 1986; SCHRAFFORDT KOOPS et al. 1983; DI FILIPPO et al. 1989). At present, 10 and 13 mg/l of limb volume appears to be the maximum tolerable dose for the upper and lower limbs, respectively (WIEBERDINK 1982).

A dosimetric method has been described, based on the exchangeable blood volume determination of the perfused limb (LEJEUNE et al. 1987). This volume is calculated with the hematocrit measurement of the priming, the peripheral blood before cannulation and the mixed perfusate following cannulation. The results of this study seem to confirm the possibility of increasing the drug dosages (at least for the upper limbs) without severe toxicity. However, few dose-escalating studies have been conducted thus far (Table 19.2).

At a temperature below 40°C, it seems possible to increase the dose up to 14 mg/l. At higher tissue temperatures (41.5°C or more) 12 mg/l of limb volume should not be exceeded as unacceptable limb toxicity may occur (DI FILIPPO et al. 1993).

Other antineoplastic drugs have been utilized for regional perfusion in either mono- or polychemotherapy regimens. The different drugs employed and their maximum tolerable doses for the upper and lower limbs are reported in Table 19.3. Other drugs such as vindesine, mitoxantrone, and ifosfamide have also been employed but the number of patients treated with these drugs is too small to allow evaluation of their efficacy.

The most common drug combination has been L-PAM plus actinomycin D, although this association has been mostly used for treatment of soft tissue limb sarcomas.

19.2.3.5 Treatment Scheduling

The most effective administration modality for L-PAM during isolating perfusion is still to be established. The pharmacokinetics of L-PAM are complex. However, all of the studies conducted on the half-life curve of L-PAM in the perfusate have revealed that the distribution is biphasic. Mean half-lives of approximately 5 min for the first phase and of up to 50 min for the second phase were observed by BRIELE et al. (1987).

On the basis of these results and the claim that bolus injection causes greater toxicity, some authors prefer to deliver the drug by fractionated doses (STOTTER et al. 1987; HAFSTROM et al. 1984; MINOR et al. 1985). Regardless of the administration modality, it is important to inject the drug into the perfusional circuit when the tumor temperature reaches the preestablished level: a preclinical study demonstrated that only the simultaneous association of heat and drugs can lead to an additive or synergistic effect (NATALI et al. 1983).

Table 19.2. Hyperthermic perfusion with L-PAM: phase I studies

Authors	Evaluable patients	Temperature (°C)	Drug dose	MTD
WIEBERDINK et al. (1982)	90	37–38	<7–13 mg/l	10 mg/l
BODDIE et al. (1992)	23	>39.4	10–16 mg/l	14 mg/l
SCOTT et al. (1992)	26	37–39	1.5–1.75 mg/kg	1.75 mg/l
DI FILIPPO et al. (1993)	23	41.5–41.8	10–14 mg/l	12 mg/l

MTD, maximum tolerable dose

Table 19.3. Reported dosages for hyperthermic (40°C) perfusion for limb tumors

Authors	Drug	Limb. dosage
AIGNER (1988)	L-PAM	Arm, 10 mg
	CDDP	Leg, 15 mg/l
DI FILIPPO et al. (1991a,b)	CDDP	Leg, 3.2 mg/kg
	Dx	Arm, 0.7 mg/kg
		Leg, 1.4 mg/kg
Fletcher (1989)	CDDP	Arm, 6 mg/kg
		Leg, 6.3 mg/kg
Ghussen et al. (1989)	L-PAM	Arm, 1 mg/kg (80 mg limit)
		Leg, 1.5 mg/kg (100 mg limit)
International Cooperative Group	L-PAM	Arm, 13 mg
		Leg, 10 mg
LEJEUNE et al. (1987)	Stages I and II	
	L-PAM	Arm, 20 μg/ml
	L-PAM	Leg, 40 μg/ml
	Stage III	
	L-PAM	Arm, 30 μg/ml
	L-PAM	Leg, 60 μg/ml
PFEFFERKORN and DILDOCHER (1982)	DTIC	Arm, 1 g/m^2
		Leg, 2 g/m^2
WIEBERDINK et al. (1982)	L-PAM	10 mg

CDDP, cisplatin; DTIC, deticene; L-PAM, L-phenylalanine mustard; Dx, doxorubicin

Interestingly, some pharmacokinetic studies have shown a greater drug uptake in the tumor and skin than in the subcutaneous fat. This could account for the high therapeutic index obtained by regional perfusion, the greater drug uptake being achieved in the tumor and in the area of potential melanoma spread, i.e., in the skin.

19.2.3.6 Temperature Levels

Experimental studies have shown that hyperthermia enhances the cytotoxic effect of L-PAM (NATALI et al. 1983). In clinical practice, some authors have reported higher survival rates with higher temperature levels (CAVALIERE et al. 1980; GHUSSEN et al. 1989). We demonstrated that a minimum tumor temperature of 41.5°C must be reached and maintained during regional perfusion to obtain a higher complete response rate which directly influences locoregional control and survival (DI FILIPPO et al. 1989).

Despite the satisfactory results obtained by "true" hyperthermia (i.e., tissue temperature greater than 41.5°C), some authors claim that such high temperatures can cause unacceptable toxicity (SCHRAFFORDT KOOPS et al. 1983; KROON 1988). However, recent studies confirm that high response rates are directly related to a 41°–42°C temperature level, which results in no major complications (DI FILIPPO et al. 1989; GHUSSEN et al. 1989).

19.3 Treatment Toxicity

Standardization of the perfusion technique and technological improvements have lowered the rate of serious complications. Slight or moderate edema, skin erythema, and pain in the perfused limb are the most common symptoms, and resolve within approximately 15 days. Vascular complications occur more rarely and, in most cases, can be treated and cured with standard therapies.

Table 19.4 reports only the *most serious complications* of HAP, such as operative mortality, the number of required amputations and limb functionality impairment. The incidence of each of these has been calculated in a total of 2996 patients. The overall rates of operative mortality, amputation, and limb functionality impairment were 0.7%, 1%, and 4.2%, respectively. These figures can be considered quite satisfactory and emphasize the safety of HAP.

Table 19.4. Toxicity in limb melanoma patients treated with HAP

Authors	Patients	Operative mortality	Amputation required	Limb functionality impairment
CAVALIERE et al. (1993)	290	–	4	4
DIDOLKAR et al. (1986)	25	–	–	–
GHUSSEN et al. (1989)	53	–	–	–
JANOFF et al. (1982)	122	–	1	1
JONSON et al. (1983)	68	–	–	1
KREMENTZ (1986)	870	9	8	38
LEJEUNE et al. (1983)	23	–	–	–
MARTIN et al. (1982)	158	2	2	5
MIKHAIL et al. (1984)	165	–	3	13
REGE et al. (1983)	39	1	1	1
SKENE et al. (1990)	91	1	1	–
STEHLIN et al. (1984)	392	3	4	2
STORM et al. (1985)	26	–	–	–
SUGARBAKER and MCBRIDE (1976)	213	1	–	8
TONAK et al. (1984)	154	3	1	13
VAGLINI et al. (1983)	32	–	2	7
WAGNER (1976)	245	–	2	30
Total	2966	0.7%	1%	4.2%

19.4 Results in Specific Diseases

19.4.1 Melanoma

The M.D. Anderson Hospital classification has been adopted by all the investigators who employ the technique of perfusion.

19.4.1.1 Stage I Melanoma

The role of HAP in the treatment of stage I limb melanoma has still not been defined. As Table 19.5 demonstrates, contrasting results have been reported in retrospective studies that have compared surgery and HAP.

STEHLIN et al. (1984) and REGE et al. (1983) reported higher survival rates in patients treated with perfusion. By contrast, FRANKLIN et al. (1988), comparing two groups of 238 and 227 patients, observed no differences in terms of 5-year survival between those treated with surgery and those submitted to HAP (82% and 83%, respectively). The only randomized study, conducted by GHUSSEN et al. (1989), showed a statistically significant advantage of perfusion in terms of 5-year survival ($P = 0.02$) but the number of patients compared (18 vs 19) does not permit a definite conclusion.

A multicenter prospective randomized study on melanoma with a thickness greater than 1.5 mm is currently being conducted (WHO/EORTC). Seven hundred and seventy-four paitents were included, of whom 724 are evaluable. Three hundred and sixty-six were treated with HAP and 358 with surgery (wide excision) (LEJEUNE et al. 1993). Node dissection was considered optional in the participating centers but once the choice was made, the individual center was required always to use the same treatment.

The median follow-up of the patients is 39 months. The disease-free interval is longer in the hyperthermia-treated group ($P = 0.007$). In terms of overall survival, however, no significant difference has been found. Different rates of locoregional relapse have been observed in patients not treated with elective lymph node dissection. The lymph node metastasis, in-transit metastasis, and local recurrence rates were 13.5%, 1.5%, and

Table 19.5. Five-year survival in stage I melanoma: surgery vs HAP

Authors	Surgery % (no. of pts.)	HAP % (no. of pts.)	P
Nonrandomized studies:			
FRANKLIN et al. (1988)	82 (238)	83 (227)	0.9
REGE et al. (1983)	63 (72)	91 (39)	NS
STEHLIN et al. (1984)	71 (67)	85 (70)	
Randomized studies:			
GHUSSEN et al. (1989)	– (18)	– (19)	0.02

2%, respectively, in the HAP group versus 21.9%, 6%, and 3.3% in the control arm.

The results of this trial will serve to define the treatment of choice for primary limb melanoma.

19.4.1.2 Stage II–III Melanoma

The results obtained with HAP are reported in terms of tumor response, locoregional control, and survival.

19.4.1.2.1 Tumor Response. Table 19.6 reports the objective tumor response rates obtained in 424 patients treated with HAP. These results have been stratified in relation to the tissue temperature utilized during the perfusional treatment.

The highest objective response rates were always obtained at 41°C or more. In fact, the objective response rates ranged from 48% to 83% for temperatures between 37°C and 40°C and from 81% to 91% at temperatures between 41°C and 42°C. A similar observation applies with regard to the complete responses obtained with HAP, as Table 19.7 illustrates. In this case as well, higher complete response rates were observed in patients treated at temperatures greater than 41°C: 26%–38% versus 50%–80%.

Aside from the relationship between tissue temperature during perfusion and the objective or complete response rate, the results obtained are certainly better than those achieved with chemotherapy, however this is administered (systemically, intra-arterially, or by normothermic perfusion) (Figs. 19.4–19.7).

19.4.1.2.2 Locoregional Control. Unfortunately, the data regarding locoregional control are not always reported in the literature and, from the few data available, the disease stage is undoubtedly the factor which most influences locoregional disease recurrence. In fact, there is a constant decrease in locoregional control rates from stage II to stage IIIAB (Table 19.8).

Table 19.6. Stage II–III limb melanoma treated with HAP: importance of temperature for objective response

Authors		No. of pts.	OR (%)	Tissue temperature (°C)
Bulman et al.	(1980)	29	48	Normothermia
Di Filippo et al.	(1989)	117	83	41–42
Jonson et al.	(1983)	15	73	38
Kroon	(1988)	18	83	37–38
Lejeune et al.	(1983)	23	91	39–41
Rochlin et al.	(1965)	17	65	37–39
Rosin et al.	(1980)	80	62	39–40
Skene et al.	(1990)	67	78	39–40
Storm et al.	(1985)	26	81	41–42
Vaglini et al.	(1983)	32	81	41
Total		424		

OR, overall response

Table 19.7. Stage II–III limb melanoma treated with HAP: importance of temperature for complete response

Authors		No. of pts.	CR (%)	Tissue temperature (°C)
Di Filippo et al.	(1989)	117	50	41–42
Kroon et al.	(1988)	18	38.8	37–38
Lejeune et al.	(1983)	23	65	39–41
Rosin et al.	(1980)	80	26.2	39–40
Storm et al.	(1985)	26	80.7	41–42
Vaglini et al.	(1983)	32	56	41
Total		296		

CR, complete response

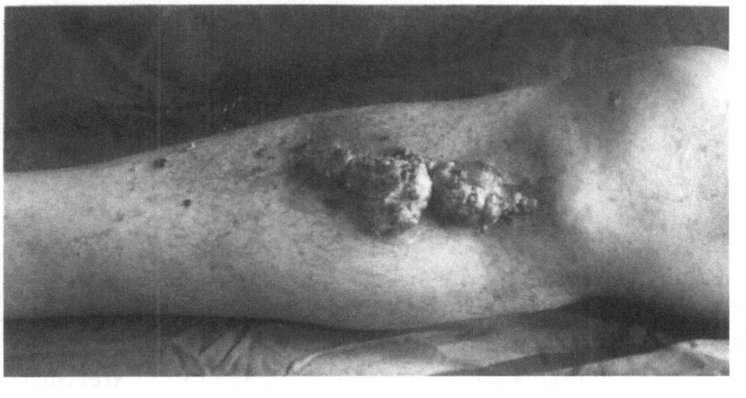

Fig. 19.4. Stage IIIA melanoma of the right leg before hyperthermic antiblastic perfusion

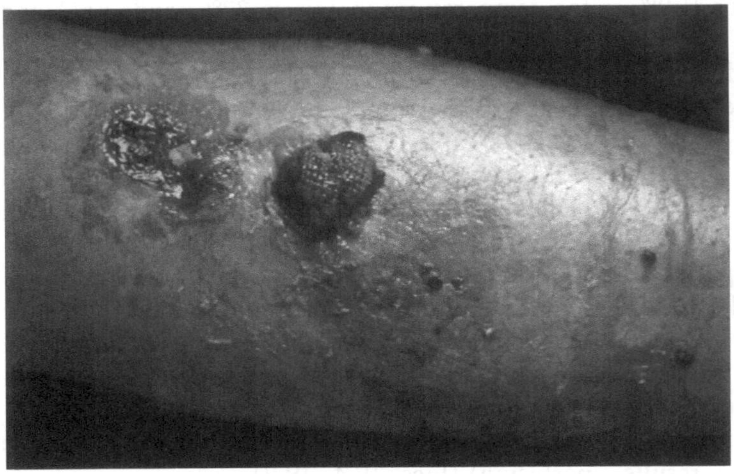

Fig. 19.5. Stage IIIA melanoma of the right leg, twelve days after the perfusion. Edema and erythema of the limb are present with disappearance of one of the large nodules

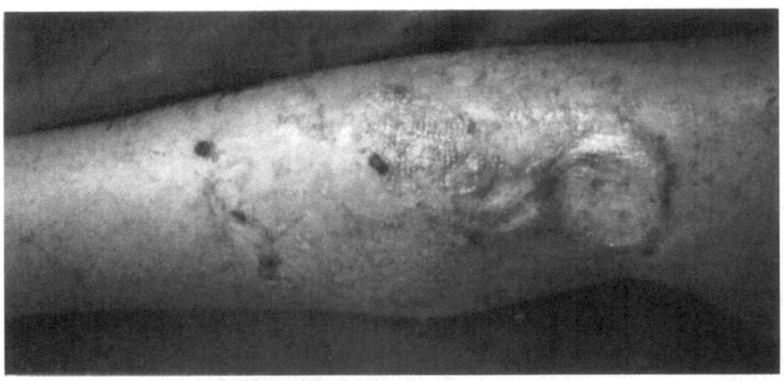

Fig. 19.6. Stage IIIA melanoma, six months after the hyperthermic antiblastic perfusion. Edema and erythema have disappeared as well as most of the metastatic nodules

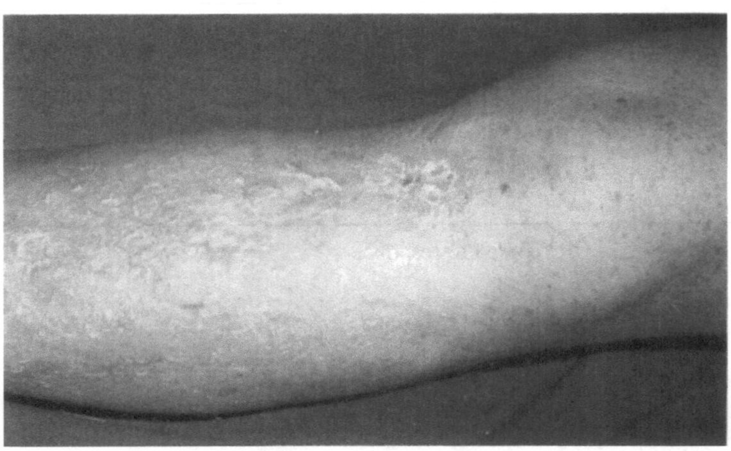

Fig. 19.7. Stage IIIA melanoma of the leg, one year after the hyperthermic antiblastic perfusion. All of the metastatic nodules have completely disappeared

19.4.1.2.3 Survival. Table 19.9 presents the 5-and 10-year survival rates of 553 patients, stratified according to the disease stage. Five-year survival rates range from 68% to 87.5% in the 146 stage II patients, from 45% to 81% in the 243 stage IIIA patients and from 31% to 45% in the 199 stage IIIAB patients. The average 5-year survival, calculated at each stage, may be considered satisfactory: 74.9% at stage II, 62.3% at stage IIIA, and 37.8% at stage IIIAB.

At the current state of the art, HAP is the treatment of choice for limb melanoma with loco-

Table 19.8. Five-year locoregional control rates in limb melanoma patients treated with HAP

Authors		Stage			Follow-up (yrs)
		II (%)	IIIA (%)	IIIAB (%)	
BAAS et al.	(1988)	76	52	57	5
DI FILIPPO et al.	(1989)	100	64.5	38.2	5
LEJEUNE et al.	(1983)	–	65	–	–
SKENE et al.	(1990)	77	70	–	5

regional spread. This is confirmed by the results of two randomized studies that compared HAP and surgery.

GHUSSEN et al. (1989) observed a statistically significant difference in terms of 5-year overall survival in favor of patients treated with HAP at both stage II and stage III (95% vs 63% at stage II, $P = 0.02$; 75% vs 30% at stage III, $P = 0.01$).

HAFSTROM et al. (1984) observed higher rates of local recurrence and of in-transit and/or lymph node metastases in the group of patients treated with surgery alone. Disease-free survival, expressed in months, was higher in those treated with perfusion than in those treated only with surgery (17 vs 10 months, $P = 0.044$). No differences were found in terms of overall survival.

19.4.2 Soft Tissue Sarcoma

In patients with soft tissue sarcomas, HAP has generally been used as neoadjuvant therapy in an attempt to reduce the neoplastic mass in order to permit the performance of conservative rather than destructive surgery.

This survey of patients treated with HAP is undoubtedly very heterogeneous in nature, because very often the perfusional treatment protocol (temperature and type of antineoplastic drug employed) varies from one center to another. Furthermore, postsurgical radiotherapy has been used in only some of the studies.

The review of the literature on HAP for the treatment of soft tissue limb sarcomas has been carried out in terms of the therapeutic scheme adopted by each individual author, the complications observed, and the results obtained.

19.4.2.1 Therapeutic Scheme

Table 19.10 presents data on the disease stage, the temperature, the type of antineoplastic drug employed, and possible combinations with radiotherapy. In this collected series of 385 patients, HAP was used only for high-grade, recurrent or locally advanced sarcomas. The temperatures generally achieved may be considered mild (39°–40°C) and the commonly employed drugs were L-

Table 19.9. Survival rates of limb melanoma patients treated with HAP

Authors	Stage	No. of patients	Survival (%) 5-year	10-year
BAAS et al. (1988)	II	36	74	63
	IIIA	47	67	45
	IIIAB	27	40	34
DAVIS et al. (1975)	II–IIIA	9	67[a]	–
DI FILIPPO et al. (1989)	II	13	87.5	87.5
	IIIA	65	56.2	56.2
	IIIAB	47	35.4	35.4
KREMENTZ et al. (1986)	II	39	68	59
	IIIA	74	45	41
	IIIAB	87	31	28
STEHLIN et al. (1984)	II	17	77	77
	IIIA	57	81	49
	IIIAB	38	45	35
WAGNER (1976)	II	41	68[a]	–

[a] Follow-up of 2–10 years

Table 19.10. Soft tissue limb sarcoma treated with HAP: clinical data and treatment protocols

Authors	Stage	No. of pts.	Protocol		
			T (°C)	Drug	XRT
HOEKSTRA et al. (1987)	I–II III	8 6	38–40	L-PAM+DACT	–
KREMENTZ et al. (1986)	–	56	40	NH_2	–
KRUGE et al. (1989)	I–II III–IV	16	?	?	+
LEBREDO et al. (1988)	I–II III–IV	25 21	40	CDDP	+ (27)
LEJEUNE et al. (1988)	T1–T3	14	39–40	L-PAM+DACT	–
LETHI et al. (1986)	I–II III–IV	32 32	>40	L-PAM+DACT	+ (29)
MCBRIDE et al. (1978)	T < 5 cm T < 5 cm	110	39	L-PAM+DACT	–
STEHLIN et al. (1984)	–	65	38–40	L-PAM+DACT	+ (65)

L-PAM, L-phenylalanine mustard; DACT, actinomycin D; CDDP, cisplatin; XRT, radiotherapy

Table 19.11. Soft tissue limb sarcoma treated with HAP: local and systemic complications

Authors	Local (%)			Systemic (%)		Mortality (%)
	Vascular	Amputation	Other	Pulmonary	Cardiac	
HOEKSTRA et al. (1987)	0	0	7.1	0	0	0
KREMENTZ et al. (1986)	9	2.4	5.7	0.8	0.8	1.6
KRUGE et al. (1989)	–	–	–	–	–	0
LEBREDO et al. (1989)	2.1	0	10.8	4	0	2
LEJEUNE et al. (1988)	0	0	35	14	7	7
LETHI et al. (1986)	1.5	1.5	4.6	1.5	0	0
MCBRIDE et al. (1978)	2.7	2.7	6.3	0.9	0	0.9
STEHLIN et al. (1984)	–	–	–	–	–	0

The overall amputation and mortality rates are 1.8% and 1.1%, respectively

PAM and actinomycin D. Only Stehlin, Lethi, Lebredo, and our own group have employed radiotherapy (STEHLIN et al. 1984; LETHI et al. 1986; LEBREDO et al. 1988; DI FILIPPO et al. 1991a).

19.4.2.2 Toxicity

Table 19.11 shows the toxicity observed in terms of rates of local and systemic complications and mortality.

The reported vascular complication rates ranged from 0% to 2.7%. The rates of other minor complications, such as erythema, edema, and pain, varied from 1.4% to 35%. The overall amputation rate was 1.8%, while the rate of systemic complications (pulmonary and cardiac) ranged from 0% to 15%. The mortality was 1.1%.

These data are very similar to those reported for the 2996 patients with melanoma and again confirm the safety of HAP.

19.4.2.3 Results

Table 19.12 reports the results obtained with HAP with and without radiotherapy, in terms of conservative surgery, local recurrence, and 5-year survival rates. The average conservative surgery rate of 93.5% should be considered satisfactory. The average local recurrence and 5-year survival rates were 14% and 69.8%, respectively. It should also be taken into account that most of the patients treated with this technique have previously relapsed and received other combined treatments (i.e., surgery and/or radiochemotherapy).

Table 19.12. Soft tissue limb sarcoma treated with HAP ± radiotherapy (XRT): clinical results

Authors	Pts.	XRT	Conservative surgery	Local relapse (%)	5-year survival (%)	Median follow-up (mos.)
Hoekstra et al. (1987)	14	–	94	7	69	>156
Krementz et al. (1986)	56	–	100	21	65	>60
Kruge et al. (1989)	16	–	–	11	64	–
Lebredo et al. (1988)	46	+	90	2	–	–
Lejeune et al. (1988)	14	–	77	31	71 (3 yr)	–
Lethi et al. (1986)	64	+	100	11	67	>60
McBride et al. (1978)	110	–	100	15	80	>60
Stehlin et al. (1984)	65	+	94	–	72.7	–

Table 19.13. Regina elena national cancer institute experience with regard to soft tissue sarcoma: distribution of patients treated with HAP according to stage and treatment protocol

Treatment	II	III	IVA	Total
Surgery	7	10	16	33
Doxorubicin i.a. infusion + excision	5	7	5	17
Radiotherapy + excision	10	5	5	20

48/70 (68.5%) at stages III–IVA; 38/70 (54.2%) recurrent cases

19.4.2.4 Clinical Experience at the Regina Elena National Cancer Institute

Eighty soft tissue sarcoma patients were treated with HAP. Eight had visceral metastases as well as local relapses and were therefore not included in any of the treatment protocols. Two treatment-related deaths occurred: one caused by a massive hemorrhage after iliac artery rupture and the other by a myocardial infarction.

Table 19.13 presents the patient characteristics (disease stage) according to the treatment protocol adopted. At the time of referral, 48 of the 70 evaluable patients (68.5%) had stage III–IVA disease and 38 (54.2%) had recurrences of previously treated sarcomas. Some developed multiple recurrences (as many as five, in several cases) after either surgery alone or multimodality treatments.

All of the patients were treated with additional therapy according to different protocols, as follows: (a) HAP plus surgery; (b) HAP plus intra-arterial doxorubicin plus surgery; or (c) HAP plus radiotherapy plus surgery.

The drug is administered when the tumor reaches a temperature of 41.5°C. L-PAM (0.8 mg/kg body weight) and actinomycin D (0.015 mg/kg body weight) were the drugs employed in the first series of 50 patients. The other 20 patients were treated with cisplatin at a dose of 3.2 mg/kg body weight.

The intra-arterial doxorubicin infusion was generally initiated 10 days after the perfusion (three cycles, 10 mg/kg for 10 days each, administered at 10-day intervals, followed by surgery). Radiotherapy was given by an external beam source within 4 weeks after the perfusion. All the patients received dosages that varied between 45 and 65 Gy, depending on local tolerance. Delayed surgery was performed 3–4 weeks later.

Regarding morbidity, only two amputations were directly related to the perfusion. Four patients had venous thrombosis which promptly recovered after standard therapy.

The clinical results obtained with HAP in relation to the treatment protocol adopted are reported in Table 19.14. The results have been evaluated in terms of conservative surgery, locoregional control, 5-year disease-free, distant disease-free, and overall survival rates.

Since the three groups of patients are well balanced in terms of disease stage, the clinical results should reflect the real effectiveness of each treatment protocol. It is readily apparent that the protocol including radiotherapy provides better results than the other two, considering each of the endpoints. In addition, limb functionality was

Table 19.14. Clinical results obtained with HAP for the treatment of soft tissue limb sarcoma

Treatment protocol	Conservative surgery (%)	Locoregional control (%)	5-yr DFS	5-yr DDFS	5-yr OS
HAP plus surgery	57.6	63.1	35.6	44.3	48
HAP plus i.a. Dx infusion plus surgery	93.7	65.7	46.7	66.7	73.3
HAP plus XRT plus surgery	100	93.3	68.1	75.4	70

Dx, doxorubicin; XRT, radiotherapy; DFS, disease-free survival; DDFS, distant disease-free survival; OS, overall survival

not impaired by these multistep protocols (Figs. 19.8–19.12).

19.4.3 Osteogenic Sarcoma

Sixty patients with osteogenic limb sarcomas have been treated with HAP at the Regina Elena National Cancer Institute. The patients may be stratified into three groups according to the treatment protocol adopted, and the effectiveness of each protocol has been evaluated in terms of tumor necrosis, locoregional control, and survival.

All the patients in the first group were submitted to HAP, routinely followed by amputation 4 weeks later. In this historical group, the treatment strategy was justified because amputation was considered mandatory at that time. Histopathological examinations revealed a high-grade of tumor necrosis (80%–100%) in all of the patients. No loco-regional relapses were observed and the 5-year disease-free (59.6%) and overall

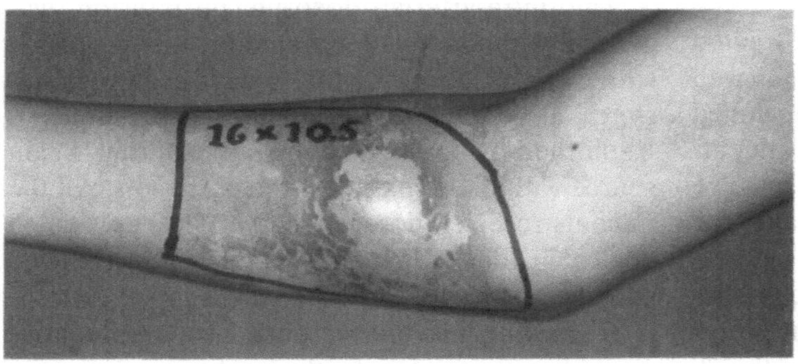

Fig. 19.8. Recurrent leiomyosarcoma of the right forearm, previously treated with surgery and radiotherapy

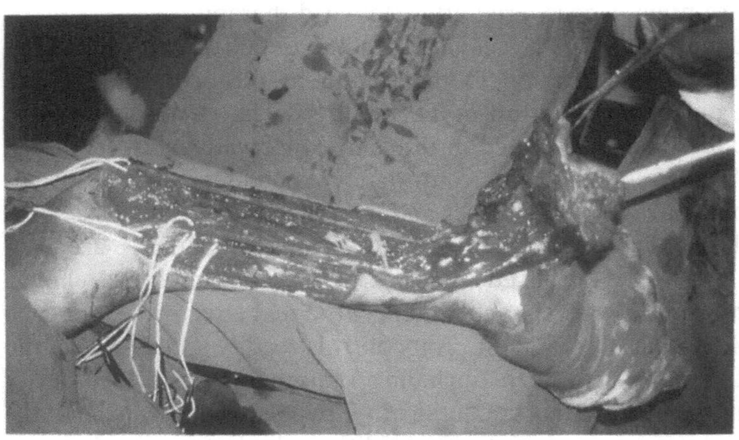

Fig. 19.9. After hyperthermic antiblastic perfusion, the tumor shrinkage permitted making a wide excision of the tumor, sparing all the major vessels and nerves of the forearm

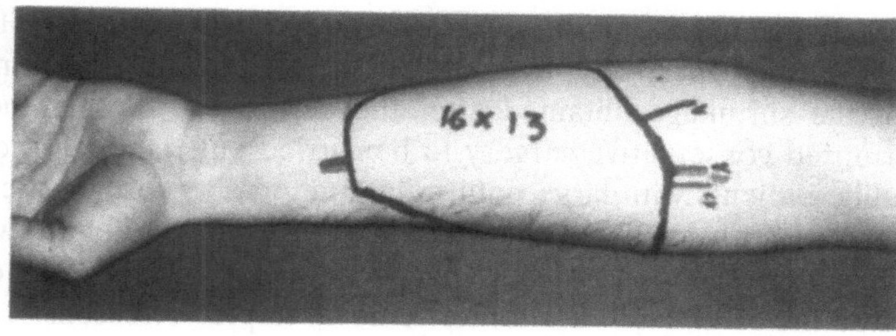

Fig. 19.10. A myocutaneous flap together with radial vessels were taken from the left forearm to cover the surgical field of the right forearm

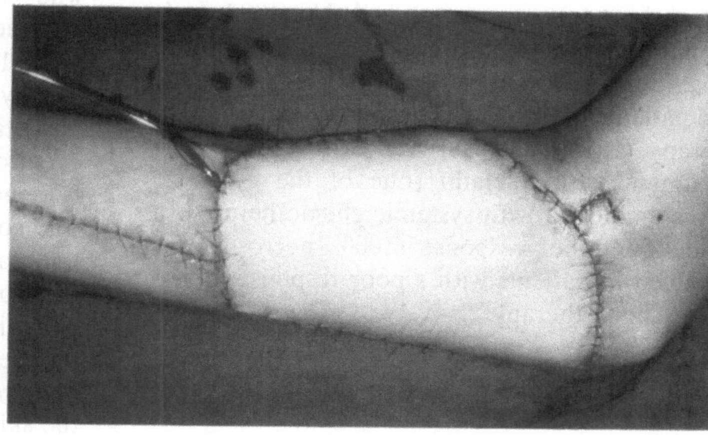

Fig. 19.11. The myocutaneous flap was implanted onto the right forearm by means of a microvascular anastomosis

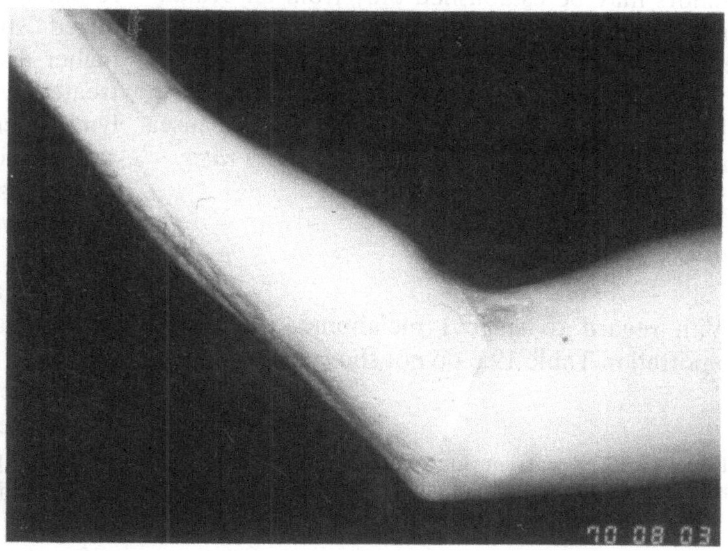

Fig. 19.12. This figure shows the right forearm, twelve months after the operation, showing a fairly good esthetic and functional result

survival (63.3%) rates should be considered satisfactory.

The results achieved in the first series of patients prompted us to modify the treatment protocol, performing conservative surgery whenever possible. In the second group, all of the patients underwent an "en bloc" resection followed by reconstruction with autoplastic bone grafts or metallic endoprostheses in collaboration with the Orthopedic Clinic of the University of Rome "La Sapienza."

The pathologically evaluated tumor necrosis was always high (80%–100%). The 5-year locoregional control rate was 96.7% (only 1 of 27 patients had a local recurrence due to the section margin being too close to the tumor). The 5-year disease-free and overall survival rates were 51.7% and 64.7%, respectively. It should be emphasized that the shrinkage obtained after the perfusion permitted conservative surgery to be carried out in nine patients with large, infiltrating tumors.

We recently modified this treatment protocol to include three cycles of systemic chemotherapy before the HAP and after tumor removal to prevent the onset of pulmonary metastases. Only five patients have entered this protocol and follow-up is too short to evaluate survival. Nonetheless, it should be stated that a grade II tumor response (according to Rosen) was achieved in three out of five patients after three cycles of systemic chemotherapy (ROSEN et al. 1982). After perfusional treatment with cisplatin (one of the cytotoxic drugs employed with systemic chemotherapy), a grade IV tumor response (100% necrosis) was obtained in patients with a poor response to systemic chemotherapy.

19.5 Discussion

The true role of HAP for the treatment of limb tumors may be established only from an evaluation of the therapeutic index: toxicity/therapeutic efficacy.

As previously stated, the toxicity reported in the various studies clearly shows that HAP causes *neither high morbidity nor high mortality rates.*

19.5.1 Melanoma

With regard to stage I melanoma, the results reported in Table 19.5 do not show a clear superiority of HAP over surgery. Neither the results of the nonrandomized retrospective studies nor those of the prospective randomized studies (even though the groups are well balanced in terms of prognostic factors) permit definitive conclusions to be drawn.

In our opinion, this is for two strictly related reasons:

1. The evaluation is not limited to those patients who can truly benefit from the perfusional treatment, i.e., those affected with melanoma of a 1.5–4 mm thickness, when the tumor usually presents a higher rate of locoregional metastases (skin and lymph nodes) than in the event of systemic spread.
2. It is not always clear whether the perfusion was conducted through the external iliac or femoral vessels. In the latter case, the area of the groin nodes is not included in the treatment and this undoubtedly limits the effectiveness of the perfusion. It is well known that lymph node relapses are more frequent than those in the skin.

It was not simply by chance that the preliminary results of the WHO/EORTC prospective randomized study showed statistically significantly higher disease-free survival rates in the patients treated with HAP who were not submitted to lymphadenectomy; in this group, a lower rate of recurrences and lymph node and/or skin metastases was observed.

However, a statistically significant difference in terms of overall survival has still not been observed and therefore only the conclusive results of this trial will be able to indicate the treatment of choice for primary limb melanomas.

As these results and randomized studies demonstrate, the possibility of improving results by optimizing the HAP treatment parameters should be considered. In fact, the results reported by different authors are diverse, there being significant variations in terms of 5-year survival in patients treated with the same technique and at the same disease stage.

19.5.2 Prognostic Factors

It has been hypothesized that factors related to both the biological aggressiveness of the tumor and the treatment are able to influence the efficacy of the perfusion and the prognosis. In order to

Table 19.15. Recurrent limb melanoma: complete response rates according to number of lesions and minimum tumor temperature

Minimum tumor temperature	% Complete tumor response
Single lesions	
≥41.5°C	100
<41.5°C	50
Multiple lesions	
≥41.5°C	28.6
<41.5°C	15

Independent prognostic parameters of tumor response in the multivariate analysis were the number of lesions ($P < 0.0001$) and the minimum tumor temperature ($P < 0.04$)

verify this hypothesis, we conducted a retrospective study on 188 patients, of whom 117 could be evaluated for tumor response. The importance of three treatment-related factors – *tumor temperature*, *drug dosage*, and *modality of administration* (bolus versus fractionated) – and of ten factors related to the characteristics of the patients and the tumor (age, sex, tumor site, number of relapses, disease stage, etc.) was evaluated in relation to the disease outcome (Di Filippo et al. 1989).

The endpoints evaluated were the rates of complete tumor response, locoregional control, and survival. With regard to complete tumor response, the multiparametric analysis, conducted with the logistic model, demonstrated that the minimum tumor temperature and the number of lesions are the prognostic factors able to influence the complete response rate to a statistically significant degree (Table 19.15). The minimum tumor temperature employed thus markedly influenced the complete tumor response in patients with the same number of lesions: 100% versus 50% in the case of single lesions and 26% versus 18% in the case of multiple lesions. This shows the need to reach and maintain a minimum tumor temperature of 41.5°C or more during the treatment.

The importance of the tumor temperature is not simply an occasional finding. In fact, from the review of the literature reported in Table 19.7, it may be observed that the complete tumor response rate is strictly correlated to the treatment temperature, the highest complete responses being observed at temperatures of 41°C or more. The modality of the drug administration does not appear to be important, while the drug dosage is only marginally important ($P = 0.08$).

To investigate further the influence of the antineoplastic drug, the proportion of complete responses was calculated within categories, defined by cross-tabulating the minimal tumor temperature and the L-PAM dose. The complete response rate after treatments performed at a minimum temperature of less than 41.5°C and at a less than standard dose was 15.4%, which rose to 20% (+4.6%) in patients treated with a higher than standard dose and to 35.3% (+19.9%) in those treated with a minimum temperature of 41.5°C or more.

The complete response rate was 59.4% (+44%) after treatments at a minimum temperature of 41.5°C or more and at a standard or greater than standard dose. The total improvement was significantly greater ($P = 0.02$) than that expected in the event of an additive relationship (+4.6% and +19.9%, i.e., 24.5%), suggesting the presence of a *synergistic effect* (Table 19.16).

19.5.3 Treatment Optimization

Thus far, L-PAM appears to be the most effective drug in the treatment of limb melanoma by HAP. Other antineoplastic drugs, either alone or in combination (thiotepa, cisplatin, deticene, vindesine, nitrogen mustard), have provided complete response rates that have never exceeded 19%. This value is certainly lower than that obtained with L-PAM, which, on average, has provided a complete response rate of 45%. Dose escalation studies at high temperatures (41°C or more) that can cause a real synergistic activity have still not been conducted in any significant number; the few that have been carried out are presented in Table 19.2.

With regard to dose escalation, Wieberdink's (1982) study established a maximum tolerable dose of 10 mg/l for temperatures between 37° and 38°C and this is the most commonly employed dosage. Boddie et al. (1992) and Scott et al. (1989) demonstrated that dosages between 14 and 15 mg/l may be employed at the same temperatures.

We conducted a dose-escalation study at higher temperatures (41.5°–41.8°C) and showed that the

Table 19.16. Recurrent limb melanoma: complete response rates according to minimum tumor temperature (I_{min}) and drug dose

I_{min}/drug dose	% Complete tumor response
I_{min} < 41.5°C Dose < SD	15.4
I_{min} < 41.5°C Dose ≥ SD	20.0 (+4.6)
I_{min} ≥ 41.5°C Dose < SD	35.3 (+19.9)
I_{min} ≥ 41.5°C Dose ≥ SD	59.4 (+44.4)

SD, standard dose

maximum tolerable dose for the lower limbs is 12 mg/l. The maximum tolerable dose was clearly lower than that employed by Boddie et al. and Scott et al. However, the use of high temperatures is more important in obtaining higher complete response rates, as is indicated by both experimental and clinical data.

In vitro experimental studies have shown that L-PAM, like other alkylating drugs, has a linear increase in efficacy in relation to the temperature level employed. Up to 40°C, the increase in efficacy is modest and the survival curve of the cells quickly reaches a plateau phase. The survival curve becomes steep only above 41°C, becoming exponential at 42°C, when a real synergistic effect is reached.

These experimental studies have been confirmed in clinical practice, both in our own experience (Tables 19.15, 19.16) and in studies reported in the literature (Table 19.7). Obviously, only with the appropriate use of these two therapeutic parameters (temperature level and drug dosage) can the highest complete response rate of 59.4% be achieved with a significant therapeutic gain, confirming truly synergistic activity.

There are basically two major arguments against the use of high temperatures: both limb toxicity and L-PAM thermoinactivation (caused by hydrolysis) are greater.

We have not observed higher local complication rates in patients treated at higher temperatures, and this experience is confirmed by other authors who employ high temperatures (LEJEUNE et al. 1983; STORM et al. 1985; VAGLINI et al. 1983). There are therefore other factors that have an important influence on toxicity, such as the peak concentration of L-PAM at the moment the drug is introduced and the blood gas analysis values (acidosis), and these should be well controlled.

With regard to the pharmacokinetics of the drug in relation to temperature. BRIELE et al.'s (1987) study clearly demonstrated that the hydrolysis of L-PAM does not present substantial modifications between 41° and 43°C.

Treatment optimization should therefore be pursued as the complete response is one of the factors with independent predictive value with respect to locoregional control, disease-free and overall survival rates, with statistically significant differences between complete and noncomplete responders (Table 19.17).

19.5.4 Soft Tissue Sarcoma

Hyperthermic antiblastic perfusion should be considered an appropriate treatment for soft tissue sarcomas, given their mode of spread. This technique, involving the entire tumor-bearing limb, should potentially treat all the tumor and possibly skip and regional metastases. The results obtained with HAP in association with surgery are quite satisfactory and are certainly better than those observed with surgery alone: with HAP the conservative surgery rates have always been high (77%–100%) and the recurrence rates relatively low (from 2%–31%), with an average 5-year survival rate of 70%.

The not completely satisfying locoregional control obtained in some studies may be due to the many patients with multiple recurrences, who are submitted to numerous surgical, radio-, and chemotherapeutic treatments. This evidently limits the potentiality of the perfusion.

High tumor temperatures and a homogeneous drug distribution cannot be attained in patients with post-surgical or radiotherapy-induced sclerosis. These two factors hamper the effectiveness of HAP because synergism is achieved only with a high tumor drug uptake in association with high temperature levels (more than 41°C).

It should also be emphasized that the drugs employed thus far during perfusion (L-PAM plus actinomycin D, CDDP, etc.) are not very active in the treatment of soft tissue sarcomas. More

Table 19.17. Recurrent limb melanoma: 5-year actuarial survival according to tumor response

Response	Locoregional control (%)	DFS (%)	OS (%)
Complete	75.2	52.2	62.6
	$P = 0.007$	$P = 0.0005$	$P = 0.0004$
Noncomplete	43.7	14.0	25.4

DFS, disease-free survival; OS, overall survival

specific drugs may increase the therapeutic efficacy of the treatment.

Radiotherapy has been included in some of the protocols and appears to demonstrate good efficacy and better results than those obtained in patients receiving other treatments (Table 19.14).

Radiotherapy may be useful in multidisciplinary protocols. Although it has a similar activity to hyperthermia and chemotherapy (alkylating drugs), it possesses some different action mechanisms that may complement the hyperthermia-chemotherapy activity by killing neoplastic cells.

19.5.5 Osteogenic Sarcoma

The role of HAP in the treatment of osteogenic sarcoma is difficult to define today for two reasons:

1. Osteogenic sarcoma, as defined by Triffeau and Mary, is a systemic, pulmonary disease that goes through a bone phase: the risk of the presence of sub-clinical pulmonary metastases is very high even at the initial stages of the disease and therefore locoregional treatment alone could be an under-treatment.
2. Systemic chemotherapy, especially with some very active drugs such as cisplatin and ifosfamide, has provided good tumor responses (necrosis rate of more than 90%) in a high number of patients, significantly improving survival.

However, there are patients with large tumors that invade the soft tissues who do not respond to systemic chemotherapy and who should therefore undergo amputation. These patients may benefit from HAP, as this technique has always provided a high necrosis rate, including in patients who do not respond to systemic chemotherapy. Moreover, a 25% limb salvage rate was obtained in patients who were candidates for amputation. This fact takes on particular importance considering that the highest incidence of osteogenic sarcoma is in the first and second decades of life and therefore the possibility of saving a limb in a young person is extremely important.

19.6 Perspectives

The possibility of improving the therapeutic efficacy of HAP is based on the optimization of the use of currently available agents and new drugs. The importance of utilizing to the utmost both hyperthermia (a minimum tumor temperature of more than 41.5°C) and L-PAM (maximum tolerable does: 14 mg/l or 1.75 mg/kg at about 39°C; 12 mg/l at a temperature of 41.5°C) has been previously stressed.

Although KROON et al. (1993) recognized the importance of a high minimum tumor temperature (41.5°C), excessive toxicity was reported at high temperatures. They therefore designed a treatment protocol foreseeing the sequential use of hyperthermia and L-PAM to utilize the two therapeutic agents at the maximum dosage. According to this protocol, hyperthermic perfusion is performed for 2 h at a tissue temperature of 42°–43°C, followed by a *normothermic* perfusion with L-PAM at a dosage of 10 mg/l, 7–10 days later. Of the 12 patients so treated thus far, 11 achieved a complete response and one patient presented a partial response. The average complete response duration was 10 months (4–24 months). Four patients later relapsed in the perfused limb (33%) at 4, 5, 5, and 18 months.

The results of this protocol appear promising in terms of complete response rates (91%). However, the short response durations and the number of locoregional recurrences indicate that the use of two separate, sequentially applied agents leads to the survival of some cell fractions that are resistant to the two agents separately. By contrast, these cells could be destroyed by the *simultaneous* use of hyperthermia and L-PAM because of the synergistic activity of this combination.

Of the new drugs that may be employed during perfusion, doxorubicin is one of the most active. This drug had never previously been utilized during perfusion because it was believed to precipitate in the presence of heparin. However, experimental data have demonstrated that this phenomenon occurs only marginally (MUCCI et al. 1991).

There are undoubtedly good reasons for employing doxorubicin during hyperthermic perfusional treatment of soft tissue limb sarcomas:

1. It is the most active cytotoxic agent against soft tissue limb sarcomas, with objective response rates ranging between 15% and 36% (complete response rate: 6%).
2. A dose-response relationship has been observed in nonrandomized studies.
3. In vivo studies have demonstrated that the simultaneous application of heat (at 41.5°C)

and doxorubicin increases the antitumor effect of the latter.
4. Its half-life during hyperthermic perfusion is 21 min versus 42 min during normothermic perfusion. The final doxorubicin tissue concentration is similar, so that the time of tumor exposure to the drug is increased with hyperthermia (DIDOLKAR et al. 1976; TATE et al. 1986).
5. Between 90% and 97% of the drug is bound to the tissue after the hyperthermic perfusion (DIDOLKAR et al. 1976).
6. Doxorubicin tissue concentrations obtained with hyperthermic perfusion are 5, 25, and 45 times greater than those obtained with normothermic perfusion, intra-arterial, and systemic infusion, respectively (DIDOLKAR et al. 1976).

On the basis of these experimental results, a phase I study of the National Registry of Implantable Systems was conducted on 23 patients (DI FILIPPO et al. 1991b). The results may be summarized as follows:

1. Hyperthermic perfusion with doxorubicin is a safe procedure.
2. The maximum tolerable dose is 0.7 mg/kg at a mean muscle temperatures of 41.4°C for the upper limbs and 1.4 mg/kg at a mean muscle temperature of 41.6°C for the lower limbs.
3. Doxorubicin has a high diffusibility rate in the perfusate (half-life of 10–20 min).
4. There is little leakage into the systemic circulation (less than 1 μg/ml) during HAP.

The results of this clinical study confirmed what had previously been demonstrated in experimental studies. Of the 23 patients treated, 16 could be evaluated for tumor response. Ten (62.5%) showed a good response (necrosis rate: 75% or more) and a minimum tumor temperature of 41°C was reached and maintained in all of these patients. Therefore, the minimum tumor temperature was also found to be important for soft tissue sarcomas treated with hyperthermic perfusion with doxorubicin.

As regards other new perspectives, the combined use of biological response modifiers and antineoplastic drugs by perfusion appears to be important.

A treatment protocol including the administration of interferon-γ (IFN-γ), tumor necrosis factor, and L-PAM has been investigated (LIENARD et al. 1993). IFN-γ stimulates neoplastic cell receptors for tumor necrosis factor, a drug with a marked antitumor activity but possessing high toxic effects when administered systemically at high doses. In addition, tumor necrosis factor has demonstrated synergistic activity if employed in combination with hyperthermia and some antineoplastic drugs, including L-PAM.

The therapeutic schedule foresees the administration of IFN-γ (1 500 000 IU/day) on the 2 days preceding the perfusion. During the perfusion, another IFN-γ dose (1 500 000 IU) is injected into the perfusional circuit and 3 or 4 mg of tumor necrosis factor for the upper and lower limbs, respectively (5–6 times the maximum tolerable systemic dose), is given. After 30 min L-PAM is administered, at a dosage of 10 mg/l of perfused limb volume.

The extremely exciting results obtained with this protocol are presented in Table 19.18. LIENARD et al.'s (1993) study is the most reliable because of the number and follow-up of the patients treated. The 90% complete response obtained in patients who often relapsed and had already been treated with perfusion is a remarkable result. If confirmed in a larger number of patients and with a longer response duration, this

Table 19.18. Limb melanoma patients treated with IFN-γ, tumor necrosis factor, and L-PAM: clinical results

Authors	No. of pts.	Response rate (%)		Median response duration (mos.)	Survival (%)
		CR	PR		
LIENARD et al. (1993)	52	90	10	12.5	74 (24 mos.)
THOMAS et al. (1993) (unpublished date)	9	100	–	11	100 (11 mos.)
VAGLINI et al. (1983)	12	68	32 (SD)	50% local relapse (2–6 mos.)	–

CR, complete response; PR, partial response

will represent a milestone for the treatment of limb melanoma.

19.7 Summary

At the current state of the art, the following conclusions may be drawn:

- HAP is the treatment of choice for locoregional spreading limb melanoma, while its role in high-risk primary melanoma has not yet been well defined.
- HAP represents an important step in the multidisciplinary treatment of soft tissue limb sarçomas.
- HAP may play a role in the treatment of osteogenic limb sarcoma when the neoplasm is at an advanced stage and a very effective neoadjuvant treatment is necessary to save the limb.

Acknowledgment. This work was partially supported by CNR grant no. 9401264PF39.

References

Aigner KR (1988) Drug filtration in high-dose regional chemotherapy. In: Aigner KR, Patt YZ (eds) Advances in regional cancer treatment: Contributions to Oncology. Karger, Basel, p 261

Baas PC, Schraffordt Koops H, Hoekstra HJ, Oosterhuis JW, Dan der Weele LT, Oldhoff J (1988) Isolated regional perfusion in the treatment of local recurrence, satellitosis and in transit metastases of melanoma of the extremities. Reg Cancer Treat 1: 33–36

Boddie AW, Briele H, Krementz E, et al. (1992) A phase I study of Melphalan in 40°C isolated limb perfusion using packed red blood cells and lactated ringer perfusate. Proceedings of the American Society of Clinical Oncology, 28th Annual Meeting, May 17–19, 1992, San Diego, CA

Briele HA, Djuric M, Sung DT, Martel T (1987) Pharmacokinetics of Melphalan in clinical isolation perfusion of the extremities. Cancer Res 45: 1885–1889

Bulman AS, Jamieson CW (1980) Isolated limb perfusion with Melphalan in the treatment of malignant melanoma. Br J Surg 67: 660–662

Cavaliere R, Giocatto EC, Giovanella BC, et al. (1967) Selective heat sensitivity of cancer cells: biochemical and clinical studies. Cancer 20: 1351–1381

Cavaliere R, Moricca, G, Di Filippo F, et al. (1980) Heat transfer problems during local perfusion in cancer treatment. Ann NY Acad Sci 335: 311–325

Cavaliere R, Di Filippo F, Giannarelli D, et al. (1993) Hyperthermic antiblastic perfusion in the treatment of local recurrence or "in transit" metastasis of limb melanoma. Seminars in Surgical Oncology 8: 372–380

Creech O Jr, Krementz ET, Ryan RF, Winblad JN (1958) Chemotherapy for cancer; regional perfusion utilizing extracorporeal circuit. Ann Surg 148: 612–632

Davis CD, Ivins JC, Soule WG (1975) Mayo Clinic experience with isolated perfusion for invasive malignant melanoma of the extremities. In: Karger S (ed) Basic properties and clinical behaviour, vol. II. Proceedings Ninth International Pigmented Cell Conference, Houston, Texas, p 379

De Cosse JJ, et al. (1966) Influence of high-pressure oxygen and chemotherapy on the AMEL hamster melanoma. Melanoma Research 3: 95

Didolkar MS, Kanter PH, Baffi RR, Schwartz HS, Lopez R, Baez N (1978) Comparison of regional versus systemic chemotherapy with Adriamycin. Ann Surg 187: 332–336

Didolkar MS, Fitzpatrick L, Jackson A, Johnston G (1986) Toxicity and complications of vascular isolation and hyperthermic perfusion with Imidazole Carboxamide (DTIC) in melanoma. Cancer 57: 1961–1966

Di Filippo F, Calabrò AM, Giannarelli D, Carlini S, Cavaliere F, Moscarelli F, Cavaliere R (1989) Prognostic variables in recurrent limb melanoma treated with hyperthermic antiblastic perfusion. Cancer 63: 2551–2561

Di Filippo F, Botti C, Giannarelli D, Graziano F, Carlini S, Cavaliere F, Cavaliere R (1991a) Thermochemotherapy for soft tissue sarcomas. In: Pinedo HM, Verweij J, Suit HD (eds) Soft tissue sarcomas: New developments in the multidisciplinary approach to treatment. Kluwer, London, pp 127–147

Di Filippo F, Cagol PP, Civalleri D, et al. (1991b) Hyperthermic perfusion with doxorubicin: phase I study. Reg Cancer Treat 4: 13

Di Filippo F, Cavaliere F, Caroli S, Petrucci F, Alimonti S, Callopoli A (1993) Hyperthermic perfusion with Melphalan: A phase I study. Melanoma Research (suppl 1): 94

Fontijne WP, Hook PH, Koops HS, Wildevuur CR (1985) Improved tissue perfusion during pressure regulated hyperthermic regional isolated perfusion. Cancer 55: 1455–1461

Franklin HR, Koops HS, Oldhoff J, Czarnetzki BM, Macher E, Kroon BBR (1988) To perfuse or not to perfuse? A retrospective comparative study to evaluate the effect of adjuvant isolated regional perfusion in patients with stage I extremity melanoma with a thickness of 1.5 mm or greater. J Clin Oncol 6: 701

Ghussen F, Nagel K, Groth W, Muller JM (1984) The limit of strain on skeletal muscle tissue during regional perfusion. Res Exp Med 184: 115–123

Ghussen F, Kruger I, Smalley RU, Groth W (1989) Hyperthermic perfusion with chemotherapy in melanoma of the extremities. World J Surg 13: 598–602

Hafstrom L, Hugander A, Jonsson PE, et al. (1984) Blood leakage and Melphalan leakage from the perfusion circuit during regional hyperthermic perfusion for malignant melanoma. Cancer Treat Rep 68: 867–872

Hoekstra HJ, Schraffordt Koops H, Molenaar WM, Oldhoff J (1987) Results of isolated perfusion in the treatment of malignant soft tissue tumor of the extremities. Cancer 60: 1703–1707

Janoff KA, Moseson D, Nohlgren J (1982) The treatment of stage I melanoma of the extremities with regional hyperthermic isolation perfusion. Ann Surg 196: 316–2323

Jolsson PE, Hafstrom L, Hugander A (1983) Results of regional hyperthermic perfusion for primary and recurrent melanoma of the extremities. Recent Results Cancer Res 86: 277–282

Klaase JM, Van Slooten GW, Benckhuijsen C, Kroon BBR (1993) Melphalan peak concentration and toxicity in regional isolated perfusion for melanoma. Melanoma Research 3: 85

Krementz ET, Knudson L (1961) The effect of increased oxygen tension on the tumoricidal effect of nitrogen mustard, Surgery 50: 266–271

Krementz ET (1986) Regional perfusion. Current sophistication; what next? Cancer 57: 416–432

Kroon BBR (1988) Regional isolation perfusion in melanoma of the limbs: accomplishments, unsolved problems, future. Eur J Surg Oncol 14: 101–110

Kroon BBR (1993) Perfusion using high dose hyperthermia and Melphalan sequentially for recurrent melanoma of the limbs. Melanoma Research 3(suppl 1): 92

Lebredo L, Woltering H, Moseley S, Bos G, Small K, Fletcher W (1988) Results of cisplatin hyperthermic isolation perfusion with dose escalation for extremity sarcomas. Reg Cancer Treat 2: 120–124

Lejeune FJ, Deloof T, Ewalenko P (1983) Objective regression of unexcised melanoma in transit metastasis after hyperthermic isolation perfusion of the limbs with Melphalan. Recent Results Cancer Res 86: 276–286

Lejeune FJ, Ghanem G (1987) A simple and accurate new method of cytostatic dosimetry in isolation perfusion of the limbs based on exchangeable blood volume determination. Cancer Res 47: 6739–6743

Lejeune FJ, Ghanem G, Lienard D (1989) Assessment of hematocrit method for dosimetry of cytostatic drugs in isolation perfusion: Reg Cancer Treat 2: 82

Lejeune FJ (1993) A randomized trial on prolongated isolation perfusion for stage I high risk (i.e., 1.5 mm thickness) malignant melanoma of the limbs an interim report. Melanoma Research 3(suppl 1): 95

Lethi PM, Moseley S, Janoff K, Stevens K, Fletcher W (1986) Improved survival for soft tissue sarcoma of the extremities by regional hyperthermic perfusion, local excision and radiation therapy. Surg Gynec Obstet 162: 149–152

Lienard D, Eggermont AMM, Schraffordt Koops H, Lejeune FJ (1993) High dose TNF-alpha, INF-gamma and Melphalan in isolation perfusion produces 90% C.R. in melanoma in transit metastases. Melanoma Research 3(suppl 1): 30

Martin H, Oldhoff J, Schraffordt Koops H (1982) Hyperthermic regional perfusion and a combination of Melphalan and Actinomycin D in the treatment of locally metastasized malignant melanoma. J Surg Oncol 20: 9–13

McBride CM, McMurtrey MJ, Copeland EM, Mickey RC (1978) Regional chemotherapy by isolation perfusion. Int Adv Surg Oncol 1: 1–9

Mikhail RA, Boddie AW, Ames FC (1984) Effect of variation of drug dosage on disease control and regional toxicity in prophylactic perfusion for stage I extremity melanoma. J Surg Oncol 27: 215–217

Minor DR, Allen R, Alberts D, Peng YM, Tardelli G, Hutchinson J (1985) A clinical and pharmacokinetic study of isolated limb perfusion with heat and Melphalan for melanoma. Cancer 55: 2638–2644

Mucci S, Mucci SJ, Crist K, Chaudhury B, Thomford N, Chaudhury P (1991) Pharmacokinetics of Doxorubicin during isolated perfusion II: loss of Doxorubicin in perfusion system. Reg Cancer Treat 4: 30

Mucci SJ, Crist K, Chaudhury B, Thomford N, Chaudury P (1991) Pharmacokinetics of Doxorubicin during isolated limb perfusion I: effect of heparin on Doxorubicin concentration. Reg Cancer Treat 4(1): 29–30

Natali PG, Zupi G, Greco C, Cavaliere R, Giacomini P, Ferrone S (1993) Effect of hyperthermia and neoplastic drugs on cell survival and antigenic profile of two melanoma cell lines. In: Spitzy KH, Karrer K (eds) Proceedings 13th International Congress Chemotherapy, Vienna, Springer, Berlin, 70 Tom 15-SE; 12-1, 12, 3, 246/18, pp 230–234

Pfefferkorn RO, Didolkar MS (1982) Regional perfusion for melanoma of the extremities. J Extraregional Tech 14: 475

Rege VB, Leone LA, Soderberg CH, Coleman GV (1983) Hyperthermic adjuvant perfusion chemotherapy for stage I malignant melanoma of the extremity with literature review. Cancer 52: 2033–2038

Rochlin DB, Smar CR (1965) Treatment of malignant melanoma by regional perfusion. Cancer 18: 1544–1550

Rosen G, Caparros B, Huvos A (1982) Preoperative chemotherapy for osteogenic sarcoma: selection of postoperative adjuvant chemotherapy based on the response of the primary tumor to preoperative chemotherapy. Cancer 49: 1221–1230

Rosin RD, Westbury G (1980) Isolated limb perfusion for malignant melanoma. Practitioner 244: 1031–1036

Schraffordt Koops (1983) Isolated perfusion of the extremities. Recent Results Cancer Res 6: 223–228

Scott RN, et al. (1989) Ph and Melphalan toxicity in human melanoma spheroids. Proceedings ICRCT, Berchtesgaden, E5

Scott RN, McKay AJ, Lingam MK, et al. (1992) Melphalan concentration and distribution in the tissue of tumor. bearing limbs treated by isolated limb perfusion. Eur J Cancer 28: 1811–1813

Skene AI, Bulman AS, Williams TR, Meirion Thomas J, Westbury G (1990) Hyperthermic isolated perfusion with Melphalan in the treatment of advanced malignant melanoma of the lower limb. Br J Surg 77: 765–767

Smith MA (1991) Influence of Doxorubicin dose intensity on response and outcome of patients with osteogenic sarcoma and Ewing's sarcoma. J Natl Cancer Inst 83: 1460–1470

Stehlin JS (1969) Hyperthermic perfusion with chemotherapy for cancer of the extremities. Surg Gynecol Obstet 129: 305–308

Stehlin JS, Giovanella BC, Gutierrez AE, De Ipoly PD, Greef PJ (1984) Fifteen years experience with hyperthermic perfusion for the treatment of soft tissue sarcoma and malignant melanoma of the extremities. Front Radiat Ther Oncol 18: 177–182

Storm FK, Morton DL (1985) Value of therapeutic hyperthermic limb perfusion in advanced recurrent melanoma of the lower extremity. Ann J Surg 150: 32–35

Stotter AT, Robinson BA, Clutterbuck RD (1987) A comparison of Melphalan levels achieved in isolated limb perfusion and systemic high dose therapy. J Exp Clin Res 6: 161–165

Sugarbaker EV, McBridge LM (1976) Survival and regional disease control after isolation perfusion for invasive stage I melanoma of the extremities. Cancer 37: 188–198

Tate PS, Djuric M, Bies J, Briele HA (1986) Pharmacokinetics of Doxorubicin in heated perfusion of canine extremities. Proceedings Annual Meeting American Associates Cancer Research (AACR) 27: 406

Tonak J, Homenberger W, Gohl J (1984) Die isolierte hypertherme Extremitaten perfusion bei malignen Melanomen und Weichgewebssarkomen. Chirurg 55: 499–504

Vaglini M, Ammatuna M, Nava M, Prada A, Rovini D, Santinami M, Cascinelli N (1983) Regional perfusion at high temperatures in the treatment of stage III–IIIB melanoma patients. Tumori 69: 585–588

Wagner DE (1976) A retrospective study of regional perfusion for melanoma. Arch Surg 111: 410–413

Wieberdink J, Benkhuizen C, Braat RP, Van Slooten EA, Olthuis GAA (1982) Dosimetry in isolation perfusion of the limb by assessment of perfused tissue volume and grading of toxicity tissue reactions. Eur J Cancer Clin Oncol 18: 905–610

Wondergem J, Stephens LC, Strebel FR, et al. (1991) Effect of Adriamycin combined with whole body hyperthermia on tumor and normal tissues. Cancer Res 51: 3559–3567

Multicenter Trials and Future Clinical Research

20 Prognostic Factors in Thermoradiotherapy Clinical Trials

G. ARCANGELI and G. GIOVINAZZO

CONTENTS

20.1 Introduction

Despite the extensive clinical experience accumulated over the past decade and the large amount of data available in the current literature, the *optimal regimen* of combined hyperthermia and radiotherapy is not yet known (MEYER et al. 1989; OVERGAARD 1989; SUGAHARA and SAITO 1989). Because of easier heat delivery and temperature monitoring, superficial hyperthermia has been more popular than interstitial or deep hyperthermia and has allowed a number of treatment combinations with radiotherapy, depending on a series of factors that may vary in different clinical situations.

The results obtained with the different treatment combinations have shown that the following variables may play an important role in the control of disease:

1. Previous radiation treatments
2. Size and depth of lesions
3. Histology and site of primary tumors and metastases
4. Planned radiotherapy schedule
5. Type of heat apparatus available
6. Planned and expected temperatures
7. Difficulty of heating and of thermometry in the specific clinical situation in question
8. The number and frequency of heat treatments

However, a retrospective evaluation and comparison of data can lead to erroneous interpretation of the results, particularly if these are not derived from site- and disease-specific clinical trials with an adequate follow-up and if the trials were not directed to test the influence of a specific variable on the endpoint under evaluation.

The variables that, with some caution, have been shown to be of a prognostic significance (ARCANGELI and YABUMOTO 1989; LUK et al. 1984; MEYER et al. 1989; VALDAGNI et al. 1988a) can be divided into two main groups: The first consists of the *intrinsic biological characteristics of tumors*, such as histology, site, and size. The second group comprises technical variables that are mainly associated with the treatment, such as the total radiation dose and fraction size, thermal parameters, the number of hyperthermia treatments, and fractionation, sequence, and timing of the two modalities.

20.2 Intrinsic Tumor Characteristics

20.2.1 Histology/Tumor Site

Although differences in thermal sensitivities have been clearly demonstrated among several experimental cell lines, the available clinical data do not show (with the exception of lymphoma, which is a radiosensitive disease) any influence of tumor histology on the response to combined radiother-

G. ARCANGELI, MD, G. Porfiri Oncology Center, Radiation Oncology Department, S. Maria Goretti Hospital, Via G. Reni, I-04100 Latina, Italy
G. GIOVINAZZO, MD, G. Porfiri Oncology Center, Radiation Oncology Department, S. Maria Goretti Hospital, Via G. Reni, I-04100 Latina, Italy

Table 20.1. Tumor control rates as a function of site/histology (series with more than 50 pts/lesions)

Authors	Squamous cell carcinoma, head and neck	Melanoma	Adenocarcinoma, breast	Sarcoma, extremity
ARCANGELI et al. (1987)	79	76	–	–
GONZALES GONZALES et al. (1986, 1988)	–	50	60	–
HOFMAN et al. (1984)	83	67	30–60	–
KAPP et al. (1990)	↑	↑	↓	↓
KIM et al. (1982)	–	82	90	100
LUK et al. (1984)	53	–	63	–
MYERSON et al. (1990)	60	55	46	50
PEREZ et al. (1987)	58	79	46	–
PEREZ et al. (1991)				
Lesions <3 cm	38	–	62	67
Lesions >3 cm	33	–	21	11
SCOTT et al. (1988)	51	–	85	–
VALDAGNI et al. (1988a,b)	50–78	75	58	43
Total	58	69	58	54

↑ means higher response
↓ means lower response

apy and hyperthermia (Table 20.1). However, some confusion in the retrospective interpretation of results from clinical studies, not specifically designed to test these parameters, arises from the fact that histology and the site of disease are mutually associated in trials with superficial hyperthermia. In fact, with the exception of melanomas, most of the published trials have been carried out on tumors of the breast/chest wall, head and neck, and extremities with histological features of adenocarcinoma, squamous cell carcinoma, and sarcoma, respectively.

Superior local control in the breast/chest wall than in the head and neck was shown by SCOTT et al. (1988) in a phase I–II RTOG study. The following phase III 81-40 RTOG study by PEREZ et al. (1991) confirmed this finding, local control being better in lesions of the chest wall and trunk/extremities than in those of the head and neck (Table 20.1). This finding, however, was limited to lesions of less than 3 cm in diameter, suggesting that, rather than being a function of histology or site of origin, local tumor control may be related to the *technical ability to heat more easily* lesions of the chest wall or extremities than those located in the neck.

In contrast, KAPP and co-workers (1990) found a significant difference in the duration of local control between a favorable group, consisting of melanomas, squamous cell carcinomas, and tumors of other histologies, and an unfavorable group, consisting of adenocarcinomas and sarcomas.

Further experience derived from specific clinical studies will likely reveal such differences and suggest the correct indication for the combined modality. To date, melanoma is the only tumor in which the response has been undoubtedly demonstrated to be better when treatment comprises the combination of hyperthermia and radiotherapy (cf. the recent randomized ESHO trial: OVERGAARD et al. 1992).

20.2.2 Tumor Status

It has been reported that previously irradiated recurrent tumors exhibit a better response than previously nonirradiated lesions (LUK et al. 1984). This finding has never been confirmed by other studies. On the other hand, because of normal tissue tolerance, previously irradiated tumors are generally treated with lower doses of radiation. The correlation between local control and radiation dose will be discussed below.

20.2.3 Tumor Size

Tumor volume has been reported to be negatively correlated with the response to radiation. Small tumors are, in general, more easily controlled than large tumors of the same histology and site. This is also in part true when radiotherapy is combined with hyperthermia, although, with this approach, the volume effect is less pronounced than with radiation alone.

Table 20.2 shows the results of some clinical trials that have looked at the volume effect. It appears that with increasing tumor volume, there is an increase in the ratio of percentage complete response after combined modality to percentage complete response after radiotherapy alone (isodose thermal enhancement ratio, i.e., TER). This means that, in spite of the greater difficulty of heating large as compared with small tumors (ARCANGELI et al. 1985; MEYER et al. 1989; OLESON et al. 1984), the addition of hyperthermia to radiotherapy is more useful for the former than for the latter lesions. This finding is better visualized in Fig. 20.1, where TER is shown as a function of tumor volume in a series of patients

Table 20.2. Complete response rates as a function of tumor volume

Authors	Tumor	volume (cm^3)	XRT + HT	XRT alone	TER
ARCANGELI et al. (1985)	Neck nodes	2–10	100	67	1.5
		13–24	60	36	1.7
		25–54	69	14	4.9
DEWHIRST (1984)	Animal tumors	<1.8	76	60	1.3
		1.8–8.3	54	60	0.9
		8.3–49	48	15	3.2
		>49	48	10	4.8
EMAMI et al. (1988)	Melanoma	<3	51	27	1.9
		>3	69	18	3.8
KIM et al. (1982)	Melanoma	<10	73	58	1.3
		>10	65	19	3.4
PEREZ et al. (1986)	Chest wall	<3	79	48	1.6
		>3	65	28	2.3
RTOG 81-04	Neck nodes	<3	38	50	0.8
	Chest wall	>3	33	30	1.1
		<3	62	40	1.6
		>3	21	28	0.8
VALDAGNI et al. (1988a,b)	Neck nodes	10–27	80	43	1.9
		32–48	85	43	2.0
		>52	85	20	4.3

XRT, radiotherapy; HT, hyperthermia; TER, thermal enhancement ratio

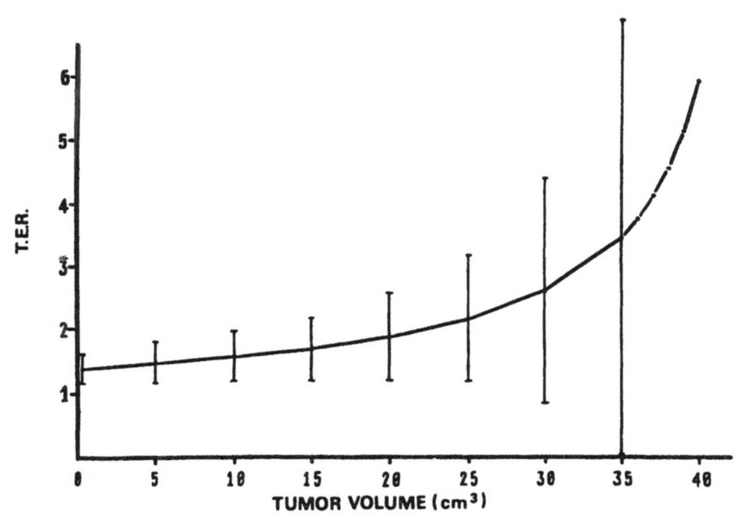

Fig. 20.1. Thermal enhancement ratio (TER) as a function of tumor volume. The *bars* are the standard deviations of TER. (From ARCANGELI et al. 1985)

with neck node metastases from head and neck cancer, treated by full doses of accelerated hyperfractionation radiotherapy alone or the same radiotherapy course plus hyperthermia at 42.5°C for 45 min given three times per week immediately after the second daily fraction of radiation (ARCANGELI et al. 1985).

However, the use of applicators not capable of heating the *whole volume* of the tumor could be responsible for a decrease in hyperthermia effectiveness and could be the reason why, in the RTOG 81-04 study, TER did not increase with the increase in tumor volume or tumor depth (PEREZ et al. 1991).

20.3 Technical Variables

20.3.1 Total Dose of Radiation

As already mentioned, hyperthermia is frequently used in patients with recurrences after full courses of radiotherapy. In these cases, because of normal tissue tolerance, radical radiation doses can rarely be given with or without concomitant hyperthermia, and the minimum dose of radiation required to obtain a satisfactory rate of complete response is still to be defined. Naturally, no limitation on total radiation doses is necessary when radiotherapy is used in combination with hyperthermia in previously untreated areas.

Table 20.3 shows the correlation of the complete response rates with the total doses of radiation, although, because of the small number of patients investigated and/or the uncertainties in the capability of heating tumors, statistical significance has not been achieved in every study.

A larger gain in response rate (an increase in TER) was observed by our group when hyperthermia was combined with nonradical, as against radical, radiation doses for the treatment of inguinal node metastases from gynecological malignancies (unpublished data). These interesting findings deserve to be confirmed by an "ad hoc" trial, and suggest that the addition of hyperthermia is more useful when radiation doses are limited by the normal tissue tolerance.

20.3.2 Size of Radiation Fractions

Two principal strategies can be followed in the application of hyperthermia according to the type of radiotherapy fractionation schedule that is planned. One strategy is to *apply hyperthermia once or twice per week, independently of radiation*, during a conventional radiotherapy course employing standard fraction sizes of 1.5–3 Gy,

Table 20.3. Tumor control rates as a function of total radiation dose

Authors	Tumor	Dose (Gy)	CR (%)	Statistical significance
EMAMI et al. (1988)	Melanoma	<30	8/21 (38)	
		>30	20/28 (71)	Yes
GONZALES GONZALES et al. (1986)	Melanoma	18	0/8	
		24–30	19/30 (63)	Yes
GONZALES GONZALES et al. (1988)	Breast recurrence	18–32	24/41 (59)	
		40–60	3/4 (75)	No
KAPP et al. (1990)	Variety	19–25	(40)	
		30–36	(82)	Yes
LUK et al. (1984)	Variety	<40	(32)	
		>40	(75)	Yes
MYERSON et al. (1990)	Variety	<45	24/44 (55)	
		>45	6/15 (40)	No
VALDAGNI et al. (1986)	Neck nodes	20–50	3/8 (38)	
		60–70	13/19 (68)	No
VAN DER ZEE (1986)	Variety	12–25	15/65 (23)	
		28–36	9/25 (36)	No
		>39	13/21 (62)	Yes

CR, complete response

utilizing the specific cytotoxic effect of heat against radioresistant, hypoxic, nutritionally deprived tumor cells. The other strategy is that of the *"quasi-simultaneous" application of the two modalities* during a hypofractionation radiotherapy course employing dose fractions of 4 or more Gy once or twice per week, utilizing the enhancement of radiation effect in heated tissues (OVERGAARD 1989).

As a matter of fact, because of the increased frequency and severity of late damage to normal tissues, hypofractionation is currently employed only for melanoma, which is believed to have a high reparative capacity and may benefit from large fractional doses of radiation.

If analysis is limited to the most representative studies of combined radiotherapy and hyperthermia for melanoma (Table 20.4), one cannot see, in general, a clear-cut influence of fraction size on complete response rates, although no comparison has been made between standard fractionation and hypofractionation radiotherapy.

Higher response rates were observed by EMAMI et al. (1988) using larger fraction sizes in groups of lesions treated with radiotherapy alone; however, such a trend could not be seen in patients treated with radiation plus hyperthermia, as if the addition of heat diminished the need for larger doses per fraction.

In contrast, a statistically significant improvement in complete response rate was observed by GONZALES GONZALES et al. (1986) when they increased the dose per fraction from 4 to 8 Gy. It is obvious that we need more specific studies to assess the value of the fraction size when radiotherapy is combined with hyperthermia.

20.3.3 Sequence and Timing of Hyperthermia and Radiation

Experimental data on the sequence and timing of the two modalities have shown that the maximum sensitization of both tumor and normal tissue is observed when heat and radiation are applied simultaneously. When an interval is introduced between the two modalities, thermal sensitization decreases more in the skin than in the tumor, where, although at a lower level, it persists for up to 24 h. When heat is applied before radiation, a prolonged sensitization is observed in the skin, slightly below that of the tumor. If radiation is given before heat, the TER of skin is markedly reduced within 1 h and disappears completely after 4 h (HILL and DENEKAMP 1979; OVERGAARD 1980).

Some of the clinical trials reported in the literature, specifically designed to test the importance of the sequence and timing of the two modalities, have at least in part confirmed the experimental findings (Table 20.5). KIM et al. (1984) observed a great increase in skin reaction when heat was applied before large radiation fractions in melanomas. Comparing immediate and delayed application of heat following each of the large radiation fractions given twice per week, an impressive correlation between clinical data and biological findings was observed by OVERGAARD and

Table 20.4. Complete responses of melanomas as a function of radiation fraction size

Authors	No. of pts/ fields	Dose (Gy)	CR (%)	Statistical significance
ARCANGELI et al. (1987)	21	5	10/13 (77)	
		6	6/8 (75)	No
EMAMI et al. (1988)	49	<5	18/30 (60)	
		>5	10/19 (53)	No
GONZALES GONZALES et al. (1986)	38	4–6	4/20 (20)	
		8	15/18 (83)	Yes
KIM et al. (1984)	50	4	16/27 (59)	
		6.6	17/23 (74)	No
VALDAGNI et al. (1988)	24	5	4/4 (100)	
		6	16/20 (80)	No

CR, complete response

Table 20.5. Sequence and timing of heat and radiation in clinical trials

Authors	No. of HTs W/T	No. of RTs W/T	Fraction size	Sequence and timing	% CR	% MD skin	Isodose TER	
							Tumor	Skin
ARCANGELI et al. (1984)	2/8	2/8	500	RT-HT	77	64	2.0	1.8
	2/8	2/8	500	RT-4-HT	67	46	1.8	1.3
	2/5[a]	2/5	600	RT-HT	87	33	2.6	1.3
	3/7	15/36	167	RT-HT	73	42	1.7	1.1
	1/5	5/25	200	RT-HT	64	43	1.8	1.2
	2/5	5/25	200	RT-HT	78	44	2.2	1.3
KIM et al. (1984)	2/10	2/10	400	HT-RT	57	NI	1.9	–
				RT-HT	63	NI	2.1	–
	1/6	1/6	660	HT-RT	75	GI	1.3	–
				RT-HT	72	I	1.2	–
					TCD_{50} (Gy)	ER_{50} (Gy)	Isoeffect TER	
							Tumor	Skin
OVERGAARD and OVERGAARD (1987)	2/3	2/3	500–1000	RT-HT	18.4	18.3	1.4	1.4
				RT-4-HT	21.2	25.2	1.2	1.0

HTs, heat treatments; RTs, radiotherapy sessions; WT, week/total; MD, moist desquamation; NI, no increase; GI, great increase; RT-4-HT, heat given 4 h after radiation; CR, complete response; TER, thermal enhancement ratio

OVERGAARD (1987) and by our group (ARCANGELI et al. 1984). Heating tumors and critical normal tissues to the same temperature, the immediate delivery of hyperthermia and radiotherapy resulted in an increased sensitization of both tumors and skin, resulting in a low therapeutic advantage. After applying hyperthermia 4 h following radiation fractions, a differential sensitizing effect in favor of the tumor was observed, resulting in a positive therapeutic ratio. The data obtained by our group (ARCANGELI et al. 1984) also showed that a positive therapeutic ratio can be obtained by cooling the skin around the tumor, or by applying hyperthermia independently of radiotherapy during a course of conventional or hyperfractionation radiotherapy.

20.3.4 Thermal Parameters

Local control and response duration are correlated with a good heating performance, no matter which method of thermal dose evaluation is used.

Several methods have been used to evaluate the quality of heat produced in tumors. A correlation of some thermal parameters with long-term response has been shown in several studies (Table 20.6). In general, a striking *correlation of minimum temperature with tumor response* and of *maximum temperature with toxicity* has been observed, although these parameters reflect the quality of heating.

Table 20.6. Thermal parameters correlated with response duration

Authors	Tumors	No. of sites	Hyperthermia parameters
ARCANGELI et al. (1985)	Neck nodes	81	Overall Eq 42.5 (from av. T in 1 tumor point)
DEWHIRST and SIM (1984)	Pet animals	117	Non-site-specific av. minimum Eq 43
KAPP et al. (1990)	Variety	179	Av. minimum tumor T (<41°C vs >41°C)
MYERSON et al. (1990)	Variety	60	SAR >25% and min T 43°C in the best HT session
OLESON et al. (1993)	Sarcomas, variety	44 105	Overall Eq 43/T_{50} Overall Eq 43/T_{90}

The amount of heating produced in tissues is better evaluated in terms of temperature applied for the cumulative duration of hyperthermic treatments according to isoeffect thermal dose formulae (FIELD 1987; SAPARETO 1987). This allows an estimate of thermal dose even when the temperature at points changes during the treatment and/or from one treatment to another.

Following this method, a thermal isoeffective dose-response relationship for different tumor volumes (Fig. 20.2) was identified by our group (ARCANGELI et al. 1987) in a clinical series of 38 neck node metastases from squamous cell carcinoma of the head and neck, treated with combined radiotherapy and hyperthermia, using a single temperature monitoring probe inserted at the base of the lesion. However, a characterization of thermal treatments that give a significant correlation with results should be based on a careful characterization of temperature distributions (LEOPOLD et al. 1989, 1992; OLESON et al. 1989). The temperatures exceeded by x% of the intratumor measurements, such as T_{90} or T_{50}, are good descriptors of temperature distributions and can be applied to the types of nonuniform temperature distributions produced by microwave applicators. Using T_{90} and T_{50} as the basis for calculating an equivalent treatment time, with T_{90} or T_{50} equal to 43°C, OLESON et al. (1993) provided thermal isoeffect dose-response curves that allowed them to estimate the sensitivity of treatment outcome to changes in thermal isoeffect dose resulting

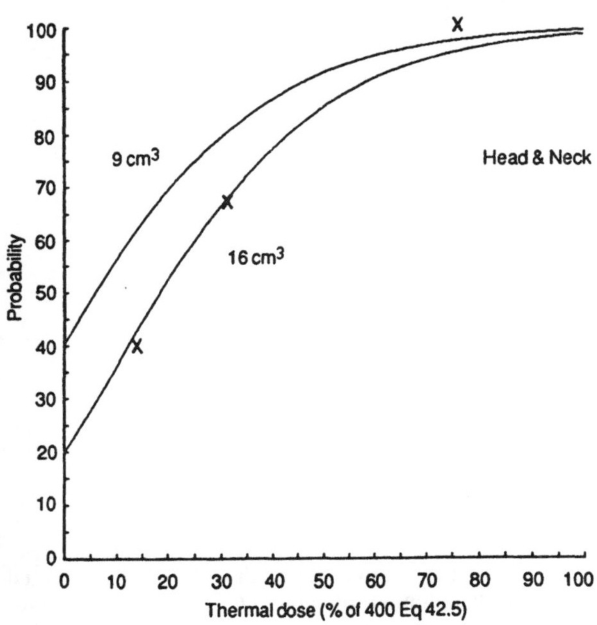

Fig. 20.2. Probability of complete response as a function of thermal isoeffect dose for two sets of tumor volumes in head and neck lesions. (From ARCANGELI et al. 1987)

from changes in treatment time or temperature. They concluded that the "thermal isoeffect dose does correlate with outcome, albeit not as strongly as cumulative minutes for superfical tumors with $T_{90} \geqslant 39.5$°C. However, the thermal dose formulation is convenient in performing calculations. . . ."

Despite the good correlation of the thermal isoeffect dose with outcome in our and Oleson et al.'s series of tumors, the applicability of thermal dose formuale to treatment of human tumors is controversial and needs to be validated by prospective clinical studies.

20.3.5 Number of Heat Treatments

There are conflicting reports regarding the optimal number of heat treatments to be applied in combination with radiotherapy (Table 21.7). The reasons for these conflicting results may consist in:

1. Inhomogeneity of samples and of treatments that is responsible for large biases between the control and the test group in the trials carried out on miscellaneous tumors (KAPP et al. 1990; KOMARNICHY et al. 1992; LINDHOLM et al. 1992; OLESON et al. 1990)
2. Lack of a control group receiving a standard treatment (i.e., radiotherapy alone) (KAPP et al. 1990; OLESON et al. 1990)
3. Too early assessment of complete response without any evaluation of local control duration (KOMARNICKY et al. 1992; OLESON et al. 1990; VALDAGNI et al. 1988b)
4. Most importantly, the inclusion of too few patients or lesions in the studies, with a consequent lack of power to show the small differences in response rates that would be expected in these trials (KOMARNICHY et al. 1992; VALDAGNI et al. 1988b)

It has been suggested that one "good" heat treatment would be sufficient to obtain the maximum effect from hyperthermia (OVERGAARD 1989). Our data in Fig. 20.2 (ARCANGELI et al. 1987) show that, to have a 90% probability of complete response in neck node metastases, 188 and 232 Eq 42.5 are required for tumors of 9 and 16 cm^3, respectively (assuming a radiotherapy dose of 60 Gy). OLESON et al. (1993) calculated the Eq min required to produce a 90% likelihood

Table 20.7. Disease outcome as a function of the number of heat treatments in randomized trials

Authors (tumors)	HT/week	Total HT	% CR	Stat. diff.	Comments
ARCANGELI et al. (1991)	0	0	13[a]		Lesions in same
(breast)	1	1	14[a]	NA	patient
	1	4	Not reached[a]		
KAPP et al. (1990)	1	2	52		No comparison
(variety)	1	6	51	NS	with RT
KOMARNICHY et al. (1992)	1	4	59		Too few lesions
(variety)	2	8	55	NS	
LEOPOLD et al. (1989)	1	5	37.5		Pathological
(soft tissue sa.)	2	10	100	<0.09	response
LINDHOLM et al. (1992)	1	3	56		Too few lesions
(variety)	2	6	69	NS	
OLESON et al. (1990)	1	?	44		No comp. with
(variety)	2	?	44	NS	RT
VALDAGNI (1988b)	2	2	86		Too few lesions
(neck nodes)	2	6	80	NS	

CR, complete response
[a] Median response duration (months)

of complete response in superficial tumors to be 186 min (assuming a radiotherapy dose of 50 Gy and a tumor volume of $100\,cm^3$). To deliver such thermal isoeffect doses in one treatment of 60 min, $T_{90} = 44.6°C$ or more would be required (OLESON et al. 1993).

It is clear that these high thermal isoeffect doses cannot be given in one single treatment with the currently available equipment for external hyperthermia, and the number of treatments necessary depends on how "good" the heating applied to the tumor is.

Our randomized study (ARCANGELI et al. 1991), carried out on a patient with multiple cutaneous metastases from breast cancer, provided a very homogenous clinical situation for the study purpose and showed a correlation of the number of heat treatments with both the regrowth delay of lesions (Fig. 20.3) and the duration of response (Fig. 20.4).

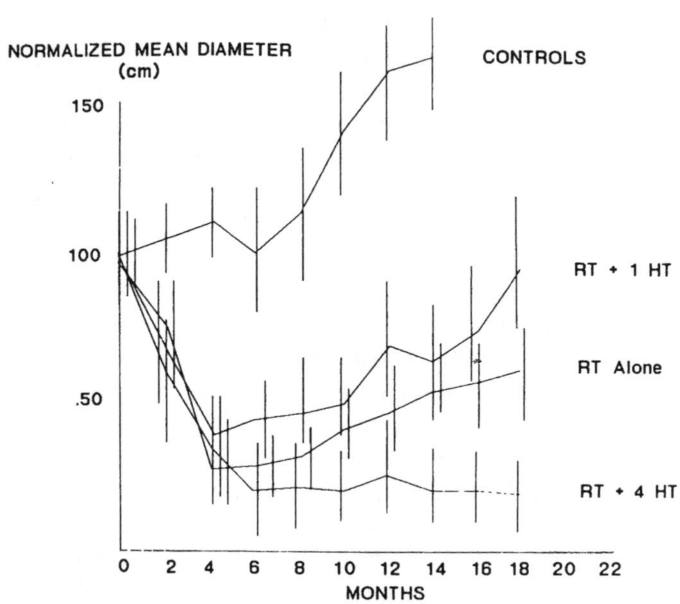

Fig. 20.3. Tumor regrowth rate of lesions treated with radiotherapy alone (*RT*), radiotherapy plus one heat treatment (*RT + 1HT*), and radiotherapy plus four heat treatments (*RT + 4HT*). *Bars* represent standard deviations. (From ARCANGELI et al. 1991)

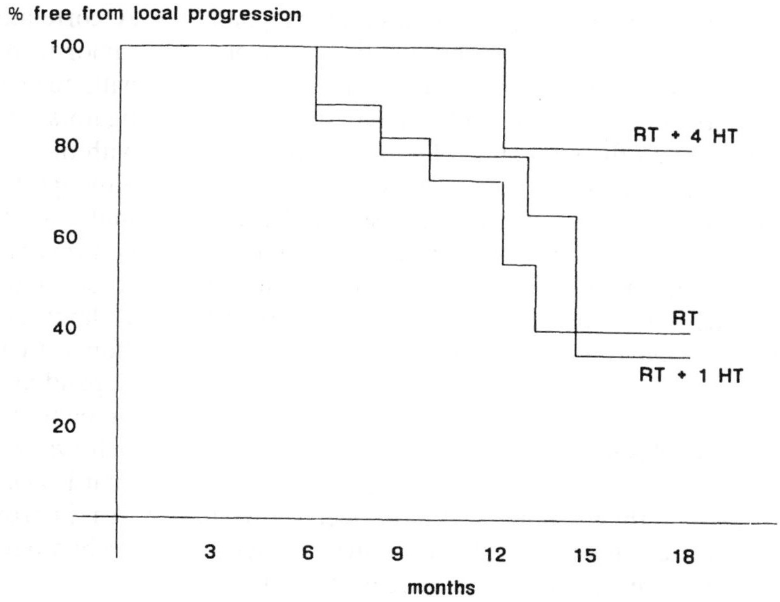

Fig. 20.4. Actuarial analysis of freedom from local progression in lesions treated with radiotherapy alone (*RT*), radiotherapy plus one heat treatment (*RT + 1HT*), and radiotherapy plus four heat treatments (*RT + 4HT*). (From ARCANGELI et al. 1991)

Three additional experimental studies analyzed the influence of the number of heat treatments in combination with fractionated radiotherapy. ZYWIETZ and JUNG (1990), in experiments on the R1H rhabdomyosarcoma of the rat, found an improvement in local control after ten, as compared with five, heat treatments given once weekly (73% vs 42%, respectively). MARINO and CIVIDALLI (1992) found a lower TCD_{50} when radiotherapy was combined with four heat treatments, rather than one, in a murine mammary carcinoma. However, MEYER et al. (1986) showed similar tumor responses for hyperthermia plus radiation when one, two, three, four, or five heat treatments were utilized.

In conclusion, although it is not possible to establish precisely an optimum regimem in terms of total number and number of heat sessions per week to be applied to a radiotherapy course, a large number of heat sessions may not be required. This is related to the temperature and temperature distribution achieved in the tumor. For a significant increase in both complete response rate and duration of response, a thermal dose of Eq min T_{90} 43 = 10 min has been considered by OLESON et al. (1993) to be a reasonable goal. Depending on the equipment available and on the individual clinical situation, this treatment could be delivered in a "few" sessions.

20.4 Univariate Versus Multivariate Analysis

Few papers examined the value of prognostic factors by means of more detailed statistical methods, such as univariate and multivariate analyses. Using various endpoints, such as the rate of complete response, local control and survival, and/or the actuarial curves for local control and survival, it is possible to determine the relative risk afforded by each variable when all variables are considered simultaneously.

By using multivariate analysis, KAPP et al. (1990) showed a significant correlation of local control with histology, radiation dose, tumor volume and Tmin >41°C.

Histology, however, was a significant prognostic factor only when the various histologies were lumped into an apparent "favorable" group (consisting of melanomas, squamous cell carcinomas and other histologies) and an "unfavorable" group (consisting of adenocarcinomas and sarcomas). Concurrent XRT dose was the most important predictive of local control, suggesting the use of the highest tolerable radiation dose in combined XRT-HT trials. The finding of the negative influence of increasing tumor volume on outcome revealed that the mean minimum tumor temperature was significantly lower in large than in small tumors, reflecting the influence of tumor size on the ability to heat tumors.

By using the multivariate logistic regression analysis, also OVERGAARD et al. (1995), in a randomized trial of the European Society of

Hyperthermic Oncology on metastatic malignant melanoma, revealed that the addition of hyperthermia to radiation, small tumor size and high radiation dose were all independent prognostic factors when the endpoints of complete response and local control were considered. However, in these patients with metastatic lesions, the Cox multivariate analysis revealed that the significant prognostic factors for the endpoint of survival were persistent local control of all known disease, being female, and a single lesion.

20.5 Conclusion

Despite all the variables that have been shown to have some influence on disease outcome, hyperthermia seems to be able to increase the effect of ionizing radiation. Further efforts should be made both to improve the currently available technology and to perform site- and disease-specific controlled clinical studies for treatment optimization.

20.6 Summary

- No clear influence of histology on the response to combined radiotherapy and hyperthermia was observed, although melanomas and squamous cell carcinomas may have a better local control than adenocarcinomas and sarcomas.
- No correlation between tumor status and local control was established.
- Local control is better in small than in large tumors of the same histology. However, since small tumors can be easily controlled by radiation alone, the addition of hyperthermia may be more useful for the large than for the small tumors.
- Significant correlation was observed between total XRT dose and local control, although a larger gain with respect to XRT alone may be observed when hyperthermia is combined with non radical as against radical XRT doses.
- No clear-cut influence of the size of radiation fractions on complete response rate was observed.
- A great increase in radiation reaction can be observed by applying heat before or concomitantly to large radiation fractions when tumors and critical normal tissues are heated to the same temperature.
- A correlation of minimum temperature with tumor response and of maximum temperature with toxicity was observed by several investigators. A good correlation of the outcome with thermal isoeffect dose was also observed, although the applicability of thermal dose formulae to treatment of human tumors is still controversial and requires specific clinical trials to be validated.
- A large number of heat sessions in combination with radiotherapy may not be required, depending on the ability of delivering a valuable amount of thermal dose in each session to achieve a cumulative thermal isoeffect dose that is necessary for a high local control rate.
- An improvement of the currently available technology and the design of appropriate site- and diseases-specific controlled clinical trials are required for treatment optimization.

References

Arcangeli G, Yabumoto E (1989) Prognostic factors in the combined treatment of tumors. In: Sugahara T, Saito M (eds) Hyperthermic Oncology 1988, vol 2. Taylor & Francis, London, p 609

Arcangeli G, Nervi C, Cividalli A, Lovisolo G (1984) Problem of sequence and fractionation in the clinical application of combined heat and radiation. Cancer Res 44: 4857s–4863s

Arcangeli G, Arcangeli GC, Guerra A, Lovisolo G, Cividalli A, Marino C, Mauro F (1985) Tumour response to heat and radiation: prognostic variables in the treatment of neck node metastases from head and neck cancer. Int J Hyperthermia 3: 207–217

Arcangeli G, Benassi M (1987) Factors and variables affecting tumor response to combined heat and radiation in head and neck. Strahlen Therapie und Onkologie 163(7): 425–427

Arcangeli G, Benassi M, Cividalli A, Lovisolo G, Mauro F (1987) Radiotherapy and hyperthermia: analysis of clinical results and identification of prognostic variables. Cancer 60: 950–956

Arcangeli G, Casale C, Colistro F, Benassi M, Lovisolo G, Begnozzi L (1991) One versus four heat treatments in combination with radiotherapy in metastatic mammary carcinoma. Int J Radiat Oncol Biol Phys 21: 1569–1574

Dewhirst MW, Sim DA (1984) The utility of thermal dose as a predictor of tumor and normal tissue response to combined radiation and hyperthermia. Cancer Res 44: 4772s–4780s

Emami B, Perez CA, Konefal J, et al. (1988) Thermoradiotherapy of malignant melanoma. Int J Hyperthermia 4: 373–381

Field SB (1987) Studies relevant to a means of quantifying the effects of hyperthermia. Int J Hyperthermia 3: 291–296

Gonzales Gonzales D, van Dijk JDP, Blank LECM, Rumke P (1986) Combined treatment with radiation

and hyperthermia in metastatic melanoma. Radiother Oncol 6: 105–113
Gonzales Gonzales D, van Dijk JDP, Blank LECM (1988) Chest wall recurrences of breast cancer: results of combined treatment with radiation and hyperthermia. Radiother Oncol 12: 95–103
Hill SA, Denekamp J (1979) The response of six mouse tumours to combined heat and X-rays: implications for therapy. Br J Radiol 52: 209–218
Hofman P, Lagendjik JJW, Schipper J (1984) The combination of radiotherapy with hyperthermia in protocolized clinical studies. In: Overgaard J (ed) Hyperthermic Oncology 1984, vol 1. Taylor & Francis, London, p 379
Kapp DS, Petersen IA, Cox RS, et al. (1990) Two or six hyperthermia treatments as an adjunct to radiation therapy yield similar tumor responses: results of a randomized trial. Int J Radiat Oncol Biol Phys 19: 1481–1495
Kim JH, Hahn EW, Ahmed SA (1982) Combination hyperthermia and radiation therapy for malignant melanomas. Cancer 50: 478–482
Kim JH, Hahn EW, Ahmed SA, Kim YS (1984) Clinical study of the sequence of combined hyperthermia and radiation therapy of malignant melanoma. In: Overgaard J (ed) Hyperthermic Oncology 1984, vol 1. Taylor & Francis, London, p 387
Komarnichy L, Engin K, Tupchong L, et al. (1992) Randomized trial of one-weekly vs twice-weekly hyperthermia treatments in thermoradiotherapy of superficial tumors. In: Gerner EW (ed) Hyperthermic Oncology 1992, vol 1. Taylor & Francis, London, p 373
Leopold KA, Harrelson JM, Prosnitz LR, Samulski TV, Dewhirst MW, Oleson JR (1989) Preoperative hyperthermia and radiation for soft tissue sarcomas: advantages of two vs one hyperthermia treatments per week. Int J Radiat Oncol Biol Phys 16: 107–115
Leopold KA, Dewhirst MW, Samulski TV, et al. (1992) Relationship among tumor temperature, treatment time and histopathological outcome using preoperative hyperthermia with radiation in soft tissue sarcomas. Int J Radiat Oncol Biol Phys 22: 989–998
Lindholm CE, Kjellen E, Nilson P (1992) A randomized trial on one versus two hyperthermia sessions per week combined with low-dose radiotherapy in superficial malignant tumors. In: Gerner EW (ed) Hyperthermic Oncology 1992, vol 1. Taylor & Francis, London, p 372
Luk KH, Pajak TF, Perez CA, Johnson RJ, Corner N, Dobbins T (1984) Prognostic factors for tumor response after hyperthermia and radiation. In: Overgaard J (ed) Hyperthermic Oncology 1984, vol 1. Taylor & Francis, London, p 353
Marino C, Cividalli A (1992) Combined radiation and hyperthermia: effects of the number of heat fractions and their interval on normal and tumor tissues. Int J Hyperthermia 8: 771–781
Meyer JL, Van Kersen I, Hahn GM (1986) Tumor responses following multiple hyperthermia and X-ray treatments: role of thermotolerance at the cellular level. Cancer Res 46: 5691–5695
Meyer JL, Kapp DS, Fessenden P, Hahn GM (1989) Hyperthermic oncology: current biology, physics and clinical results. Pharmacol Ther 42: 251–258
Myerson RJ, Perez CA, Emami B, Straube WS, Kuske RR, Leybovich LB, von Gerichten D (1990) Tumor control in long-term survivors following superficial hyperthermia. Int J Radiat Oncol Biol Phys 18: 1123–1129
Oleson JR, Sim DA, Manning MR (1984) Analysis of prognostic variables in hyperthermia treatment of 161 patients. Int J Radiat Oncol Biol Phys 10: 2231–2239
Oleson JR, Dewhirst MW, Harrelson JM, Leopold KA, Samulski TV, Tso CY (1989) Tumor temperature distributions predict hyperthermia effect. Int J Radiat Oncol Biol Phys 16: 559–570
Oleson JR, Leopold KA, Samulski TV, et al. (1990) Results of a phase II trial of HT + RT. Proceedings of the 38th annual meeting of the Radiation Research Society, New Orleans, abstract no. Ak-8
Oleson JR, Samulski TV, Leopold KA, Clegg ST, Dewhirst MW, Dodge RK, George SL (1993) Sensitivity of hyperthermia trial outcomes to temperature and time: implications for thermal goals of treatment. Int J Radiat Oncol Biol Phys 25: 289–297
Overgaard J (1980) Simultaneous and sequential hyperthermia and radiation treatment of an experimental tumor and its surrounding normal tissue in vivo. Int J Radiat Oncol Biol Phys 6: 1507–1517
Overgaard J (1989) The current and potential role of hyperthermia in radiotherapy. Int J Radiat Oncol Biol Phys 16: 535–549
Overgaard J, Overgaard M (1987) Hyperthermia as an adjunct to radiotherapy in the treatment of malignant melanoma. Int J Hyperthermia 3: 483–501
Overgaard J, Gonzales Gonzales D, Hulshof MCCM, Arcangeli G, Dahl O, Hella O, Bentzen SM (1995) Randomised trial of hyperthermia as adjuvant to radiotherapy for recurrent or metastetic malignant melanoma. The Lencet 345: 540–543
Perez CA, Kuske RR, Emami B, Fineberg B (1986) Irradiation alone or combined with hyperthermia in the treatment of recurrent carcinoma of the breast in the chest wall. A nonrandomized comparison. Int J Hyperther 2: 179–187
Perez CA, Emami B, Hederman MA, Straube W, von Gerichten D, Fox S (1987) Clinical results of irradiation combined with local hyperthermia in superficial tumors. Proceedings of the 35th annual meeting of the Radiation Research Society, Atlanta, p 18
Perez CA, Pajak T, Emami B, Hornback NB, Tupchong L, Rubin P (1991) Randomized phase III study comparing irradiation and hyperthermia with irradiation alone in superficial measurable tumors. Am J Clin Oncol 14: 133–141
Sapareto SA (1987) Thermal isoeffect dose: addressing the problem of thermotolerance. Int J Hyperthermia 3: 297–307
Scott R, Gillespie B, Perez CA, et al. (1988) Hyperthermia in combination with definitive radiation therapy: results of a phase I/II RTOG study. Int J Radiat Oncol Biol Phys 15: 711–716
Sugahara T, Saito M (1989) Hyperthermic oncology 1988, vols 1, 2. Taylor & Francis, London
Valdagni R, Kapp DS, Valdagni C (1986) N3 (TNM-UICC) metastatic neck nodes managed by combined radiation therapy and hyperthermia: clinical results and analysis of treatment parameters. Int J Hyperthermia 2: 189–200
Valdagni R, Liu FF, Kapp DS (1988a) Important prognostic factors influencing outcome of combined radiation and hyperthermia. Int J Radiat Oncol Biol Phys 15: 959–972
Valdagni R, Amichetti M, Pani G (1988b) Radical radiation alone versus radical radiation plus microwave hyperthermia for N3 (TNM-UICC) neck nodes: a prospective

randomized clinical trial. Int J Radiat Oncol Biol Phys 15: 13–24

van der Zee J, van Putten WLJ, van den Berg AP, van Rhoon GC, Hooley JLW, Broekmeyer-Reurink MP, Reinhold HS (1986) Retrospective analysis of the response of tumors in patients treated with a combination of radiotherapy and hyperthermia. Int J Hyperthermia 2: 337–349

Zywietz F, Jung H (1990) Response of the R1H tumor to fractionated radiotherapy and hyperthermia: dependence on number and application period of heat treatments. Strahlenther Oncol 8: 540–541

21 Considerations for Hyperthermia Clinical Trials Design

M.W. Dewhirst

CONTENTS

21.1 Introduction

This author has been fortunate to be involved in a number of activities in the United States, primarily at Duke University Medical Center, Durham, North Carolina, over the past several years that have related directly to the issue of clinical trial design considerations for hyperthermia. First, I conducted or participated in three veterinary clinical trials that tested the value of *hyperthermia as an adjuvant to radiotherapy* (Dewhirst et al. 1984; Gillette et al. 1987; Gillette-McChesney et al. 1992). Second, I have been involved in the development of clinical trials and analysis of data from human studies conducted at Duke over the past 9 years (Leopold et al. 1989, 1992, 1993; Oleson et al. 1989, 1993). The major focus of the Duke clinical trials has been the development of a robust and *quantifiable dosimetry for hyperthermia*. Because of our research interest in dosimetry, we have been active in national efforts to standardize hyperthermia practice for multi-institutional trials.

M.W. Dewhirst, DVM, PHD, Tumor Microcirculation Laboratory, Department of Radiation Oncology, Duke University Medical Center, P.O. Box 3455, Durham, NC 27710, USA

The first step in achieving standardization required consensus in treatment documentation and patient selection criteria. The Hyperthermia Task Force was commissioned in 1989 by the Radiation Therapy Oncology Group (RTOG) to work on these goals and a series of quality assurance documents for the conduct of hyperthermia clinical trials resulted from that effort (Dewhirst et al. 1990; Waterman et al. 1991; Emami et al. 1991; Sapozink et al. 1991). More recently, I participated in the preparation of a position statement by the Intersociety Council on Radiation Oncology, which addresses the unique problems that have been encountered in the United States in the development of new technologies for cancer therapy (Dewhirst et al. 1993). This chapter is focused on major issues that need to be controlled and important questions that need to be addressed in the continued clinical testing of hyperthermia. Some of the concepts discussed are unique to the scientific-economic system that exists in the United States, but many of the concepts are also broadly applicable to conduct of hyperthermia clinical trials in any setting.

21.2 Historical and Economic Perspective

21.2.1 Historical Issues

Clinical testing of hyperthermia began in the late 1970s, largely based on rather compelling evidence from in vitro and in vivo murine studies that it might be a powerful adjuvant to radiation therapy (Dewey et al. 1977; Overgaard 1989). It became clear rather early that the treatment held promise. Perhaps the most compelling evidence for its efficacy were the results of a number of matched lesion studies that demonstrated enhanced response rates for heat combined with radiation compared to radiation alone (Overgaard 1985). The enthusiasm surrounding these trials resulted in rapid movement toward phase III testing. The first randomized human clinical trial, sponsored by the RTOG, was initiated in 1981 (RTOG 81-04). The intent of the trial was to compare the efficacy of radiation alone with that of hyperthermia plus radiation in the treatment of recurrent and/or locally advanced superficial lesions.

When the results of RTOG 81-04 were finally analyzed, there was *no demonstrated therapeutic benefit for hyperthermia* (PEREZ et al. 1989). However, initiation of this trial was premature. At the time that the trial was conceived there were no standards for quality assurance, no methods for writing or verifying a treatment prescription, and no methods to optimize hyperthermia treatment. Thermometry was very rudimentary and/or nonexistent, typically consisting of one or two measured points. In some patients no thermometry was performed at all. It was widely recognized then and now that temperatures are nonuniform and the use of a single thermometry point to describe the temperature distribution within the tumor volume and prescribe the whole heat treatment did not reflect the reality of how the treatment was actually being delivered. In the application of brachytherapy a radiation oncologist commonly will prescribe the dose to be delivered, relative to a certain margin around the implant volume, with the knowledge that all tissue within that volume is subjected to a higher dose than that prescribed at the margin. In addition, certain limits are usually followed regarding the range of doses to be accepted within the implant volume. It would be totally unacceptable to write a prescription based on an arbitrary point within the implant volume, rather than insisting on detailed knowledge of the three-dimensional radiation dose distribution. Yet so far common practice in hyperthermia has been to do just that.

21.2.2 Economic Constraints

The early matched lesion studies also stimulated considerable commercial interest. By 1984 there were at least a dozen companies worldwide that had entered into the production and testing of hyperthermia equipment. Commercialization was welcomed by the scientific community in the United States because it was generally perceived that Food and Drug Administration (FDA) approval of this modality would stimulate technology development as well as establish the modality as being reimbursable by insurance. It was believed that recovery of some of the cost of treatment by scientific investigators would further stimulate clinical testing of the modality. In retrospect, this strategy was ill-conceived and several devastating economic consequences of early FDA approval have greatly handicapped further development of the modality, at least in the United States. First, the equipment was inadequately designed to heat most tumors. Power deposition was not adequate, i.e., nonuniform across applicators, and generally only a small portion of any applicator emitted enough power to heat even small superficial tumors. Thermometers had been engineered to minimize interference with microwave fields, but there were far too few of them available with any commercial device to adequately sample the temperatures achieved in the heated tumor volume. Many clinicians (both in the private sector and in the academic community) who invested in this early technology quickly discovered that it was difficult to heat tumors with this equipment and abandoned the method. Subsequent lack of sales impeded additional equipment development from the commercial side. Adding to these problems, procedures for obtaining FDA premarket approval of these types of devices were very expensive and virtually eliminated any technology development once the prototypical devices made it through the system. In summary, *the premarket approval of prototypical commercial equipment was counterproductive*. Lagging sales and the cost of getting even these simple devices through the FDA virtually eliminated the further commercial development of the technology.

The approval of hyperthermia by the FDA backfired in terms of insurance reimbursement as well. In the USA, the Health Care Finance Administration (HCFA) sets policy regarding which medical procedures will be considered reimbursable by Medicare. Generally, private insurance companies follow those guidelines for their own reimbursement policies as well. As soon as premarket approval was gained, HCFA was petitioned to establish policy for reimbursement of hyperthermia treatment and it was approved for those tumors that were specifically included in the product labels (e.g., superficially accessible tumors that were recurrent or locally advanced, with or without prior radiotherapy). Reimbursement codes were recommended by the American College of Radiology and approved by the American Medical Association to establish means of payment. It was generally believed that this step would be an economic boon for hyperthermia and that significant technology development would shortly follow. The major block to this theory was that the fees were set too low to cover the costs of treatment. *Lack of adequate third-party reimbursement* limited enthusiasm for clinical use of hyperthermia, reduced sales, and resulted in stagnation in commercial development of the technology. In addition, modern standards for application and documentation of this technology are far more expensive than these early estimates anticipated and unfortunately, the likelihood that reimbursement fees will be upgraded are remote, particularly considering the current climate of containing escalating health costs in the United States and other Western countries.

One would like to believe that economic factors such as those discussed above would not have an impact on the conduct of human clinical trials, but unfortunately they do. The cost of conducting hyperthermia clinical trials is not insignificant, and successful conduct of human trials in the United States in the future will require careful pooling of institutional resources, third-party coverage, federal grant funds, and funds from private enterprise. *Sources of adequate funding to pay for future human clinical trials are of fundamental importance for the future development of hyperthermia and without such sources the scientific issues, which will be discussed below, become of moot importance.*

21.3 Scientific Issues

21.3.1 Quality Assurance Documents for Multi-institutional Trials

The failure of RTOG 81-04 to show a therapeutic benefit for hyperthermia was not necessarily a definitive proof of lack of treatment value for hyperthermia. As has been discussed by Perez et al. (1989), the trial was conducted *without proper safeguards for quality assurance* regarding patient selection procedures or documentation of treatment delivered. It is likely that the majority of patients received inadequate therapy, which reduced the probability of observing a therapeutic advantage in the overall patient group (Oleson et al. 1993). This assertion was supported by the observation that a therapeutic advantage was only observed in a subset of tumors that were <3 cm in diameter. The RTOG responded to this problem by commissioning the development of quality assurance documents that have set the standard for the use of hyperthermia in the United States. The first document which began this process was published in 1989 (Shrivastava 1989). Similar efforts were ongoing in Europe (Hand et al. 1989). More recent guidelines have been published as a result of the RTOG Hyperthermia Quality Assurance Task Force (Dewhirst et al. 1990; Emami et al. 1991; Sapozink et al. 1991; Waterman et al. 1991). These more recent documents present updated thinking about quality assurance, particularly in regard to thermometry and applicator selection. The clinical thermometry recommendations seen in the earlier RTOG publication (Shrivastava 1989) are not compatible with these newer recommendations. The recommendations for accuracy in temperature measurement, power meters, safety, measurement of power deposition (specific absorption rate, SAR), and general guidelines regarding the type of data needed for the conduct of hyperthermia trials remain valid, however. The newest documents served two purposes: (a) they established rules for application and treatment verification, and (b) they represented a consensus for the hyperthermia community. Thus, the *standards have become widely adopted* in the conduct of single-institution and multi-institutional studies.

The RTOG quality assurance documents covered the use of all known superficial applicator technologies, including microwave and ultrasound for superficial tumors, interstitial hyperthermia with microwave antennas, radiofrequency heating and hot source techniques, and hyperthermia for deep-seated tumors with annular phased arrays and capacitive radiofrequency. Guidelines for thermometry were relatively standardized across all heating technologies. Scanned focused and phased array ultrasound systems and multielement microwave devices were not specifically considered in these documents, and additional attention will need to be paid to them as they are more fully implemented into clinical testing. In the following discussion emphasis will be placed on superficial microwave applicators, for illustrative purposes. However, similar principles apply for any hyperthermia device. Comparisons between RTOG and European guidelines will be made.

21.3.1.1 Guidelines for Thermometry

Guidelines for thermometry for U.S. and European trials are quite similar (Table 21.1). First, there are specifications on accuracy and minimization of measurement artifact. Selection of proper thermometry is influenced by the type of heating device (e.g., fiberoptic or high-resistance thermistors for microwave vs thermocouples for ultrasound). Guidelines have also been established for how many measurements need to be made in tumors. In European Society of Hyperthermic Oncology (ESHO) trials, a minimum of three points (center, edge, and deep aspect) is required (HAND et al. 1989). In the United States, the guidelines are more stringent, requiring multipoint thermometers or thermal mapping within preplaced catheters (DEWHIRST et al. 1990). The RTOG guidelines were made more stringent because: (a) it was recognized that more than three points would be needed to adequately describe the true temperature distribution; and (b) because of the recognition that distortions in the estimate of the true temperature distribution will occur if catheter orientation strategies are not standardized (EDELSTEIN-KESHET et al. 1989). For bulky tumors, the RTOG guidelines specify that thermometry catheters cross the geometric center of a tumor (Figs. 21.1, 21.2), within certain tolerances.

Given the difficulty in determining tumor boundaries visually or by palpation, it has been recommended that thermometry catheter placement be verified with computerized tomography (CT), magnetic resonance imaging (MRI), or ultrasonography (US). ESHO also requires radiological verification of thermometry placement. The distance between measurements in catheters has been set by the RTOG to be between 0.5 and 1.0 cm (depending on tumor size) and a minimum of three thermometry catheters is required, except in the case of deep-seated tumors, where anatomical access may restrict the number of catheters to only one. The frequency of measurements for a given site has also been established. The RTOG requires a measurement

Table 21.1. Comparison of microwave quality assurance requirements, ESHO vs RTOG trials for superficial bulky (>1.5 cm depth) malignancies

Parameter	ESHO	RTOG
1. Thermometry		
a) Characteristics		
Nonperturbing	Yes	Yes
Accuracy	±0.2°C	±0.2°C
Calibrate vs traceable standard	Yes	Yes
Good thermal contact with tissue	Yes	Yes
b) Use in clinic		
Measurement frequency	Every min	Every 10 min
No. of points in tumor	3 points (multipoint catheter recommended)	3 catheters, many points/catheter (required)
Position verification	CT, US recommended	CT, US, MRI required
Position requirements	Center, edge, deep base	Geometrical catheter orientation (Figs. 21.1, 21.2)
2. Applicators		
a) Characterization		
Applicator/bolus is single unit	Yes	Yes
Determine SAR of each unit	Yes	Yes
SAR characteristics	Effective field size (EFS)[a] Penetration depth (PD)[a]	25% iso-SAR relative to max SAR in Phantom
b) Applicator selection	Tumor margin covered by EFS and PD	Tumor margin covered by 25% iso-SAR line

[a] Effective field size = 50% iso-SAR contour at 1 cm depth, in muscle phantom; penetration depth = distance below 1 cm depth in phantom at which SAR is at least 50% of 50% iso-SAR at 1 cm depth

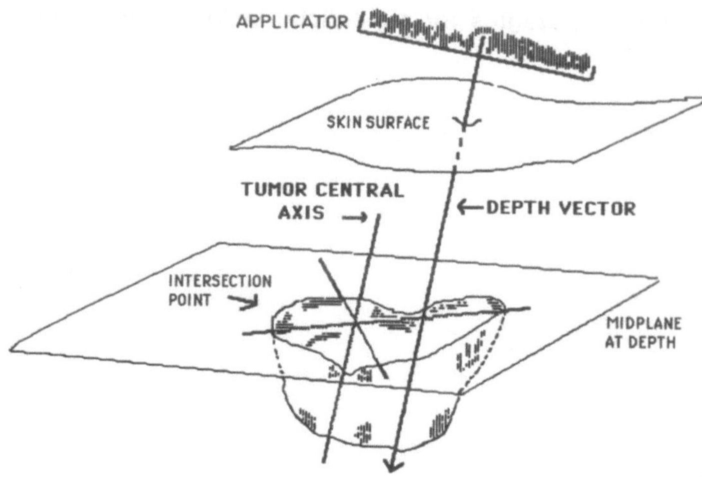

a

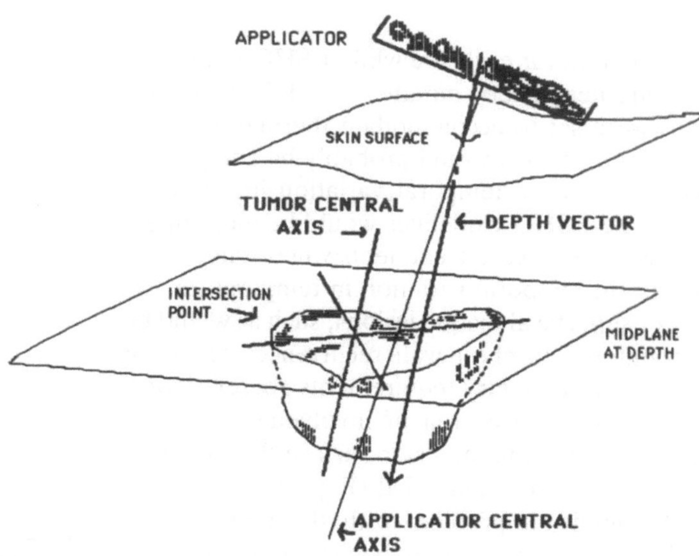

b

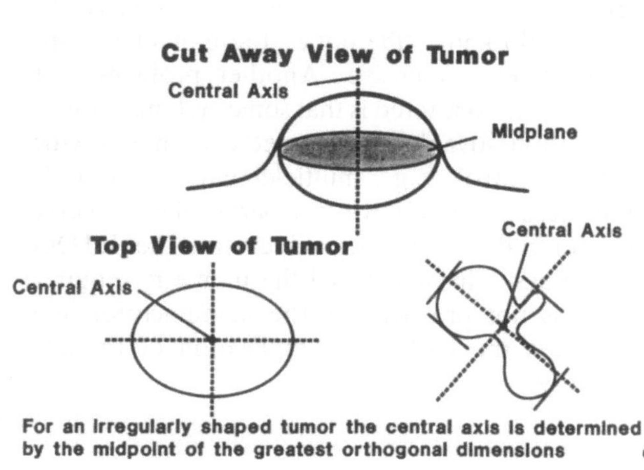

c

Fig. 21.1a–c. Descriptive terms for tumor geometry. These features are used to identify the orientation of thermometry catheters. The features are independent of the applicator position. The goal of this geometric strategy is to devise an applicator-independent, but tumor shape- and size-dependent, means of introducing thermometry catheters. The *midplane at depth* is an imaginary plane perpendicular to and bisecting the tumor dimension along the depth vector (defined below). The *tumor central axis* is a line traversing the tumor in its greatest lateral orthogonal dimensions perpendicular to the midplane and parallel or coincident with the depth vector. An *intersection point* is that point at which two catheters cross or are in close proximity to each other. The *depth vector* is a vector pointing normal to the skin surface at the point of intersection of the surface and the applicator central axis and extending to the greatest depth of the tumor. The *applicator central axis* may not be parallel with the depth vector if the applicator is not coplanar with the tissue surface (see **b**). (From DEWHIRST et al. 1990)

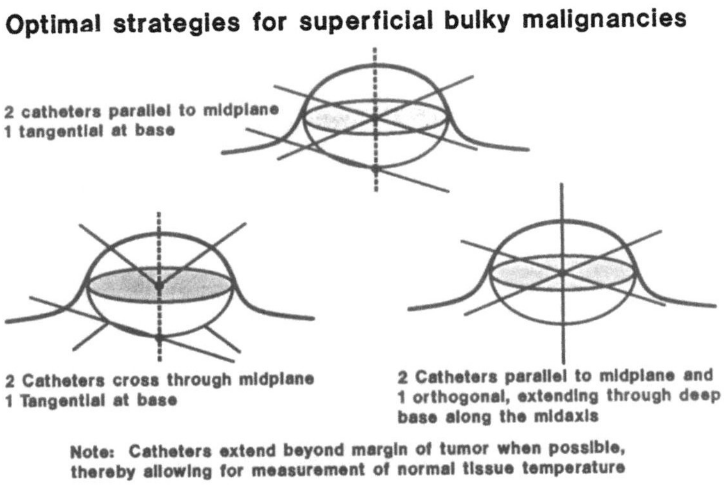

Fig. 21.2. The goal of catheter orientation is to have an intersection point of two catheters in close proximity to the intersection between the tumor central axis and the midplane at depth. A third catheter can be used to measure temperature at the greatest depth of the tumor. (From DEWHIRST et al. 1990)

every 10 min for each site while ESHO requires a measurement every minute. The RTOG guidelines were set to accommodate thermal mapping techniques, which would probably be adequate if there were little temporal variation in temperature. The ESHO guidelines would be more likely to accurately record treatments where there were significant temporal variation in temperature.

For superficial plaque lesions, such as would be encountered in chest wall recurrences of breast cancer, thermometry requirements are set according to the surface area of involvement. In this case, subcutaneous and skin surface thermometry catheters are recommended (Fig. 21.3).

A significant problem with the RTOG thermometry requirements has been that thermometry systems that can comply with the regulations are not readily available commercially. Only one commercial thermal mapping system is available (BSD Corporation, Salt Lake City, Utah, USA) and multipoint fiberoptic thermometers are prohibitively expensive. Another problem that has been encountered is that some systems require static (nonmovable) thermometers for multisector power control (e.g., multielement ultrasound). For these types of devices separate thermometry is required to be compatible with the RTOG guidelines. This additional thermometry requirement is not provided by the manufacturer and increases the cost and complication of therapy delivery.

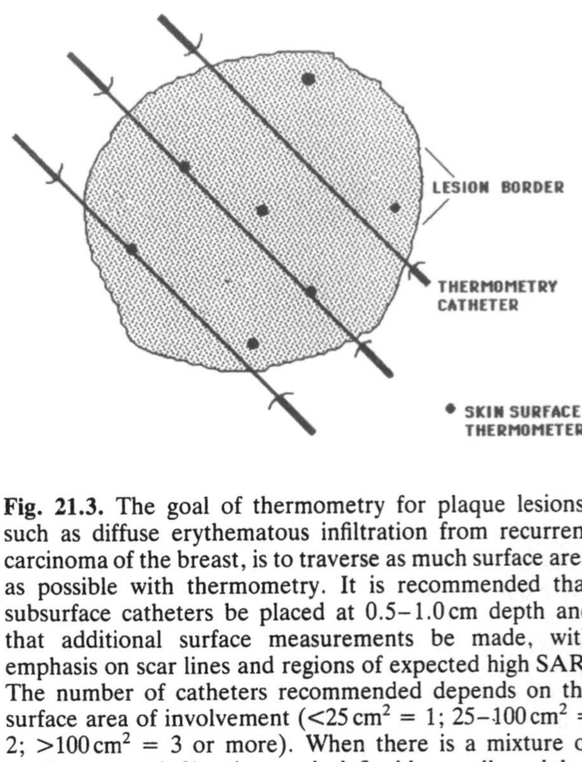

Fig. 21.3. The goal of thermometry for plaque lesions, such as diffuse erythematous infiltration from recurrent carcinoma of the breast, is to traverse as much surface area as possible with thermometry. It is recommended that subsurface catheters be placed at 0.5–1.0 cm depth and that additional surface measurements be made, with emphasis on scar lines and regions of expected high SAR. The number of catheters recommended depends on the surface area of involvement ($<25\,cm^2 = 1$; $25–100\,cm^2 = 2$; $>100\,cm^2 = 3$ or more). When there is a mixture of erythematous infiltration and definable small nodules, then the catheters should traverse beneath as many of the nodules as possible. (From DEWHIRST et al. 1990)

21.3.1.2 Guidelines for Applicator Selection

It is important to choose an applicator that has power deposition (SAR) patterns that are large enough to cover the entire tumor volume. An important contribution made by the Hyperthermia

Physics Quality Assurance Contract Group [funded by the National Cancer Institute (NCI)] as well as others was the observation that the performance of various commercial hyperthermia applicatiors varied significantly, even for the same device. Thus, both RTOG and ESHO guidelines require that all applicators be tested prior to use in the clinic. An additional problem with microwave applicators was the fact that the size of the usable SAR pattern was small relative to the size of the applicator and the usable dimension became even smaller with depth. For microwave applicators the SAR pattern was strongly influenced by the thickness and characteristics of the coupling bolus. In order to control for these problems it was recommended that the power deposition pattern of each applicator/bolus unit be measured in a standard phantom. The resultant data would be used to establish the largest tumor that could be treated with that applicator/bolus system. The current RTOG recommendation is that the tumor margin must be covered by at least the 25% of maximum iso-SAR. Similar requirements are made for the ESHO trials. Methods to easily select applicator/bolus systems for a given tumor were developed by the RTOG, based on the measured phantom data (Fig. 21.4). The aforementioned requirement meant that a procedure for measuring applicator SAR patterns had to be established that could be either used at each participating institution or at a centralized testing facility.

21.3.1.3 Treatment Documentation

Quality assurance (QA) also includes the accurate documentation and recording of all pertinent patient selection and treatment data. The RTOG recommended that multi-institutional trials have *quality assurance officers* who could assist in assuring compliance by examining patient selection

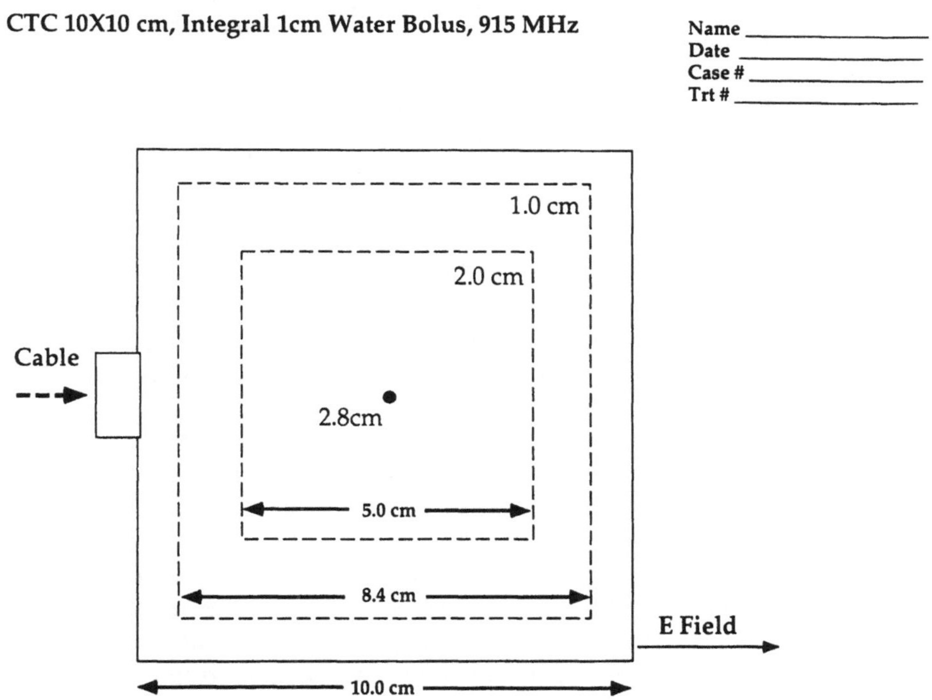

Fig. 21.4. Applicator/bolus transparency overlay for treatment documentation. This type of diagram can be drawn to scale for any applicator/bolus combination for which the SAR patterns are characterized and copied onto transparent sheets. The *solid line* represents the physical dimensions of the applicator housing. The *inner dashed lines* approximate the shape of the 25% of maximum iso-SAR lines at 1.0, 2.0, and 2.8 cm depth. In order to be within RTOG guidelines, a tumor treated with this device cannot be larger than 8.4 cm diameter at 1.0 cm depth and 5.0 cm diameter at 2 cm depth, and cannot be deeper than 2.8 cm. The transparent version of this diagram can be used to document the treatment setup, including the dimensions of the tumor at the surface, position of skin surface thermometers, presence of ulcers or scar lines, and entry point and trajectory of thermometry catheters. Documentation can easily be made by placing the transparency over the treatment field and marking the appropriate information on the sheet

documents and treatment data. In addition, regular QA checks would be performed on data from participating centers to check for missing data and noncompliance problems.

It was recognized that this level of QA would be substantial and that any multi-institutional trial would need substantial monetary support for a QA and data management center as well as support for QA at individual participating institutions. Any efforts that could be made up-front to reduce the level of complexity in QA would result in better compliance and accuracy in data recording as well as considerable cost and time savings. An important problem that was encountered in this regard was that the type of data required to be recorded by the commercial devices in order for them to be operated was not what was needed for the clinical trials. Furthermore, most institutions participating in such trials already had their own databases and there was understandable reluctance to abandon the institutional database for one that they were not familiar with. In addition, there would be considerable overlap between what was already being recorded at each institution and what was required by protocol. To this end, a *hyperthermia data file standard* was developed that allowed for conversion of single institution databases or commercial device treatment data to a standard format for transfer to a data processing center (SAPARETO and CORRY 1989). A PC-based program was developed that would assist the operator in identifying missing data and in accurately recording treatment data required by protocol. The database can be adapted for the specific requirements of any protocol. A second part of the solution has been the development of a universal operating system that would be compatible with all hyperthermia systems (Corry, personal communication). This type of system would allow for universality in control system software, such that all systems would appear the same to the operator at the treatment console. Another cost savings measure that was adopted was to reduce the amount of hand recording of treatment data. An earlier attempt to establish QA for treatment documentation required very detailed recording of treatment and thermometry parameters, such as orientation of applicator relative to a patient coordinate system, thickness of bolus, etc. (SHRIVASTAVA 1989). The more recent standards are more easily documented, since the selection of applicator/bolus combinations and methods for thermometry are standardized. Such standardization allows for the use of visual documentation methods rather than detailed recording of this type of setup data.

21.3.1.4 Quality Assurance Training

A final strategy that was adopted by the RTOG was the initiation of training sessions. In these sessions, hands-on demonstrations were used to teach individuals involved in the actual performance of treatment how to record important data, comply with thermometry standards, select appropriate hyperthermia applicators, etc. The training sessions were required even for institutions with considerable experience since prior experience would not necessarily qualify a participant to be familiar with the specific requirements of the multi-institutional protocol. These efforts required up-front funds to pay for travel of participants to the training center, but it was reasoned that the investment would pay for itself in terms of reducing inaccuracies in patient selection, data recording, and noncompliance. It was found that even personnel who had been practicing hyperthermia for many years benefited from these training sessions. An organizational diagram demonstrating how QA procedures could be implemented for multi-institutional studies is shown in Fig. 21.5.

21.3.1.5 Standardization in Prescription Writing and Data Reporting

A final issue that desperately needs standardization is in the prescription and reporting of clinical thermometry data. An examination of any two papers on hyperthermia will reveal every possible combination of thermal parameters to describe the treatment delivered. Even more confusing is the fact that the same terms are often used to describe parameters that are derived dissimilarly from the database. *It is the contention of this author that standards for prescription writing and data reporting should be agreed upon by the international hyperthermia community and that the parameters chosen should be those that have been shown to consistently carry prognostic significance in terms of antitumor effect or in terms of predicting normal tissue tolerance*. Examples of appropriate descriptors of tumor data would include T_{min}, cumulative minutes T_{90} exceeding a threshold temperature, and the cumulative T_{90} converted to equivalent minutes at a standard temperature, such as 43°C.

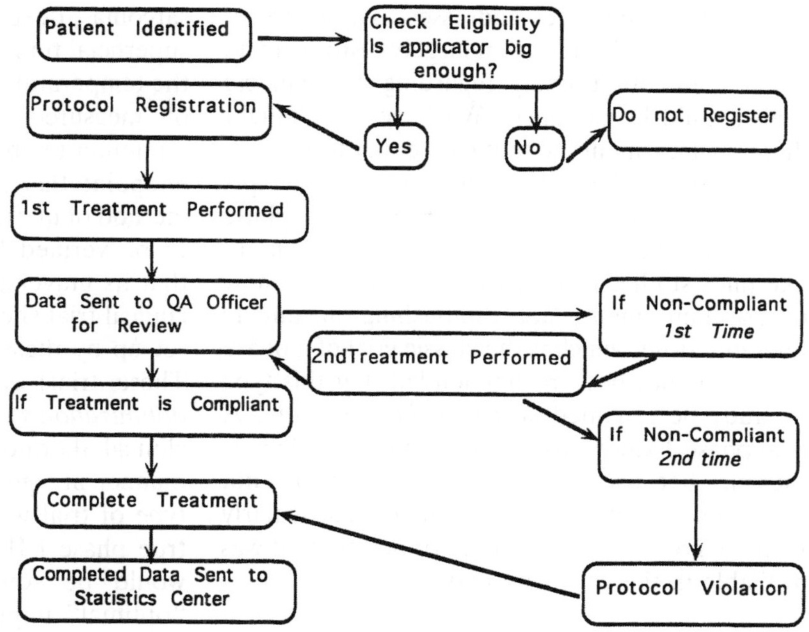

Fig. 21.5. Schema for QA implementation in multi-institutional trials. This schema was adopted by the RTOG Hyperthermia Quality Assurance Task Force. It allows for feedback from the QA officer to the participating institution to verity that essential QA features of a given trial are being followed for each patient. QA features that would be checked include choice of proper applicator/bolus unit (based on SAR coverage of tumor volume), thermometry coverage of treatment area (catheter orientation and number and location of surface probes), etc.

Treatment prescriptions should be written to reflect actual practice and not an unattainable or unquantifiable goal. For example, a typical treatment prescription that specifies that all temperature sensors exceed 43°C for 1 h is a totally unachievable goal and does not reflect actual practice. Alternatively, a treatment prescription that states that 90% of all measured points exceed 41.5°C is an achievable goal that carries prognostic significance (OLESON et al. 1993).

All manuscripts that are submitted should include at least the agreed upon set of parameters, although additional ones could be added at the discretion of the authors as long as they are completely and unambiguously described. This issue is described more fully in Chap. 6 in volume 1.

21.3.2 Questions That Need to Be Asked in Hyperthermia Clinical Trials

21.3.2.1 Restructuring Clinical Trial Designs for Hyperthermia

Once all of the above-described QA is in place, the obvious question that needs to be asked is what types of trials need to be conducted? In a recent position statement, the Intersociety Council on Radiation Oncology posed this question and some answers regarding the future for clinical trials of hyperthermia and radiation (DEWHIRST et al. 1993). The basic premise of that essay was the belief that the most important issue facing the ultimate test of hyperthermia in a randomized clinical trial is to first demonstrate that the majority of patients in the hyperthermia arm of the study will receive *the best hyperthermia treatment that is possible*. If this goal is not achieved, the likelihood that a significant difference will be observed in a randomized study between thermoradiotherapy and radiotherapy is prohibitively diminished (OLESON et al. 1993). In order to make such a determination, it is necessary to understand how to unambiguously and quantitatively measure the "dose" of hyperthermia that is delivered. This capability will allow us to write a *quantitative and verifiable prescription for hyperthermia*.

21.3.2.2 Device Evaluation Studies

Unfortunately, the goal of understanding how to quantitate or prescribe hyperthermic treatment has usually not been an important goal in clinical studies, and in fact has often been ignored completely or has only been addressed as a side issue. The reason for this has been largely historical and is based on our training regarding how clinical trials should be designed. We have been taught that new treatment modalities are first tested in a phase I study. Many of us called our first attempts to use prototypical hyperthermia equipment phase I studies, when in fact those studies were more like pilot studies in which we were learning how to use equipment, not establishing maximally tolerated dose, which is the classic goal of a phase I study. It has been recommended that this type of study be renamed *device evaluation study*. A true phase I study has never been done in hyperthermia because until recently we could not accurately quantitate the treatment, particularly with the grossly inadequate thermometry that was available in the early and middle 1980s.

21.3.2.3 Thermal Dosimetric Evaluation Studies

In spite of a lack of real phase I data, a number of institutions moved into what has been called phase II testing. Classically, phase II testing utilizes the maximally tolerated dose and looks to establish response. What many investigators have been doing, however, is examining the relation between some measure of temperatures achieved and treatment outcome. This is not a phase II study, and it has been suggested that these studies be renamed *thermal dosimetric evaluation studies*.

21.3.2.4 Thermal Dosimetric Optimization Studies

Recent advances in our ability to interpret thermometry data have placed us in the position of being able to prescribe how to deliver optimal hyperthermia treatment. The concept involves using a descriptor of the measured temperature distribution, most commonly the 10th percentile, or T_{90}, or the 50th percentile, or T_{50}. The validity of the descriptor is dependent upon following rigorous QA in thermometry, as defined by the RTOG, and more than three measured points per tumor are needed to perform this type of analysis (preferably 10–20 points). In a recent analysis of temperature distribution data, OLESON and coworkers (1993) demonstrated that the T_{90} descriptor is strongly and consistently correlated with treatment outcome for patients with soft tissue sarcomas, deep-seated lesions, and miscellaneous superficial tumor sites. This method of describing the temperature distribution is superior to the use of measured temperature minimum, because minimum temperature is a statistically ill-defined endpoint that cannot be easily identified. This method of quantitating treatment delivered needs to be verified by other investigators, but given that its universality can be determined, the next clinical trial should test whether the thermal goal set up by these previous trials can be achieved. These trials can be called *thermal dosimetric optimization studies*. More specific details on how clinical thermometry data are analyzed in this manner are given in Chap. 6 in volume 1. This type of trial would be somewhat analogous to a true phase I-II study, since the optimal therapy would be sought in all patients. The term "optimal" implies that the therapy delivered is maximally tolerable, and the response rate would be that predicted from the dosimetric evaluation studies outlined above. For example, it can be seen in Fig. 21.6 that a T_{90} of at least 10 cumulative equivalent minutes at 43°C (for one treatment of heat per week) is needed to increase the probability for response from 10% to 50% for patients with soft tissue sarcomas.

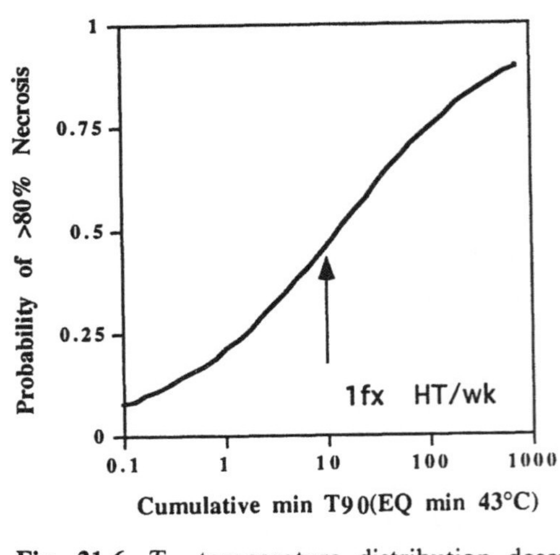

Fig. 21.6. T_{90} temperature distribution descriptor converted to equivalent minutes at 43°C. In this analysis, a T_{90} was calculated for each minute of treatment and the resulting temperature was converted to equivalent minutes at 43°C, using the formulation developed by SAPARETO and DEWEY (1984). The advantage of this method of presentation of the data is that it combines both temperature and time, allowing for performance of sensitivity analyses relating to optimization of therapy. Data based on analyses previously published (OLESON et al. 1993)

Separate analysis demonstrated that the achievement of this thermal goal was not associated with increased risk of normal tissue complications. A thermal dosimetric optimization study would test the hypothesis that the response rate in an equivalent group of patients would be at least 50%, if the target T_{90} of 10 cumulative equivalent minutes at 43°C were achieved in the majority of the group. It would also verify that this response rate could be achieved without high risk for complications.

21.3.2.5 Phase III Studies

It is recommended that *phase III studies* be initiated only after methods are developed that allow for optimal treatment of the majority of tumors of a selected type. Sites for which adequate technology currently exists to achieve T_{90}s >40.5°–41.0°C may include glioblastoma multiforme and pelvic tumors treated with *interstitial heating methods* and recurrent chest wall lesions treated with *multielement arrays*. Dosimetric optimization studies have yet to be reported for any of these sites, however.

21.4 Conclusions

Throughout the text of this chapter there are numerous references to problems that have been encountered in the conduct of clinical trials over the past 15 years. These comments should not be interpreted as reflecting a lack of enthusiasm about the future role for hyperthermia as an effective treatment modality. As with all new science, mistakes will be made along the way. Those scientists who learn from the mistakes are the ones most likely to succeed in the long run. It is my belief that the hyperthermia community has learned from its mistakes and that progress has been and will continue to be made.

The advent of clinically verifiable methods for writing treatment prescriptions for hyperthermia, as has been presented (OLESON et al. 1993), indicates that we have an unprecedented opportunity to move forward with the rational development of technologies and strategies for optimizing hyperthermia therapy. These analyses set the standard for equipment performance, establish how to deliver effective therapy (i.e., set standards of practice), and ultimately may have some impact on reimbursement for treatment. The ability to write a hyperthermia treatment prescription is as important to establishing the legitimacy of hyperthermia as the development of a radiation dose unit was for the development of radiation therapy. The technological and methodological tools to move from patient pain as the thermometer to an identifiable dosimetry is analogous to moving from erythema dose to the rad in radiation therapy and maximizes our opportunities to perform adequate tests of its value as an effective treatment modality.

21.5 Summary

- Factors that detracted from the success of early Phase III trials in the United Sates to compare the efficacy of thermoradiotherapy to radiotherapy alone
  - Lack of adequate quality assurance for thermometry, applicatory selection, equipment performance.
  - Inadequate financial support for conduct of necessary clinical trials
  - Financial pressure from vendors to conduct proof-of-efficacy trials to establish third-party reimbursement
- Establishment of quality assurance measures by Radiation Oncology Therapy Group and European Society for Hyperthermic Oncology
  - Equipment performance criteria
  - Rules for acquisition of thermometric data
  - Rules for hyperthermia device selection
  - Mechanisms for assurance of accuracy in data recording and patient selection
  - Standards for computerized data acquisition
- New concepts in hyperthermia clinical trial design
  - Trials in which new devices are being evaluated should be called Device Evaluation Studies, not Phase I trials.
  - Trials in which the relationship between measured temperatures and treatment outcome is sought should be called dosimetric evaluation trials, not Phase II studies.
  - Current trials should focus on dose optimization studies (analogous to traditional Phase I-II studies), which will determine whether an optimal thermal dose, as established from dosimetric evaluation trials, can be achieved in the majority of patients.

- Future Directions
  - There is a need to establish world-wide consensus on standardization of thermal dosimetry reporting.
  - New Phase III trials should await results of dose optimization studies so that "best" hyperthermia therapy can be offered to all patients enrolled on trial.

References

Dewey WC, Hopwood LE, Sapareto SA, Gerweck LE (1977) Cellular responses to combinations of hyperthermia and radiation. Radiology 123: 463–474

Dewhirst MW, Sim DA, Grochowski KJ (1984) Thermal influence on radiation induced complications vs tumor response in a phase II randomized trial. In: Overgaard J (ed) Hyperthermic oncology. Taylor and Francis, London, pp 313–316

Dewhirst MW, Phillips TL, Samulski TV et al. (1990) RTOG quality assurance guidelines for clinical trials using hyperthermia. Int J Radiat Oncol Biol Phys 18: 1249–1259

Dewhirst MW, Griffin TW, Smith AR, Parker RG, Hanks GE, Brady LW (1993) Intersociety Council on Radiation Oncology essay on the introduction of new medical treatments into practice. J Natl Cancer Inst 85: 951–957

Edelstein-Keshet L, Dewhirst MW, Oleson JR, Samulski TV (1989) Characterization of tumour temperature distributions in hyperthermia based on assumed mathematical forms. Int J Hyperthermia 5: 757–777

Emami B, Stauffer P, Dewhirst MW et al. (1991) RTOG quality assurance guidelines for interstitial hyperthermia. Int J Radiat Oncol Biol Phys 20: 1117–1124

Gillette EL. McChesney SL, Dewhirst MW, Scott RJ (1987) Response of canine oral carcinomas to heat and radiation. Int J Radiat Oncol Biol Phys 13: 1816–1867

Gillette-McChesney S, Dewhirst MW, Gilette EL et al. (1992) Response of canine soft tissue sarcomas to radiation or radiation plus hyperthermia: a randomized phase II study. Int J Hypperthermia 8: 309–320

Hand JW, Logenclijk JJ, Bach Andersen J, Bolomey JC (1989) Quality assurance guidelines for ESHO protocols. Int J Hyperthermia 5: 421–428

Leopold KA, Harelson J, Prosnitz L, Samulski TV, Dewhirst MW, Oleson JR (1989) Preoperative hyperthermia and radiation for soft tissue sarcomas: advantage of two vs one hyperthermia treatments per week. Int J Radiat Oncol Biol Phys 16: 107–115

Leopold KA, Dewhirst MW, Samulski TV et al. (1992) Relationships among tumor temperature, treatment time and histopathological outcome using preoperative hyperthermia with radiation in soft tissue sarcomas. Int J Radiat Oncol Biol Phys 22: 989–998

Leopold KA, Dewhirst MW, Samulski TV et al. (1993) Cumulative minutes with T_{90} greater than $TEMP_{index}$ is predictive of response of superficial malignancies to hyperthermia and radiation. Int J Radiat Oncol Biol Phys 25: 841–847

Oleson JR, Dewhirst MW, Harrelson JM, Leopold KA, Samulski TV, Tso CY (1989) Tumor temperature distributions predict hyperthermia effect. Int J Radiat Oncol Biol Phys 16: 559–570

Oleson JR, Samulski TV, Leopold KA et al. (1993) Sensitivity of hyperthermia trial outcomes to temperature and time: implications for thermal goals of treatment. Int J Radiat Oncol Biol Phys 25: 289–297

Overgaard J (1985) Rationale and problems in the design of clinical studies. In: Overgaard J (ed) Hyperthermic oncology 1984. Taylor & Francis, London, pp 325–338

Overgaard J (1989) The current and potential role of hyperthermia in radiotherapy. Int J Radiat Oncol Biol Phys 16: 535–549

Perez CA, Gillespie B, Pajak T, Hornback NB, Emami B, Rubin P (1989) Quality assurance problems in clinical hyperthermia and their impact on therapeutic outcome: a report by the Radiation Therapy Oncology Group. Int J Radiat Oncol Biol Phys 16: 537–558

Sapareto SA, Corry PM (1989) A proposed standard data file format for hyperthermia treatments. Int J Radiat Oncol Biol Phys 16: 613–627

Sapareto SA, Dewey WC (1984) Thermal dose determination in cancer therapy. Int J Radiat Oncol Biol Phys 10: 787–800

Sapozink MD, Corry PM, Kapp DS et al. (1991) RTOG quality assurance guidelines for clinical trials using hyperthermia for deep seated malignancy. Int J Radiat Oncol Biol Phys 20: 1109–1115

Shrivastava P (1989) Hyperthermia quality assurance guidelines. Int J Radiat Oncol Biol Phys 16: 571–587

Waterman FM, Dewhirst MW, Fessenclen P et al. (1991) RTOG quality assurance guidelines for clinical trials using hyperthermia administered by ultrasound. Int J Radiat Oncol Biol Phys 20: 1099–1107

22 Review of Biostatistical Methods and Interpretation of Hyperthermia Clinical Trials

D. MACHIN and J. WHALEY

CONTENTS

22.1 Introduction

Chapter 21 has reviewed topics connected with the design requirements for hyperthermia clinical trials. The object of this chapter is to review some of the *statistical methodology* required to assist in the interpretation of such trials. Emphasis is given to estimation of measures of the relative effect of the treatments under comparison in a (randomised) trial together with associated confidence intervals. We describe how these can be calculated for situations where it is relevant to compare two proportions and we describe in some detail how this is adapted when comparisons have to be adjusted for variables which describe prognostic characteristics of the patients. We point out that it is usually more efficient (statistically) to record, for example, the exact time that a complete remission has occurred following commencement of treatment, rather than noting its presence or absence at a particular fixed time point. This approach permits survival time comparisons to be made between patient groups. We also use specific clinical examples to focus the discussion.

D. MACHIN, PhD, Medical Research Council Cancer Trials Office, 5 Shaftesbury Road, Cambridge, CB2 2BW, UK

J. WHALEY, BVM&S, Medical Research Council Cancer Trials Office, 5 Shaftesbury Road, Cambridge, CB2 2BW, UK

22.2 Example of a Randomised Trial

The Radiation Therapy Oncology Group (RTOG) report a randomised phase III trial comparing irradiation and hyperthermia with irradiation alone in superficial measurable tumours (PEREZ et al. 1991). The design of this trial is summarised in Fig. 22.1. Thus, all eligible patients receive 8 × 4 Gy fractions of radiotherapy and those randomised to hyperthermia receive their heat treatment immediately after each fraction of radiotherapy. A complete response (CR) is defined as the complete disappearance of all tumour at the treated site and the time to CR is measured from start of treatment.

In this trial 307 patients were randomised, 250 with single lesions and 57 with multiple lesions. The analysis reported (and the one we will use for illustration) concerns 236 patients with single lesions and Table 22.1 summarises the CR rates observed by treatment group, site and size of tumour.

22.3 Estimating Response Rates

Suppose for the moment we confine our attention to head and neck patients in Table 22.1 whose tumours were greater than 3 cm and who had received radiotherapy alone as treatment. The proportion of CRs in this subgroup is estimated by $P = 14/46 = 0.3043$ or 30%. To assess the reliability of P we need to calculate a confidence interval (CI) for the CR. Loosely speaking, a 95% CI establishes a plausible range of values for the (true) population value of the CR although there remains a 1 in 20 (5%) chance that the real

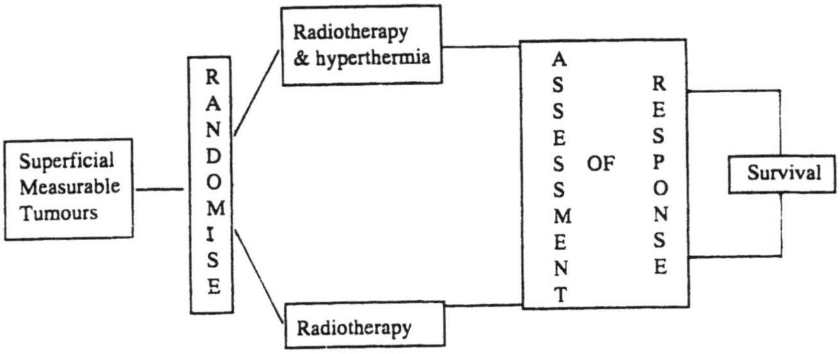

Fig. 22.1. Design of a randomised phase III trial to evaluate the addition of hyperthermia to radiotherapy (after PEREZ et al. 1991)

Table 22.1. Observed complete response (CR) rate by treatment, site and tumour size and associated exact 95% confidence intervals (data from PEREZ et al. 1991)

Site	Size	Treatment	Number of patients with			CR rate P% (R/N)	95% CI*
			CR R	No CR N-R	Total N		
Head and neck	<3 cm	Radiotherapy	7	7	14	50.00	23.04–76.96
	<3 cm	Radiotherapy + hyperthermia	3	5	8	37.50	8.52–75.51
	>3 cm	Radiotherapy	**14**	**32**	46	30.43	17.74–45.75
	>3 cm	Radiotherapy + hyperthermia	**15**	**30**	45	33.33	20.00–48.95
Breast and chest wall	<3 cm	Radiotherapy	4	6	10	40.00	12.16–73.76
	<3 cm	Radiotherapy + hyperthermia	8	5	13	61.54	31.58–86.14
	>3 cm	Radiotherapy	8	21	29	27.59	12.73–47.24
	>3 cm	Radiotherapy	6	23	29	20.69	7.99–39.72
Trunk and extremities	<3 cm	Radiotherapy	0	4	4	00.00	0.00–60.24
	<3 cm	Radiotherapy + hyperthermia	4	2	6	66.67	22.28–95.67
	>3 cm	Radiotherapy	2	12	14	14.29	1.78–42.81
	>3 cm	Radiotherapy + hyperthermia	2	16	18	11.11	1.38–34.71
All sites and sizes		Radiotherapy	35	82	117	29.91	
		Radiotherapy + hyperthermia	38	81	119	31.93	
All patients			73	163	236		

* Exact CI, not that calculated following the method described in Sect. 22.3

value falls outside this range. The true or population CR could only be determined if *all* the patients with this disease were treated with the same radiotherapy schedule and their response assessed. A more careful and detailed definition of a CI is given by GARDNER and ALTMAN (1989).

The expression for an approximate 95% CI for P is:

$$P - 1.96 \times SE(P) \text{ to } P + 1.96 \times SE(P), \quad (22.1)$$

where $SE(P) = [P(1 - P)/N]^{1/2}$, is the estimated standard error (SE) of the CR rate and N is the sample size, that is, the number of patients in the particular group (see Table 22.1).

The SE for the head and neck patients who received radiotherapy alone with tumours greater than 3 cm is therefore, $SE(P) = (0.3043 \times 0.6957/46)^{1/2} = (0.004602)^{1/2} = 0.0678$. Hence the 95% CI for the CR rate is:

$$0.3043 - (1.96 \times 0.0678) \text{ to } 0.3043 + (1.96 \times 0.0678),$$

or from 0.1713 (17%) to 0.4373 (44%).

Thus, despite the fact that this group of patients is the largest group in Table 22.1, there remains considerable uncertainty concerning the true CR rate to radiotherapy alone in such patients. For example, this CI is not inconsistent with a CR rate of 20%. Neither is it inconsistent with a CR rate as high as 40%. There is even more uncertainty with respect to the true CR rates in the smaller patient subgroups.

It is worth noting that as the number of patients in the group, N, increases, the SE decreases and consequently the width of the CI decreases. One method of determining the appropriate study size is to specify the width of the CI in advance, using a reasoned guess for P the CR rate. Using this given width one can then back-calculate to obtain a value for N. This provides a guide to the appropriate number of patients required when discussing all aspects of the projected design of the trial.

It has become something of a convention to calculate 95% CIs rather than, say, 99% CIs, but it is *only* a convention. If a 99% CI is required, all that is necessary is to change the 1.96 in the expression above to 2.58, then it is always wider than the corresponding 95% CI because this change increases the chance of this range including the true (population) value. For the head and neck patients with tumours greater than 3 cm the 99% CI is 0.1294 to 0.4792 or 13% to 48%.

The expression used for the CI is really only applicable if N, the size of the group, is reasonably large and its use would not be advisable with $N < 10$. However, CIs can be calculated for small groups but by using special tables of the binomial probabilities, for example, those in Geigy Scientific Tables (1991), volume 2, pp 89–102. Thus, for the eight head and neck patients with tumours <3 cm receiving radiotherapy and hyperthermia, of whom three responded to give an estimated CR rate $P = 0.375$ (38%), the exact 95% CI is 8.52–75.51 or 9%–76%. For the four patients in the trunk/extremities <3 cm tumours subgroup receiving radiotherapy alone no CRs were observed and the tables give the 95% CI as 0%–60.24%. This suggests that we cannot exclude the possibility of a CR rate of as high as 60% for this group. The CIs given in Table 22.1 are those extracted from the above statistical tables. They are quoted to 2 decimal places to facilitate comparisons with the corresponding tabular entry. It is worth noting that, in contrast to the CIs calculated using Eq. 22.1, these exact CIs are not symmetric about P. This will always be the case unless $P = 0.5$ precisely.

22.4 Treatment Comparisons of Response Rates

There is a presumption in the Perez et al. (1991) trial, and in many other trials, that site and lesion size could affect prognosis and CR rates and that is why they are reported separately. If this is indeed the case, then random allocation to treatment should take these prognostic (stratifying) variables into account. This would ensure that approximately equal numbers of patients in each group would receive the two therapies. In Table 22.1 there is good balance between these therapies within the larger lesion sites, where there are also more patients, but more disparity in the smaller lesion groups, which also have few patients. The published report of the trial indicates that stratification for type, histology, size and site of lesion was included in the randomisation process. The imbalance of numbers may be accounted for by the exclusion from the published analysis of all patients with multiple lesions, and, for a variety of reasons, of 14 of the 250 remaining patients.

In order to make sensible treatment comparisons it is important to *compare "like patients" with "like patients" who differ only in the randomised therapy allocated*. Thus in Table 22.1 we can compare radiotherapy alone and radiotherapy with the addition of hyperthermia in, for example, the group of head and neck patients with lesions >3 cm. (We make some comment on subgroup analysis later, when we also describe a combined analysis of all the data of Table 22.1.) The CR rate observed for those patients receiving radiotherapy followed by hyperthermia in this patient subgroup is $P_{RTH} = 15/45 = 0.3333$ and, for those not receiving hyperthermia, $P_{RT} = 14/46 = 0.3043$, as we have previously observed. To estimate the value of hyperthermia following radiotherapy, it is necessary to calculate the difference in CR rates given by $d = P_{RTH} - P_{RT} = 0.3333 - 0.3043 = 0.0290$ or 2.9%. If there is no effect of hyperthermia in addition to that given by radiotherapy alone then we would expect the value of d to be zero. Although here we observe a small benefit for hyperthermia of almost 3%, we need to be satisfied that this is not merely a random departure from a (true) zero difference if we are to make even modest claims for the addition of hyperthermia to this modality. To assess the reliability of d we require the associated CI. This has a similar structure to that for P given by Eq. 22.1. It is:

$$d - 1.96 \times SE(d) \text{ to } d + 1.96 \times SE(d), \quad (22.2)$$

where $SE(d) = \{P_{RTH}(1 - P_{RTH})/N_{RTH} + P_{RT}(1 - P_{RT})/N_{RT}\}^{1/2}$.

For our example, $SE(d) = \{(0.3333 \times 0.6667/45) + (0.3043 \times 0.6957/46)\}^{1/2} = (0.009540)^{1/2} = 0.0977$. Thus the 95% CI for d is:

$$0.0290 - (1.96 \times 0.0977) = -0.1625 \text{ to}$$
$$0.0290 + (1.96 \times 0.0977) = +0.2205, \text{ or}$$
$$-16\% \text{ to } +22\%.$$

In view of this wide interval there remains considerable uncertainty about the value of the addition of hyperthermia since, as the CI of the difference is, for example, consistent with both an advantage for, and a disadvantage to, hyperthermia of 15%.

22.5 Odds Ratio

We have indicated in the above that it is necessary to take account of the various patient subgroups in a stratified analysis. To do this most efficiently (see below) one can use multiple regression techniques. Essentially these relate the individual patient response to therapy (CR, No CR) not only to the actual therapy received but also to the patient's own characteristics such as site and size of initial tumour and any other variables potentially influencing prognosis.

Before describing these statistical techniques it is useful to introduce the odds ratio (OR) as an alternative measure of relative treatment efficacy to d, the difference in proportions of CRs. From Table 22.1 we can see that the odds of a patient with head and neck cancer of size >3 cm responding with radiotherapy is 14:32, that is 14 respond and 32 do not. The odds for those patients of the same type receiving radiotherapy and hyperthermia is 15:30, that is, 15 respond and 30 do not. The ratio of these two odds is termed the odds ratio (OR). Thus, for these patients, we have OR = {(15/30)/(14/32)} = 1.14. An OR of greater than unity implies benefit to hyperthermia as it indicates a better odds of response in patients so treated.

Algebraically the OR is expressed as:

$$OR = \frac{P_{RTH}(1 - P_{RT})}{(1 - P_{RTH})P_{RT}}. \quad (22.3)$$

The ORs for the other patient groups are calculated in a similar way except that for trunk/extremities in lesions <3 cm the ratio is infinite because of the CR of 0% with radiotherapy alone.

If the addition of hyperthermia confers no benefit (or detriment) then the OR = 1 for all patient groups. This is equivalent to $d = 0$ referred to earlier. For technical reasons we use the format 22.2 to calculate a CI but use $\log_e(OR)$ in place of d rather than the OR itself. The expression for the SE is:

$$SE[\log(OR)] = [1/a + 1/b + 1/c + 1/d]^{1/2},$$

where a, b, c and d are the cells of a typical 2 × 2 table indicated in bold in Table 22.1. Finally, the expression for the 95% CI for OR, [= exp{log(OR)}], is obtained by exponentiating the upper and lower CI on this scale. Thus a 95% CI for OR is:

$$\exp\{\log(OR) - 1.96 \times SE[\log(OR)]\} \text{ to}$$
$$\exp\{\log(OR) + 1.96 \times SE[\log(OR)]\}. \quad (22.4)$$

Table 22.2 gives the estimated ORs and 95% CIs calculated for the (five) patient subgroups using the above expression. It is clear from Table 22.2 that there are rather different estimates of the value of hyperthermia as an addition to radiotherapy amongst the six patient groups represented. Thus two indicate an advantage, one of which is substantial, for the addition of hyperthermia, whilst three suggest that it is of detriment. There is considerable uncertainty surrounding

Table 22.2. Comparisons (ORs) of the effect of the addition of hyperthermia to radiotherapy in six site by lesion size patient subgroups (data from PEREZ et al. 1991). The table also includes the adjusted ORs calculated from a logistic regression of all the data

Site	Lesion size	OR	95% CI	From logistic regression OR_{LR}
Head and neck	<3 cm	0.60	0.10–3.54	1.18
	>3 cm	1.14	0.47–2.76	0.44
Breast/chest wall	<3 cm	2.40	0.44–12.98	0.94
	>3 cm	0.68	0.20–2.30	0.35
Trunk/ extremities	<3 cm	–[a]		0.47
	>3 cm	0.75	0.09–6.11	0.17

[a] Cannot be estimated since there are 0 (zero) responses in one subgroup

each estimate and the overlapping CIs tend to indicate that no subgroup can rule out the possibility suggested by any of the others. For example, the data are all consistent with an OR = 1.5 advantage to hyperthermia.

It is worth noting in the randomised trial described by SHARMA et al. (1989, Table 6) in 50 patients with carcinoma of the cervix that there is an implication that there is a differential effect in tumours of different sizes. Thus they state, following tests of statistical significance, that $p < 0.05$ for tumours >4 cm and $p > 0.05$ for tumours 2–4 cm in size, implying a benefit of hyperthermia in one group but not the other. In fact the estimated effects of hyperthermia from each group are $OR_{2-4\,cm} = 3.00$ and $OR_{>4\,cm} = 2.97$, respectively, and these are almost identical. Hence both these subgroups are supportive of the value of hyperthermia. Using the methods described below a stratified analysis gives a combined OR = 2.98 with a 95% CI as 0.65–13.69. The latter leaves considerable doubt concerning the true efficacy and suggests that the statistical significance (see below) in the 2–4 cm subgroup in favour of hyperthermia reported by the authors is probably spurious. There is no convincing evidence that there is a differential effect on tumours of different sizes. This also emphasises the need to give exact p-values when reporting statistical tests and also the value of a confidence interval. Both these points are stressed by GARDNER and ALTMAN (1989).

22.6 Logistic Regression

As we have indicated, in a randomised trial, other variables beside the allocated treatment may influence outcome. It is important therefore to check whether any imbalance of these variables between the treatment groups influences the estimate of the relative treatment benefit. Such a multivariable analysis will often result in a more reliable estimate of the treatment effect and is usually advised. Thus an approach to the analysis of Table 22.1 is to use logistic regression in which we specify a linear model of the log odds for the patient groups. Thus we write:

$$\log[P/(1 - P)] = b_0 + b_1(\text{Treatment}) + b_2(\text{Tumour Size}) + b_3(\text{Tumour Site}), \quad (22.5)$$

where $P/(1 - P)$ is the odds.

If hyperthermia treatment brings no benefit, and neither tumour size nor site has any influence on P, the proportion of patients who achieve CR, then each of the regression coefficients b_1, b_2 and b_3 in the above model will have a value zero. In this situation the CR rate (irrespective of whether hyperthermia is added or not) is estimated from all patients by $P = 73/236 = 0.3093$ (31%), from which $1 - P = 0.6907$ and this would give $b_0 = \log[0.3093/0.6907] = \log[0.4478] = -0.8033$ in the above logistic regression equation.

For further details of such models see ALTMAN (1991). They require specialist computer programs to fit such as those of EGRET (SERC 1990), which are readily available.

For our example, we have to modify Eq. 22.5 since there are three (as opposed to two) tumour sites. It becomes:

$$P/(1 - P) = \exp\{b_0 + b_1x_1 + b_2x_2 + b_3x_3 + b_4x_4\}, \quad (22.6)$$

where $x_1 = 0$ for radiotherapy alone, $x_1 = 1$ for radiotherapy with hyperthermia, $x_2 = 0$ for tumours <3 cm and $x_2 = 1$ for tumours >3 cm. To cope with the three categories of tumour site we state for head and neck patients $x_3 = x_4 = 0$, for breast/chest wall $x_3 = 1, x_4 = 0$ and for trunk $x_3 = 0, x_4 = 1$. Once this model is fitted to the data we have estimates of b_0, b_1, b_2, b_3 and b_4.

To compare treatments with the OR, but now adjusted for differences between patient groups, we calculate OR_{LR} using Eq. 22.3 but with the estimates of the numerator and denominator obtained from the regression equation 22.6 with the appropriate values of x_1, x_2, x_3 and x_4 in the numerator and denominator. The numerator corresponds to the addition of hyperthermia; hence $x_1 = 1$ and the denominator radiotherapy alone; hence $x_1 = 0$. Thus:

$$OR_{LR} = \frac{\exp\{b_0 + b_1 + b_2x_2 + b_3x_3 + b_4x_4\}}{\exp\{b_0 + b_2x_2 + b_3x_3 + b_4x_4\}}$$

In this ratio all but the term involving b_1 divide out and so, the treatment effect is estimated by:

$$OR_{LR} = \exp\{b_1\}.$$

This provides us with an estimate of the effect of hyperthermia as an addition to radiotherapy adjusted for, that is irrespective of, tumour site and size. This technique effectively adjusts all patients to have the same prognostic characteristics.

In a similar way $\exp\{b_2\}$ compares small and large lesions, and $\exp\{b_3\}$, $\exp\{b_4\}$ breast/chest and trunk/extremities with head and neck sites. The results of a full analysis using EGRET are summarised in Table 22.3. The estimated OR_{LR} = 1.18 is in favour of hyperthermia but the associated CI of 0.66–2.08 is wide. It is, however, narrower than any of those given in Table 22.2. The analysis also shows that tumour size is a significant determinant of response with the larger tumours doing less well since OR_{LR} = 0.37 and the associated CI does not include unity. There is also a suggestion of fewer responses in the breast/chest wall group and even fewer in the trunk/extremities diagnostic group as compared to patients with head and neck tumours. The latter CI excludes (just) the null hypothesis value of unity.

The advantage of the logistic regression method is that it considers *the whole structure of the data set as one*, and in this way smooths out chance variations in CRs as a consequence of small numbers. In addition the ORs can be combined multiplicatively and this permits an estimate of the odds of achieving CRs with hyperthermia in any subgroup relative to small head and neck tumours receiving radiotherapy alone. Thus, for example, for trunk/extremities of <3 cm (see the 0/4 group of Table 22.1) the estimated OR = 1.18 × 1 × 0.40 = 0.472 (see Table 22.2). This provides us with an estimate for the OR for this patient group which we did not have previously! It indicates that such patients are less likely to respond.

22.7 Survival Comparisons

The major outcome variable in some studies is the time between successive critical events. The time to CR (the second critical event) is measured from the date of randomisation (the first critical event). The time, t, between the two events is often referred to as a survival time as the techniques used to analyse such data have often been applied to patient survival times following diagnosis of cancer. An analysis using actual time to achieve a CR rather than comparing patients achieving or not achieving a CR at a certain (fixed) time is usually more statistically efficient.

Perez et al. (1991) record the time to achievement of CR in their patients, and those who did not respond were followed until they were either lost to follow-up or died. Such non-responding patients therefore failed to achieve a CR within the time that they were observed in the trial. For these, we have a censored time to CR, which we denote by $t+$. All we know is that while under observation they had not responded. However, we can make use of these censored data when comparing the rate of CR in the two treatment groups.

For illustration suppose we restrict the observation time for the patients of Perez et al. (1991) to 3 months. Thus we record the time to CR in those who respond before 3 months, and note the censored response time in those who either die, are lost to follow-up or who are still alive but have not responded by 3 months.

The so-called Kaplan-Meier CR curves for the two randomised groups of patients whose tumours are <3 cm, are shown in Fig. 22.2, for the first 3 months (see Perez et al. 1991, Fig. 3A). The displayed curves suggest that the patients receiving the hyperthermia respond more rapidly (at a greater rate) than those receiving radiotherapy alone.

Suppose all the 28 patients receiving radiotherapy have a CR then there will be 28 CR

Table 22.3. Logistic regression analysis of the tumour response data of Perez et al. (1991)

Variable		Regresion coefficient	Standard error SE	OR_{LR}	95% CI
Constant	b_0	0.062	0.348		
Radiotherapy		0	–	1	
Radiotherapy + hyperthermia	b_1	0.162	0.291	1.18	0.66–2.08
Size <3 cm		0	–	1	
>3 cm	b_2	−0.989	0.326	0.37	0.20–0.70
Head and neck		0	–	1	
Breast/chest	b_3	−0.220	0.320	0.80	0.43–1.50
Trunk/ extremities	b_4	−0.906	0.452	0.40	0.17–0.98

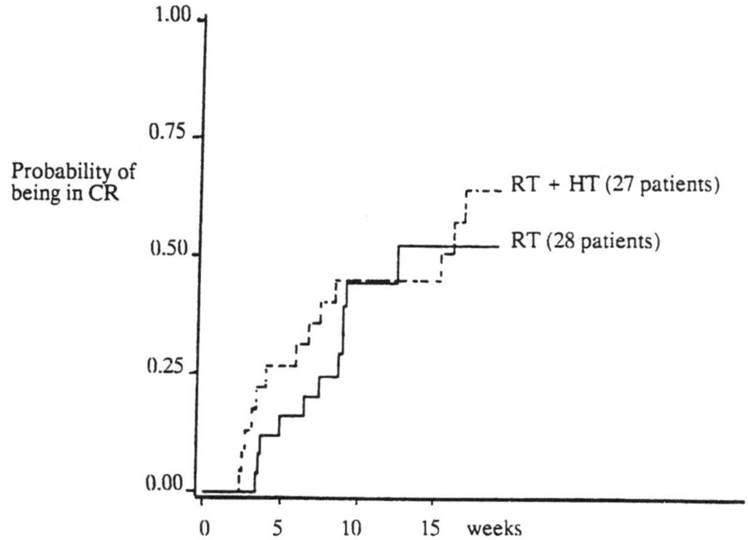

Fig. 22.2. Probability of being in complete response by treatment group in patients with tumours <3 cm (after PEREZ et al. 1991)

recovery times. These data can then be represented in a cumulative (response) survival curve as follows. First the individual CR times are ordered from smallest to largest. Then beginning at time 0, we move along horizontally until we reach the day of the shortest CR time (approximately at 3½ weeks). At that time we move upwards with a step equal to one patient. This step will be 1/28 or 0.0357 on the probability scale. The horizontal move then recommences until week 4, when there is another step upwards at the time the next patient achieves a CR, followed by a horizontal move until the next recovery time. This process continues until the very last (and longest) CR time, to complete the survival curve. A similar process applies to the 27 patients who also receive hyperthermia.

It is clear, however, that the steps are not equal in height and neither does the curve reach completion at 1 (28 times the step of 0.0357) on the vertical axis. The first may be explained by two (or more) patients having exactly the same CR times and so there would be a double (or greater) step at that point. A second reason is the presence of patients with censored observations, $t+$, in that they have not (as yet) achieved a CR. Figure 22.2 makes use of these censored times and such patients account, in part, for the differing step sizes. Details of the precise method of calculating the Kaplan-Meier or Product Limit estimates of the survival curves are given in, for example, CAMPBELL and MACHIN (1993). One useful summary statistic is the *median CR time*, which is the time by which half the patients have achieved a CR. This is calculated from the cumulative survival curve by drawing a line parallel to the time axis and noting at which time this cuts the survival curve. For the radiotherapy alone group the line cuts the cumulative time to CR curve at approximately 3 months. The median time for those patients receiving hyperthermia is approximately 4 months.

The relationship between the CR rate in the two groups may be summarised by the hazard ratio (HR), which is similar to the OR introduced earlier. In essence to estimate the HR the CR times of all the patients within the two groups separately are first calculated. The observed total number of CRs, $O_{RTH} + O_{RT}$, in both groups is then divided up in the ratio of the total (censored and non-censored) response times observed in each group. This gives the expected number of responses, E_{RTH} and E_{RT}, in each group. Exact details are given by ALTMAN (1991), who also describes how formal statistical comparisons are made using the logrank test.

The ratios O_{RTH}/E_{RTH} and O_{RT}/E_{RT} compare the observed with the expected CR rates. Finally:

$$HR = (O_{RTH}/E_{RTH})/(O_{RT}/E_{RT}). \qquad (22.7)$$

A value of HR = 1 would indicate that the rate at which CR occurred in both treatment groups was the same.

For technical reasons a CI for the HR is obtained first by obtaining a CI for $\log_e(HR)$ using the expression 22.4 given earlier, where HR replaces OR, as appropriate. In this situation:

$$SE(\log_e HR) = \{1/(1/E_{RTH} + 1/E_{RT})\}^{1/2}.$$

Table 22.4. Summary of rate of CRs in patients with recurrent breast cancer by treatment received

Treatment	No. of patients	No. achieving CR			Hazard ratio
		Observed	Expected	Ratio	
Radiotherapy + hyperthermia	N_{RTH}	O_{RTH}	E_{RTH}	O_{RTH}/E_{RTH}	$\frac{O_{RTH}/E_{RTH}}{O_{RT}/E_{RT}}$
Radiotherapy	N_{RT}	O_{RT}	E_{RT}	O_{RT}/E_{RT}	
Total	N	O	E		

The effect of prognostic factors such as site and lesion size on the time to CR can be investigated using Cox's proportional hazards model (see CHRISTENSEN 1987) in a similar manner to that for logistic regression

The results of survival (time to CR) studies are often summarised in the format of Table 22.4 together with the associated CI for the HR. However, to calculate the expected number of events and the CI we require the individual patient CR times and since these are not usually given in the literature we are unable to give an example for a published hyperthermia trial.

22.8 Subgroup Analysis

We have shown that it is important to analyse the results of a trial taking due account of prognostic variables and patient subgroups. The object of such an analysis is to give a clear and unbiased interpretation of the main design question concerning relative treatment efficacy. It is not relevant to examine statistical significance within these subgroups in the hope of identifying a group of patients who are particularly responsive to therapy. It goes without saying that because of random variation, even in the situation when in fact no difference in treatment efficacy exists, there will be some groups that respond favourably to one therapy and these will be balanced (offset) by those groups favouring the other. We would not be surprised if one of two patients with apparently the same prognosis fails to respond while the other responds. Equally we should not take as evidence of a differential effect one (small) subgroup of patients doing better with hyperthermia than without.

Of course, once the results of a randomised clinical trial of an appropriate size are available, we should examine the data carefully – perhaps to suggest hypotheses for the next trial. However, these hypotheses need external support (rather than merely internal evidence from our own trial) before they can be taken as serious suggestions for further work.

On a statistical point if six subgroups are examined for statistical significance (Table 22.2) [for a detailed discussion of statistical significance see CAMPBELL and MACHIN (1993)] at test size $\alpha = 0.05$, then the true significance level $\alpha' = 1 - (1 - \alpha)^6 = 0.26$. Thus if one of these six subgroups has $p = 0.05$ exactly (just significant!) then in fact the *true* p-value is nearer 0.26, which is far from significant. To correct for the six comparisons a simple rule is to declare subgroup differences only significant if the p-value is less than $\alpha/6$, that is $0.05/6 = 0.008$ in this case. With this rule there will be far fewer subgroup comparisons that are "significant"! An alternative is to multiply the p-value obtained by, in this case, 6 to obtain a revised value which can then be compared with 0.05.

22.9 Multiple Lesions

In certain circumstances patients presenting with multiple lesions will be suitable for testing both therapies. Thus, in a patient with two lesions both lesions should first be assessed for suitability for either therapy. If they are both suitable, then all that is necessary is first to specify a particular (target) lesion and to randomise the treatment allocation to that lesion; the other lesion automatically gets the other therapy. The individual lesions are then assessed for CR status.

If both lesions show a CR then these lesions contribute no information on the difference between the treatment modalities. In such circumstances it is also good to record the time when any

CRs occur. In this way the treatment corresponding to the lesion with the earlier (quicker) response will be preferred for that individual. An analysis for similar circumstances has been described by FRANCE et al. (1991). Unfortunately the analysis of the trial conducted by OVERGAARD et al. (1995), which treated 134 metastatic or recurrent lesions in 70 patients with malignant melanoma, does not distinguish between patients with multiple lesions and those with single lesions. As a consequence, it is not possible to know if the claimed benefit of hyperthermia over radiotherapy alone is really established for this disease. This type of design is best avoided.

22.10 Design Implications

It should be stated that the analysis of a clinical trial should reflect the *main objectives of the trial* so that the basic design is of paramount importance. For example, we have been somewhat dismissive of the small numbers within subgroups of Table 22.1. However, had this study been designed as a series of parallel phase II trials our view might be different. In such trials [see MACHIN and CAMPBELL (1987) for a brief description], we often specify a minimum CR rate as a target (often set at 20%) below which response there would be little biological or clinical interest. One strategy, the GEHAN (1961) design, is to recruit $n = 14$ patients of a particular type, say, trunk and extremities with tumours >3 cm, and observe the total CRs (r). This number of patients ensures that the probability of observing zero (that is, $r = 0$) CRs, if indeed the CR rate is 20%, is less than 0.05. If $r = 1$ or more a second group of m patients is recruited. If $r = 1$ then $m = 1$, if $r = 2$ (as is observed in our example) then $m = 6$. The maximum extra number of patients required is if $r \geqslant 3$ when $m = 11$. The final group size is $N = n + m = 20$ for our example, in which a total of R ($\geqslant 2$) responses are observed. This strategy ensures a SE(P) of 10% if the CR rate is indeed equal to the target 20%. Although we use the Gehan design here as a guide rather than a rule, it does suggest that the numbers in certain site by size combinations in Table 22.1 are far from sufficient even for phase II purposes.

It is also important to emphasise that the definitions of which patients go into which patient subgroups have to be made with care. Thus we might question whether it is really appropriate to classify trunk and extremities as one group since by so doing we are implying the therapies are equally effective at all sites within the group. We need to be really sure that a CR is clearly and objectively defined and can be assessed in all patients.

22.11 Size of a Randomised Trial

It is important to determine as precisely as possible at the design stage of a trial the number of patients that should be recruited and we have already referred to this in several places. If the numbers recruited are too small they may be insufficient to answer reliably the question posed. On the other hand, if too large then some patients may receive an inferior treatment unnecessarily.

Patient numbers depend critically on the size of the difference between treatments that will be observed. Clearly, if we knew this difference we would not conduct the trial as we would know the answer to the question posed. All we can do at the design stage is make a reasonable guess of the size of the effect. For example, this anticipated effect may be expressed as the difference δ between two proportions or the size of an OR as appropriate.

As well as the anticipated benefit there are two statistical requirements that need to be specified at the design stage. These are the pre-specified significance level, α, to be used in the subsequent calculation of CIs, and the power usually termed $1 - \beta$. The null hypothesis postulates that there is no difference between treatments and β is the probability of not rejecting this null hypothesis when the stated anticipated benefit exists. For example, if the anticipated benefit is to increase the response rate from 30% with radiotherapy alone to 45% by the addition of hyperthermia, we set for the design $\pi_{RT} = 0.30$ and $\pi_{RTH} = 0.45$ so that $\delta = 0.15$ and we would wish to detect this with our trial. Here the notation π rather than P for the response rate is used because the former refers to the value anticipated before the trial is conducted, the latter the value calculated once the trial has been completed.

The number of patients required, N, is given by

$$N = \frac{2(z_{1-\alpha} + z_{1-\beta})^2\{\pi_{RT}(1-\pi_{RT}) + \pi_{RTH}(1-\pi_{RTH})\}}{\delta^2} \quad (22.8)$$

where $z_{1-\alpha}$ and $z_{1-\beta}$ are values obtained from tables of the normal distribution.

It is usual to set $\alpha = 0.05$ and to have $1 - \beta = 0.9$ (or more), these imply $z_{1-\alpha} = z_{0.95} = 1.96$ and $z_{1-\beta} = z_{0.90} = 1.28$. Then with these and $\pi_{RT} = 0.30$, $\pi_{RTH} = 0.45$, $\delta = 0.15$, substituted in equation (22.8) we need approximately $N = 450$ patients. Half of these will be randomised to radiotherapy alone the other half will receive hyperthermia in addition.

If the anticipated benefit δ is 0.1 rather than 0.15 then $N \approx 1000$ patients is required. Thus a much larger trial would be needed to detect this smaller difference. **Small** trials can only detect **large** differences and in most examples in cancer therapy it is small rather than large treatment differences that are usually observed.

Details of sample size requirements for other situations are provided by MACHIN and CAMPBELL (1987).

22.12 Practical Considerations

In the assessment of the clinical value of hyperthermia much stress has rightly been laid on the importance of *quality assurance* in the techniques of heat delivery and thermometry. This level of quality assurance must also be applied to all data gathered in any clinical trial. It is therefore important to consider how the data generated in any study are to be collected, collated and ultimately analysed. It is also essential to define clearly in a trial protocol the *response categories* and objective response criteria to be used before contemplating any data management activities.

Data management is the task of ensuring that the data upon which the statistical analysis of a trial is based are as accurate, up to date and complete as possible. Data management starts at the protocol development stage in the development of a trial and continues to the final publication of the results, encompassing Form design, Randomisation, Establishment of a database, Data checking, Data entry and finally Retrieval of the required data for analysis.

Forms must be designed to enable the essential data to be recorded by the clinician with no possibility of errors or omissions, at the same time minimising the chance of error in transferring the data from form to database. For example, where time intervals are required, for instance time since start of treatment to achieve a CR, actual dates are preferable to a question simply asking for a number of days, as a simple computer calculation can remove the chance of errors by clinician or data manager (see below for computer checking).

While the current trend is toward the collection of a minimum of data, enough information must be collected, whether or not it is needed for the final analysis, to enable essential data items to be confirmed. For example, in trials for superficial tumours, the response of the target lesions must not only be recorded according to the agreed response categories, but the individual measurements must be given so evaluation of the response can be verified.

A computerised database is an essential ingredient for the management of a clinical trial. Thus the COMPACT software package (COMPACT Steering Committee 1991) was developed specifically for cancer trials and is designed to cope with the storage and handling of large amounts of data involving lengthy follow-up. It acts as an interface between the trial data and standard statistical software packages enabling "flat" files to be generated for analysis. Data management is greatly facilitated by the range and consistency checking which can be incoorporated into the database, with the creation of a "problems" file recording all deviations from predetermined conditions or ranges of values.

Retrieval of data may be required during the course of a trial for interim analyses. The importance of keeping the trial database as complete and up to date as possible at all times is therefore particularly important. Data sent promptly from clinician to data manager are more likely to be accurate, and the possibility of bias arising from the principle that "bad news travels fast" is kept to a minimum.

It is important to identify a suitable statistical package for analysis, although specialist advice on this may have to be sought because some of the statistical methods that are required may not be included. Confidence intervals, for example, are not generated by some packages. One of the dangers of using any statistical package is that the software will produce numbers and statistics in response to whatever data have been entered and analysis requested. It is easy to be seduced into carrying out numerous analyses without considering whether the procedures chosen are appropriate. An understanding of the data being analysed is essential.

Finally, a useful checklist for points to consider in the design of a trial and the subsequent reporting are given by GARDNER et al. (1989).

22.13 Summary

- Comparative trials should be randomised and patients assessed for inclusion before the randomisation is effected.
- A clear protocol containing key information should be written for all trials.
- Where appropriate definitions of, for example, CR and how and when it is determined need to be stated.
- Trials should be large enough to answer the question posed. The steps taken to estimate the size should be carefully documented.
- The estimates of treatment response rates and any treatment difference summary, for example, OR or HR, should be reported together with associated CIs.
- Analysis should take account of any imbalance in important prognostic variables between the treatment options.
- Subgroup analyses, unless specifically defined a priori, are likely to involve small groups and are potentially misleading.
- If lesions, as opposed to patients, are randomised then the analysis should reflect this. It will be misleading to report them otherwise.
- Before conducting a randomised clinical trial or any major study, care should be taken to ensure that an appropriate data base is available and that it will interface with the statistical package that is to be used for analysis.

References

Altman DG (1991) Practical statistics for medical research. Chapman and Hall, London

Campbell MJ, Machin D (1993) Medical statistics: a common sense approach, 2nd edn. Wiley, Chichester

Christensen E (1987) Multivariate survival analysis using Cox's regression model. Hepatology 7: 1346–1358

COMPACT Steering Committee (1991) Improving the quality of data in clinical trials in cancer. Br J Cancer 63: 412–415

France LA, Lewis JA, Kay R (1991) The analysis of failure time data in crossover studies. Stat Med 10: 1099–1113

Gardner MJ, Altman DG (1989) Estimation rather than hypothesis testing: confidence intervals rather than p-values. In: Gardner MJ, Altman DG (eds) Statistics with confidence. BMJ, London, pp 6–19

Gardner MJ, Machin D, Campbell MJ (1989) Use of check lists in assessing the statistical content of medical studies. In: Gardner MJ, Altman DG (eds) Statistics with confidence. BMJ, London, pp 101–108

Gehan EA (1961) The determination of the number of patients required in a preliminary and a follow-up trial of a new chemotherapeutic agent. J Chronic Dis 13: 346–353 (see also Tables 11.1 and 11.2 of Machin and Campbell 1987)

Geigy Scientific Tables (1991), vol 2. Introduction to statistics. Statistical tables and mathematical formulae. Ciba-Geigy, Basle, Switzerland

Machin D, Campbell MJ (1987) Statistical tables for the design of clinical trials. Blackwell, Oxford

Overgaard J, Gonzalez Gonzalez D, Hulshof MCCM, Arcangeli G, Dahl O, Mella O, Bentzen SM, for European Society for Hyperthermic Oncology (1995) Randomised trial of hyperthermia as adjuvant to radiotherapy for recurrent or metastatic malignant melanoma. Lancet 345: 540–543

Perez CA, Pajak T, Emami B, Hornback NB, Tupchong L, Rubin P (1991) Randomised phase III study comparing irradiation and hyperthermia with irradiation alone in superficial measurable tumours. Am J Clin Oncol 14: 133–141

SERC (1990) EGRET reference manual: first draft. Statistics and Epidemiology Research Corporation, Seattle

Sharma S, Patel FD, Sandhu APS, Gupta BD, Yadav NS (1989) A prospective randomised study of local hyperthermia as a supplement and radiosensitizer in the treatment of carcinoma of the cervix. Endocuriether Hypertherm Oncol 5: 151–159

23 Standardized Thermoradiotherapy Treatment Documentation

S.A. Sapareto, R.G.F. Knol, P.M. Corry, and M.H. Seegenschmiedt

CONTENTS

23.1 Introduction

The development of a treatment modality requires a cooperative effort of many investigators, clinicians, and technologists for the purpose of demonstrating safety and efficacy. In order to ensure reproducibility, appropriate quality assurance (QA) methods must be developed and employed. It is the purpose of this chapter to describe efforts that have been made to develop standards for data in clinical hyperthermia trials and to propose additional components that will continue to allow the acceptance and use of these standards.

S.A. Sapareto, PhD, Department of Radiation Oncology, Good Samaritan Regional Medical Center, 1111 East McDowell Road, Phoenix, AZ 85006, USA

R.G.F. Knol, Department of Radiation Research, City of Hope National Medical Center, Duarte, CA 91010, USA

P.M. Corry, PhD, Department of Radiation Oncology, William Beaumont Hospital, Royal Oaks, MI 48073-6769, USA

M.H. Seegenschmiedt, MD, Department of Radiation Oncology, University of Erlangen-Nürnberg, Universitätsstraße 27, D-8520 Erlangen, FRG

Standards can be of most benefit in clinical hyperthermia if used for (a) *defining nomenclature*, particularly for thermal analysis, and (b) for *storage of treatment information and documentation*. While the latter has been previously defined in the Hyperthermia Data Standard (HDS), because of its complexity, a method for evaluation and validation is essential. A special computer program, HDSGen, has been developed for this purpose and is described here, also.

23.2 Standards in Nomenclature

Much of the required nomenclature of use in clinical hyperthermia trials is similar to that of conventional cancer therapy and has already been developed. These include the International Classification of Diseases for Oncology (ICD-O, 1976), Systematized Nomenclature of Medicine (SNOMED; Cote 1984), and Tumor, Node, Metastasis (TNM 1985) classification schemes. An area particular to clinical hyperthermia, however, which has not been developed, is that of *thermal treatment assessment*. To date, numerous methods of analyzing thermal treatments have been proposed and used. Unfortunately, even though identified with the same terminology, differences exist in the methods used by various investigators to calculate these thermal descriptive parameters. Often these differences are not well documented and can lead to erroneous comparisons of "apples with oranges." A good example of this is the difference between thermal isoeffect dose (TID) as calculated in Europe (Field and Morris 1983) and in the United States (Sapareto and Dewey 1984). In Europe, the TID is calculated using a factor of 6 below a temperature break point of 42.5°C whereas in the United States a factor of 4 below a breakpoint of 43°C is used. While in most cases, particularly at temperatures above 43°C, there are no differences between these two calculations, differences will be found when temperatures are in the range of 41°–43°C. The significance of these differences has not been investigated: however, at the very least they should be documented and acknowledged. By providing unequivocal definitions with distinct nomenclature, we hope to clarify some of these differences and prevent future "Babylonian confusion."

23.2.1 Thermal Parameter Definitions

A number of thermal descriptive parameters have been reported in the literature to demonstrate correlations with response or toxicity. These can be broken down into three specific groups: *basic data*, *standard statistics* and *thermal analysis parameters*.

The basic or raw data values comprise those values that are actually measured such as temperature, time and number of thermoprobes. These fundamental data sets are essential for any further statistical or thermal modeling analysis. The terminology used to describe these values is straightforward and, for the most part, consistent throughout the literature. However, the standard use of subscripts will reduce ambiguity and clarify usage.

Standard statistical parameters are those that can be derived from the raw or basic data using well-established statistical definitions. These parameters would include averages, standard deviations, medians, minimums, maximums, etc. While we here attempt to define the more common and clinically useful of these parameters, there are many others which can be derived.

The final set of parameters has, for the most part, been derived from various thermal models in an attempt to relate the thermal history to assessable thermal damage. These parameters, as such, all incorporate an analysis of both time and temperature in their calculation and invariably require a nonlinear function of temperature. While a number of parameters have been proposed, the list provided here represents those which have demonstrated correlations with response or toxicity in animal or clinical studies with varying degrees of success. In order to clarify the formulas of such methods, we propose here a list of defined nomenclatures for the more common and likely useful of these parameters and we encourage the use of these standard nomenclatures.

The above described hyperthermia data parameters are listed below with descriptions in Tables 1–7 divided into basic data, time scaling, and specific thermal parameters respectively.

Table 23.1. Temperature and power data sets for typical hyperthermia treatments

Definitions	Units	Descriptions
$T_n(\mathbf{r},t)$	°C	Measured temperature of thermoprobe number n at location $\mathbf{r} = (x,y,z) = (r,\varphi,z)$ and at time t derived from HDS files or similar protocols
N		Number of all used thermoprobes where $n \in N$
N_{Tumor}		Number of thermoprobes in tumor
N_{Normal}		Number of thermoprobes in normal tissue
N_{Skin}		Number of thermoprobes on skin
N_{Other}		Number of thermoprobes somewhere else
		Finally, we distinguish: $N = N_{Tumor} + N_{Normal} + N_{Skin} + N_{Other}$
$P_l(\mathbf{r},t)$	W	Amount of power output of applicator number l at location $\mathbf{r} = (x,y,z) = (r,\varphi,z)$ and at time t derived from HDS files or similar protocols
L		Number of all installed applicators with: $l \in L$
$t = m \cdot \Delta\tau$	s	Running time of measurement
M		Number of measurement intervals with $m \in M$
$\Delta\tau = \Delta\tau^{on}_{Power} + \Delta\tau^{off}_{Power}$	s	Measurement interval, e.g., $\Delta\tau = 15\,s$
$\Delta\tau^{on}_{Power}$	s	Measurement interval with power output, e.g, $\Delta\tau^{on}_{Power} = 13\,s$
$\Delta\tau^{off}_{Power}$	s	Measurement interval without power output, e.g, $\Delta\tau^{off}_{Power} = 2\,s$

Table 23.2. Specific time points and time scales for temperature data evaluation

Definitions	Units	Descriptions
t_{init}	s	Beginning of hyperthermia treatment $\exists l \in L : P_l(t_{init}) \neq 0$
t_{init}^{steady}	s	Beginning of *steady state level* when manifest in temperature slope, otherwise using the following definition: $t_{init}^{steady} = t_{init} + 10\,\text{min}$
t_{end}^{steady}	s	End of *steady state level* End of hyperthermia treatment All generators and applicators are off: $P_l(t_{end}^{steady}) = 0, \forall l \in L$
t_{end}	s	End of temperature measurement
$\Delta t^{steady} = t_{end}^{steady} - t_{init}^{steady}$	s	Duration of *steady state level*
$\Delta t_{treat}^{total} = t_{end}^{steady} - t_{init}$	s	Duration of hyperthermia treatment
$\Delta t_{measure}^{total} = t_{end} - t_{init}$ or: $\Delta t_{measure}^{total} = M \cdot \Delta\tau$	s s	Duration of temperature measurement
$\Delta t_{power}^{on} = M \cdot \Delta\tau_{power}^{on}$	s	Duration of power output

Table 23.3. Minimum, maximum, and mean values of measured temperature data of hyperthermia treatments. Averages are either time-*averaged* or sensor *mean*

Definitions	Units	Descriptions
$T_n^{peak} = \max_{t \in \Delta t^{steady}} T_n(t)$	°C	Highest measured temperature at thermoprobe *n*
$T_n^{gap} = \min_{t \in \Delta t^{steady}} T_n(t)$	°C	Lowest measured temperature at thermoprobe *n*
$T_{max}^{mean} = \frac{\sum_{n=1}^{N} T_n^{peak}}{N}$	°C	Mean maximum temperature of all *N* thermoprobes in *steady state level* (T^{90} = maximum temperature which 90% of the probes achieve)
$T_{min}^{mean} = \frac{\sum_{n=1}^{N} T_n^{gap}}{N}$	°C	Mean minimum temperature of all *N* thermoprobes in *steady state level* (T^{50} = maximum temperature which 50% of the probes achieve)
$T_n^{av} = \frac{\sum_{t=t_{init}^{steady}}^{t_{end}^{steady}} T_n(t)}{\Delta t^{steady} \cdot \Delta\tau^{-1}}$	°C	Averaged temperature of thermoprobe *n* in *steady state level*
$T_{max}^{av} = \max_{n \in N} T_n^{av}$	°C	Maximum averaged temperature involving all *N* thermoprobes in *steady state level*
$T_{min}^{av} = \min_{n \in N} T_n^{av}$	°C	Minimum averaged temperature involving all *N* thermoprobes in *steady state level*
$T^{mean}(t) = \frac{\sum_{n=1}^{N} T_n(t)}{N}$	°C	Mean temperature of all *N* thermoprobes at a certain time *t*
$T_{init}^{mean} = T^{mean}(t_{init})$	°C	Mean temperature of all *N* thermoprobes at the beginning of hyperthermia treatment
$T_{end}^{mean} = T^{mean}(t_{end})$	°C	Mean temperature of all *N* thermoprobes at the end of temperature measurement
$T_{total}^{av\,mean} = \frac{\sum_{t=t_{init}}^{t_{end}^{steady}} \sum_{n=1}^{N} T_n(t)}{N \cdot \Delta t_{treat}^{total} \cdot \Delta\tau^{-1}}$	°C	Mean averaged temperature of all measured temperature values and all *N* thermoprobes during hyperthermia treatment Δt_{treat}^{total}
$T_{steady}^{av\,mean} = \frac{\sum_{t=t_{init}^{steady}}^{t_{end}^{steady}} \sum_{n=1}^{N} T_n(t)}{N \cdot \Delta t^{steady} \cdot \Delta\tau^{-1}}$	°C	Mean averaged temperature of all measured temperature values and all *N* thermoprobes during *steady state level* Δt^{steady}

Table 23.4. Integrated time intervals describing temperature distributions of hyperthermia treatments

Definitions	Units	Descriptions
$ITI_n^{43} = \sum_{t=t_{init}^{steady}}^{t_{end}^{steady}} \Delta\tau\Theta(T_n(t) - 43°C)$	min	Integrated time intervals in *steady state level* where thermoprobe *n* indicates temperatures exceeding 43°C
$ITI_{max}^{43} = \max_{n \in N} TI_n^{43}$	min	Longest integrated time intervals in *steady state level* of all *N* thermoprobes exceeding 43°C
$ITI_{min}^{43} = \min_{n \in N} TI_n^{43}$	min	Shortest integrated time intervals in *steady state level* of all *N* thermoprobes exceeding 43°C
$ITI_{mean}^{43} = \frac{\sum_{n=1}^{N} TI_n^{43}}{N}$	min	Mean integrated time intervals in *steady state level* of all *N* thermoprobes exceeding 43°C

Analogue definitions: ITI_n^{40}, ITI_n^{41}, ITI_n^{42}
Analogue definitions for minimum, maximum, and mean values: $ITI_{min}^{T_{ref}}$, $ITI_{max}^{T_{ref}}$, and $ITI_{mean}^{T_{ref}}$

Table 23.5. Statistical Thermal Dose Concept using Combined Thermal Variables.

Definitions	Units	Descriptions
T_{10}	°C	Temperature exceeded by 10% of all measured temperatures of all N thermoprobes in *steady state level.* T_{10} is statistically the 90% Percentile.
Analogue definitions are given for:		
T_{20}	°C	is statistically the 80% Percentile.
T_{50}	°C	is statistically the 50% Percentile.
T_{80}	°C	is statistically the 20% Percentile.
T_{90}	°C	is statistically the 10% Percentile.
$ITI_{mean}^{T_{90} \leq T_{index}} = \frac{\sum_{n=1}^{N} ITI_n^{T_{90} \geq T^{index}}}{N}$	min	Mean Integrated Time Intervals, within the Index Temperature is exceeded by 90% of all measured temperatures of all *N* thermoprobes in *steady state level*.

Analogue definitions are possible: $ITI_{mean}^{T_{50} \leq T_{index}}$, $ITI_{mean}^{T_{10} \leq T_{index}}$, etc.

Table 23.6. Biological motivated definition of thermal isoeffect dose [in equivalent minutes at T_{ref} = 43°C (minEq43)] used for ESHO protocols (see Dunlop et al. 1986; Hand et al. 1989)

Definitions	Units
$TID_n^{43} = TID^{43}\left(\Delta t_{measure}^{end}, T_n(t)\right) = \sum_{t=t_{init}}^{t_{end}} \Delta t_{eq43}(T_n(t))$	min
is the calculated thermal isoeffect dose at thermoprobe *n*	
with $\Delta t_{eq43}(T_n(t)) = \begin{cases} 2^{(T_n(t)-43°C)} \cdot \Delta\tau: T_n(t) \geq T_{trans} \\ 2^{(T_{trans}-43°C)} 6^{(T_n(t)-T_{trans})} \cdot \Delta\tau: T_n(t) < T_{trans} \end{cases}$	
where T_{trans} = 42.5°C is the assumed transition temperature and $\Delta\tau$ = 15 s the measurement interval	

Examples for constant temperatures T_n:
$TID^{43}(\Delta t_{measure}^{end} = 9\,\text{min}, T_n = 41°C) = TID^{43}(\Delta t_{measure}^{end} = 26\,\text{s}, T_n = 43°C)$
$TID^{43}(\Delta t_{measure}^{end} = 15\,\text{s}, T_n = 45°C) = TID^{43}(\Delta t_{measure}^{end} = 1\,\text{min}, T_n = 43°C)$

Table 23.7. Further definitions of thermal isoeffect dose for ESHO protocols and at Duke University (see OLESON et al. 1993)

Definitions	Units	Descriptions
$TID^{43}_{max} = \max_{n \in N} TID^{43}_{n}$	min	Highest calculated thermal isoeffect dose of all thermoprobes N in minEq43
$TID^{43}_{min} = \min_{n \in N} TID^{43}_{n}$	min	Lowest calculated thermal isoeffect dose of all thermoprobes N in minEq43
$ITI^{43}_{mean} = \frac{\sum_{n=1}^{n=N} TID^{43}_{n}}{N}$	min	Mean calculated thermal isoeffect dose of all thermoprobes N in minEq43
CEM 43 $T_{90} = \Sigma(\Delta t)R^{(43-T)}$	min	Cumulative equivalent minutes at a T_{90} converted to 43°C with: Δt = time increments that thermal data is acquired during treatment T bar = average temperature over time interval Δt R = 0.25 for T < 43°C; 0.5 for T ≥ 43°C

Analogue definitions for thermal isoeffect dose are possible for different reference temperatures T_{ref} = 40°C, 41°C, and 42°C
Analogue indices are recommended: TID^{40}_{n}, TID^{41}_{n}, and TID^{42}_{n}
Analogue definitions for minimum, maximum, and mean values: $TID^{T_{ref}}_{min}$, $TID^{T_{ref}}_{max}$, and $TID^{T_{ref}}_{mean}$

23.2.2 Data Storage Standards: HDS Version 2.0

We have previously proposed a standard file format, the Hyperthermia Data Standard (HDS Version 1.0) (SAPARETO and CORRY 1989), for collection and transport of all hyperthermia data. This standard provides a method of organization and identification of data which might be collected for and during a clinical hyperthermia treatment. The data are identified as *keywords* followed by values and are organized into *segments* for the various groups of data. The nine initially defined segments in HDS Version 1.0 included /VERSION, /IDENT, /TEXT, /TUMOR, /HSETUP, /FORMAT, /DATA, /FOLLOWUP, and /ANALYSIS. In the process of developing software to use the standard, we have realized that a number of significant changes have become essential for functionality and simplicity. Because of several required incompatibilities with Version 1.0, this version has been designated 2.0 (SAPARETO et al., in press). Although substantially the same as the first version, several new items have been added to Version 2.0 to better fit standard practice and the needs of clinical protocols. In addition, some changes have been made to previously defined items, thus precluding upward compatibility between the two versions. Significant changes include: elimination of the /FORMAT segment and the addition of /EVALUATION and /RSETUP segments. The /EVALUATION segment documents general patient criteria and eligibility; the /RSETUP segment contains the Radiation setup information. The standard was adopted by the Radiation Therapy Oncology Group (RTOG) for use in all hyperthermia clinical trials (DEWHIRST et al. 1990) and has been endorsed by the American Society of Therapeutic Radiology and Oncology (ASTRO), the North American Hyperthermia Society (NAHS), and the European Society of Hyperthermic Oncology (ESHO).

HDS Version 2.0 defines a standard yet flexible format for documenting clinical hyperthermia treatments. Considerable effort has been made to solicit input from those expected to use this standard format, both by correspondence and in a workshop held at the 8th Annual Meeting of the North American Hyperthermia Group (Philadelphia, 1988). In general, all comments and recommendations have been addressed in one way or another and most have been incorporated into this standard. In Version 2.0, an attempt has been made to address the limitations of Version 1.0 by adding new segments for documentation of radiation treatments and patient evaluation. In addition, keywords for the /FOLLOWUP and /ANALYSIS segments as well as a few others have been added so that these can be used for current and future clinical protocols. The most important change to the standard precluding upward compatibility is the elimination of /FORMAT segment and the use of specific keywords for entering data (i.e., temperatures, powers, etc.) in the /DATA segment. However, programmers who write to this standard will find that this new structure is significantly more simple to use.

Every effort has been made to allow for all anticipated uses of this format. For example, the expected use of *pullback thermometry mapping techniques* can easily be documented by considering each pullback location as a fixed measurement location. Likewise, the expected increased use of power multiplexing of interstitial radiofrequency and microwave systems can be addressed by assuming each implant as an applicator or string of applicators. The $SEQ keyword was specifically defined for these techniques. In addition, we have added a new keyword $TRACK to expedite documentation of catheters that will be mapped. Nevertheless, it is anticipated that problems and unforeseen uses (e.g., electronically focused ultrasound) will become apparent with future implementation of this standard format. However, since new keywords and segments may be defined at any time, users may design their own improvements. All users are encouraged to contact the authors about any future problems and possible solutions.

The primary purpose for this standard is the exchange of data with the deliberate sacrifice of data compactness for the ease of reading and debugging, particularly important in the development of a standard. This ease more than outweighs the increase in file size. In order to implement this standard, it is expected that those who have developed computerized documentation of clinical hyperthermia treatments, particularly all commercial manufacturers, will provide computer programs for conversion of their own formats into this standard. Indeed, there have been encouraging efforts in this area. We urge the clinical hyperthermia community to request and encourage the rapid implementation of this standard format by all commercial manufacturers.

The need for improvements in the documentation of clinical hyperthermia treatments is apparent from the clinical studies which have been published, including the recent report of an RTOG cooperative trial (Perez et al. 1991). By providing a mechanism for documenting all of the information recommended by the Hyperthermia Quality Assurance Committee of the American College of Radiology and approved by several organizations (Shrivastava et al. 1989,) hopefully, this standard will actually encourage the collection of these data. As can be seen from the definition of more than 60 standard keywords, the amount of data collectible is enormous, precluding the likelihood of any manual collection of this information. However, by using computerized forms with predefined or automated keyword value assignments, this task would become far simpler and more manageable. The implementation of this data format hopefully will be an important catalyst in much needed improvements in documenting and assessing clinical hyperthermia treatments (Oleson 1989). However, the success of this format and its ability to foster advances in clinical hyperthermia will depend on the acceptance and utilization of this standard by the clinical and scientific communities.

23.3 Validation of Standards

While the benefits of a standard file format for documenting clinical hyperthermia data are obvious, the acceptance and use of such a standard are by no means guaranteed. For such a standard to be useful, methods must be available to verify that any user-generated data file, in fact, adheres to the standard unambiguously. To perform such a task it was decided to develop a computer program that could read and verify any HDS file. In addition, features to create or edit HDS files were also included. For this purpose a PC-based program, HDSGen, has been developed. HDSGen Version 1.0 is written under MS-DOS and utilizes a customized menu-driver allowing for the optional use of a mouse. Since formal HDS data requirements may constitute only a subset of requirements of individual institutes, the package allows for the presence of user-defined data sequences, as supported by the standard.

The software package HDSGen validates information in HDS data files against an associated base format given in an HDS *definition* file. The purpose of definition files is to define data structures, referred to as segments and keywords and related indices and arguments, that are allowed in HDS data files.

Like HDS data files, information in definition files is grouped into *segments* and, within these, into *keywords*. Declaration of a segment or keyword name in a definition file indicates that the use of a segment or keyword with that particular name is permitted in HDS data files. Declarations take indices and arguments which define their value or scope in data files. The presence of indices and arguments in data files can be declared to be optional or required. Indices can take free or interval restricted integer values. Arguments may take alphanumeric, free or interval restricted numeric and choice-list restricted values.

Definition files can be tailored to conform to specific requirements, e.g., protocols. For this purpose, a set of index and argument declarators and rules was developed, shown in Appendix A. With these declarators and rules, the definition file excerpted in Appendix B was created. Finally, Appendix C shows a partial HDS data file validated against the definition file in Appendix B.

23.4 HDSGen Software

To facilitate creation, modification, and validation of HDS data sequences, the PC software package HDSGen Version 1.0 has been developed. To standardize and simplify interaction with software, a mouse/keyboard driven menu system was designed. The resulting package provides interaction between the user and HDS segment and keyword structures through *menu screens*. Menu screens are segment-oriented collections of descriptive text and *fields* for each of the indices and arguments of the keyword structures contained in the segment. Fields have (a) display, (b) display and selection or display, (c) selection, entry, and edit function.

Menu screens are contained in specially generated files. Changes in HDS definition files do not automatically generate the appropriate changes in the accompanying menu screens.

23.4.1 Validation of Data Files

The validity of the contents of data files with respect to HDS Version 2.0 can be verified by activating this option. Any discrepancy is reported in an error file, which can be examined upon termination of HDSGen. Attention has been given to the legibility and clarity of error files created.

23.4.2 Display of Data Files

A validation of the data file contents is performed. Any discrepancy between the file content and the Standard is reported in an error file. Information found to be in accordance with the Standard is displayed. No edit functions are provided.

23.4.3 Creation and Modification of Data Files

New data files can be created and edited through this option. Existing data files are, after an initial validation, available for editing. To allow for uninterrupted data entry, minimal validation procedures are active during editing, since newly entered partial segment/keyword indices and arguments are not necessarily coherent and/or complete and thus in accordance with the Standard. Upon completion of data entry, proper validation of the data file contents is required.

Data are entered by means of menu screens. To guide and restrict the entry of notably choice-list options, "*PopUp*" boxes were designed to assist data entry procedures. PopUp boxes overlay the menu screen and provide a list of fixed choices. Upon selection, the element chosen is automatically entered into the appropriate field of the menu screen.

Certain data file elements require a specialized display. For these data types, e.g., thermometry data, a special menu screen is used. While most edit screens are user modifiable, because of its complexity and uniqueness, this one edit screen is not readily modifiiable by users. The program has been presented at annual meetings of the North American Hyperthermia Society and the European Society for Hyperthermic Oncology and has been distributed to interested researchers. It is available from the authors.

23.5 Summary

- A standardization of nomenclature for documenting hyperthermia treatment parameters is presented to improve communication in published literature.
- The Hyperthermia Data Standard (HDS) Version 2.0 can provide a universal means of storing and transferring complete documentation of hyperthermia treatments.
- A computer program HDSGen Version 1.0 has been written to allow creation, editing and

verification of HDS Version 2.0 files. Its structure and use are described in this chapter.

- The HDSGen program can be used to provide some verification of the completeness of protocol data and can be used for the submission of protocol data for multi-institutional trials.

Acknowledgments. This work was supported in part by PHS grants CA-51189 and CA-44550 awarded by the National Cancer Institute, US Public Health Service.

References

Cote RA (ed) (1984) SNOMED: Systematized Nomenclature of Medicine, vol I and II, 2nd edn. Skokie, College of American Pathologists

Dewhirst MW, Phillips TL, Samulski TV (1990) RTOG quality assurance guidelines for clinical trials using hyperthermia. Int J Radiat Oncol Biol Phys 18: 1249–1259

Dunlop PRC, Hand JW, Dickinson RJ, Field SB (1986) An assessment of local hyperthermia in clinical practice. Int J Hyperthermia 2: 39–50

Field SB, Morris CC (1983) The relationship between heating time and temperature: its relevance to clinical hyperthermia. Radiother Oncol 1: 179–186

Hand JW, Lagendijk JJW, Bach Andersen J, Bolomey JC (1989) Quality assurance guidelines for ESHO protocols. Int J Hyperthermia 5: 421–428

International Classification of Diseases for Oncology (ICD-O) (1976) World Health Organization, Geneva

Oleson J (1989) Editorial: If we can't define the quality, can we assure it? Int J Radiat Oncol Biol Phys 16: 879–880

Oleson JR, Samulski TV, Leopold KA, Clegg ST, Dewhirst MW, Dodge RK, George SL (1993) Sensitivity of hyperthermia trial outcomes to temperature and time: implications for thermal goals of treatment. Int J Radiat Oncol Biol Phys 25: 289–297

Perez CA, Pajak T, Emami B, Hornback NB, Tupchong L, Rubin P (1991) Randomised phase III study comparing irradiation and hyperthermia with irradiation alone in superficial measurable tumours. Am J Clin Oncol 14: 133–141

Sapareto SA, Corry PM (1989) A proposed standard data file format for hyperthermia treatments. Int J Radiat Oncol Biol Phys 16: 613–627

Sapareto SA, Dewey WC (1984) Thermal dose determinations in cancer therapy. Int J Radiat Oncol Biol Phys 10: 787–800

Sapareto SA, Knol RGF, Corry PM (in press) The standard data file format for hyperthermia treatments: HDS Version 2.0. Int J Radiat Oncol Biol Phys

Shrivastava P, Luk K, Oleson J (1989) Hyperthermia quality assurance guidelines. Int J Radiat Oncol Biol Phys 16: 571–588

TNM Atlas (1985) Illustrated guide to the TNM/pTNM Classification of malignant tumors, 2nd edn. Spiessl B, Hermanek P, Scheibe O, Wagner G (eds). Springer, Berlin Heidelberg New York

Appendix A. Rules, Index and Argument Declarators for HDS Definition Files

Rules:

1. Optional indices and arguments have declarators placed between "[" and "]".
2. Required indices and arguments have declarators placed between "(" and ")".
3. Only segment and keyword declarators can have indices.
4. "Choice list" argument declarators have their elements separated by "|".
5. Declaration order of segment/keyword arguments is reflected in data files.
6. Required segments/keywords in data files have declarators preceded by "!".

Index and argument declarators:

INT/INT a-b	Free/interval a-b restricted integer number
NUM/NUM a-b	Free/interval a-b restricted real number
IORANGE/ IORANGE a-b	Free/ interval a-b restricted range or number
IRANGE/ IRANGE a-b	Free/interval a-b restricted range
TIME	Time field (HH:MM:SS)
DATE	Date field (MM/ DD/YYYY or DD/MM/ YYYY)
TEXT	Any (alpha-) numeric text
"*literal text*"	Text restricted to the pattern *literal text*

Note: HH = hour; MM = minutes; SS = seconds; DD = day; MM = month; YYYY = year

Appendix B. Excerpt of the /HSETUP Segment from an HDS Definition File

/HSETUP[INT 1-99],(TEXT),(DATE)
;Hyperthermia setup #, patient id., date of setup

$HEATSYS,(TEXT),(TEXT),[TEXT],[TEXT]
;Heat. sys. manufacturer, model, serial id., description

$OPER,(TEXT)
;Hyperthermia equipment operator

$HMODALITY,("MW"|"RF"|"US"),[TEXT]
;Heating modality: MW, RF, or US, description

$TINTERVAL,(TIME)
;Time interval between heat and other modality

$APPLCATOR[IORANGE 1-99],(TEXT),(TEXT),[TEXT],[TEXT]
:Appl. #, manufacturer, model, serial id., description

$APPSIZE[IORANGE 1-99],(NUM),(NUM),[TEXT]
:Appl. #, aperture size *x*, aperture size *y*, description

$APPLOC[INT 1-99],(NUM −25.0 −25.0),(NUM −25.0 −25.0),(NUM −25.0 −25.0)
:Appl. #, *x*,*y*,*z* location with respect to center of tumor

$APPORIENT[IORANGE 1-99],(INT 0−360),(INT 0−360),[INT 0−360],[INT 0−360]:
;Appl. #, rotation, orientation, tilt direction, tilt angle

....

....

!$END
;End of this segment (required keyword)

NOTE: ";" semicolon is standard nomenclature in computer programming designating comments

Appendix C. Partial HDS Data File Validated with Definition File in Appendix B

/HSETUP1, 910005-12, 07/07/1991
$TINTERVAL, 00:12:00
$OPER, H. Ray
$HEATSYS, Custom built, 915 MHz/16 chx/100 Watt
$HMODALITY, MW, 915 MHz non-coherent continuous heating
$APPLICATOR1−3, Custom built, Waveguide, 915 MHz TE10 type I ceramic
$APPLICATOR4, Custom built, Waveguide, 915 MHz TE10 type II ceramic
$APPSIZE1, 60.0, 60.0, mm.
$APPSIZE4, 90.0, 90.0, mm.
$APPSIZE2−3, 60.0, 60.0, mm.
$APPORIENT1−4, 0, 90
$APPLOC1, −3.0, 3.0, 1.0
$APPLOC2, 3.0, 3.0, 0.5
$APPLOC3, 4.5, −4.5, 1.0
$APPLOC4, −3.0, −3.0, 0.5
.....
.....
$END

24 Appendix: Tabulation of Parameters for Hyperthermic Data Evaluation*

J. ERB and M.H. SEEGENSCHMIEDT

Table 24.1. Basic data protocol for hyperthermia treatments I: Temperature data, number and location of thermosensors

Definition	Unit	Description
$T_n(\mathbf{r},t)$	°C	Measured temperature of thermosensor number n at location $\mathbf{r} = (x,y,z) = (r,\varphi,z)$ and at time t derived from HDS files or similar protocols
N	1	Number of all used thermosensors where $n \in N$ Additional information on thermosensor location is given by:
N_{Tumor}	1	Number of thermosensors in tumor
$N_{Boundary}$	1	Number of thermosensors at tumor boundary
N_{Normal}	1	Number of thermosensors in normal tissue
N_{Skin}	1	Number of thermosensors on skin
N_{Other}	1	Number of thermosensors elsewhere
		Finally, we have: $N = N_{Tumor} + N_{Boundary} + N_{Normal} + B_{Skin} + N_{Other}$

Table 24.2. Basic data protocol for hyperthermia treatments II: power data, number and location of applicators

Definition	Unit	Description
$P_l(\mathbf{r},t)$	W	Amount of power output of applicator number l at location $\mathbf{r} = (x,y,z) = (r,\varphi,z)$ and at time t derived from HDS files or similar protocols
L	1	Number of installed and powered applicators. resulting in: $l \in L$

Table 24.3. Basic data protocol for hyperthermia treatments III: time and temperature measurement intervals

Definition	Unit	Description
$t = m \cdot \Delta\tau$	s	Running time of measurement
M	1	Number of measurement intervals with $m \in M$
$\Delta\tau = \Delta\tau^{on}_{Power} + \Delta\tau^{off}_{Power}$	s	Temperature measurement interval, e.g., $\Delta\tau = 15\,\mathrm{s}$
$\Delta\tau^{on}_{Power}$	s	Measurement interval with power output, e.g., $\Delta\tau^{on}_{Power} = 13\,\mathrm{s}$
$\Delta\tau^{off}_{Power}$	s	Measurement interval without power output, e.g., $\Delta\tau^{on}_{Power} = 2\,\mathrm{s}$

* This work was supported by the Deutsche Forschungsgemeinschaft (grants: Fi 371/2-1 and Se 525/4-2), by the Sophie-Wallner Foundation, and by the Johannes and Frieda Marohn Foundation at the University Erlangen-Nürnberg.

J. ERB, PhD, Institute of Medical Physics, University of Erlangen-Nürnberg, Krankenhausstraße 12, D-91054 Erlangen, FRG
M.H. SEEGENSCHMIEDT, MD, Department of Radiation Oncology, University of Erlangen-Nürnberg, Universitätsstraße 27, D-91054 Erlangen, FRG

Table 24.4. Time scaling I: typical time points of hyperthermia treatments

Definition	Unit	Description
t_{init}	min	Beginning of hyperthermia treatment $\exists l \in L: P_l(t_{init}) \geqslant 0$
t_{init}^{steady}	min	Beginning of steady state level when manifest in temperature slope, otherwise using the following definition: $t_{init}^{steady} = t_{init} + 10\,\text{min}$
t_{end}^{steady}	min	End of steady state level End of hyperthermia treatment All generators and applicators are off: $P_l(t_{end}^{steady}) = 0, \forall l \in L$
t_{end}	min	End of temperature measurement

Table 24.5. Time scaling II: time scales for temperature data evaluation

Definition	Unit	Description
$\Delta t^{init} = t_{init}^{steady} - t_{init}$	min	Initial period before reaching steady state level
$\Delta t^{steady} = t_{end}^{steady} - t_{init}^{steady}$	min	Duration of steady state level
$\Delta t_{treat}^{total} = t_{end}^{steady} - t_{init}$	min	Duration of hyperthermia treatment
$\Delta t_{measure}^{total} = t_{end} - t_{init}$ or $\Delta t_{measure}^{total} = M \cdot \Delta\tau$	min	Duration of temperature measurement
$\Delta t_{power}^{on} = M \cdot \Delta\tau_{power}^{on}$	min	Duration of power output

Table 24.6. Induction time evaluation

Definition	Unit	Description
$t_{max\ ind}^{Tumor\ 38}$	s	Observed maximum induction time to raise all thermosensors in tumor above equal 38°C
Analogue definitions are: $t_{max\ ind}^{Tumor\ 39}$, $t_{max\ ind}^{Tumor\ 40}$, $t_{max\ ind}^{Tumor\ 41}$, $t_{max\ ind}^{Tumor\ 42}$, and $t_{max\ ind}^{Tumor\ 43}$.		
$t_{max\ ind}^{Boundary\ 38}$	s	Observed maximum induction time to raise all thermosensors at the tumor boundary above equal 38°C
Analogue definitions are: $t_{max\ ind}^{Boundary\ 39}$, $t_{max\ ind}^{Boundary\ 40}$, $t_{max\ ind}^{Boundary\ 41}$, $t_{max\ ind}^{Boundary\ 42}$, and $t_{max\ ind}^{Boundary\ 43}$.		
$t_{max\ ind}^{Normal\ 38}$	s	Observed maximum induction time to raise all thermosensors in normal tissue above equal 38°C
Analogue definitions are: $t_{max\ ind}^{Normal\ 39}$, $t_{max\ ind}^{Normal\ 40}$, $t_{max\ ind}^{Normal\ 41}$, $t_{max\ ind}^{Normal\ 42}$, and $t_{max\ ind}^{Normal\ 43}$.		

Table 24.7. Average slope data evaluation

Definition	Unit	Description
$\Delta T_{\Delta t^{init}}^{Tumor}$	$\frac{°C}{min}$	Mean increase in temperature of all thermosensors in tumor within intial period Δt^{init}
$\Delta T_{\Delta t^{init}}^{Boundary}$	$\frac{°C}{min}$	Mean increase in temperature of all thermosensors at tumor boundary within intial period Δt^{init}
$\Delta T_{\Delta t^{init}}^{Normal}$	$\frac{°C}{min}$	Mean increase in temperature of all thermosensors in normal tissue within intial period Δt^{init}
$\Delta T_{t_1-t_2}^{Tissue}$	$\frac{°C}{min}$	Mean change in temperature of all thermosensors in tissue between two time points t_1 and t_2, observation starting at time t_1
Examples: ΔT_{18-22}^{Tumor}, $\Delta T_{18-22}^{Boundary}$, $\Delta T_{18-22}^{Normal}$		

Table 24.8. Maximum, minimum and mean peak temperatures

Definition	Unit	Description
$T_n^{peak} = \max_{t \in \Delta t^{steady}} T_n(t)$	°C	Highest measured temperature at thermosensor n
$T_n^{gap} = \min_{t \in \Delta t^{steady}} T_n(t)$	°C	Lowest measured temperature at thermosensor n
$\overline{T_{max}} = \frac{\sum_{n=1}^{N} T_n^{peak}}{N}$	°C	Mean maximum temperature of all N thermoprobes at steady state level
$\overline{T_{min}} = \frac{\sum_{n=1}^{N} T_n^{gap}}{N}$	°C	Mean minimum temperature of all N thermoprobes at steady state level

Examples: $\overline{T_{min}}^{Tumor}$, $\overline{T_{max}}^{Tumor}$, $\overline{T_{min}}^{Boundary}$, $\overline{T_{max}}^{Boundary}$, $\overline{T_{min}}^{Normal}$, $\overline{T_{max}}^{Normal}$.

Table 24.9. Averaged temperatures

Definition	Unit	Description
$\langle T_n \rangle = \frac{\sum_{t=t_{init}^{steady}}^{t_{end}^{steady}} T_n(t)}{\Delta t^{steady} \cdot \Delta \tau^{-1}}$	°C	Time averaged temperature of thermosensor n at steady state level
$\langle T_{max} \rangle = \max_{n \in N} \langle T_n \rangle$	°C	Maximum time averaged temperature involving all N thermosensors at steady state level
$\langle T_{min} \rangle = \min_{n \in N} \langle T_n \rangle$	°C	Minimum time averaged temperature involving all N thermosensors at steady state level

Table 24.10. Mean temperatures

$\overline{T}(t) = \frac{\sum_{n=1}^{N} T_n(t)}{N}$	°C	Mean temperature of all N thermosensors at a certain time t
$\overline{T_{init}} = \overline{T}(t_{init})$	°C	Mean temperature of all N thermosensors at the beginning of hyperthermia treatment
$\overline{T_{end}} = \overline{T}(t_{end})$	°C	Mean temperature of all N thermosensors at the end of temperature measurement

Examples: $\overline{T}(t)^{Tumor}$, $\overline{T}(t)^{Boundary}$, $\overline{T}(t)^{Normal}$.

Table 24.11. Mean time averaged temperatures

Definition	Unit	Description
$\langle \overline{T} \rangle_{total} = \frac{\sum_{t=t_{init}}^{t_{end}^{steady}} \sum_{n=1}^{N} T_n(t)}{N \cdot \Delta t_{treat}^{total} \cdot \Delta \tau^{-1}}$	°C	Mean time averaged temperature of all measured temperature values and all N thermosensors during hyperthermia treatment Δt_{treat}^{total}
$\langle \overline{T} \rangle_{steady} = \frac{\sum_{t=t_{init}^{steady}}^{t_{end}^{steady}} \sum_{n=1}^{N} T_n(t)}{N \cdot \Delta t^{steady} \cdot \Delta \tau^{-1}}$	°C	Mean time averaged temperature of all measured temperature values and all N thermosensors at steady state level Δt^{steady}

Examples: $\langle \overline{T} \rangle_{steady}^{Tumor}$, $\langle \overline{T} \rangle_{steady}^{Boundary}$, $\langle \overline{T} \rangle_{steady}^{Normal}$

Table 24.12. Maximum and minimum thermosensor I: Definition

Definition	Unit	Description
$n_{max} = \{n \mid \max_{n \in N}^{t \in \Delta t^{steady}} T_n(t)\}$	1	Number of maximum thermosensor: sensor which detected a momentary maximum of all collected temperatures at steady state level involvig all N sensors
$n_{min} = \{n \mid \min_{n \in N}^{t \in \Delta t^{steady}} T_n(t)\}$	1	Number of minimum thermosensor: sensor which detected a momentary minimum of all collected temperatures at steady state level involving all N sensors

Table 24.13. Maximum and minimum thermosensor II: temperature data

Definition	Unit	Description
$T_{max}^{peak} = T_{n_{max}}^{peak} = \max^{t \in \Delta t^{steady}} T_{n_{max}}(t)$	°C	Highest temperature at steady state level measured using thermosensor n_{max}
$T_{min}^{peak} = T_{n_{min}}^{peak} = \max^{t \in \Delta t^{steady}} T_{n_{min}}(t)$	°C	Highest temperature at steady state level measured using thermosensor n_{min}
$T_{min}^{gap} = T_{n_{min}}^{gap} = \min^{t \in \Delta t^{steady}} T_{n_{min}}(t)$	°C	Lowest temperature at steady state level measured using thermosensor n_{min}
$T_{max}^{gap} = T_{n_{max}}^{gap} = \min^{t \in \Delta t^{steady}} T_{n_{max}}(t)$	°C	Lowest temperature at steady state level measured using thermosensor n_{max}

Table 24.14. Maximum and minimum thermosensor III: temperature parameters using hyperthermia temperature data of maximum thermosensor n_{max} and minimum thermosensor n_{min} only. Furthermore, there exists a characteristic difference: $\langle T_{n_{min}} \rangle \neq \langle T_{min} \rangle$ and $\langle T_{n_{max}} \rangle \neq \langle T_{max} \rangle$ (see also Table 24.9)

Definition	Unit	Description
$\langle T_{n_{max}} \rangle = \dfrac{\sum_{t=t_{init}^{steady}}^{t_{end}^{steady}} T_{n_{max}}(t)}{\Delta t^{steady} \cdot \Delta\tau^{-1}}$	°C	Time averaged temperature of sensor number n_{max} at steady state level
$\langle T_{n_{min}} \rangle = \dfrac{\sum_{t=t_{init}^{steady}}^{t_{end}^{steady}} T_{n_{min}}(t)}{\Delta t^{steady} \cdot \Delta\tau^{-1}}$	°C	Time averaged temperature of sensor number n_{min} at steady state level

Table 24.15. Lowest and highest '10 Minutes-Temperatures' using hyperthermia temperature data of all maximum and minimum thermosensors

Definition	Unit	Description
$T_{max}^{10} = \max_{\bar{t} \in \Delta t^{steady}} \left(\dfrac{\sum_{t=\bar{t}}^{\bar{t}+10\,min} T_{n_{max}}(t)}{10\,min \cdot \Delta\tau^{-1}} \right)$	°C	Higest temperature within 10 min at sensor number n_{max} including T_{max}^{peak}
$T_{min}^{10} = \min_{\bar{t} \in \Delta t^{steady}} \left(\dfrac{\sum_{t=\bar{t}}^{\bar{t}+10\,min} T_{n_{min}}(t)}{10\,min \cdot \Delta\tau^{-1}} \right)$	°C	Lowest temperature within 10 min at sensor number n_{min} including T_{min}^{gap}

Table 24.16. Thermal quality I: parameters to describe thermal quality of hyperthermia treatments

Definition	Unit	Description
$TQ^{43}_{peak} = \frac{\sum_{n=1}^{N} \Theta(T_n^{peak} - 43°C)}{N}$	%	Percentage of all observed N thermosensors at steady state level, for which maximum temperature values exceed 43°C
$TQ^{43}_{gap} = \frac{\sum_{n=1}^{N} \Theta(T_n^{gap} - 43°C)}{N}$	%	Percentage of all observed N thermosensors at steady state level, for which minimum temperature values exceed 43°C
$\overline{TQ^{43}} = \frac{\sum_{n=1}^{N} \Theta(\langle T_n \rangle - 43°C)}{N}$	%	Percentage of all observed N thermosensors at steady state level, for which time averaged temperature values exceed 43°C

Table 24.17. Thermal quality II: parameters to describe thermal quality of hyperthermia treatments

Definition	Unit	Description
$TQ^{43} = \frac{\sum_{t=t_{init}^{steady}}^{t_{end}^{steady}} \sum_{n=1}^{N} \Theta(T_n(t) - 43°C)}{\sum_{t=t_{init}^{steady}}^{t_{end}^{steady}} \sum_{n=1}^{N} T_n(t)}$	%	Percentage of all observed N thermosensors at steady state level, for which temperature values exceed 43°C

Analogue definitions: TQ^{40}, TQ^{41}, TQ^{42}

Analogue definitions for peak, gap and mean values following Tab. 24.16 are possible: TQ^{Tref}_{peak}, TQ^{Tref}_{gap} and $\overline{TQ^{Tref}}$

Table 24.18. Integrated time intervals I: integrated time intervals for evaluation of hyperthermia treatments

Definition	Unit	Description
$ITI^{43}_n = \sum_{t=t_{init}^{stead}}^{t_{end}^{steady}} \Delta\tau \; \Theta(T_n(t) - 43°C)$	min	Integrated time intervals at steady state level where thermosensor n indicates temperatures exceeding 43°C
$ITI^{43}_{max} = \max_{n \in N} ITI^{43}_n$	min	Longest integrated time intervals at steady state level of all N thermosensors exceeding 43°C
$ITI^{43}_{min} = \min_{n \in N} ITI^{43}_n$	min	Shortest integrated time intervals at steady state level of all N thermosensors exceeding 43°C

Table 24.19. Integrated time intervals II: minimum, maximum and mean values

Definition	Unit	Description
$\overline{ITI^{43}} = \frac{\sum_{n=1}^{N} ITI^{43}_n}{N}$	min	Mean integrated time intervals at steady state level of all N thermosensors exceeding 43°C

Analogue definitions: ITI^{40}_n, ITI^{41}_n, ITI^{42}_n

Analogue definitions for minimum, maximum and mean values: ITI^{Tref}_{min}, ITI^{Tref}_{max} and $\overline{ITI^{Tref}}$

Table 24.20. Thermal isoeffect dose in equivalent minutes at $T_{ref} = 43°C$ (minEq43) used for ESHO protocols (See DUNLOP et al. 1986; HAND et al. 1989)

Definition	Unit
$TID_n^{43} = TID^{43}(\Delta t_{measure}^{total}, T_n(t)) = \sum_{t=t_{init}}^{t_{end}} \Delta t_{eq43}(T_n(t))$	min
is the thermal isoeffect dose at thermosensor n,	
with $\Delta t_{eq43}(T_n(t)) = \begin{cases} 2^{(T_n(t)-43°C)} \cdot \Delta T: & T_n(t) \geq T_{trans} \\ 2^{(T_{trans}-43°C)} 6^{(T_n(t)-T_{trans})} \cdot \Delta T: & T_n(t) < T_{trans} \end{cases}$	
where $T_{trans} = 42.5°C$ is the assumed transition temperature and $\Delta\tau = 15$ s is the measurement interval	
Examples for constant temperatures T_n:	
$TID^{43}(\Delta t_{measure}^{total} = 9\,\text{min}, T_n = 41°C) = TID^{43}(\Delta t_{measure}^{total} = 26\,\text{s}, T_n = 43°C)$	
$TID^{43}(\Delta t_{measure}^{total} = 15\,\text{s}, T_n = 45°C) = TID^{43}(\Delta t_{measure}^{total} = 1\,\text{min}, T_n = 43°C)$	

Table 24.21. Thermal isoeffect dose II: definitions

Definition	Unit	Description
$TID_{max}^{43} = \max_{n \in N} TID_n^{43}$	min	Highest thermal isoeffect dose of all thermosensors N in minEq43
$TID_{min}^{43} = \min_{n \in N} TID_n^{43}$	min	Lowest thermal isoeffect dose of all thermosensors N in minEq43
$\overline{TID^{43}} = \frac{\sum_{n=1}^{n=N} TID_n^{43}}{N}$	min	Mean thermal isoeffect dose of all thermosensors N in minEq43
Analogue definitions for thermal isoeffect dose are also possible for different reference temperatures $T_{ref} = 40°C$, 41°C and 42°C.		
Analogue indices are recommended: TID_n^{40}, TID_n^{41} and TID_n^{42}.		
Analogue definitions for minimum, maximum and mean values: $TID_{min}^{T_{ref}}$, $TID_{max}^{T_{ref}}$ and $\overline{TID^{T_{ref}}}$.		

Table 24.22. Effective tissue perfusion rate: Tissue perfusion rate w_{eff} is an effective value, which depends on metabolic heat production, heat conductivity and blood perfusion. v_{perf}^{eff} is equal to blood perfusion rate v_{perf}, if heat conductivity and metabolism are neglected (ROEMER et al. 1985 and SAMULSKI et al. 1987)

Definition	Unit
$w_{eff} = -\frac{\rho_{tissue} \cdot c_{tissue}}{c_{blood} \cdot (t - t_{end}^{steady})} \cdot \ln\left(\frac{T_n(t) - T_{body}}{T_n(t_{end}^{steady}) - T_{body}}\right)$	$\frac{\text{kg}}{\text{m}^3 \cdot \text{s}}$
Time runs from $0 < t - t_{end}^{steady} \leq 120$ s after generator power off,	
where $T_{body} = 37°C$ is the baseline temperature	
with $\rho_{blood} = 1000 \frac{kg}{m^3}$, $\rho_{tissue} = 1070 \frac{kg}{m^3}$	
and $c_{blood} = 4186 \frac{W \cdot s}{kg \cdot K}$, $c_{tissue} = 3470 \frac{W \cdot s}{kg \cdot K}$	
$v_{perf}^{eff} = \frac{w_{eff}}{\rho_{blood} \cdot \rho_{tissue}}$	$\frac{\text{m}^3}{\text{kg} \cdot \text{s}}$ or $\frac{6 \cdot 10^6\,\text{ml}}{100\,\text{g} \cdot \text{min}}$

Table 24.23. Linear Perfusion Rate (LAGENDIJK et al. 1988 and FELDMANN et al. 1992)

Definition	Unit
$w_{lin} = \frac{\rho_{tissue} \cdot c_{tissue}}{c_{blood} \cdot (t - t_{end}^{steady})} \cdot \left(\frac{T_n(t) - T_{body}}{T_n(t_{end}^{steady}) - T_{body}}\right)$	$\frac{kg}{m^3 \cdot s}$
Time runs from $0 < t - t_{end}^{steady} \leq 120$ s after generator power off,	
where $T_{body} = 37°C$ is the baseline temperature	
with $\rho_{blood} = 1000 \frac{kg}{m^3}$, $\rho_{tissue} = 1070 \frac{kg}{m^3}$	
and $c_{blood} = 4186 \frac{W \cdot s}{kg \cdot K}$, $c_{tissue} = 3470 \frac{W \cdot s}{kg \cdot K}$	
$v_{perf}^{lin} = \frac{w_{lin}}{\rho_{blood} \cdot \rho_{tissue}}$	$\frac{m^3}{kg \cdot s}$ or $\frac{6 \cdot 10^6 \, ml}{100 \, g \cdot min}$
These values produce the following numeric formula:	
$v_{perf}^{lin} = \frac{6000}{T_n(t_{end}^{steady}) - T_{body}} \cdot \frac{T_n(t) - T_{body}}{t - t_{end}^{steady}}$	$\frac{ml}{100 \, g \cdot min}$

Table 24.24. Mean time averaged initial and final changes in temperature

Definition	Unit	Description
$\Delta T_{init} = \frac{\langle \bar{T} \rangle_{steady} - \overline{T_{init}}}{t_{init}^{steady} - t_{init}}$	°C	Mean temperature increase of all N thermosensors from beginning of hyperthermia treatment (generator power on) until steady state level
$\Delta T_{washout} = \frac{\langle \bar{T} \rangle_{steady} - \overline{T_{end}}}{t_{end} - t_{init}^{steady}}$	°C	Mean temperature decrease of all N thermosensors from end of steady state level (generator power off) until end of temperature measurement

Table 24.25. Basis for a statistical thermal dose concept: temperature frequency distribution and density

Definition	Unit	Description
T_{10}	°C	Temperature exceeded by 10% of all measured temperatures of all N thermosensors at steady state level. T_{10} is statistically the 90% percentile
Analogue definitions are given for:		
T_{20}	°C	is statistically the 80% percentile
T_{50}	°C	is statistically the 50% percentile
T_{80}	°C	is statistically the 20% percentile
T_{90}	°C	is statistically the 10% percentile

Table 24.26. Combination I: statistical thermal dose concept and thermal parameter T_{index}

Definition	Unit	Description
$\mathrm{ITI}_n^{T_{90} \geqslant T_{index}} = \sum_{t=t_{init}^{steady}}^{t_{end}^{steady}} \Delta\tau\,\Theta(T_n(t) - T_{index})$	min	Integrated time intervals where 90% of all measured temperatures exceed the index temperature T_{index} using thermosensor n at steady state level
Analogue definitions are possible: $\mathrm{ITI}_n^{T_{50} \geqslant T_{index}}$, $\mathrm{ITI}_n^{T_{10} \geqslant T_{index}}$, etc.		

Table 24.27. Combination II: statistical thermal dose concept and thermal parameter T_{index}

Definition	Unit	Description
$\overline{\mathrm{ITI}^{T_{90} \geqslant T_{index}}} = \dfrac{\sum_{n=1}^{N} \mathrm{ITI}_n^{T_{90} \geqslant T_{index}}}{N}$	min	Mean integrated time intervals where 90% of all measured temperatures exceed the index temperature T_{index} when using all N thermosensors at steady state level
Analogue definitions are possible: $\overline{\mathrm{ITI}^{T_{50} \geqslant T_{index}}}$, $\overline{\mathrm{ITI}^{T_{10} \geqslant T_{index}}}$, etc.		

Table 24.28. Standard deviation I: Description of a hyperthermia treatment characterizing stability of temperatures during steady state level

Definition	Unit	Description
$\langle T_n \rangle = \dfrac{\sum_{t=t_{init}^{steady}}^{t_{end}^{steady}} T_n(t)}{\Delta t^{steady} \cdot \Delta\tau^{-1}}$	°C	Time averaged temperature of thermosensor n at steady state level Δt^{steady}
$\langle \sigma_n \rangle = \dfrac{1}{\dfrac{\Delta t^{steady}}{\Delta\tau} - 1} \sqrt{\sum_{t=t_{init}^{steady}}^{t_{end}^{stady}} \left(T_n(t) - \langle T_n \rangle\right)^2}$	°C	Standard deviation of thermosensor n at steady state level Δt^{steady}

Table 24.29. Standard deviation II: Description of a hyperthermia treatment characterizing stability of temperatures during steady state level

Definition	Unit	Description
$\bar{T}(t) = \dfrac{\sum_{n=1}^{N} T_n(t)}{N}$	°C	Mean temperature of all N thermosensors at time t
$\bar{\sigma}(t) = \dfrac{1}{N-1} \sqrt{\sum_{n=1}^{N} \left(T_n(t) - \bar{T}(\mathrm{t})\right)^2}$	°C	Standard deviation of all N thermosensors at time t

Table 24.30. Standard deviation III: Description of a hyperthermia treatment characterizing stability of temperatures during steady state level

Definition	Unit	Description
$\langle \bar{T}_n \rangle_{steady} = \frac{\sum_{t=t_{init}^{steady}}^{t_{end}^{steady}} \sum_{n=1}^{N} T_n(t)}{N \cdot \Delta t^{steady} \cdot \Delta\tau^{-1}}$	°C	Mean time averaged temperature of all measured temperatures using all N thermosensors at steady state level Δt^{steady}
$\langle \bar{\sigma} \rangle_{steady} = \frac{1}{N \cdot \frac{\Delta t^{steady}}{\Delta\tau} - 1} \sqrt{\sum_{t=t_{init}^{steady}}^{t_{end}^{steady}} \sum_{n=1}^{N} \left(T_n(t) - \langle \bar{T} \rangle_{steady}\right)^2}$	°C	Standard deviation of all measured temperatures using all N thermosensors at steady state level Δt^{steady}

References

Dunlop PRC, Hand JW, Dickinson RJ, Field SB (1986) An assessment of local hyperthermia in clinical practice. Int J Hyperthermia 2: 39–50

Feldmann HJ, Molls M, Hoederath A, Krümpelmann S, Sack H (1992) Blood flow and steady state temperatures in deep-seated tumors and normal tissues. Int J Radiat Oncol Biol Phys 23: 1003–1008

Hand JW, Lagendijk JJW, Bach Andersen J, Bolomey JC (1989) Quality assurance guidelines for ESHO protocols. Int J Hyperthermia 5: 421–428

Lagendijk JJW, Hofman P, Schipper J (1988) Perfusion analyses in advanced breast carcinoma during hyperthermia. Int J Hyperthermia 4: 479–495

Roemer RB, Fletcher AM, Cetas TC (1985) Obtaining local sar and blood perfusion data from temperature measurements: steady state and transient techniques compared. Int J Radiat Oncol Biol Phys 11: 1539–1550

Samulski TV, Fessenden P, Valdagni R, Kapp DS (1987) Correlations of thermal washout rate, steady state temperatures, and tissue type in deep seated recurrent or metastatic tumors. Int J Radiat Oncol Biol Phys 13: 907–916

[illegible]

References

[illegible]

Subject Index

List of Contributors

MITSUYUKI ABE, MD
Director
Kyoto National Hospital
Fushimi-Ku
Kyoto 612
Japan

F. AMBESI IMPIOMBATO, MD
Istituto Regina Elena
Per Lo Studio e La Cura Dei Tumori
291, Viale Regina Elena
00161 Rome
Italy

MAURIZIO AMICHETTI, MD
Istituto per La Ricerca Scientifica e Tecnologica
38 100 Trento
Italy

MICHELE ANZA, MD
Istituto Regina Elena
Per Lo Studio e La Cura Dei Tumori
291, Viale Regina Elena
00161 Rome
Italy

GIORGIO ARCANGELI, MD
G. Porfiri Oncology Center
Radiation Oncology Department
S. Maria Goretti Hospital
Via G. Reni
04100 Latina
Italy

MELVIN A. ASTRAHAN, MD
Department of Radiation Oncology
Kenneth Norris Jr. Cancer Hospital
and Research Institute
1441 Eastlake Avenue, Room 34
P.O. Box 33804
Los Angeles, CA 90033-0804
USA

LUC BAERT, MD
Professor and Chairman
Department of Urology
University of Leuven
St. Pieter's Hospital
Brusselsestraat 69
3000 Leuven
Belgium

JOAN M.C. BULL, MD
Division of Oncology
The University of Texas at Houston Medical School
University of Texas
P.O. Box 20708
6431 Fannin Road
Houston, TX 77225
USA

ALFREDO CALLOPOLI, MD
Istituto Regina Elena
Per Lo Studio e La Cura Dei Tumori
291, Viale Regina Elena
00161 Rome
Italy

A. CAPUA, MD
Istituto Regina Elena
Per Lo Studio e La Cura Dei Tumori
291, Viale Regina Elena
00161 Rome
Italy

SANDRO CARLINI, MD
Istituto Regina Elena
Per Lo Studio e La Cura Dei Tumori
291, Viale Regina Elena
00161 Rome
Italy

Francesco Cavaliere, MD
Istituto Regina Elena
Per Lo Studio e La Cura Dei Tumori
291, Viale Regina Elena
00161 Rome
Italy

Renato Cavaliere, MD
Professor, Istituto Regina Elena
Per Lo Studio e La Cura Dei Tumori
291, Viale Regina Elena
00161 Rome
Italy

T.A. Colacchio, MD
Professor of Surgery
Section of General Surgery
Dartmouth-Hitchcock Medical Center
Lebanon, NH 03756
USA

Peter M. Corry, PhD
Department of Radiation Oncology
William Beaumont Hospital
Royal Oaks, MI 48073-6769
USA

Piotr Debicki, MD
Department of Radiation Oncology
Kenneth Norris Jr. Cancer Hospital
and Research Institute
1441 Eastlake Avenue, Room 34
P.O. Box 33804
Los Angeles, CA 90033-0804
USA

Mark W. Dewhirst, DVM, PhD
Department of Radiation Oncology
Tumor Microcirculation Laboratory
Duke University Medical Center
P.O. Box 3455
Durham, NC 27710
USA

Franco Di Filippo, MD
Istituto Regina Elena
Per Lo Studio e La Cura Dei Tumori
291, Viale Regina Elena
00161 Rome
Italy

F. d'Oleire, MD
Department of Human Oncology
The University of Wisconsin
Madison, WI 53792
USA

Jürgen Erb, PhD
Institute of Medical Physics
University of Erlangen-Nürnberg
Universitätsstraße 27
91054 Erlangen
Germany

Horst-Jürgen Feldman, MD
Klinik und Poliklinik für Strahlentherapie
und Radiologische Onkologie
der Technischen Universität München
Klinikum rechts der Isar
Ismaninger Straße 22
81675 München
Germany

Paul T. Finger, MD
Director, The Ocular Tumor Service
The New York Eye and Ear Infirmary
310 E. 14th Street
New York, NY 10003
USA
and
Chief, The Division of Ocular Tumor and
Orbital Disease
North Shore University Hospital
300 Community Drive
Manhasset, NY 11030
USA

Rosa Garinei, MD
Istituto Regina Elena
Per Lo Studio e La Cura Dei Tumori
291, Viale Regina Elena
00161 Rome
Italy

Frederic A. Gibbs, Jr., MD
Department of Radiation Oncology
University of Utah
50 North Medical Drive
Salt Lake City, UT 84132
USA

GIUSEPPE GIOVINAZZO, MD
G. Porfiri Oncology Center
Radiation Oncology Service
S. Maria Goretti Hospital
Via G. Reni
04100 Latina
Italy

DIONISIO GONZÁLEZ GONZÁLEZ, MD
Academish Medisch Centrum
Department of Radiation Oncology
Meibergdreef 9
1105 AZ Amsterdam
The Netherlands

W. HAVERS, MD
Universitätskinderklinik Essen
Hufelandstraße 55
45147 Essen
Germany

MASAHIRO HIRAOKA, MD
Department of Radiology
Faculty of Medicine
Kyoto University
Kyoto 606
Japan

ROLF D. ISSELS, MD, PhD
GSF-Institut für Klinische Hämatologie
Institut für Klinische Hämatologie
Marchioninistraße 25
81377 München
Germany
and
Klinikum Großhadern
Medizinische Klinik III
Marchioninistraße 15
81377 München
Germany

K. KITAMURA, MD
Dept. of Surgery II
Kyushu University
3-1-1, Maidashi, Higashi-ku
Fukuoka, 812
Japan

GUNTHER KLAUTKE, MD
Klinik und Poliklinik für Strahlentherapie
Universität Erlangen-Nürnberg
Universitätsstraße 27
91054 Erlangen
Germany

ROBERT G.F. KNOL
Department of Radiation Research
City of Hope National Medical Center
Duarte, CA 91010
USA

KENNETH LEOPOLD, MD
Department of Radiation Oncology
Duke University Medical Center
P.O. Box 3085-154
Durham, NC 27710
USA

DAVID MACHIN, PhD
Medical Research Council Cancer Trials Office
5 Shaftesbury Road
Cambridge, CB2 2BW
United Kingdom

JENS OVERGAARD, MD
Department of Experimental
Clinical Oncology
Danish Cancer Society
Norrebrogade 44
8000 Aarhus C
Denmark

PASQUALE PERRI, MD
Istituto Regina Elena
Per Lo Studio e La Cura Dei Tumori
291, Viale Regina Elena
00161 Rome
Italy

ZBIGNIEW PETROVICH, MD
Professor and Chairman
Department of Radiation Oncology
Kenneth Norris Jr. Cancer Hospital
and Research Institute
1441 Eastlake Avenue, Room 34
P.O. Box 33804
Los Angeles, CA 90033-0804
USA

Angelo Psaila, MD
Istituto Regina Elena
Per Lo Studio e La Cura Dei Tumori
291, Viale Regina Elena
00161 Rome
Italy

Ralf van Heek-Romanowski, MD
Universitätskinderklinik Essen
Hufelandstraße 55
45147 Essen
Germany

T.P. Ryan, MD
Section of General Surgery
Dartmouth-Hitchcock Medical Center
Lebanon, NH 03756
USA

Stephen A. Sapareto, PhD
Department of Radiation Oncology
Good Samaritan Regional Medical Center
1111 East McDowell Road
Phoenix, AZ 85006
USA

M. Schiratti, MD
Istituto Regina Elena
Per Lo Studio e La Cura Dei Tumori
291, Viale Regina Elena
00161 Rome
Italy

Johannes Schorcht, MD
Klinik und Poliklinik für Strahlentherapie
Universitätsklinikum Carl Gustav Carus
der TU Dresden
Fetscherstraße 74
01307 Dresden
Germany

M. Heinrich Seegenschmiedt, MD
Klinik und Poliklinik für Strahlentherapie
Universität Erlangen-Nürnberg
Universitätsstraße 27
91054 Erlangen
Germany

Ralph Seidel, MD
Klinik und Poliklinik für Strahlentherapie
Universität Erlangen-Nürnberg
Universitätsstraße 27
91054 Erlangen
Germany

Penny K. Sneed, MD
Department of Radiation Oncology
University of California
P.O. Box 0226
San Francisco, CA 94143
USA

Paul R. Stauffer, MD
Department of Radiation Oncology
University of California
San Francisco, CA 94143-0226
USA

Baldassarre Stea, PhD, MD
Department of Radiation Oncology
University of Arizona Health Sciences Center
Tucson, AZ 85724
USA

Keizo Sugimachi, MD
Professor, Department of Surgery II
Kyushu University
3-1-1, Maidashi, Higashi-ku
Fukuoka, 812
Japan

Riccardo Valdagni, MD
Case di Cura San Pio X
Division of Radiation Oncology
Via F Nava 31
20159 Milano
Italy

Jacoba van der Zee, MD, PhD
Hyperthermia Oncologist
Department of Hyperthermia
Dr. Daniel Den Hoed Cancer Center
Groene Hilledijk 301
3075 EA Rotterdam
The Netherlands

CLARE C. VERNON, MA, FRCR
Clinical Oncologist
Department of Clinical Oncology
Hammersmith Hospital
Ducane Road
London W12 OHS
United Kingdom

JILL WHALEY, BVM & S
Medical Research Council Cancer Trials Office
5 Shaftesbury Road
Cambridge, CB2 2BW
United Kingdom

MICHAEL ZIMMERMANN, PhD
Isotopen-Technik
Dr. Sauerwein GmbH
Bergische Straße 16
42781 Han
Germany

Contents of Volume 1

MEDICAL RADIOLOGY – Diagnostic Imaging and Radiation Oncology

Titles in the series already published

Lung Cancer
Edited by C. W. SCARANTINO

Innovations in Radiation Oncology
Edited by H. R. WITHERS and L. J. PETERS

Radiation Therapy of Head and Neck Cancer
Edited by G. E. LARAMORE

Gastrointestinal Cancer - Radiation Therapy
Edited by R. R. DOBELBOWER, Jr.

Radiation Exposure and Occupational Risks
Edited by E. SCHERER, C. STREFFER, and K.-R. TROTT

Radiation Therapy of Benign Diseases – A Clinical Guide
S. E. ORDER and S. S. DONALDSON

Innovations in Diagnostic Imaging
Edited by J. H. ANDERSON

Interventional Radiation Therapy Techniques – Brachytherapy
Edited by R. SAUER

Radiopathology of Organs and Tissues
Edited by E. SCHERER, C. STREFFER, and K.-R. TROTT

Concomitant Continuous Infusion Chemotherapy and Radiation
Edited by M. ROTMAN and C. J. ROSENTHAL

Radiology of the Upper Urinary Tract
Edited by E. K. LANG

Intraoperative Radiotherapy – Clinical Experiences and Results
Edited by F. A. CALVO, M. SANTOS, and L. W. BRADY

The Thymus – Diagnostic Imaging, Functions, and Pathologic Anatomy
Edited by E. WALTER, E. WILLICH, and W. R. WEBB

Radiotherapy of Intraocular and Orbital Tumors
Edited by W. E. ALBERTI and R. H. SAGERMAN

Interstitial and Intracavitary Thermoradiotherapy
Edited by M. H. SEEGENSCHMIEDT and R. SAUER

Interventional Neuroradiology
Edited by A. VALAVANIS

Non-Disseminated Breast Cancer Controversial Issues in Management
Edited by G. H. FLETCHER and S. H. LEVITT

Current Topics in Clinical Radiobiology of Tumors
Edited by H.-P. BECK-BORNHOLDT

Practical Approaches to Cancer Invasion and Metastastes: A Compendium of Radiation Oncologists' Responses to 40 Histories
Edited by A. R. KAGAN with the assistance of R. J. STECKEL

Radiology of the Pancreas
Edited by A. L. BAERT, co-edited by G. DELORME

Radiation Therapy in Pediatric Oncology
Edited by J. R. CASSADY

Radiology of the Lower Urinary Tract
Edited by E. K. LANG

Radiation Therapy Physics
Edited by A. R. SMITH

Late Sequelae in Oncology
Edited by J. DUNST AND R. SAUER

Mediastinal Tumors. Update 1995
Edited by D. E. WOOD and C. R. THOMAS JR.

Thermoradiotherapy and Thermochemotherapy Volume 1 Biology, Physiology, and Physics
Edited by M. H. SEEGENSCHMIEDT, P. FESSENDEN, and C. C. VERNON

Thermoradiotherapy and Thermochemotherapy Volume 2 Clinical Applications
Edited by M. H. SEEGENSCHMIEDT, P. FESSENDEN, and C. C. VERNON

MIX
Papier aus verantwortungsvollen Quellen
Paper from responsible sources
FSC® C105338

If you have any concerns about our products,
you can contact us on
ProductSafety@springernature.com

In case Publisher is established outside the EU,
the EU authorized representative is:
Springer Nature Customer Service Center GmbH
Europaplatz 3, 69115 Heidelberg, Germany

Printed by Libri Plureos GmbH
in Hamburg, Germany